Table of Contents

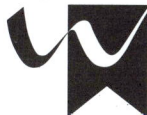

IARC
2007

This Handbook was made possible thanks
to the generous
funding by the
Ministère de la Santé, de la Jeunesse
et des Sports

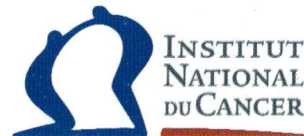

Liberté • Égalité • Fraternité
RÉPUBLIQUE FRANÇAISE

MINISTÈRE DE LA SANTÉ,
DE LA JEUNESSE
ET DES SPORTS

INSTITUT
NATIONAL
DU CANCER

International Agency for Research on Cancer

The International Agency for Research on Cancer (IARC) was established in 1965 by the World Health Assembly, as an independently financed organization within the framework of the World Health Organization. The headquarters of the Agency are in Lyon, France.

The Agency conducts a programme of research concentrating particularly on the epidemiology of cancer and the study of potential carcinogens in the human environment. Its field studies are supplemented by biological and chemical research carried out in the Agency's laboratories in Lyon and, through collaborative research agreements, in national research institutions in many countries. The Agency also conducts a programme for the education and training of personnel for cancer research.

The publications of the Agency contribute to the dissemination of authoritative information on different aspects of cancer research. Information about IARC publications, and how to order them, is available via the Internet at: http://www.iarc.fr/.

This publication represents the views and opinions of an IARC Working Group on Reversal of Risk after Quitting Smoking, which met in Lyon, France, 13–20 March 2006.

Funding

The IARC Tobacco Control Handbooks are generously funded by the Ministère de la Santé, de la Jeunesse et des Sports, France.

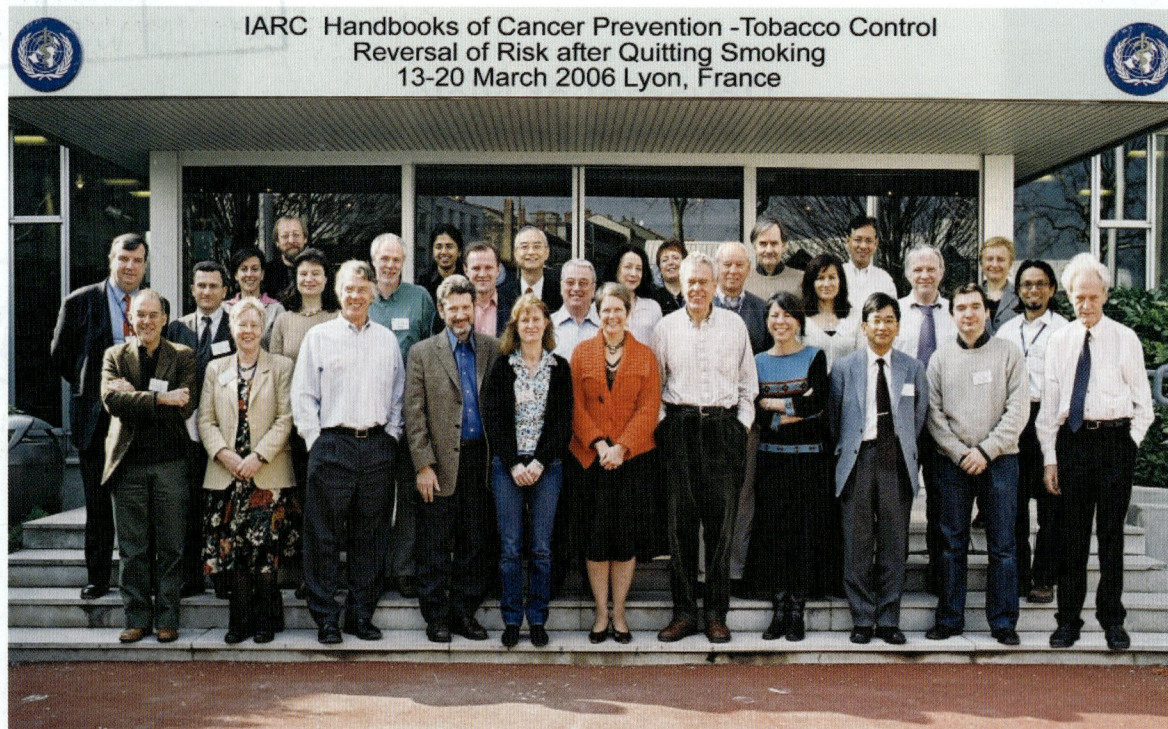

IARC Handbooks of Cancer Prevention -Tobacco Control
Reversal of Risk after Quitting Smoking
13-20 March 2006 Lyon, France

Published by the International Agency for Research on Cancer,
150 cours Albert Thomas, 69372 Lyon Cedex 08, France

Distributed by
WHO Press, World Health Organization, 20 Avenue Appia, 1211 Geneva 27, Switzerland (tel: +41 22 791 3264;
fax: +41 22 791 4857; email: bookorders@who.int).

Format for bibliographic citation:

IARC (2007). IARC Handbooks of Cancer Prevention, Tobacco Control, Vol. 11: Reversal of Risk After Quitting Smoking.
Lyon, France

IARC Library Cataloguing-in-Publication Data

Reversal of Risk After Quitting Smoking/IARC Working Group on Reversal of Risk after Quitting Smoking (2007: Lyon, France)

(IARC Handbooks of Cancer Prevention; 11)

1. Neoplasms – prevention & control   2. Risk Assessment   3. Smoking – adverse
effects   4. Smoking Cessation   I. IARC Working Group on Reversal of Risk after
Quitting Smoking   II. Series

ISBN 978 92 832 3011 6   (NLM Classification QZ 39)
ISSN 1027-5622

Dedication

This report is dedicated to Richard Doll (1912-2005), one of the epidemiologists who, around the middle of the 20th century, showed that smoking was 'a cause, and a major cause' of lung cancer, and helped identify the other main diseases caused by smoking. He was also the founding editor of Cancer in Five Continents, the periodic International Agency for Research on Cancer (IARC) publication that documents the worldwide variation in cancer incidence rates. The final results from his 50-year prospective study (1951-2001) of smoking and death among British doctors showed that about half of all smokers are eventually killed by their habit, that smokers lose about 10 years of life expectancy, and that stopping smoking at ages 60, 50, 40 or 30 gains respectively about 3, 6, 9 or almost the full 10 years of life expectancy. Richard Doll smoked for 20 years, stopping at age 37 when his first clear results emerged, and is pictured here at age 91, at the press conference where he announced the 50-year results. During his final year he travelled widely and lectured, on cancer, in five continents.

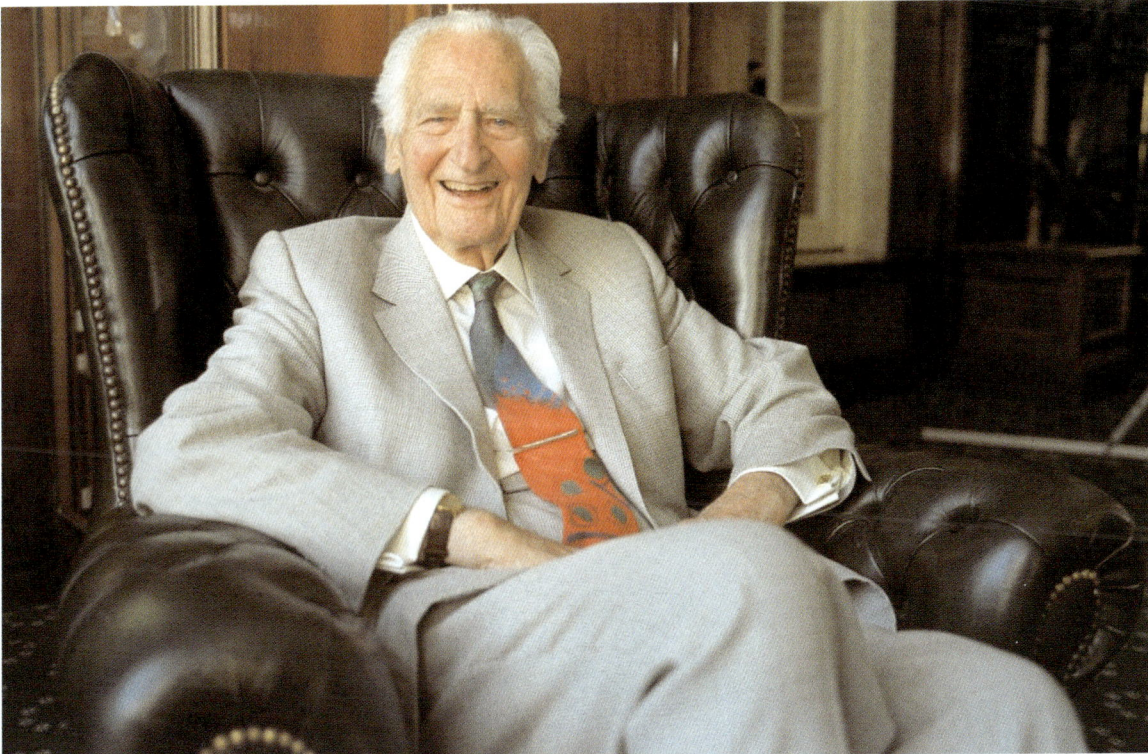

Source: Michael Crabtree, copyright Troika Photos

List of Participants

David M. Burns (Chairman)
University of California at San Diego
School of Medicine
1545 Hotel Circle So, Suite 310
San Diego, CA 92108
USA

Sarah C. Darby
Cllinical Trials Service Unit
University of Oxford
Richard Doll Building
Roosevelt Drive
Oxford OX3 7LF
United Kingdom

Nina S. Godtfredsen
Medical Department Ifael
Bispebjerg Hospital
Bispebjerg Bakke 23
2400 Copenhagen NV
Denmark

Prakash C. Gupta
Healis-Sekhsaria Inst. for Public Health
Plot No. 28, Sector 11
CBD Belalpur
601/B Great Eastern Chambers
Navi Mumbai
India

Trevor Hansel
Airway Diseases Section
National Heart & Lung Institute
Imperial College School of Medicine
Royal Brompton Campus
Dovehouse Street
SW3 6LY London
United Kingdom

Martin Jarvis
Cancer Research UK
Health Behaviour Unit
Dept of Epidemiol. & Public Health
University College London
2-16 Torrington Place
London WC1E 6BT
United Kingdom

Anne Marie Joseph
Veterans Affairs Medical Center
Section of General Internal Medicine
Center for Chronic Dis. Outcome Res.
One Veterans Drive
Minneapolis, MN 55417
USA

Pekka Jousilahti
National Public Health Institute
Dept Epidemiol. & Health Promotion
Mannerheimintie 166
00300 Helsinki
Finland

Tai Hing Lam
Dept. of Community Medicine
 & Unit for Behavioural Sciences
University of Hong Kong Medical Centre
Faculty of Medicine Building
21 Sassoon Road, Pokfulam
Hong Kong Special Administrative Region
China

Carlo La Vecchia
Laboratory of General Epidemiology
Ist. Ricerche Farmacologiche
Mario Negri
via Eritrea, 62
20157 Milano
Italy

Patrick Maisonneuve
European Institute of Oncology
Epidemiology Unit
Via Ripamonti 435
Milan 20141
Italy

Richard Peto
Clinical Trials Service Unit
University of Oxford
Richard Doll Building
Roosevelt Drive
Oxford OX3 7LF
United Kingdom

Eva Prescott
Rigshospitalet
Department of Cardiology
Blegdamsvej 9
2100 Copenhagen 0
Denmark

Chris Robertson
Statistics and Modelling Science
Strathclyde University
Glasgow G1 1XH
United Kingdom

Tomotaka Sobue
Res. Center for Cancer Prev. &
Screening
National Cancer Center
Statistics and Cancer Control Division
5-1-1 Tsukiji Chuo-ku
Tokyo 104-0045
Japan

Michael Thun
American Cancer Society
Epidemiology & Surveillance Research
1599 Clifton Road NE
Atlanta, GA 30329-4251
USA

Melvyn Tockman
Molecular Screening and Population Studies
H. Lee Moffitt Cancer Center & Research Institute
12902 Magnolia Drive
Tampa, FL 33612
USA

Representatives
Yumiko Mochizuki
Tobacco Free Initiative (TFI)
WHO
Switzerland

Poonam Dhavan
TFI
WHO
Swizterland

Sylviane Ratte
Department of Prevention
National Cancer Institure (INCa),
France

IARC Secretariat
Robert Baan
Julien Berthiller
Paolo Boffetta
Vincent Cogliano
Carolyn Dresler (Responsible Officer)
Silvia Franceschi
Vendhan Gajalakshmi
Nigel Gray
María León (Co-Responsible Officer)
Amir Sapkota
Béatrice Secrétan
Kurt Straif

Technical Assistance
Karima Abdedayem (Secretarial)
Catherine Bénard (Secretarial)
John Daniel (Editor)
Roland Dray (Graphics)
Georges Mollon (Photography)
Annick Rivoire (Bibliography)
Josephine Thévenoux (Layout)

Acknowledgements

The Working Group acknowledges the significant contribution to the work presented in this Handbook by the following individuals:

Jill Boreham (CTSU, Oxford, UK), Cristina Bosetti (Mario Negri Institute, Milan, Italy), SY Chan (Department of Community Medicine, University of Hong Kong, Hong Kong, China), Lindsay Hannan and Jane Henley (American Cancer Society, Atlanta, USA), Jane Hayman and Vicki White (Cancer Victoria, Australia), Kota Katanoda and Tomomi Marugame (National Cancer Center, Tokyo, Japan), Cecily Ray (Healis Sekhsaria Institute for Public Health, Navi Mumbai, India), XY Sai, B Wang, ZZ Wang, D Xiao, and Professor YP Yan (The Fourth Military Medical University, Xi'an, China).

The IARC secretariat is grateful to Mathieu Boniol, Min Dai, and Jacques Ferlay and to the staff of the Libraries at the International Agency for Research on Cancer, Lyon and the World Health Organization, Geneva for their invaluable help.

Preface

Why a Handbook on Reversal of Risk After Quitting Smoking?

The International Agency for Research on Cancer (IARC) Handbooks of Cancer Prevention have added Tobacco Control as a new area of prevention for their reviews. Tobacco use is a preponderant risk factor in the causation of many cancer types, and numerous scientific and public health responses have evolved to address this hazard.

Tobacco smoking causes cancer of the lung, oral cavity, nasal cavity and nasal sinuses, pharynx, larynx, oesophagus, stomach, pancreas, liver, rinary bladder, kidney and uterine cervix, and myeloid leukaemia (IARC, 2004). In addition to cancer, smoking causes cardiovascular diseases (coronary heart disease, cerebrovascular disease, atherosclerosis, and abdominal aortic aneurysm), respiratory diseases (chronic obstructive pulmonary disease, acute respiratory illnesses including pneumonia, respiratory effects *in utero* and during childhood and adolescence), reproductive effects (reduced fertility, pregnancy complications, fetal death and stillbirths, low birth weight) and other morbid conditions (US Department of

Health and Human Services, 2004). Despite these known health effects, about 1.3 billion people worldwide smoke (WHO, 2006), making tobacco use the single major avoidable cause of disease and mortality worldwide. Irrefutably, the potential for prevention is vast.

Given the number of current smokers worldwide, promoting tobacco abstinence becomes paramount. To this end, characterizing the changes in morbidity and mortality risks occurring after cessation provides valuable support. This body of knowledge has been already covered in part by several publications (U.S. Surgeon General's Report, 1990; IARC Monograph 83, 2004). Why, then, revisit the argument?

Cancer, chronic obstructive pulmonary disease and vascular diseases represent the three main causes of smoking-attributable deaths worldwide. The *Handbook* will review and assess the scientific literature to generate an updated, more complete characterization of the changes in risk of cancer, cardiovascular and chronic obstructive lung diseases following smoking

cessation by asking specific questions to drive the review: Does the risk of developing or dying from each of these diseases decrease after smoking cessation? What is the time course of the change in risk? Does the risk return to that of never smokers with long durations of cessation? The volume will also identify instances when no data are available to respond to these queries.

The main goal of the *Handbook* is to provide scientific evidence critically appraised on the health benefits of smoking cessation for public health and public policy decisions. We hope its evaluation will help promote and support widespread efforts leading to tobacco abstinence. The Handbook Meeting and the concomitant evaluation of the evidence took place in Lyon in March of 2006, in a year that saw the WHO Framework Convention on Tobacco Control's first Conference of the Parties in Geneva in February and the Tobacco or Health Conference in Washington DC in July, all laudable efforts on different fronts with the common objective of arresting the tobacco epidemic.

References

IARC (2004). *IARC Monographs on the Evaluation of Carcinogenic Risks to Humans, Vol. 83, Tobacco Smoke and Involuntary Smoking.* Lyon, IARCPress.

United States Department of Health and Human Services (USDHHS) (1990). *The Health Benefits of Smoking Cessation. A Report of the Surgeon General.* Rockville, MD, Centers for Disease Control, Office on Smoking and Health.

United States Department of Health and Human Services (USDHHS) (2004). *The Health Consequences of Smoking. A Report of the Surgeon General.* Atlanta, GA, Centers for Disease Control and Prevention, Office on Smoking and Health.

WHO (2006) Why is tobacco a public health priority? World Health Organization, Date Accessed: October 18,2006. Last Update: 2006. Available from: http://www.who.int/ tobacco/ health_priority

Health Benefits of Stopping Smoking

Introduction and Overview

Cigarette smoking is responsible for more than four million deaths each year worldwide (IARC, 2004). Cigarette smoking causes lung cancer, bladder cancer, cervical cancer, esophageal cancer, kidney cancer, laryngeal cancer, leukemia, oral cancer, pancreatic cancer, and stomach cancer. It also causes abdominal aortic aneurysm, peripheral vascular disease, atherosclerosis, cerebrovascular disease, coronary heart disease, chronic obstructive pulmonary disease, fetal deaths and stillbirths, low birth weight and complications of pregnancy (IARC, 2004; USDHHS, 2004).

Prevention of tobacco use, particularly smoking initiation among adolescents, is the only way to completely eliminate tobacco-related morbidity and mortality. However, there is a long lag time between the onset of smoking and manifestation of the diseases which result from smoking, other than those associated with pregnancy. So, even if no individual began smoking from this point forward, it would still require several decades before these prevention efforts would result in reduced death rates from tobacco related diseases.

Cessation of cigarette smoking by those who are currently smoking cigarettes does offer the prospect of reducing tobacco-related deaths and disease morbidity in the near term, and this effect has been recognized for several decades. With prolonged abstinence, most of the increased risk that would have accrued with continuing smoking is avoidable, even for smokers who have three or more decades of smoking history.

This International Agency for Research on Cancer (IARC) *Handbook* reviews in detail the evidence that exists to define and quantify the changes in risk following cessation for many of the diseases caused by smoking. It also identifies gaps in our understanding of the benefits of cessation for specific diseases and where new opportunities for productive research exist. Perhaps most importantly, information presented in this Handbook identifies that declines in lung cancer death rates currently occurring in developed countries may slow or even stop unless increased rates of cessation can be achieved among current populations of smokers.

The differences in risk that occur with smoking cessation and continued abstinence for the most common cancers and lung and vascular diseases associated with smoking are described in this volume. It examines the biological changes in disease mechanisms that follow cessation and how the timing of these changes might be expected to translate into changes in rates of disease occurrence, understanding that this translation is likely to be different for cancers, vascular diseases and chronic obstructive pulmonary disease (COPD).

Difficulties in measuring cessation and abstinence in epidemiological studies, and how these difficulties can bias the observations of disease rates in former smokers, are also considered.

The scientific evidence for each disease is examined in detail in order to answer three questions:

1. Is the risk of disease lower in former smokers than in current smokers?
2. What is the time course of the reduction in risk with continued abstinence?
3. Does the risk return to that of never smokers after long periods of abstinence?

This handbook attempts to present a comprehensive review of the evidence on the changes in disease risks following cessation, but it does not attempt to exhaustively list or discuss every study which has published data on former smokers. Where large numbers of studies are available, as in the case of studies which examine lung cancer in former smokers, representative studies are cited to support the conclusions; other studies are cited when they contribute substantively to expanding the understanding of the questions being discussed. This approach avoids repetitive discussion of similar findings and hopefully will result in a more readable and understandable volume.

The handbook also does not examine many of the diseases or conditions where injury or death has been established as causally related to smoking, most notably complications of pregnancy. In addition, we do not examine issues of improved quality of life or prolongation of survival following cancer diagnosis, both of which have been demonstrated to be positively associated with smoking cessation (Gritz et al., 2005).

Changes in overall mortality following cessation

Most of the studies discussed in this handbook examine a single disease entity or closely related diseases. For the smokers who quit in these studies, however, it is important to note that the benefits of cessation are not limited to the single disease being examined but are spread across all of the diseases caused by cigarette smoking. Thus, the examination of changes in disease-specific risks contained in this volume are accurate descriptions of the changes in risk for that individual disease, but they dramatically underestimate the total benefit of cessation, the sum of the risk reductions for each of the specific diseases caused by tobacco smoking.

Data from the British Physicians Study have been used to estimate the lifetime risks of smoking and the amount of that risk that can be avoided by cessation and continued abstinence at different ages (Doll et al., 2004). Figure 1 presents the data from these analyses which estimate the cumulative mortality for smokers and never smokers beginning at different ages. These cumulative mortality curves describe the fraction of those alive at given ages who survive at each older age up to age 100 years. The survival of smokers is contrasted with that estimated for smokers who quit at

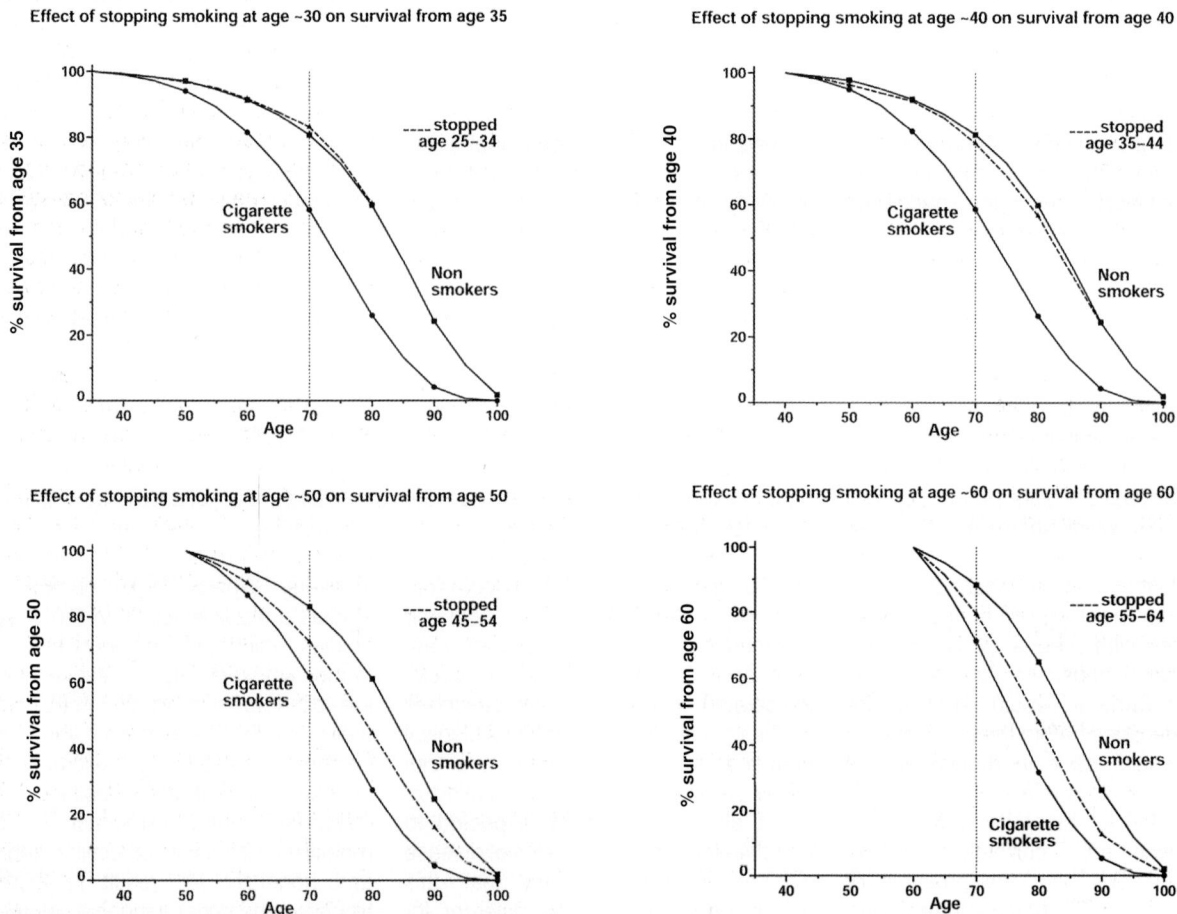

Figure 1. Effects on survival of stopping smoking at age 25–34, age 35–44, age 45–54 and age 55–64
Dotted line corresponds to the survival of those stopping smoking
Reproduced with permission from Doll et al., BMJ 2004; 328: 1519–1527

the age where the curves begin; thus the curve for former smokers (dotted line) describes amount of smoking-related mortality that the smoker can avoid by quitting at that age.

Figure 1 makes the value of cessation clear and demonstrates that the vast majority of smoking-caused mortality is avoidable by quitting prior to age 45 years. Even at older ages, a substantial fraction of the excess mortality due to smoking can be avoided by quitting.

Examining the differences in mortality from all causes among smokers and never smokers offers the most inclusive estimate of the magnitude of the risks associated with smoking and, correspondingly, the proportion of that risk that can be avoided by quitting. Overall mortality, however, also includes causes of death that result from lifestyles or behavioral traits found more commonly among smokers than among nonsmokers, rather than being caused by smoking directly. Smokers have higher cause-specific death rates from cirrhosis of the liver, accidents and homicides than do nonsmokers, but these increases are felt to be largely or entirely caused by factors other than smoking. Cirrhosis may be more common in smokers because smokers are more likely to be heavy consumers of alcohol than nonsmokers. These associated, but not caused, excess deaths lead to a small overestimate of the excess mortality caused by smoking.

Alcohol use, risk-taking and other disease-causing behaviors do not necessarily change following cessation, and therefore estimation of the reductions in risk with cessation would seem to be less likely to be influenced by these factors. However, former smokers may also differ from current smokers in these lifestyle and risk-taking behaviors, raising the possibility that the slight overestimate of the risk of smoking may also be accompanied by a slight overestimate of the benefits of cessation

when all-cause mortality rates are examined.

Even when the concerns about over estimation of the smoking risks and benefits of cessation with all-cause mortality are considered, change in all-cause mortality remains the best summary measure of the benefits of cessation.

Defining cessation

According to results of the Current Population Surveys (CPS) carried out in the United States between 1992 and 1999 and reported by Burns *et al.* (2003), thirty to forty percent of those who were daily smokers one year prior to the survey report making a serious attempt to quit in the past year, about 8 percent of all those who were daily smokers one year ago currently report being abstinent at the time of the survey, about 5% report being abstinent for 3 or more months, and about 2-3% of all smokers achieve long-term abstinence in any given year (Burns *et al.*, 1997). Many smokers who successfully quit smoking have made multiple unsuccessful attempts to quit in the past. These observations suggest that cessation is a process rather than a point in time, and smokers may act repetitively on a desire to quit by making a cessation attempt, but they may have intervals between attempts where they are less interested in cessation. An important corollary of these observations is that smoking status defined at a specific point in time is not a uniformly accurate measure of subsequent smoke exposure. Current smokers may quit and former smokers may relapse. The inaccuracy of former smoking status assessment is greatest for recent quitters, and the inaccuracy of current smoking status assessment is greatest for those who are farthest from their last assessment of smoking status. For smokers who are within several years of their date of cessation, regular

assessment of their smoking status is needed during follow-up to confirm whether they have remained abstinent or relapsed back to smoking since their smoking status was last recorded. Current smokers also need regular assessment of their smoking status to assess whether they have quit. It is only after smokers have been abstinent for long durations that their likelihood of relapse becomes small.

In prospective epidemiological analyses, cessation is usually defined as a single point in time, and that point in time is conceptualized as the point when all cigarette smoking exposures stopped. The observed rates of disease for former smokers are then often presented with the assumption that smoking exposure stopped for all individuals in the group and therefore the rates in that group accurately reflect what happens to risk when smokers become abstinent. The time point for cessation is usually self-reported, and the individual is assumed to have remained abstinent unless evidence to the contrary is available. This set of observations and assumptions is likely to be valid for individuals with long durations of abstinence, but it is in conflict with what is known about cessation behavior for shorter durations of abstinence.

Among smokers with long periods of continued abstinence, the date of last smoking regularly can be used as a measure of the point where exposure changed. However, when examining the effects of shorter-term cessation, the problems of assessing the end of exposure for prospective epidemiological studies are more complicated. In any baseline evaluation of smoking status, those who have recently quit are at high likelihood of relapsing back to smoking, and that likelihood persists with a declining probability for several years following cessation. In following a group of recent quitters for disease outcomes, it is then reasonable to assume that some substantial fraction of those defined as former smokers by the baseline evaluation will relapse back to active smoking early in the follow-up. Continued inclusion of these relapsed smokers in the former smoker category will lead to an underestimate of the benefits of quitting, since the former smoker group on which the estimate is based is composed of both relapsed current smokers and abstinent former smokers. The longer the follow-up period without interval re-evaluation of smoking status, the larger will be the misclassification of the smoking status of those who had quit in the few years preceding the baseline evaluation.

Misclassification of smoking status for recent former smokers leads to an overestimate of the risk of disease among recent former smokers, just as continuing cessation activity after the baseline evaluation leads to an underestimate of the risks of continuing smoking. The magnitude of these mis-estimations increases as the interval between evaluations of smoking status increases. It is still possible to assess whether rates are lower among former smokers even with the misclassification, since the former smoker category will still contain a higher fraction of abstinent former smokers than the continuing smoker category. Misclassification is largely a problem in assessing the timing of the decline, and the magnitude of the decline in the first few years following cessation, in prospective studies which have infrequent or absent interval evaluation of smoking status.

An additional problem in defining cessation for epidemiological analyses is that cessation attempts and cessation success are not uniformly spread through the population. They vary with age, education and income, race/ ethnicity and a variety of other individual characteristics that also influence disease outcomes. The relationship of these factors to cessation attempts may also be different from the relationship with cessation success. For example, some surveys show that cessation attempts decline with age (Burns, 2000), but that long-term cessation success increases with age (Burns *et al.,* 1997).

Differences between countries in the disease burden of the tobacco epidemic

Death rates from tobacco related disease vary markedly from country to country. These differences are largely determined by differences in the rates of smoking initiation two to seven decades earlier and rates of cessation five and more years prior to the year of the death rate. As a result, differences in current smoking prevalence for a given year in different countries may not match differences in lung cancer rates in the same year. These differences have been described as falling into four stages of the tobacco epidemic (Lopez *et al.,* 1994) (Figure 2). The pattern of smoking behavior common in most developed countries of the Americas and northern Europe is one in which smoking initiation increased rapidly in men in the early decades of the last century and in women a few decades later. Cessation began to occur during the second half of the last century. Lung cancer rates are now falling for men in these countries and the increase in rates for women is leveling off or also falling (represented by the United Kingdom at Stage 4 in Figure 2). In the eastern European countries,

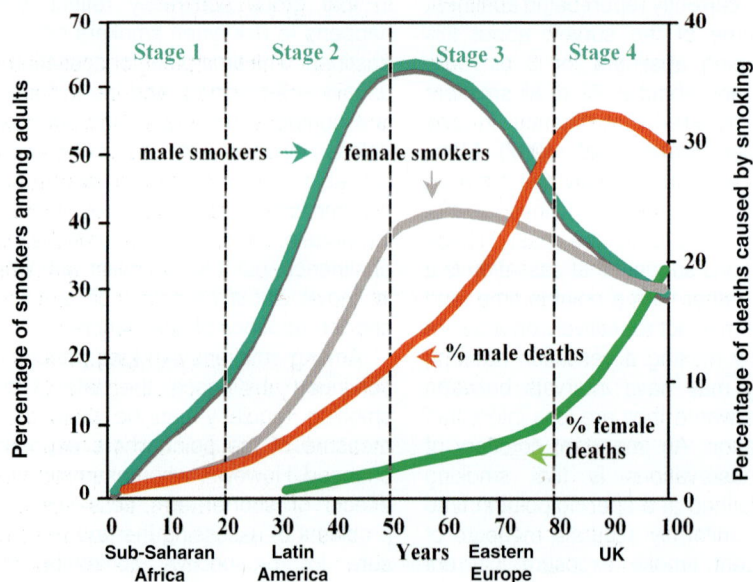

Figure 2. Stages of the tobacco epidemic

Death rates from tobacco related disease vary markedly from country to country. These differences are largely determined by differences in the rates of smoking inititiation two to seven decades earlier and rates of cessation five and more years prior to the year of the death rate. As a result, differences in current smoking prevalence for a given year in different countries may not match differences in lung cancer rates in the same year. These differences have been described as falling into four stages of the tobacco epidemic (Reproduced with permission from Lopez *et al.,* 1994).

smoking prevalence remains high for men because there are lower rates of cessation, and women are either continuing heavy smokers or increasing in prevalence. Lung cancer rates are continuing to rise among both males and females in these countries (Stage 3 in Figure 2).

Earlier stages in the tobacco epidemic are also reflected by patterns of use in Asia, Latin America and some countries in southern Europe (Stage 2 in Figure 2). Smoking is high among men and until recently was low among women. Aggressive marketing of cigarettes to women has led to a relatively recent rapid rise in female smoking prevalence. The net result of this pattern is a high rate of lung cancer in men with a much lower rate of lung cancer among women in comparison to men and in comparison to that which one would expect if current female smoking prevalence rates had existed over the past several decades. In these areas, an epidemic of lung cancer among women will begin to appear in the next decades.

The earliest stage in the tobacco epidemic is represented by countries in sub-Saharan Africa (Stage 1 in Figure 2), where tobacco use was uncommon among both men and women until recently. The rates of lung cancer and other tobacco related diseases are low due to both the low prevalence of smoking in the past and the low life expectancy of the population. As cigarette marketing and smoking prevalence increase, these countries are likely to begin down the path of the tobacco-related disease epidemic observed over the last century in the developed world. It is hoped that the recent adoption and entry into force of the international Framework Convention on Tobacco Control may enable these countries, and others around the world, to avoid the tragic experiences of the developed world with tobacco use and its subsequent disease burden.

The stage of the tobacco epidemic in a specific country is an important consideration when examining evidence on disease risks produced by smoking and correspondingly the benefits of cessation for the population of that country. For countries where the epidemic is in an early stage, prevalence may have increased but the disease risks will not be evident, and there will therefore be little demonstrable benefit of cessation at a population level. Even when the tobacco epidemic is well underway, the magnitude of the damage caused by smoking and the magnitude of the benefits of cessation are likely to be substantially underestimated. This reality has important public policy considerations. For very legitimate reasons, policymakers in a country prefer to have risk data that have been developed based on studies of populations of that country. However, when a country is in the early stages of the tobacco epidemic, studies done in the country will substantively underestimate the damage that will be caused in the near future in the population of that country. These studies will also underestimate the benefits of cessation for future population risks. Both of these underestimates may lead to poorly informed decisions on the appropriate allocation of scarce public health resources to tobacco control programs.

The evidence presented in this volume expands the understanding of the phases of the tobacco epidemic by examining the timing of the changes in rates of initiation and cessation for several countries and the impact of differences in the timing on lung cancer rates. In the United States and the United Kingdom, reductions in the rate of smoking initiation occurred roughly simultaneously with increases in rates of smoking cessation. That is, as the peak prevalence of smoking by birth cohort began to decline in sequential birth cohorts, rates of smoking cessation

began to increase in the same calendar year periods. However, for other countries such as Japan, a decline in peak prevalence has not occurred, and cessation has increased modestly or not at all. These differences in cessation help explain some of the differences between Japan and the USA in lung cancer death rates that are not explained by the differences in peak prevalence. Consideration of differences in both rates of initiation and rates of cessation, rather than simply current smoking prevalence, may improve our understanding of what determines the differences in observed lung cancer rates between men and women, and between countries.

Describing changes in risk following cessation

Changes in risk following cessation can be examined using a variety of metrics and comparison groups. Relative risks (RR) are the ratio of the rates of disease in two groups. The likelihood of developing or dying of disease for populations of former smokers can be compared either to current smokers or to never smokers. When risks for former smokers are compared to current smokers, the numerical value of the relative risk ratio declines to below 1.0 as a demonstration of lower risk for former smokers compared with current smokers. When risks for former smokers are compared with never smokers, the numerical value of the relative risk ratio commonly remains above 1.0 as a demonstration that the risk in former smokers remains elevated compared to never smokers. It is the same experience in former smokers that is compared to current and to never smokers, but the difference given by this comparison offers different insights about the risk that remains following cessation.

Actual rates of disease, either age-specific or age-standardized rates, in populations of former smokers can also be compared to those of current or never smokers. The rates can be compared directly (for example, rates of disease in former smokers compared to current smokers) or the rate of disease in never smokers can be subtracted from that of current smokers to calculate the excess rate of disease caused by smoking in the smokers. Disease rates in former smokers can also be expressed as an excess rate by subtracting the rate of disease occurring in never smokers of similar ages. The excess rate in former smokers can be compared with that of continuing smokers to examine the fraction of the excess disease rate produced by smoking that remains after specified durations of cessation.

Rates of disease in smokers can also be expressed as a cumulating fraction of the population of smokers who develop or die from all causes or from a specific disease. The cumulative risk of disease for those who quit at different ages can then be compared to the cumulative risk for continuing smokers. This comparison allows a better understanding of the amount of smoking-related disease that is avoidable with cessation at different ages. This form of comparison also provides a clearer picture of the burden of disease occurring in populations of current and former smokers.

While all of these ways of describing the changes following cessation are expressing the same observed change in risk, each is capable of enhancing in different ways our understanding of the reality of disease risk for former smokers.

Comparisons with continuing smokers have particular relevance for individuals who are considering quitting smoking or who are currently abstinent, since they reflect the choice actually available to the smoker: to stop or to continue smoking. The comparison of former smoker risk to that of continuing smokers defines the alternative pathways of future risk available to the smoker contemplating cessation. For this comparison to be an accurate depiction of the alternative risks, the former smokers must be compared to continuing smokers with similar ages and intensities of smoking, and the duration of smoking for the current smokers should equal the sum of the duration of smoking of the former smokers plus the duration of abstinence; that is, the duration is that which would occur if the smoker continues to smoke.

In contrast, if the question being considered is how long the risk produced by smoking remains elevated for former smokers or how large is the persistent excess risk, then it is easier to consider the evidence as a comparison of the risks for former smoker to those of never smokers.

Because relative risks are the ratio of disease frequencies in two populations, they are powerfully influenced by the rates of disease in the reference population. With diseases such as coronary heart disease (CHD), where multiple factors can independently cause the disease, observed rates of disease may be high among never smokers and increase steeply with age. This effect of the disease rate in the reference population on relative risk means that the same burden of disease caused by smoking will generate a larger relative risk when the rate of disease occurrence among never smokers is low, as it is for lung cancer, than it will when the rate of disease occurrence among never smokers is high, as it is for CHD. As a result, relative risks must be considered carefully or they may present a distorted picture of the relationship between smoking behavior and disease risk. For example, smoking-related relative risks for CHD decline with advancing age, as

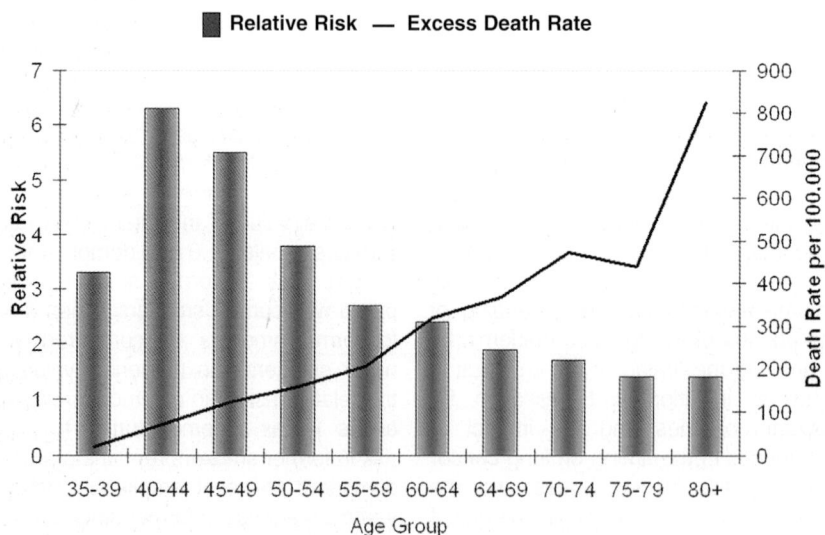

Figure 3. Relative risks and excess mortality rates for coronary heart disease among male cigarette smokers at different ages.
Adapted from Thun *et al.* (1997).

depicted by the vertical bars in Figure 3 (Thun *et al.*, 1997). These relative risks are greatest at younger ages and decline steeply with advancing age. In contrast, the actual excess death rate (the death rate in smokers minus the death rate in never smokers) increases with age as depicted in the solid line in Figure 3. Both the decline in relative risk with age and the increase in excess risk with age are accurate descriptions of the change in risk with age, but they describe different aspects of that change in risk.

Relative risk helps us understand the fraction of disease attributable to smoking in a population. With an increasing rate of CHD among never smokers as they age, the proportion of all CHD caused by smoking makes up a smaller fraction of the total CHD occurring in the population.

Excess rates of disease help us appreciate the absolute magnitude of the disease burden produced by smoking. As smokers age, the cumulative damage caused by smoking grows and is manifest as an increasing excess death rate.

The different considerations for relative and absolute risks are important in considering the studies of former smokers presented in this volume. The relative risks for former smokers with increasing durations of abstinence cannot reasonably be expected to exceed the risks for continuing smokers or to drop below the risks for never smokers. With relative risks of 3 for continuing smokers, as are commonly found in studies of CHD, the relative risks for former smokers compared to never smokers can only vary between 2.99 and 1, and the relative risks compared to continuing smokers cannot drop below 0.33. For a disease like lung cancer where the relative risks in continuing smokers commonly exceed 10, the range of relative risks expected in comparisons with never smokers is

larger (e.g. 9.99 to 1.0) and for comparisons with continuing smokers the relative risks could drop as low as 0.1. Thus the same reduction in burden of disease following cessation might give the appearance of a smaller change in relative risk for CHD than for lung cancer.

Additionally, trying to define whether a residual increased risk remains following long durations of abstinence is likely to be more difficult for CHD than for lung cancer due to the differences in the magnitude of the relative risks. For example, if ten percent of the risk produced by smoking remains after long durations of abstinence, the expected relative risk for lung cancer would still be 2.0, whereas the expected relative risk for CHD would be 1.2, a level that might be difficult to define with confidence. This may be true, even though the absolute decline in death rates for the two diseases may be similar and the residual risk with long durations of abstinence, in absolute rates of disease occurrence, could also be similar for the two diseases. This reality of risk estimation could create a circumstance where it is possible to define whether there is a persistent elevated risk of lung cancer for former smokers of long duration, while the same magnitude of disease burden for CHD was difficult to separate from the risk of never smokers with confidence.

Comparisons of relative risks may also be potentially misleading when two studies of the same disease in former smokers are compared with one another if the populations of former smokers differ in age. Relative risks for active smokers are lower at older ages for most smoking-related diseases (Thun *et. al.*, 1997). The same lowering of relative risks with increasing age will occur for former smokers since they are the result of the same rising rate of disease with age among never smokers. Therefore, one would expect a lower relative risk for both current and former smokers in

studies of individuals with higher mean ages, and care should be taken when examining the results for former smokers from different studies of the same disease to carefully consider the effects of differences in age of the population examined on both relative and absolute disease risks.

Short-term changes following cessation: exposure measure and physiological responses

Considerable attention is paid in this volume to the biological changes that occur with cessation and which underlie the changes in observed risk. The inhalation, deposition, absorption, metabolism and excretion of the several thousand constituents of smoke produce both acute and, if the exposure is sustained, chronic changes in human physiology, metabolism, organ structure, and biochemical and cellular function that reflect the gradual progression toward disease manifestation. In a similar fashion, once the exposure stops, there is clearance of smoke constituents from the body with reversal of their acute effects, slowing of the progression and potential reversal of the damage at the cellular and organ level. These changes underlie the changes in risk that occur following cessation.

The disappearance of smoke constituents from the body differs by constituent. Nicotine is rapidly metabolized within minutes and even its metabolic products are largely gone within days. Carbon monoxide disappears even more rapidly. It is exhaled as it becomes unbound from hemoglobin and clears with a half-life of hours. Most of the carcinogens present in smoke require metabolic activation to be toxic, while other constituents such as free radicals may be present only for short periods of time. Hemoglobin-carcinogen adducts, which are suggested markers of carcinogen exposure, are cleared slowly, consistent with turnover of the red cells and the hemoglobin they contain. This raises a concern that DNA adducts may persist for long periods of time in cells that continue replicating indefinitely, such as the basal cell layer of the respiratory epithelium. Persistence of these adducts may offer continued opportunity for replicative errors and progression of the carcinogenic process even after cessation of smoke exposure.

Oxidation and inflammation are injuries that have been broadly implicated in the mechanistic pathways of many diseases including cancer, vascular disease and chronic lung disease. While the exposures that cause these changes will disappear rapidly following cessation, the consequences of those exposures persist. The time course of the reversal of oxidation and inflammation following cessation are not well described, and the factors that lead to persistence of these processes once the exposure ceases are also not well understood. Factors that seem important include the extent and duration of the resultant injury. For example, changes in small airway function of the lung, a marker of inflammation in those airways, reverse within a year of smoking cessation among individuals with short smoking histories (USDHHS, 1984). However, once inflammation has been present for longer durations or has caused structural changes in the lung, it may not fully reverse even with long durations of abstinence. A similar picture is beginning to emerge with the endothelial changes that are important parts of the mechanism of vascular injury and disease, and which are described in the section on vascular mechanisms in this volume. Changes occur rapidly with smoke exposure and are present at very low exposure doses; but when they are due to short-term exposure, they also reverse rapidly. The extent of injury that can be present and

still reverse is not clear, and the potential of significant injury to partially or fully heal following cessation is also uncertain at this point.

Problems in measuring change in risks following cessation for different diseases

With perhaps the exception of complications of pregnancy which appear to disappear if smoking stops by the end of the first trimester, increased risk of incidence and death from the major diseases caused by smoking persists for multiple years following cessation. While we treat the initial manifestation of new disease as if it were an acute event, it is usually the result of a process of progressive injury and organ change over several decades. The underlying level of injury present at cessation, and the momentum of the process of injury, defines the rate of disease manifestation following cessation, in contrast to the absence of new disease observed with acute infectious diseases once exposure to the agent ceases. One should expect that the timing and extent of reductions in the risk of a given disease following cessation might then differ for the different disease processes.

The defining event for a cancer is likely to be the transformation of an individual cell into a cancer cell, and there is little evidence to suggest that cessation can reverse that transformation as opposed to reducing the rate at which such transformations occur in the future. A substantial interval, likely several years, is then required before the single cell can divide and grow into a tumor large enough to be detected; an additional interval is usually present between detection and death from the tumor. One would not expect a difference between smokers and former smokers in the rate of lung cancer incidence or death until at least the most rapidly

growing lung cancers present at time of cessation had time to complete the process of growth to detection or death. Once the most rapidly growing tumors had fully manifested, and assuming a reduced rate of new carcinogenic transformation following cessation, lung cancer rates in continuing smokers and former smokers would begin to diverge. Cancers present at the time of cessation would continue to manifest with a declining frequency over time as slower-growing tumors reach a size where they are detected. Thus, one would not expect a difference in lung cancer risk between smokers and former smokers until two or more years following cessation. The subsequent risk would be a mix of the rate of new carcinogenic transformation and a declining contribution of cancers present at the time of cessation as ones with slower doubling times eventually become manifest.

The pathophysiological processes by which smoking causes vascular disease would be expected to result in a very different time course of changing risk following cessation compared to cancers. Smoking causes atherogenesis with chronic progressive development of plaque and other changes in the vascular wall. It also is a powerful determinant of the endothelial and thrombotic processes that cause acute infarction. The endothelial and thrombotic processes can reverse relatively rapidly, and this rapid reversal would be expected to result in a rapid decline in the risk of acute events. The excess atherosclerosis produced by smoking would contribute to an increased risk of acute events for a more prolonged period, as other factors will continue to promote atherogenesis as the individual ages. This bimodal mechanistic effect would also be expected to produce more rapid and dramatic benefits in those with pre-existing disease, since they have atherosclerotic change sufficient to cause disease without further progression and the predominant effect would be the reversal of endothelial changes and thrombosis.

The pattern of change following cessation with COPD is again different. COPD is a disease where substantial lung injury is present before the disease can be detected and where the disease progresses slowly over many years before causing death. The later stages of the disease involve structural remodeling of the lung, much of which is irreversible. Cessation can slow disease progression, but does not lead to lung regeneration. In this setting, the greatest opportunity to alter disease risk is for those with mild disease, where slowing of lung function decline may prevent the development of disease symptoms. In those with extensive disease, slowing of disease progression may be less evident since so little lung function remains to be preserved.

An additional concern in measuring the change in risk following cessation is that cessation may occur due to the presence of disease symptoms or following disease diagnosis. This phenomenon is often referred to as reverse causality and is one reason why lung cancer death rates are higher among former smokers than among continuing smokers for the first few years after cessation. Reverse causality results when the population of recent quitters is enriched with patients with lung cancer who quit following diagnosis. This group of smokers who quit following diagnosis with lung cancer will obviously have a very high lung cancer death rate in the next few years. Combining them with smokers who quit prior to developing lung cancer will spuriously elevate the rate of disease in former smokers above that of continuing smokers for the first few years after cessation.

Since survival with lung cancer is relatively short among those who die of the disease, the overestimate of lung cancer rates among former smokers is evident for only a few years following cessation. However, both COPD and CHD have many patients who are alive for a decade or more following onset of their disease. Most of these individuals will have been advised to quit following diagnosis, and many have followed that advice. Once again, individuals who quit following onset of disease enrich the population of former smokers with individuals who have evident disease and who will have a relatively high mortality from that disease. Because survival with CHD or COPD is relatively long, the effect of this enrichment on disease rates is likely to persist for much longer and lead to an overestimate of disease rates among former smokers even ten or more years after cessation. Retrospective studies of first onset of disease in relation to the timing of quitting smoking may be less influenced by these biases.

The effects of reverse causation are likely to be present for many cancers and may persist in analyses of the first several years of cessation. Some studies examine cessation with categories of duration of abstinence that are very broad—for example those who have been abstinent for 10 years or less and 10 years or more. In a category of abstinence this broad, the effect of reverse causation may be masked because the risk for all of the individuals in the category is less than that of continuing smokers. Combining the first few years of abstinence, where reverse causation is present, with a an interval of 5 to 10 years of abstinence, where reverse causation is not likely to be a problem, does not eliminate the effect of reverse causation, it only masks it and underestimates the benefits of cessation for those who do not have a diagnosis at the time of cessation.

Defining the questions

The three questions addressed for each disease are intended to highlight different aspects of the risks following cessation.

1. **Is the risk of disease lower in former smokers than in otherwise similar current smokers?**

This question is the most general and the one where most of the diseases examined will have some evidence. In examining that evidence, particularly in comparing across studies, it is important to carefully weigh the factors that influence the metric used to assess risk in former smokers. Comparisons of former smokers must adjust for the intensity and duration of smoking prior to cessation in order to make comparisons with smokers or across studies. It is less commonly recognized that mean duration of abstinence, and the distribution of the duration of abstinence, are critical characteristics of former smokers that define risk, and that vary dramatically across studies of different populations or of the same population at different points in time.

If the relative risk of a disease for smokers is low in the population examined, the decline in relative risk must also be smaller. This is a factor when comparing studies of populations in countries that are in different stages of the tobacco epidemic, studies where there are different levels of other causes of smoking related diseases, and studies where the age distribution of the former smokers examined are substantively different.

2. **What is the time course of the reduction in risk with continued abstinence or, among otherwise similar former smokers, does the risk of disease lower with more prolonged abstinence?**

How soon a change in risk is evident, and how rapid the decline in risk relative to continuing smokers occurs, are important concerns of smokers who are quitting and are common questions asked by smokers of their care providers. They are also important questions for health care planning and cost effectiveness analyses of tobacco control activities.

3. Does the risk return to that of never smokers after long periods of abstinence?

For many diseases, only a modest amount of data is available to address this question because of the long durations of abstinence required to examine the question and the large sample sizes needed to define with precision low levels of risk. It addresses whether the damage caused by smoking persists forever, or whether the accelerated progression toward disease produced by smoking is reversible or can be overtaken by other exposures and injuries as individuals age. As those smokers who quit in response to the tobacco control interventions of the 1970s and 1980s achieve periods of abstinence of 20 years and more, answering questions on the risk that remains for this group becomes more important. However, answering the question is complicated by the reality that the only way that one can have a longer duration of abstinence is to have a shorter duration of smoking. Long durations of smoking preclude long durations of abstinence and vice versa. The relative and excess risks of disease produced by smoking increase dramatically as the duration of smoking increases, but it is difficult to demonstrate increased levels of risk for durations of smoking less than 10-15 years. This raises a concern in evaluations of long durations of abstinence. The low levels of risk observed with long durations of abstinence may be due to short durations of smoking rather than long durations of abstinence.

Interpretation of the Absence of Data
For many of the questions raised and the diseases examined, there are scant data to examine. It would be inappropriate to suggest that, in the absence of data, no statement can be made about the benefits of cessation for that disease. Demonstration of a causal link between smoking and a given disease carries with it the strong presumption that stopping smoking will alter the smoker's subsequent risk. In the absence of evidence to the contrary, it would seem reasonable that diseases with similar mechanisms would respond to cessation with a similar time course and residual risk. The purpose of examining each question for each disease is to stimulate research and analyses on cessation, and the gaps identified should not be mistaken for a statement that cessation is without benefit for those diseases where gaps in the evidence exist.

Summary and assesment of the evidence

When assessing risk reduction within the first two years after smoking cessation, certain methodological issues of particular concern, including reverse causation and constancy of smoking habits, complicate interpretation of the data. Assessment of risk reduction following long term abstinence is less subject to these methodological concerns and can rely more on the very large observational cohort studies available to shed light on the issue. These methodological challenges in studying the effects of cessation are pertinent to all of the diseases covered in the Handbook and were acknowledged when examining the available evidence.

Lung Cancer
A large number of epidemiologic studies have compared lung cancer risk in persons who stop smoking with the risk of those who continue. The major published studies show lower lung cancer risk in former than in current smokers. The absolute annual risk of developing or dying from lung cancer does not decrease after stopping smoking. Rather, the principal benefit from cessation derives from avoiding the much steeper increase in risk that would result from continuing to smoke. Within five to nine years after quitting, the lower lung cancer risk in former compared with otherwise similar current smokers becomes apparent and diverges progressively with longer time since cessation. There is a persistent increased risk of lung cancer in former smokers compared to never smokers of the same age, even after a long duration of abstinence. Stopping smoking before middle age avoids much of the lifetime risk incurred by continuing to smoke. Stopping smoking in middle or old age confers substantially lower lung cancer risk compared with continuing smokers.

The full benefits of smoking cessation and hazards of continued smoking are underestimated, at least in absolute terms, in studies of populations where the maximum hazards of persistent lifetime smoking have not yet emerged. Individuals and policymakers who live in countries where lung cancer risk is still increasing should recognize that the maximum hazard from continuing to smoke—and the maximum benefits from cessation—have not yet been reached. Studies of cessation in these circumstances will seriously underestimate the long-term benefits of cessation.

Laryngeal Cancer
Four cohort studies and at least 15 case-control studies have reported information on smoking cessation and laryngeal cancer. These studies indicate that the risk of laryngeal cancer is considerably reduced in former smokers compared with current smokers. The relative risk steeply decreases with time since stopping smoking, with reductions

of about 60% after 10 to 15 years since cessation, and even larger after 20 years. The favourable effect of stopping smoking is already evident within a few years after cessation. However, after stopping smoking, former smokers still have elevated risks of laryngeal cancer as compared to never smokers for at least twenty years.

Oral Cancer

The results of four cohort studies and at least 25 case-control studies on oral and pharyngeal cancers have shown the risk for former smokers to be intermediate between those of never smokers and current smokers. In studies where risks were analysed by duration of abstinence, there was generally a decreasing relative risk with increasing duration of abstinence compared with continuing smokers. In several studies, the risk remained elevated compared with never smokers during a second decade of abstinence, but reached the level of never smokers thereafter.

Oesophageal Cancer

The results from at least 10 cohort and 10 case-control studies indicate that former smokers have a lower risk than current smokers of squamous-cell oesophageal cancer. Most investigations have shown that the risk of oesophageal cancer remains elevated many years (at least 20) after cessation of smoking. After 10 years since cessation of smoking, former smokers still have twice the oesophageal cancer risk of never smokers.

A few studies have investigated the effect of smoking cessation on adenocarcinoma, indicating no clear reduction of risk. The data on oesophageal adenocarcinoma are too limited, however, to provide adequate inference on the relation with time since smoking cessation.

Stomach Cancer

Epidemiological studies show that former smokers have a lower risk for stomach cancer than do current smokers. Increasing number of years since cessation and younger age at cessation were associated with decreasing risk in comparison with continuing smokers in most studies.

Liver Cancer

The risk of cancer of the liver appears to be lower in former than in current smokers, but the data are inconsistent across geographic areas. There is inadequate information to assess the effect of time since cessation.

Pancreatic Cancer

The risk of pancreatic cancer is lower in former than in current smokers. Based on the limited evidence, the risk declines with time since cessation compared to continuing smokers, but remains higher than that in never smokers for at least 15 years after cessation.

Bladder Cancer

The risk of cancer of the bladder is lower in former than in current smokers. The relative risk declines with time since cessation in comparison with continuing smokers, but remains higher than that for never smokers for at least 25 years after cessation.

Renal Cell Cancer

The risk of renal cell cancer is lower in former than in current smokers. Based on limited evidence, the relative risk declines with time since cessation in comparison with continuing smokers, but remains higher than that for never smokers for at least 20 years after cessation.

Cervical Cancer

The risk of squamous cell carcinoma of the cervix is lower in former smokers than in current smokers. Following cessation, the risk in former smokers rapidly decreases to the level of never smokers.

Myeloid Leukemia

The risk of myeloid leukemia may be lower in former smokers than in current smokers, but available data are inconsistent. There is inadequate information to assess the effect of duration of abstinence.

Nasopharyngeal and Sinonasal Cancer

The risk in former smokers seems to be lower than in current smokers for nasopharyngeal carcinoma. There is inadequate information to assess the effects of duration of abstinence.

For sinonasal carcinoma as well there is inadequate information to assess the effect of abstinence.

Coronary Heart Disease (CHD)

Cigarette smoking is a major cause of coronary heart disease. The risk is manifest both as an increased risk for thrombosis and as an increased degree of atherosclerosis in coronary vessels. The cardiovascular risk caused by cigarette smoking increases with the amount smoked and with the duration of smoking. Former smokers have considerably reduced risk of CHD compared to smokers.

Evidence from studies of patients with manifest CHD point toward a relative risk reduction in the order of 35% compared with continued cigarette smokers of similar accumulated exposure within the first two to four years of smoking cessation. Findings from case-control studies and cohort studies of subjects without diagnosed CHD are compatible with this conclusion and point toward a similar relative risk reduction following smoking cessation.

Some studies of prolonged abstinence find the risk to be similar to never smokers after 10 to 15 years of abstinence, whereas others find a persistent increased risk of 10-20% even after 10 to 20 years. The main methodological issue in this type of study is misclassification of both current and former smoking status with prolonged follow-up without re-assessment of smoking status. An additional issue is self-selection of former smokers. Taking these methodological issues into account, the body of evidence suggests that the risk of CHD with long-term abstinence approaches the risk of never smokers asymptotically. The risk reduction is observed after controlling for other major risk factors.

Cerebrovascular Disease

Smoking is a cause of stroke. Data from large prospective studies revealed that current smokers have a relative risk of 1.5 to 4 for stroke compared with never-smokers. Former smokers have markedly lower risk compared to current smokers.

Studies that have assessed the effect of duration of abstinence on stroke risk report a marked risk reduction by two to five years after cessation, and the relative risk decreases for up to 15 years after cessation. In some studies, the risk returns to that of never smokers by five to ten years, but other studies report small increased risks even after 15 years of abstinence; all of these studies show a lower risk for former smokers than for continuing smokers. The risk reduction is observed after controlling for other major risk factors.

There is inadequate evidence to assess the effect of smoking cessation on the long-term prognosis among cerebrovascular disease patients.

Abdominal Aortic Aneurysm (AAA)

Prospective cohort and screening studies show that the risk of death from, and prevalence of, AAA is large (RR: 4.0-8.0) in current smokers compared with never smokers. The magnitude of this relative risk is greater than that observed in other forms of CVD for current smokers. Former smokers have a lower risk of AAA

than do continuing smokers. The limited data that address the relationship between the duration of cessation and risk of AAA suggest that cessation is associated with a slow decline in risk that continues for at least 20 years after stopping smoking. The risk remains greater than that of a never smoker, even after a prolonged duration of abstinence. This pattern is different from that observed in patients with coronary heart disease and cerebrovascular disease in that the risk remains significantly higher than that of never smokers. In patients with an established diagnosis of AAA, the single published intervention study concludes that former smoking status is associated with reduced all-cause mortality and AAA rupture compared with continued smoking.

Peripheral Artery Disease (PAD)

Data that address the time course of the change in risk with cessation are very limited, and the time course is different for populations with and without clinically evident disease.

In populations without clinically evident disease

Current smoking is a major cause of PAD. Former smokers have a reduced risk compared with current smokers. In former smokers without clinical evidence of disease, the reduction in risk of development of disease occurs over an extended period (at least 20 years), but the time course of reduction in risk is poorly characterized. Prospective cohort studies suggest that the relative risk of PAD in former smokers remains greater than that of never smokers even after long duration of abstinence (at least 20 years).

In populations with clinically evident disease

In patients with clinical evidence of PAD, the evidence suggests an improvement in clinical outcomes among former smokers compared to continuing smokers. PAD patients who stop smok-

ing experience complication rates that are similar to those who are classified as nonsmokers in the studies in a relatively short period of time following cessation (within one to five years), and the rates are substantially below those of continuing smokers. However, studies in patients with clinically evident PAD often classify smoking status as current smoker, ex-smoker and 'non-smoker', with non-smokers including never smokers and smokers who stopped before the beginning of follow-up. The evidence as a whole suggests there are important benefits of smoking cessation for patients with established PAD.

Chronic Obstructive Pulmonary Disease (COPD)

Former smokers have lower risk of accelerated loss of lung function and COPD-related morbidity and mortality than do continuing smokers.

Evidence from cross-sectional and longitudinal studies shows that symptoms of chronic bronchitis (chronic cough, mucus production and wheeze) decrease rapidly within a few months after smoking cessation. Prevalence of these symptoms is the same as that reported by never smokers within five years of sustained smoking abstinence. With respect to lung function loss, cohort studies of the general population show that the accelerated decline in FEV_1 observed in current smokers reverts to the age-related rate of decline seen in never smokers within 5 years of smoking cessation. In people diagnosed with mild to moderate COPD, an increase in FEV_1 during the first year after smoking cessation has been observed; in following years, the rate of decline in FEV_1 in sustained quitters has been half the rate of that observed in continuing smokers.

Data on lung capacity and hospital admission for patients with severe COPD are limited, but available evidence suggests that smoking cessation results in a reduction in excess lung function loss and a decrease in risk of hospitalization for COPD in comparison with continuing smokers. Evidence from several long-term studies indicates a substantial reduction in mortality risk in former smokers compared with continuing smokers. Assessment of risk reduction for COPD mortality following smoking cessation is complex because of reverse causality. For example, there is a persistent increased risk of COPD mortality with long duration of abstinence.

COPD in China

China is the world's largest producer of tobacco and cigarettes, with the world's largest number of smokers and largest number of tobacco deaths (about 1 million per year). Of all the diseases contributing to tobacco-related mortality, the most numerically significant is COPD, constituting 45% of tobacco-related deaths. Hence, China has the world's largest number of COPD deaths due to smoking, about 450 000 per year.

Evidence from 17 studies in the Chinese medical literature on the effects of cessation in COPD, though limited in quality and quantity, supports the finding that among middle-aged asymptomatic subjects, smoking cessation delayed the decline of FEV_1 when compared with continuing smokers. The decline became similar to that in never smokers after cessation for six years or more. In young and healthy smokers, the benefits of smoking cessation (improvements in FEV_1, or decline relative to continuing smokers) can be observed after cessation for a few months. Among subjects with chronic cough and phlegm but no COPD, cessation for at least one month to eight years delayed decline of FEV_1 and reduced the risk of developing COPD compared with that of continuing smokers. Whereas smoking can clearly increase the risk of COPD deaths, the benefits of cessation on COPD mortality have not been observed in the Chinese population. Instead, studies found excess risk among older quitters, probably due to reverse causality. It is not clear why Chinese never smokers have a much higher prevalence of COPD than those in North America; possible explanations are poor indoor air quality from burning of biomass and/or genetic differences. In addition, there is a common belief among the Chinese public that smoking cessation may be harmful in smokers with COPD. Smokers who already have serious COPD, diagnosed or undiagnosed by a doctor, may appear to die from COPD soon after quitting smoking (reverse causality). Because of the higher proportion of COPD among the total tobacco death toll in China, smoking cessation on a large scale is likely to result in greater long-term effects on COPD morbidity and mortality than for other diseases, such as lung cancer and ischaemic heart disease.

References

Burns D, Lee L, Shen Z, et al. (1997). Cigarette smoking behavior in the United States. In: Burns DM, Garfinkel L, Samet J, eds. *Changes in Cigarette-Related Disease Risks and Their Implication for Prevention and Control*. US DHHS, NIH, NCI: 13-112.

Burns D (2000). Smoking cessation: Recent indicators of what's working at a population level. In: Burns D, Shopland D, eds., *Population Based Smoking Cessation: Proceedings of a Conference on What Works to Influence Cessation in the General Population*. USDHHS, NIH, NCI, NIH: 1-23.

Burns D, Major J, Anderson C, et al. (2003) Changes in cross-sectional measures of cessation, numbers of cigarettes smoked per day, and time to first cigarette –

California and national data. In Burns D, ed., Those who Continue to Smoke: Is Achieving Abstinence Harder and Do We Need to Change Our Interventions? USDHHS, NIH, NCI, NIH: 101-125.

Doll R, Peto R, Boreham J, et al. (2004). Mortality in relation to smoking: 50 years' observations on male British doctors. *BMJ,* 328(7455):1519.

Gritz ER, Dresler C, Sarna L (2005). Smoking, the missing drug interaction in clinical trials: ignoring the obvious. *Cancer Epidemiol Biomarkers Prev,* 14(10):2287-2293.

IARC (2004). *IARC Monographs on the Evaluation of Carcinogenic Risks to Humans, Vol. 83, Tobacco Smoke and Involuntary Smoking.* Lyon, IARCPress.

Lopez AD, Collishaw NE, Piha T (1994). A descriptive model of the cigarette epidemic in developed countries. *Tob Control,* 3:242-247.

Thun MJ, Myers DG, Day-Lally C, et al. (1997). Age and the exposure-response relationships between cigarette smoking and premature death in Cancer Prevention Study II. In: *Changes in Cigarette-Related Disease Risks and Their Implications for Prevention and Control* NIH Publication No1 97-4213: 383-476.

United States Department of Health and Human Service (USDHHS) (1984). *The Health Consequences of Smoking: Chronic Obstructive Lung Disease*. A Report of the Surgeon General. Rockville, MD, U.S. Dept. of Health and Human Services, Public Health Service, Office on Smoking and Health; Washington, D.C.

United States Department of Health and Human Service (USDHHS) (2004). *The Health Consequences of Smoking. A Report of the Surgeon General*. Atlanta, GA, U. S. Department of Health and Human Services, Centers for Disease Control and Prevention, Office on Smoking and Health.

Is There Sufficient Evidence to Address Questions on the Effects of Smoking Cessation on Risk of Disease?

1. **Risk for Former Smokers:** Is there sufficient evidence to determine whether the risk of disease is lower in former smokers than in otherwise similar current smokers?

2. **Risk with Prolonged Abstinence:** Is there sufficient evidence to determine whether, among otherwise similar former smokers, the risk of disease is lower with more prolonged abstinence?

3. **Residual Increased Risk:** Is there sufficient evidence to determine whether the risk returns to that of never smokers after long periods of abstinence?

Disease	Risk for Former Smokers (1)	Risk with Prolonged Abstinence (2)	Residual Increased Risk (3)
Cancers			
Lung cancer	■	■	■
Laryngeal cancer	■	■	■
Oral cancer	■	■	■
Squamous cell esophageal cancer	■	■	■
Esophageal adenocarcinoma	□	□	□
Stomach cancer	■	⊠	□
Liver cancer	⊠	□	□
Pancreatic cancer	■	■	⊠
Bladder cancer	■	■	■
Renal cancer	■	⊠	□
Cervical cancer	■	■	■
Myeloid leukemia	+/-	□	□
Nasopharyngeal cancer	⊠	□	□
Sinonasal cancer	□	□	□
Vascular Disease			
CHD incidence and death in subjects without established disease	■	■	■
CHD incidence and death in those with clinical evident disease	■	■	Not applicable
Cerebrovascular disease incidence and death for those without established disease	■	■	⊠
Cerebrovascular disease incidence and death for those with clinical disease	□	□	Not applicable
Aortic aneurysm incidence and death for those without established disease	■	⊠	⊠
Aortic aneurysm incidence and death for those with clinical disease	■	□	Not applicable
PAD incidence and death for those without established disease	■	⊠	⊠
PAD incidence and death for those with clinical disease	⊠	⊠	Not applicable
Lung Disease			
Cough and phlegm production	■	■	■
Decline in FEV_1 in healthy subjects	■	■	■
Decline in FEV_1 for those with mild/moderate disease	■	■	Not applicable
Decline in FEV_1 for those with severe disease/Morbidity	■	■	Not applicable
Mortality from COPD	■	■	⊠

Level of evidence to address questions:

■ Adequate: The evidence is adequate to draw a clear conclusion on the question; ⊠ Limited: The evidence to answer the question is suggestive; the interpretation is considered by the Working Group to be credible, but chance, bias, confounding or other factors cannot be adequately evaluated; +/- Conflicting: The data provide conflicting answers to the question; □ Absence of Observations: There is an absence of data or data are inadequate to address the question.

FEV_1: Forced expiratory volume in one second; CHD: Coronary Heart Disease; PAD: Peripheral Artery Disease

The Hazards of Smoking and the Benefits of Stopping:
Cancer Mortality and Overall Mortality

This *Handbook* is concerned with the health benefits of smoking cessation and, in particular, with the full eventual effects of cessation on life expectancy. It is chiefly concerned not with how to achieve cessation, but merely with the health benefits that smokers can expect if they do stop—and stay stopped—in comparison with the hazards that they would face if they were to continue. In general, for smokers who stop before middle age the resulting difference in life expectancy is about 10 years. This conclusion comes chiefly from studies of males in populations where the full hazards of smoking are already apparent, but it is likely to apply approximately equally to females and to populations where the hazards are not yet fully apparent, as young smokers in those populations will eventually experience substantial hazards if they continue.

Different sections of the main report deal separately (citing full references) with the eventual effects of smoking, and of smoking cessation, on particular conditions such as cancers of the lung, mouth, pharynx, larynx, oesophagus, stomach, liver, pancreas, kidney, bladder or cervix, heart disease, stroke, other vascular diseases and chronic obstructive lung disease. This Introductory section, however, stands back from such detail and summarises the eventual effects of smoking, and the eventual effects of smoking cessation, on overall mortality and on lung cancer mortality (or on the total cancer mortality attributed to smoking, most of which involves lung cancer). As long as due allowance is made for the remarkably long delay between cause and full effect, reliable quantitative conclusions emerge about the hazards that will eventually be faced by those in their 20s, 30s or 40s who have been habitual cigarette smokers since early adult life if they continue to smoke and, correspondingly, about the eventual benefits for such persistent smokers of stopping permanently.

Smoking is extraordinarily destructive (Table 1). Cigarette smoking is common in many populations, and where the

---

Table 1.   Main findings for the individual who becomes a habitual cigarette smoker in adolescence or early adult life

The risk is big

– About half are eventually killed by smoking, if they continue.
  [Among persistent cigarette smokers, male or female, the overall relative risk of death is greater than 2 throughout middle age and well into old age. Thus, among smokers of a given age more than half of those who die in the near future would not have done so at never smoker death rates.]
– On average, smokers lose about 10 years of life.
  [This average combines a zero loss for those not killed by tobacco, and an average loss of much more than 10 years for those who are killed by it.]

Those killed in middle age (35-69 years of age) can lose many years of life

– Some of those killed in middle age might have died soon anyway, but others might have lived on for another 10, 20, 30 or more good years.
– On average, those killed in middle age lose about 20 years of never smoker life expectancy.

Stopping smoking works

– Even in early middle age, those who stop (before they have incurable lung cancer or some other fatal disease) avoid most of their risk of being killed by tobacco.
– Stopping before middle age works even better.
– Those who have habitually smoked cigarettes since early adult life but stop at 60, 50, 40 or 30 years of age gain, respectively, about 3, 6, 9 or almost the full 10 years of life expectancy, in comparison with those who continue to smoke.

Main reference: Doll *et al.* (2004)

habit has been widespread among young adults for many decades, about half of all persistent cigarette smokers are eventually killed by it, unless they stop. Bidi smoking ('bidis' consist of a small amount of tobacco wrapped in the leaf of another plant), which is common in parts of Asia, probably causes similar risks (Gajalakshmi et al., 2003). Cigarette smoking causes relatively few deaths before about 35 years of age, but it causes many deaths in middle age (here defined as 35–69 years) and at older ages. Although some of those killed by tobacco in middle age might have died soon anyway, many could have lived on for another 10, 20, 30 or more good years. Those who stop

smoking in early middle age, however (before they have incurable lung cancer or some other fatal disease), avoid most of their risk of being killed by tobacco, and stopping before middle age is even more effective, gaining on average about an extra 10 years of life.

Effects of cessation on lung cancer mortality and on all-cause mortality in Europe and North America

Lung cancer is one of the main diseases caused by smoking. Even though it accounts for less than half of all smoking-attributed mortality, when the

lung cancer death rates among persistent cigarette smokers, former smokers and never smokers are compared, the relative risks are so extreme that the long-term hazards of smoking and benefits of stopping can be seen particularly clearly. Figures 1–3 compare, for men in Western Europe, Eastern Europe and North America, the lung cancer rates in continuing smokers, never smokers, and former smokers who stopped at about 30, 40 or even 50 years of age (although the risks among continuing smokers are slightly under-estimated in the North American study–see Figure 3). In each population the hazards of persistent cigarette smoking are substantial, and in each population the former smokers

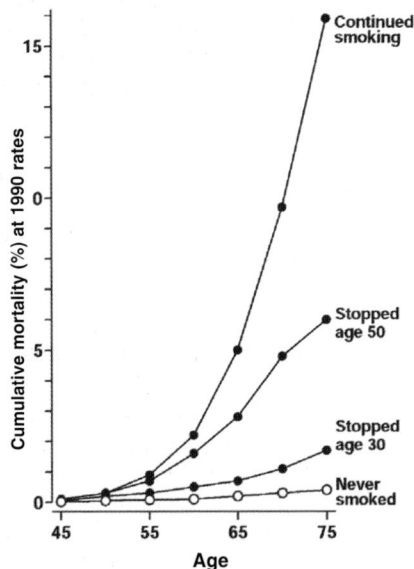

Figure 1. Lung cancer mortality (%) in UK males at 1990 death rates by smoking status

Only selected smoking categories are displayed (never, stopped within 5 years of stated age, continued), and almost all smokers had used cigarettes.

In each age range the relative risks match those in a case-control study of smoking, and an appropriately weighted average of the absolute risks matches the national lung cancer death rate.

Reproduced with permission from Peto et al. (2000).

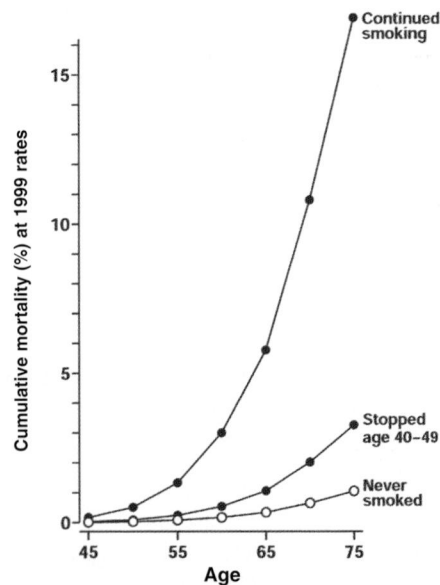

Figure 2. Lung cancer mortality in Polish males at 1999 death rates by smoking status

Only selected smoking categories are displayed (never, stopped within 5 years of stated age, continued), and almost all smokers had used cigarettes.

In each age range the relative risks match those in a case-control study of smoking, and an appropriately weighted average of the absolute risks matches the national lung cancer death rate.

Reproduced with permission from Brennan et al. (2006).

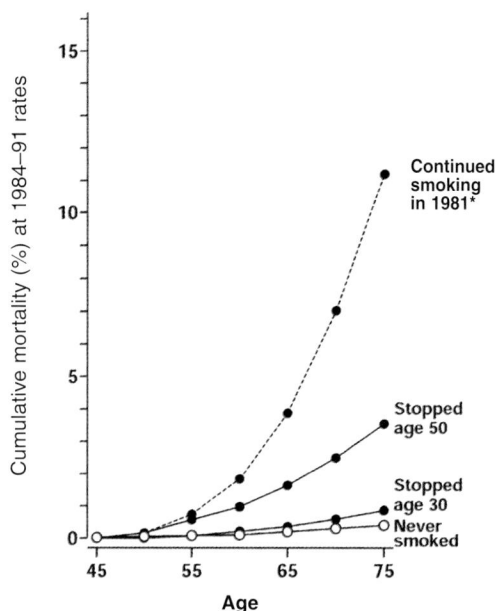

Figure 3. Lung cancer mortality in US males, 1984–91, by smoking status in 1981: ACS CPS–II prospective study

Only selected smoking categories are displayed (never, stopped within 5 years of stated age, continued), and almost all smokers had used cigarettes.

From the American Cancer Society (ACS) CPS-II 10-year prospective study of one million adults, omitting the earlier years (1981–83). *Re-survey of a sub-sample suggested that about half of those who were continuing to smoke in 1981 stopped during the 1980's but that few who had stopped by 1981 would restart. Data provided in 2006 by M. Thun, personal communcation.

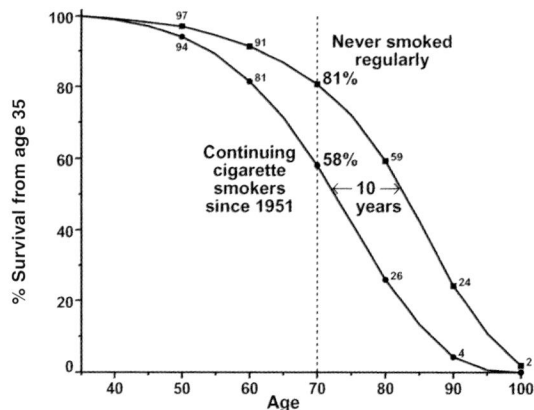

Figure 4. Survival from age 35: continuing cigarette smokers vs never smokers

50-year prospective follow-up (1951-2001) of mortality in relation to smoking among male British doctors born 1900-1930. Men were asked in 1951, and again every few years until 2001, what they smoked. Few never smokers or ex-smokers became smokers, but many smokers became ex-smokers. Analyses are by habit last reported. Among men born 1900-1930, the continuing smokers (and ex-smokers) would on average have started at about 18 years of age, and smoked about 20 cigarettes per day.

Reproduced with permission from Doll *et al.* (2004).

still have some excess risk many years after stopping. There is, however, a large absolute difference between the eventual risks in those who stop at about 30 to 50 years of age and in those who continue smoking. This is true for lung cancer, and it is also true for overall mortality (see below)—indeed, during the first decade or two after stopping smoking, the absolute mortality difference may well be much greater for other diseases than for lung cancer.

British males born in the 20th century were the first large population in which many began to smoke substantial numbers of cigarettes in early adult life, and continued to do so. The lifelong effects of persistent cigarette smoking, and the corresponding benefits of stopping, can therefore be illustrated by the experience of male British doctors born during the first few decades of the 20th century (1900–1930) and followed prospectively throughout the last half of it (1951–2001). Their smoking habits were ascertained in 1951 and every few years thereafter, and their mortality was monitored reliably. Figure 4 compares cigarette smokers with never smokers, showing the 10-year decrease in life expectancy. During middle age (35-69) 19% of the never smokers and 42% of the cigarette smokers died (i.e. the respective probabilities of survival were 81% and 58%), and much of this absolute difference of 23% in mortality was actually caused by smoking. For, it mainly involved differences in the numbers dying from diseases that can be caused by smoking (lung cancer, heart disease, chronic lung disease, etc.); most of the participants had much the same profession (as all were male doctors who had been on the UK Medical Register in 1951); and there were no material differences between smokers, former smokers and never smokers in mean alcohol consumption or obesity.

Figure 5 shows, however, that those who stopped at around 40 (35-44) years of age lost only about 1 year of life expectancy instead of 10 years, even though they had already smoked cigarettes for a mean of some 20 years before stopping. On average, the life expectancy gained by stopping at about 60, 50, 40 or 30 years of age, in comparison with those who continued, was, respectively, about 3, 6, 9 or almost the full 10 years in this study. Other studies indicate that those who smoke until 30 years of age and then stop do have a small but significant excess risk of lung cancer in old age (Figures 1-3), but agree that cessation avoids most of the excess mortality among continuing smokers.

The study of mortality in relation to smoking among British doctors assessed the effects of men who had not yet developed a life-threatening disease stopping before middle age or during middle age, but other studies have shown that even after the onset of disease cessation may well remain important (Table 2).

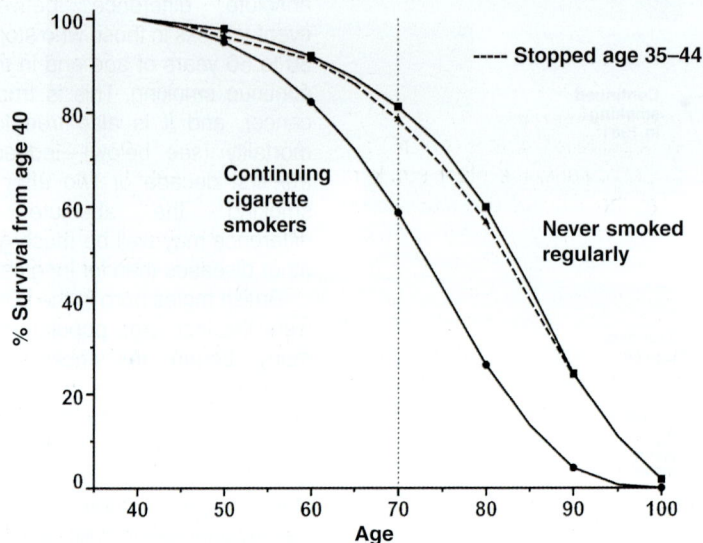

Figure 5. Survival from age 40: continuing cigarette smokers vs never smokers vs smokers who stopped at about age 40

50-year prospective follow-up (1951–2001) of mortality in relation to smoking among male British doctors born 1900-1930. Men were asked in 1951, and again every few years until 2001, what they smoked. Few never smokers or ex-smokers became smokers, but many smokers became ex-smokers. Analyses are by habit last reported. Among men born 1900–1930, the continuing smokers (and ex-smokers) would on average have started at about 18 years of age, and smoked about 20 cigarettes per day. Dotted line corresponds to the survival of those stopping smoking.

Reproduced with permission from Doll *et al.* (2004).

Table 2. Effects of cessation at different ages

Time of stopping smoking	Effect on later risk of death from smoking
Before middle age, e.g. at about age 20–30	Avoids nearly all of the future mortality from tobacco in middle and old age
During middle age, e.g. at about 40–50, but before major disease onset	Avoids much hazard over the next few decades, but some hazard remains
After the onset of life-threatening disease	Rapid benefit (particularly for vascular mortality), unless the existing disease causes death

Main reference: present volume

Under-estimation of eventual hazards of smoking and benefits of stopping in many studies of other populations

Cigarette consumption was low worldwide in 1900, but among men in many developed countries such as the United Kingdom or United States it increased substantially during the first few decades of the 20th century (IARC, 2004). In recent decades it has also increased substantially among women in many developed countries and among men in many developing countries, including China. When in a particular population there is an upsurge of cigarette smoking among young adults, it may be about 30 or 40 years before the main upsurge of tobacco deaths in middle age is seen, and then another 20 years before the main upsurge of tobacco deaths in old age.

The United Kingdom was the first major country in the world to experience a large increase in lung cancer from cigarette smoking. Even in Britain, however, it is only among men born early in the 20th century, many of whom started in youth the habit of smoking substantial numbers of cigarettes, that we can assess directly the full hazards of continuing to do so throughout adult life, and, correspondingly, the full long-term benefits of stopping at various ages. That is why the results for such men (Figures 4 and 5) are particularly relevant to predicting the future worldwide health effects of current smoking patterns, and the eventual importance of cessation, particularly before middle age. For, even in populations where there is not yet a high death rate from smoking (because relatively few who are now in middle or old age have been habitual cigarette smokers throughout adult life), many of those who start smoking cigarettes nowadays do so in adolescence or early adult life, as did many of the British doctors described in Figures 4 and 5, so the

young smokers in those populations will eventually also face substantial risks in middle and old age if they continue to smoke, and have much to gain from prompt cessation.

Many previous epidemiological studies of smoking and disease took place in populations where the middle-aged or, particularly, the older smokers had not at the time of the study been smoking substantial numbers of cigarettes throughout adult life, and where the national lung cancer rates in middle or old age were still relatively low, or rising steeply. This is true for many previous studies of men and may well be true for all previous studies of women. The risks found by comparing the smokers and the former smokers (or never smokers) in those studies may therefore greatly underestimate the risks that the younger cigarette smokers of today will eventually face if they continue. Hence, in those previous studies the apparent absolute benefits after 20, 30 or more years of cessation are likely to be substantially less than the absolute benefits that the younger cigarette smokers of today could gain from cessation (in comparison with the risks they would otherwise face if they were to continue).

In many studies the proportional excess mortality in middle and old age from smoking is greater among male than among female smokers, but this may be chiefly because they smoked cigarettes more intensively when young than the female smokers did. If, however, smoking cigarettes throughout adult life eventually produces about as great a proportional increase in female as in male overall death rates, then in terms of years of life expectancy lost or gained the eventual hazards of persistent cigarette smoking (and the corresponding benefits of cessation) may well be about as great for women as for men.

Likewise, among men in developing countries such as China, the hazards

that younger cigarette smokers will eventually face in middle and old age may well be substantially greater than the risks now seen among Chinese smokers in middle and old age (Peto *et al.*, 1999). Indeed, for any cigarette smoker, male or female, in any part of the world who started smoking substantial numbers of cigarettes when young and has continued doing so, the eventual hazards may well be similar: about half will be killed by their habit unless they stop, and cessation before age 40 (or, better, before age 30) would avoid most of that risk. In any population in the world, therefore, the prevalence of cigarette (or bidi) smoking among young adults can be used as a proxy to predict the eventual future impact of smoking on mortality in that population several decades hence if those who now smoke continue to do so, and to predict the corresponding importance for those who now smoke of prompt cessation.

Contrasting national trends in tobacco-attributed mortality at ages 35–69

In many countries the trends in cigarette smoking and, more recently, in cessation have been so extreme that they have dominated the recent national trends in cancer mortality and in overall mortality, at least among middle-aged men. The United Kingdom, Poland and the USA offer three contrasting examples of this (Figures 6–11).

In the United Kingdom (Figures 6 and 7), cigarette smoking became widespread during the first few decades of the 20th century among men, and around the middle of the century among women. By the 1960s the male death rates attributed to tobacco in the United Kingdom were among the worst in the world, with smoking causing more than half of the cancer mortality and almost

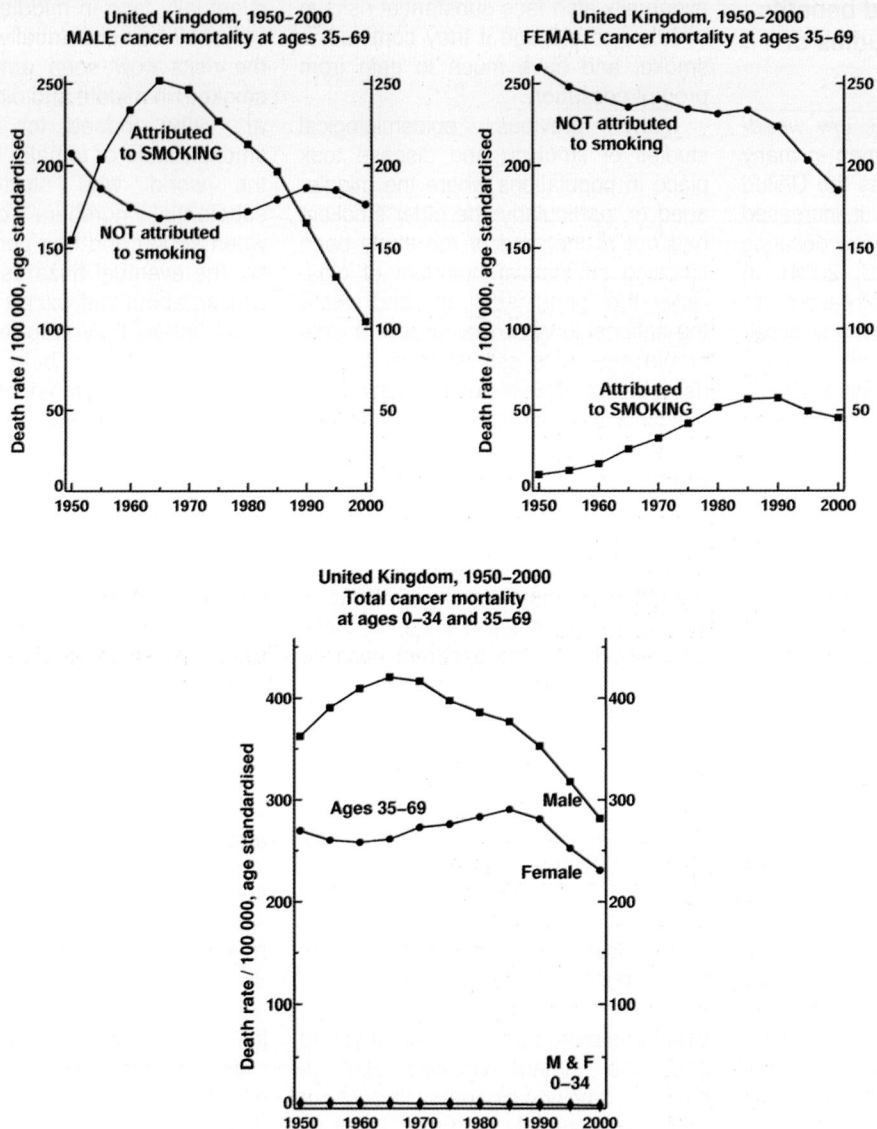

**United Kingdom, 1950–2000
MALE cancer mortality at ages 35–69**

Attributed to SMOKING

NOT attributed to smoking

**United Kingdom, 1950–2000
FEMALE cancer mortality at ages 35–69**

NOT attributed to smoking

Attributed to SMOKING

**United Kingdom, 1950–2000
Total cancer mortality
at ages 0–34 and 35–69**

Ages 35–69

Male

Female

M & F
0–34

Figure 6. United Kingdom, 1950–2000. Total annual cancer mortality rates at ages 0–34 and 35-69 years, with the total male and total female rates at ages 35–69 years subdivided into the parts attributed, and not attributed, to smoking

Rates are calculated from WHO mortality data and UN population estimates, and are standardised to a uniform age distribution (so the standardised rate for a 35-year age range is the mean of the 7 rates in the component 5-year age ranges). In the absence of other causes of death, an annual rate of death of R per 100 000 would correspond to a 35-year probability of death of 1-exp(–35R/100 000). Thus, a rate of 300 would correspond to a probability of 10%.

The mortality attributed to smoking is estimated indirectly from the national mortality statistics (using the absolute lung cancer rate as a guide to the fraction of the deaths from other causes, or groups of causes, attributable to smoking).

From Peto *et al.* (1992, 1994). Update of figures, covering the period 1950–2000, available on www.deathsfromsmoking.net.

1950–2000: UNITED KINGDOM

Population risk of dying at ages 0–34

Population risk of a 35-year-old dying at ages 35–69 from smoking (shaded) or from any cause (shaded and white)

*e.g., at year 2000 male death rates out of 100 men aged 35, 25 would die before age 70 (with 6 of these deaths attributed to smoking)

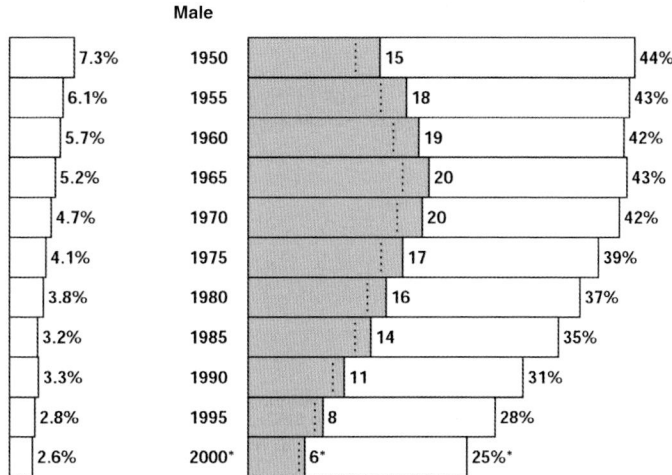

Male

Risk 0–34	Year	Shaded	Total
7.3%	1950	15	44%
6.1%	1955	18	43%
5.7%	1960	19	42%
5.2%	1965	20	43%
4.7%	1970	20	42%
4.1%	1975	17	39%
3.8%	1980	16	37%
3.2%	1985	14	35%
3.3%	1990	11	31%
2.8%	1995	8	28%
2.6%	2000*	6*	25%*

Note: Most of those killed by smoking would otherwise have survived beyond age 70, but a minority (shaded area to right of dotted line) would have died by 70 anyway

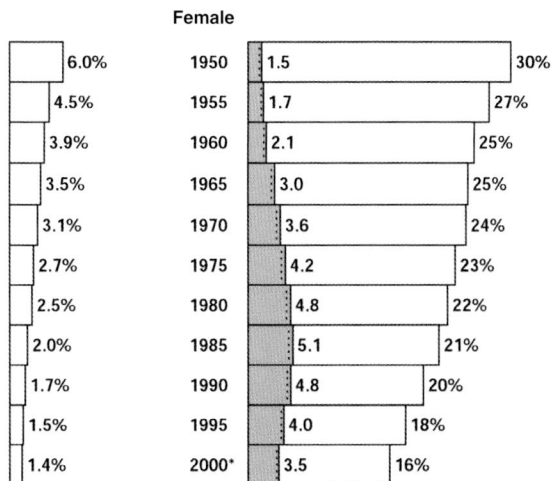

Female

Risk 0–34	Year	Shaded	Total
6.0%	1950	1.5	30%
4.5%	1955	1.7	27%
3.9%	1960	2.1	25%
3.5%	1965	3.0	25%
3.1%	1970	3.6	24%
2.7%	1975	4.2	23%
2.5%	1980	4.8	22%
2.0%	1985	5.1	21%
1.7%	1990	4.8	20%
1.5%	1995	4.0	18%
1.4%	2000*	3.5	16%

Figure 7. United Kingdom, 1950–2000. Probabilities of death at ages 0–34 and 35–69 at the death rates of particular calendar years, with the male and female probabilities of death from smoking at ages 35-69 shaded

Rates are calculated from WHO mortality data and UN population estimates, and are standardised to a uniform age distribution (so the standardised rate for a 35-year age range is the mean of the 7 rates in the component 5-year age ranges).

The mortality attributed to smoking is estimated indirectly from the national mortality statistics (using the absolute lung cancer rate as a guide to the fraction of the deaths from other causes, or groups of causes, attributable to smoking).

From Peto *et al.* (1992, 1994). Update of figures, covering the period 1950–2000, available on www.deathsfromsmoking.net.

Poland, 1965–2000
MALE cancer mortality at ages 35–69

Poland, 1965–2000
FEMALE cancer mortality at ages 35–69

Poland, 1965–2000
Total cancer mortality
at ages 0–34 and 35–69

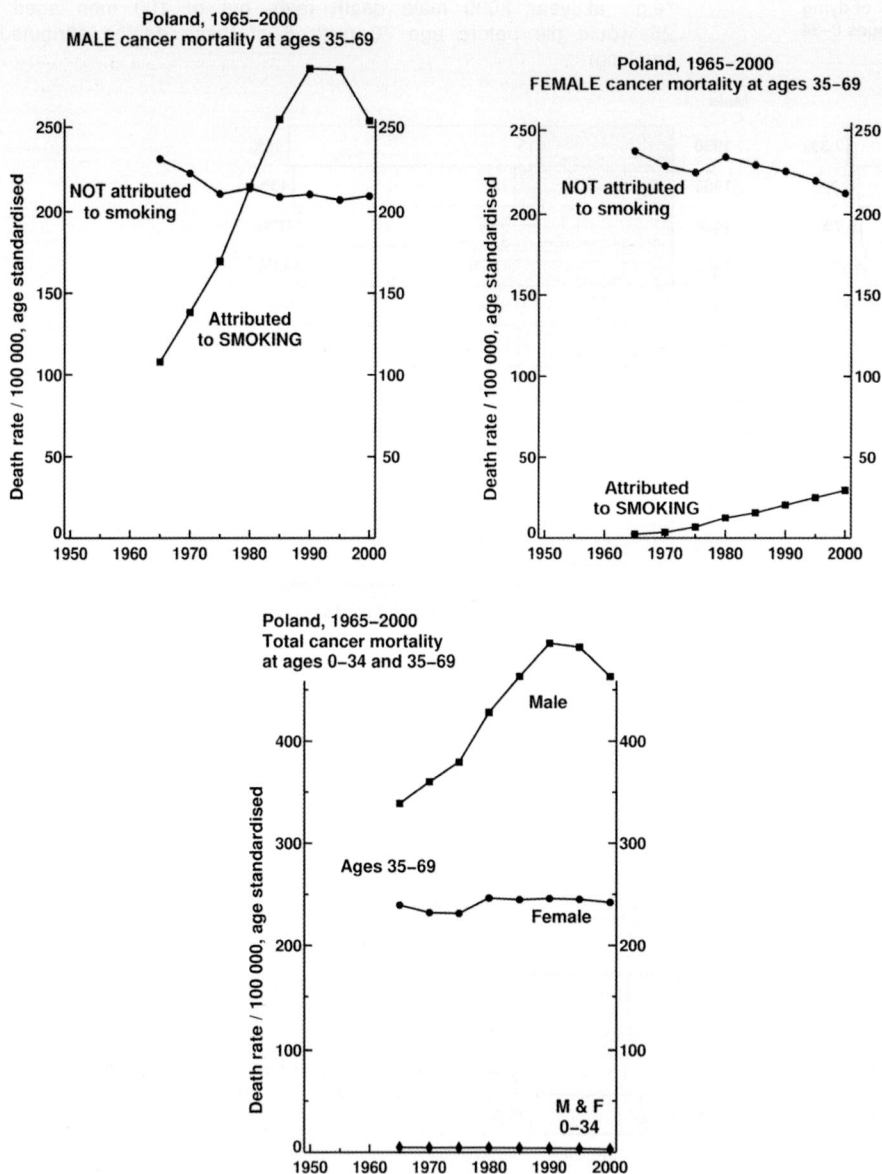

Figure 8. Poland, 1965–2000. Total annual cancer mortality rates at ages 0–34 and 35-69 years, with the total male and total female rates at ages 35-69 years subdivided into the parts attributed, and not attributed, to smoking

Rates are calculated from WHO mortality data and UN population estimates, and are standardised to a uniform age distribution (so the standardised rate for a 35-year age range is the mean of the 7 rates in the component 5-year age ranges). In the absence of other causes of death, an annual rate of death of R per 100 000 would correspond to a 35-year probability of death of 1-exp (–35R/100 000). Thus, a rate of 300 would correspond to a probability of 10%.

The mortality attributed to smoking is estimated indirectly from the national mortality statistics (using the absolute lung cancer rate as a guide to the fractionof the deaths from other causes, or groups of causes, attributable to smoking).

1955–2000: POLAND

Population risk of dying at ages 0–34

Population risk of a 35-year-old dying at ages 35–69 from smoking (shaded) or from any cause (shaded and white) *e.g., at year 2000 male death rates out of 100 men aged 35, 41 would die before age 70 (with 16 of these deaths attributed to smoking)

MALE

Population risk of dying at ages 0-34	Year	Shaded	Total
15.6%	1955	6	44%
10.4%	1960	8	40%
8.5%	1965	9	39%
8.0%	1970	12	41%
7.3%	1975	13	41%
6.9%	1980	16	46%
5.9%	1985	19	46%
5.7%	1990	20	47%
4.7%	1995	19	45%
3.7%	2000*	16*	41%*

Note: Most of those killed by smoking would otherwise have survived beyond age 70, but a minority (shaded area to right of dotted line) would have died by 70 anyway

FEMALE

Population risk of dying at ages 0-34	Year	Shaded	Total
12.1%	1955	0.2	31%
7.3%	1960	0.3	26%
5.6%	1965	0.4	25%
4.9%	1970	0.5	24%
4.1%	1975	0.8	23%
3.5%	1980	1.5	24%
3.0%	1985	2.0	24%
2.7%	1990	2.3	23%
2.3%	1995	2.5	21%
1.7%	2000*	2.6	19%

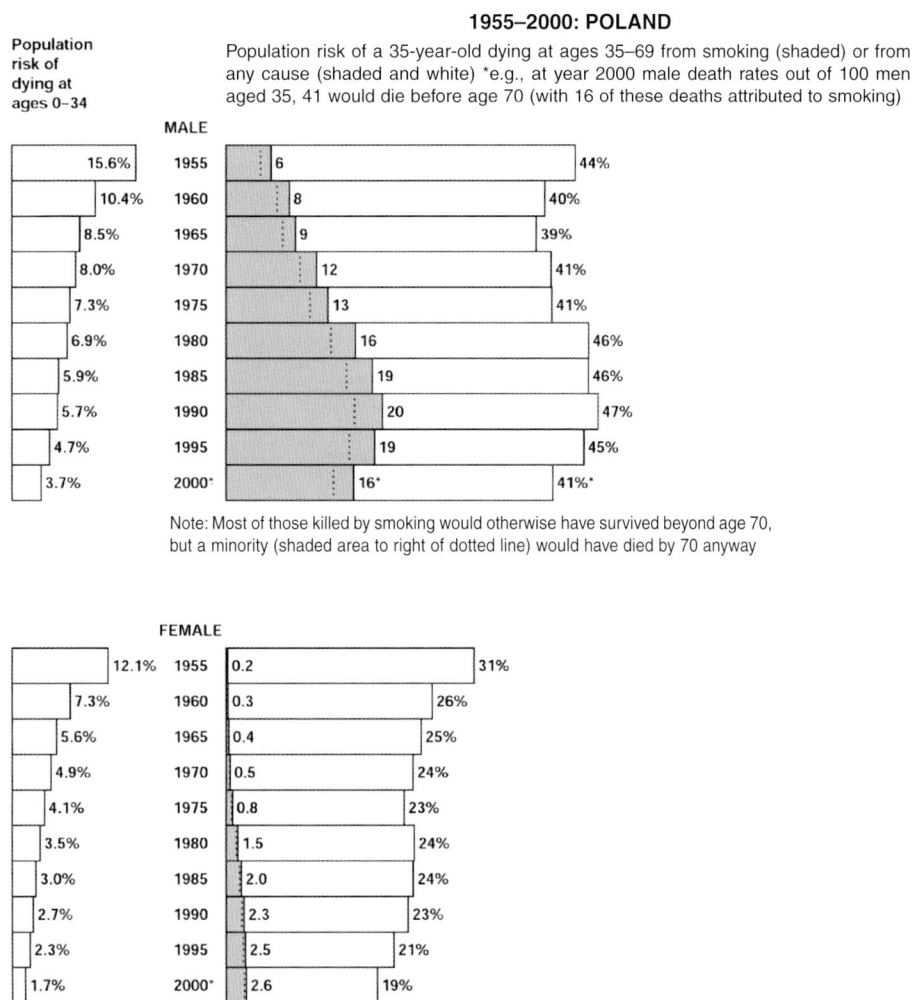

Figure 9. Poland, 1955–2000. Probabilities of death at ages 0-34 and 35-69 at the death rates of particular calendar years, with the male and female probabilities of death from smoking at ages 35-69 shaded

Rates are calculated from WHO mortality data and UN population estimates, and are standardised to a uniform age distribution (so the standardised rate for a 35-year age range is the mean of the 7 rates in the component 5-year age ranges).

The mortality attributed to smoking is estimated indirectly from the national mortality statistics (using the absolute lung cancer rate as a guide to the fraction of the deaths from other causes, or groups of causes, attributable to smoking).

From Peto *et al.* (1992, 1994). Update of figures, covering the period 1950–2000, available on www.deathsfromsmoking.net.

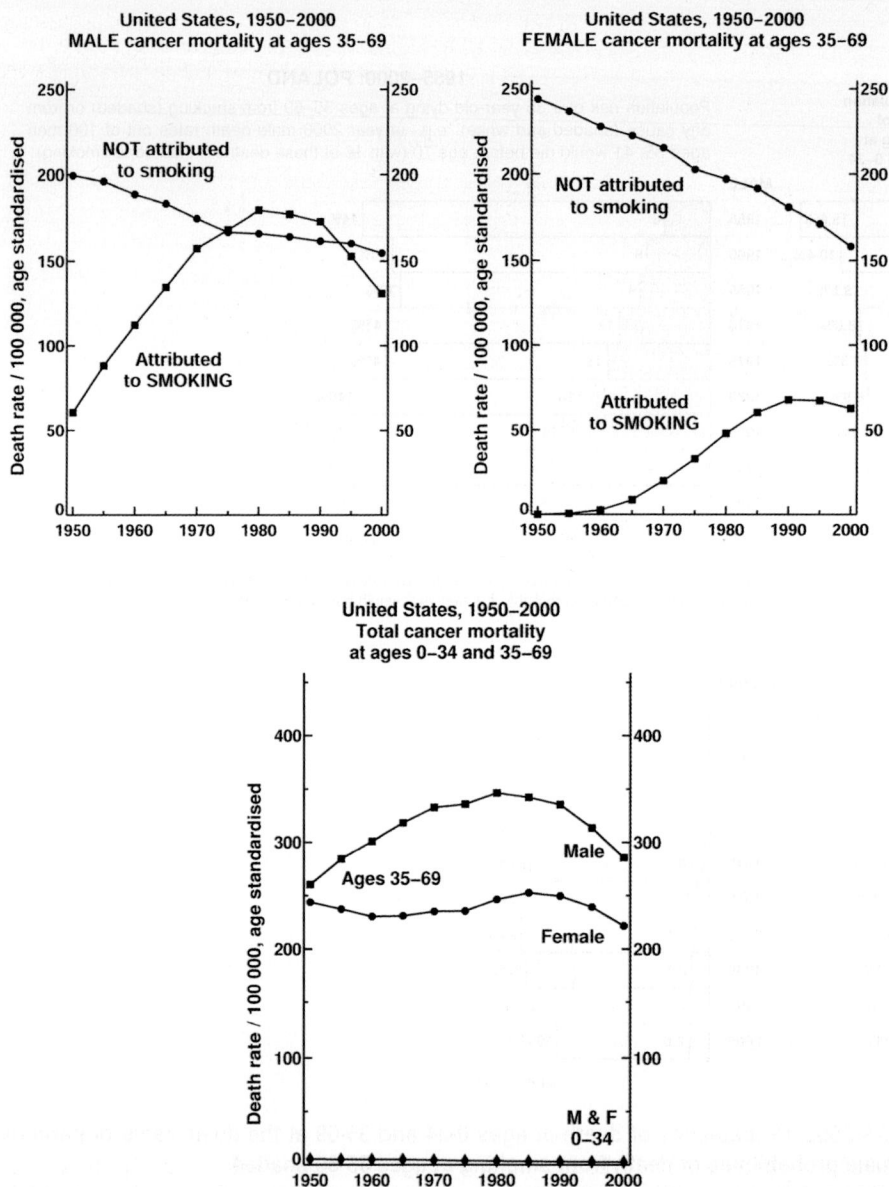

Figure 10. USA, 1950-2000. Total annual cancer mortality rates at ages 0–34 and 35-69 years, with the total male and total female rates at ages 35-69 years subdivided into the parts attributed, and not attributed, to smoking

Rates are calculated from WHO mortality data and UN population estimates, and are standardised to a uniform age distribution (so the standardised rate for a 35-year age range is the mean of the 7 rates in the component 5-year age ranges). In the absence of other causes of death, an annual rate of death of R per 100 000 would correspond to a 35-year probability of death of 1-exp (-35R/100 000). Thus, a rate of 300 would correspond to a probability of 10%.

The mortality attributed to smoking is estimated indirectly from the national mortality statistics (using the absolute lung cancer rate as a guide to the fraction of the deaths from other causes, or groups of causes, attributable to smoking).

From Peto *et al.* (1992, 1994). Update of figures, covering the period 1950–2000, available on www.deathsfromsmoking.net

1950–2000: UNITED STATES

Population risk of a 35-year-old dying at ages 35–69 from smoking (shaded) or from any cause (shaded and white) *e.g., at year 2000 male death rates out of 100 men aged 35, 27 would die before age 70 (with 8 of these deaths attributed to smoking)

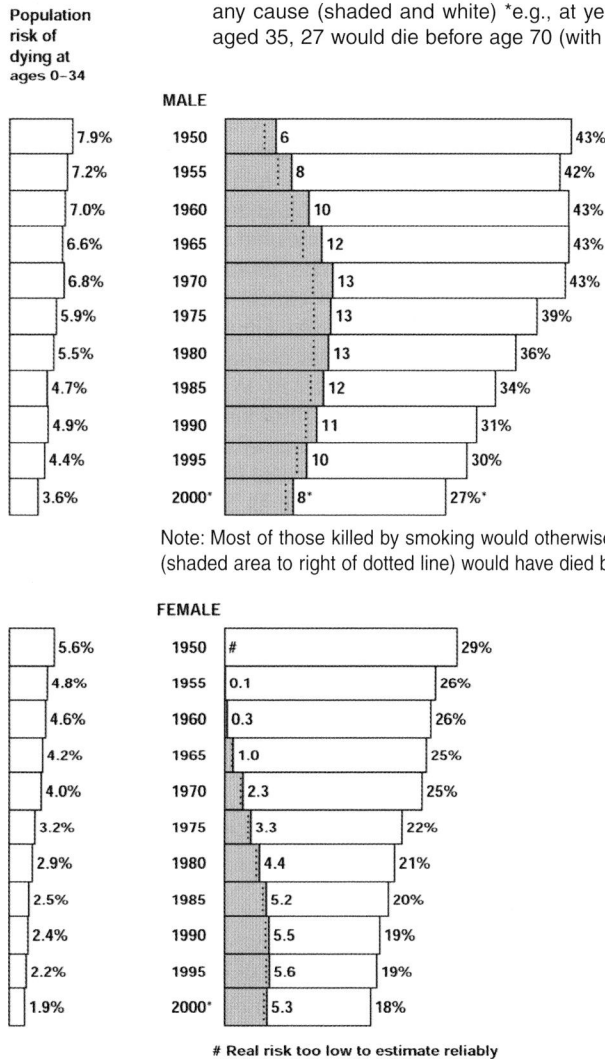

Population
risk of
dying at
ages 0-34

MALE

Population risk 0-34	Year	Smoking (shaded)	Any cause
7.9%	1950	6	43%
7.2%	1955	8	42%
7.0%	1960	10	43%
6.6%	1965	12	43%
6.8%	1970	13	43%
5.9%	1975	13	39%
5.5%	1980	13	36%
4.7%	1985	12	34%
4.9%	1990	11	31%
4.4%	1995	10	30%
3.6%	2000*	8*	27%*

Note: Most of those killed by smoking would otherwise have survived beyond age 70, but a minority (shaded area to right of dotted line) would have died by 70 anyway

FEMALE

Population risk 0-34	Year	Smoking (shaded)	Any cause
5.6%	1950	#	29%
4.8%	1955	0.1	26%
4.6%	1960	0.3	26%
4.2%	1965	1.0	25%
4.0%	1970	2.3	25%
3.2%	1975	3.3	22%
2.9%	1980	4.4	21%
2.5%	1985	5.2	20%
2.4%	1990	5.5	19%
2.2%	1995	5.6	19%
1.9%	2000*	5.3	18%

Real risk too low to estimate reliably

Figure 11. USA, 1950-2000. Probabilities of death at ages 0-34 and 35-69 at the death rates of particular calendar years, with the male and female probabilities of death from smoking at ages 35-69 shaded

Rates are calculated from WHO mortality data and UN population estimates, and are standardised to a uniform age distribution (so the standardised rate for a 35-year age range is the mean of the 7 rates in the component 5-year age ranges).

The mortality attributed to smoking is estimated indirectly from the national mortality statistics (using the absolute lung cancer rate as a guide to the fraction of the deaths from other causes, or groups of causes, attributable to smoking).

From Peto *et al.* (1992, 1994). Update of figures, covering the period 1950–2000, available on www.deathsfromsmoking.net.

half of the overall mortality among men in middle age, and the death rates from smoking among women were rising. Over the past few decades, however, there has been widespread cessation, a substantial decrease in the male death rates and, more recently, some decrease in the female death rates from smoking in the UK. Had UK female smokers all continued smoking, there could well have been a substantial rise in the UK female death rates from smoking in recent decades instead of the moderate decrease actually seen.

In Poland (Figures 8 and 9), the main increase in cigarette smoking took place around the middle of the century among males, and was followed by a large increase in tobacco-attributed mortality during the second half of the century (to levels comparable with those seen earlier in the UK). However, a decrease in smoking during the 1990s has been associated with the start of a decrease in this mortality. Women have thus far been less severely affected than men in Poland, although young Polish women who smoke will also face substantial hazards if they do not stop.

In the USA (Figures 10 and 11), a rapid increase in tobacco-attributed mortality among males was still in progress when it was halted (before the cancer or overall death rates from smoking were as high as they had been in the United Kingdom, and would become in Poland) by a substantial decrease in cigarette consumption over the past few decades. Since 1970 male lung cancer mortality in early middle age has fallen substantially, and male lung cancer mortality at later ages is beginning to do likewise. The death rate from smoking among women in the USA was still very low in 1950, but it rose rapidly and by the 1990s the female death rates attributed to smoking in the USA were among the worst in the world, although (as in men in the USA) the rise was

eventually halted by a decrease in cigarette consumption. Again, had US female smokers all continued smoking, there could well have been a substantial rise in recent decades in the US female death rates from smoking.

The methods used in these three populations to estimate smoking-attributed mortality, past and present, are indirect, so the absolute death rates in Figures 6-11 are somewhat uncertain (although they cannot be greatly in error for smoking-attributed cancer mortality, as most of this involves lung cancer), and some of the recent changes in the overall mortality attributed to smoking may be due to factors other than cessation, such as changes in other causes of vascular disease, or in its treatment. Nevertheless, the overall patterns should be reasonably trustworthy, confirming the enormous potential relevance of smoking cessation to overall mortality rates in such countries, and the practicability of substantial changes accumulating over a period of several years. This is true both in populations where smoking is already a major cause of death and in populations where it is not, but where it could become so if current smoking patterns persist.

Worldwide trends

Worldwide, about 100 million people a year reach adult life. Based on present smoking patterns about 50% of the young men and 10% of the young women will start to smoke, and most will continue. Of those who continue to smoke cigarettes or bidis, whether in Asia, America, Africa or Europe, about half will eventually be killed by their habit (unless they die before middle age of something else). Hence, if more than 20 million of these 30 million new smokers a year continue smoking cigarettes, and do not stop, and half of those who do so are killed by it, then

eventually more than 10 million people per year will be killed by tobacco.

Based on current smoking patterns, worldwide annual mortality from tobacco is likely to rise to about 10 million per year (i.e. 100 million per decade) by around the year 2030 (Peto *et al*, 1994, 2001), and will rise somewhat further in later decades. Tobacco is therefore expected to cause about 150 million deaths in the first quarter of the twenty-first century and 300 million in the second quarter. Predictions for the third and, particularly, the fourth quarter of the century are inevitably more speculative. However, if over the next few decades about 30% of the young adults become persistent cigarette or bidi smokers and about half who do are eventually killed by it, then about 10–15% of adult mortality in the second half of the century will be due to tobacco smoking (probably implying more than 500 million deaths due to tobacco in the second half of the century; Table 3).

The number of tobacco deaths predicted to occur before 2050 cannot be greatly reduced unless a substantial proportion of the adults who have already been smoking for some time give up the habit. A decrease over the next decade or two in the proportion of

Table 3. Projected numbers of deaths from tobacco during the 21st century, if current smoking patterns persist	
Period (years)	**Tobacco deaths (millions)**
2000-2024	~150
2025-2049	~300
2050-2099	>500
Total, 21st century	~1000
20th century, for comparison	~100

Source: Peto & Lopez (2001)

children who become smokers will not have its main effects on mortality until the middle and second half of the century. The effects of adult smokers quitting on deaths before 2050 and of young people not starting to smoke on deaths after 2050 will probably be approximately as follows:

- *Quitting:* If many of the adults who now smoke were to give up over the next decade or two, thus halving global cigarette consumption per adult by the 2020s, this would prevent about one-third of tobacco-related deaths in the 2020s and would almost halve tobacco-related deaths thereafter. Such changes could avoid about 20 or 30 million tobacco-related deaths in the first quarter of the century and

could avoid 100 million in the second quarter.

- *Not starting:* If, by progressive reduction over the next decade or two in the global uptake rate of smoking by young people, the proportion of young adults who become smokers were to be halved by the 2020s, this would avoid hundreds of millions of deaths from tobacco after 2050. It would, however, avoid almost none of the 150 million deaths from tobacco in the first quarter of the century, and would probably avoid 'only' about 10 or 20 million of the 300 million deaths from tobacco in the second quarter of the century.

Thus, using widely practicable ways of helping large numbers of young people not to become smokers could avoid

hundreds of millions of tobacco-related deaths in the middle and second half of the twenty-first century, but not before. In contrast, widely practicable ways of helping large numbers of adult smokers to quit (preferably before middle age, but also in middle age) might avoid one or two hundred million tobacco-related deaths in the first half of this century. Large numbers of deaths during the second half of the century could also be avoided if many of those who, despite warnings, still start to smoke in future years could be helped to stop before they are killed by the habit. Such calculations suggest that the effect of quitting could be more rapidly apparent on a population scale than the effects of not starting to smoke. Both, however, are of great importance.

References

Brennan P, Crispo A, Zaridze D, et al. (2006). High cumulative risk of lung cancer death among smokers and nonsmokers in Central and Eastern Europe. *Am J Epidemiol* 164(12): 1233-1241.

Doll R, Peto R, Wheatley K, et al. (1994). Mortality in relation to smoking: 40 years' observations on male British doctors. *BMJ*, 309(6959):901–911.

Doll R, Peto R, Boreham J, et al. (2004). Mortality in relation to smoking: 50 years' observations on male British doctors. *BMJ*, 328(7455):1519-1527.

Gajalakshmi V, Hung RJ, Mathew A, et al. (2003). Tobacco smoking and chewing, alcohol drinking and lung cancer risk among men in southern India. *Int J Cancer*, 107(3):441-447.

IARC (2004). *IARC Monographs on the Evaluation of Carcinogenic Risks to Humans, Vol. 83, Tobacco Smoke and Involuntary Smoking.* Lyon, IARCPress.

Peto R, Lopez AD, Boreham J, et al. (1992). Mortality from tobacco in developed countries: indirect estimation from national vital statistics. *Lancet,* 339(8804):1268–1278.

Peto R, Lopez AD, Boreham J, et al. (1994). *Mortality from Smoking in Developed Countries 1950-2000: Indirect Estimates from National Vital Statistics.* Oxford, Oxford University Press.

Peto R, Lopez AD, Boreham J, et al. (1996). Mortality from smoking worldwide. *Br Med Bull,* 52(1):12–21.

Peto R, Chen ZM, Boreham J (1999). Tobacco--the growing epidemic. *Nat Med*, 5(1):15-17.

Peto R, Darby S, Deo H, et al. (2000). Smoking, smoking cessation, and lung cancer in the UK since 1950: combination of national statistics with two case-control studies. *BMJ,* 321(7257):323-329.

Peto R, Lopez AD (2001). Future worldwide health effects of current smoking patterns. In: Koop CE, Pearson C, Schwarz MR, eds., *Critical issues in Global Health.* New York, Jossey-Bass: 154–161.

Websites

Deaths from smoking
http://www.deathsfromsmoking.net

Mechanistic Understandings of: Lung Cancer, Cardiovascular Diseases and Chronic Obstructive Pulmonary Disease

Tobacco Smoking Carcinogenesis and the Biology of Persistent Lung Cancer Risk

Introduction

Biomarkers of Gene Damage

Tobacco smoking has been causally associated with the development of human cancers of the lung, oral cavity, naso-, oro-, and hypopharynx, nasal cavity and paranasal sinuses, larynx, oesophagus, stomach, pancreas, liver, kidney (body and pelvis), ureter, urinary bladder, uterine cervix and bone marrow (acute myeloid leukemia) (IARC 1986, 2004). More than one in every 5 cancer deaths in the world in the year 2000 were caused by smoking, making it possibly the single largest preventable cause of cancer mortality (Ezzati et al., 2005). This section will focus on gene expression in the lung following cessation of cigarette smoking.

Tobacco smoke is a complex mixture that may lead to cancer through several mechanisms. Included among the 10^{10} particulates/ml and 4800 compounds of tobacco smoke (Hoffmann & Hecht, 1990) are 66 carcinogens evaluated by the International Agency for Research on Cancer (IARC) as having 'sufficient evidence for carcinogenicity' in laboratory animals or humans (Hoffmann et al., 2001). Of these, polycyclic aromatic hydrocarbons and the tobacco-specific nitrosamine 4-(methylnitrosamino)-1-(3-pyridyl)-1-butanone (NNK) are likely to play major roles (Hecht, 1999a). In addition, inducers of reactive oxygen species (ROS) like NO, NO_2, peroxynitrite and nitrosamines initiate, promote or amplify oxidative DNA damage (Church & Pryor, 1985; Zhang et al., 2002).

Several points may be summarized from the comprehensive review of tobacco carcinogenicity and its mechanism within the recent IARC Monograph volume 83 (IARC, 2004). Cells oxygenate most carcinogens using cytochrome P450 enzymes to convert carcinogens into an excretable form (Guengerich & Johnson, 1997). Excretion of oxygenated carcinogens may be facilitated by Phase II enzymes such as glutathione S-transferases (Beland & Kadlubar, 1985). However, some electrophilic oxygenated carcinogens seek the electrons on DNA and form covalently bound adducts. Six tobacco smoke carcinogens have been demonstrated to form DNA adducts in human tissues: benzo[a]pyrene (BaP) (IARC, 1983, 1987), 4-(N-nitrosomethylamino)-1-(3-pyridyl)-1-butanone (NNK) (IARC, 1985; Hecht et al., 1994), N-nitrosodimethylamine (NDMA) (IARC, 1978; Shuker & Bartsch, 1994), N'-nitrosonornicotine (NNN) (IARC, 1985; Hecht et al., 1994), ethylene oxide (IARC, 1994a) and 4-aminobiphenyl (4-ABP) (IARC, 1972; Kadlubar, 1994). Nitrosamines are direct-acting, nicotine-derived carcinogens in tobacco smoke that (unlike PAH) do not require activation to form DNA adducts (Hoffmann & Hecht, 1985). DNA adducts are central to the carcinogenic process induced by these agents (Hecht, 1999a; Tang et al., 2001).

Cells can remove adducts and repair the DNA to its normal structure (Memisoglu & Samson, 2000; Pegg, 2000; Hanawalt, 2001; Norbury & Hickson, 2001). Naturally occurring polymorphisms or acquired tobacco-related damage of DNA repair genes *OGG1* (8-oxoguanine glycosylase 1), *XRCC1* (X-ray repair cross-complementing group 1), *XPC* (xeroderma pigmentosum C), XPD, XPF and XRCC3 have been associated with lower DNA-adduct repair capacity and higher risk of lung cancer (David-Beabes & London, 2001; Spitz *et al.*, 2001; Liang *et al.*, 2003; Zhou *et al.*, 2003; Ito *et al.*, 2004). Studies have shown that the levels of carcinogen-DNA adducts in the tissues of smokers exceed those of nonsmokers. Carcinogen uptake, activation and binding to cellular macromolecules including DNA are higher in smokers than nonsmokers. Serial samples from 40 heavy smokers enrolled in a smoking cessation program demonstrated a significant reduction in mean PAH-DNA and 4-ABP-Hb adducts after cessation in all persons who were cotinine-verified quitters for at least 8 months (Mooney *et al.*, 1995). The balance between metabolic activation and metabolic detoxification, as well as the efficiency of DNA repair pathways, may define cancer risk in an individual exposed to polycyclic aromatic compounds (PACs).

Persisting BaP diol-epoxide-DNA adducts (primarily with the exocyclic amino group of guanosine) can lead to replication (meiotic) errors (G:C to T:A transversions) (Law, 1990). This reaction has been shown to be responsible for activating mutations in the HRAS-1 proto-oncogene (Marshall *et al.*, 1984; Vousden *et al.*, 1986) and inactivation of the tumour suppressor gene *TP53* (Hecht, 1999b). The gene most frequently found to be mutated in smoking-associated lung tumours is TP53 (Hernandez-Boussard & Hainaut, 1998; Hainaut & Pfeifer, 2001; Hussain *et al.*, 2001; IARC, 2004). *TP53* mutations are more common in smokers than in nonsmokers, and the frequency of *TP53* mutations shows a direct correlation with the number of cigarettes smoked. *TP53* mutations are found in preneoplastic lesions of the lung, indicating that they are early events in cell transformation. The *TP53* mutation spectrum in lung tumours of smokers contains 30% GC to TA transversion, while only 10% of

TP53 mutations in nonsmoker lung cancer are of this type. Mutations at K-RAS codons 12, 13, or 61 occur in approximately 30% of lung adenocarcinomas of smokers and also are primarily GC to TA transversions (as seen in TP53) (Slebos *et al.*, 1991; Husgafvel-Pursiainen *et al.*, 1993; Westra *et al.*, 1993; Gealy *et al.*, 1999; Ahrendt *et al.*, 2001). Mutations in other genes such as *FHIT, BCL-2*, and *BAX*, loss of heterozygosity (LOH) at specific chromosomal locations and gene overexpression (*TP53, MDM2)* have also been characterized in smoking-associated tumours (IARC, 2004).

Gene expression also may be altered by epigenetic mechanisms (without change in the DNA code) (Wolffe & Matzke, 1999). For example, during development imprinted embryonic cells epigenetically regulate programs of gene expression in precursor cells and their descendants (Reik *et al.*, 2001). Methylation of cytosine located upstream of guanine (CpG dinucleotides) in the regulatory (promoter) region of specific genes results in transcriptional silencing in cancer (Laird & Jaenisch, 1996; Jones & Laird, 1999). Several studies have shown that promoter hypermethylation of critical pathway genes could identify potential biomarkers for lung cancer (Belinsky *et al.*, 1998, 2005). Recently, Baylin & Ohm (2006) have proposed that epigenetic mechanisms may lead to alteration of TP53 chromatin through the SIRT1 histone deacetylase, inhibiting its transcription and impairing the TP53 response to DNA damage. Figure 1 diagrams one pathway toward lung carcinogenesis. This model illustrates the fundamental role of nicotine addiction to the chronic presentation of carcinogens to the airway epithelium. In 10–15% of smokers, this chronic exposure leads to molecular lesions (genetic and epigenetic) which in the presence of reduced metabolic detoxification result in the reduced repair

capability and/or loss of the TP53 gate-keeper that overwhelm cellular defenses and ultimately lead to lung cancer (Hecht, 1999b; Shields, 1999).

The multistep cancer progression model

The logarithmic increase of human cancers with aging has led to the hypothesis that the development of cancer requires four to seven rate-limiting stochastic events (Armitage & Doll, 1954; Renan, 1993). The concept of multi-step carcinogenesis is supported by description of the pathology of cancer of a variety of organs that shows a stepwise morphologic progression from normalcy through invasive cancer (Foulds, 1954; Saccomanno *et al.*, 1974). This Darwinian acquisition of numerous genetic changes which confer one or another type of growth advantage has been conceptually simplified by Hanahan and Weinberg (2000) into six essential alterations in cell physiology that define progression toward malignancy: self-sufficiency in growth signals, insensitivity to growth-inhibitory signals, evasion of programmed cell death (apoptosis), limitless replication potential, sustained angiogenesis, and tissue invasion and metastasis.

Multistage tobacco-related carcinogenesis is accompanied by two corollaries: 1) cancer risk increases with duration of (smoking) exposure, and 2) interruption of carcinogenic exposure before cell transformation inhibits cancer progression. Smoking cessation, for example, confines the risk of cancer to existing damage that would persist through daughter generations until resolved by repair or apoptosis. While smoking cessation, particularly at an early age, greatly reduces the risk of subsequent lung cancer (Peto *et al.*, 2000), prolonged smoking often leads to tobacco-specific molecular lesions in the nonmalignant bronchial epithelium, similar to those found in lung cancers,

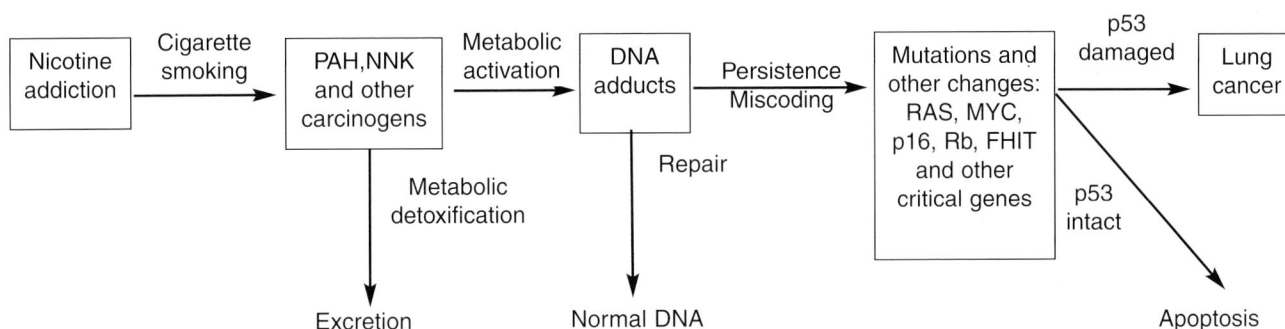

Figure 1. Steps in molecular progression to lung cancer

This model illustrates the role of nicotine addiction and the chronic presentation of carcinogens to the airway epithelium in the induction of mutations in key genes leading to lung cancer.
PAH = polycyclic aromatic hydrocarbons
NNK = 4-(methylnitrosamino)-1-(3-pyridyl)-1-butanone

Adapted from Hecht, JNCI 1999, 91: 1194–1210 by permission of Oxford University Press

that may persist for many years after smoking cessation (Wistuba et al., 1997). Progression of preneoplastic lung lesions may be held in check by activation of the DNA damage response through the ATM/ATR dependent checkpoints which depend downstream on an intact TP53 response (Bartkova et al., 2005; Gorgoulis et al., 2005).

Field carcinogenesis

The tennis-court-sized surface of the respiratory epithelium is widely affected by tobacco smoking, leading to multiple sites of epithelial and inflammatory cell stimulation and corresponding molecular changes, referred to as "field cancerization" (Slaughter et al., 1953; Strong et al., 1984). It is not surprising that chronic tobacco smoke exposure leads airway epithelial cells to alter gene expression. Even biopsies of histologically non-malignant bronchial epithelium of current and former smokers have shown genetic and epigenetic lesions similar to those

seen in lung cancer. (Thiberville et al., 1995; Wistuba et al., 1997; Belinsky et al., 1998; Caballero et al., 2001).

Autopsy studies have identified the presence of multiple sub-clinical lung cancers discovered at autopsy (Auerbach et al., 1961; Chan et al., 1989) and at lung reduction surgery (Pigula et al., 1996). Forty years ago, Auerbach et al (1961) reported a 5–6% frequency of carcinoma in situ (defined as "lesions composed entirely of atypical cells with cilia absent") increasing with cigarettes per day in the autopsies of 339 males who did not die from lung cancer. In a more recent report, 4.8% of 210 patients being evaluated for lung reduction surgery (6 women and 4 men, all heavy smokers with severe ventilatory impairment) harbored unsuspected neoplastic lesions (Pigula et al., 1996). Black (2000) places the 46 "excess" lung cancer cases detected by chest x-ray and sputum cytology screening in the Mayo Lung Project (1% of 4618 male, 45–70-year-old smokers screened) in

this category as "overdiagnosis." (Fontana et al., 1991; Marcus et al., 2000). More recently, helical CT screening of populations in New York, Minnesota and Milan have shown biopsy-confirmed lung cancer in 2–3% of the asymptomatic middle-aged male and female heavy smokers who volunteered for screening (Henschke et al., 1999; Swensen et al., 2002; Pastorino et al., 2003). Thus, from heavy smokers in the general population available for screening to severely obstructed patients considering lung reduction surgery, it is not unreasonable to suspect that 1–5% of middle-aged smokers may harbor indolent, clinically unsuspected lung cancer. This prevalence is substantially greater than the rates expected from clinical lung cancer actually presenting for treatment. These data suggest that the smoke-exposed airway epithelium of large numbers of current and former smokers contain multiple foci of transformed cells at various stages of neoplastic progression.

Tobacco-specific molecular lesions

Persistent Smoking-Induced Epithelial Gene Expression (SIEGE) in Former Smokers

Data are not yet available to describe the frequencies of combined gene mutation and epigenetic silencing in the lungs of healthy former smokers (without cancer). Nevertheless, the persistence of epithelial damage can be appreciated by an examination of gene expression in former smokers.

To describe the cigarette smoke effects on gene expression by large airway epithelial cells of healthy subjects ("the airway transcriptome"), Spira and collaborators (2004) obtained bronchial epithelial cells from brushings of the right main bronchus and defined profiles of gene expression of 93 nonsmoking and smoking subjects using the Affymetrix U133A GeneChip array. Bronchial brushings yielded 6-8 mg of total RNA that was processed, labeled and hybridized to HG-U133A arrays containing ~22,500 human transcripts. Arrays of poor quality were excluded, as were those whose "90th percentile for the $P_{(detection)}$ value was >0.05 for genes that should be detected in epithelial cells or whose 80th percentile $P_{(detection)}$ was < 0.05 for genes that should not be expressed in bronchial epithelial cells." A total of 9968 probe sets were analyzed with the Affymetrix Microarray Suite 5.0 software to provide a single weighted mean expression level for each gene. This same software was used to scale the data from each array (normalize) for interarray comparisons. Bronchoscopic specimens could not be collected on age-, race-, and gender-matched patients for the smoker vs. nonsmoker comparisons. To evaluate the effects of these imbalances on gene expression, the investigators performed a covariance analysis that showed no substantial

effect of age, gender, and race on the normal airway transcriptome (supplemental data in Table 6 at http://www.pnas.org/cgi/content/full/0401422101/DC1, Spira et al., 2004). Pearson correlation coefficients were calculated on replicate samples to evaluate variation due to technique (RNA isolated from epithelial cells of one patient was divided in half and processed separately, data not shown), spatial (right and left bronchus from same subject, $R^2 = 0.92$) and temporal sources (baseline and at 3 months from same subject, $R^2=0.85$) (supplemental data Figures 5A and 5B at http://www.pnas.org/cgi/content/full/0401422101/DC1, Spira et al., 2004). Mean expression levels for each gene were compared among smoking groups to a Student's t test probability value threshold based on a permutation analysis performed to address the multiple comparison problem inherent in any microarray analysis. A stringent multiple comparison correction and p–value threshold were selected to identify a subset of genes altered by cigarette smoking with only a small probability of having a false positive.

To facilitate other studies of the effects of cigarette smoking on "the airway transcriptome," Shah and colleagues (2005) deposited their data in the Smoking Induced Epithelial Gene Expression (SIEGE) relational database accessible through a web interface, http://pulm.bumc.bu.edu/siegeDB. The SIEGE database structure links a patient's clinical and sample data with individual gene expression values and respective gene annotations. Users of the website may perform database queries by selecting software scripts encoded through structured database query language (SQL). These allow users to write and execute user-defined SIEGE database searches (Shah et al., 2005). SIEGE conforms to the minimal information about microarray experiment (MIAME) guidelines (Brazma et al., 2001).

For this review, SIEGE was interrogated for genes differentially expressed by airway epithelial cells of all available former smokers (n=22) compared with all never smokers (n=26) with a threshold set at a p-value of 0.001, indicating a 99.99% confidence interval. Table 1 shows the demographic characteristics of the former and never smokers. The average age of the former smokers (FS) is 57 years, slightly more than half (55%) are African-American, 68% are male and the average number of years of smoking cessation is 12.5 (median 8 years). The never smokers (NS) are significantly younger (average age 34 years). Neither the gender distribution nor the greater heterogeneity of races is significantly different when comparing former to never smokers. Since the gene expression values are not age-adjusted, some component of the FS/NS differential expression may be associated with age and not to the lingering damage from smoking. Yet, since Spira (2004) had found no effect of age on the NS transcriptome, the smaller age coefficient of variation (CV) obtained in former smokers provides some reassurance that any age effect on the FS/NS differential gene expression is likely to be minor.

This query resulted in 50 differentially expressed genes, 16 overexpressed and 34 underexpressed by former smokers. These 50 genes are listed in Table 2A ranked by FS/NS expression ratio. The genes for which a functional annotation could be obtained from Entrez Gene, EASE and GO (Ashburner et al., 2000) are listed in Table 2B, classified by biological process and relative expression. From these 50 genes were identified 11 whose annotated functions might contribute to airway carcinogenesis. From their highlighted notation in Table 2B, these 11 genes primarily address cellular growth, proliferation and cell signaling. In Table 3, these 11 genes are ordered by their FS/NS expression ratio,

Table 1. Demographic and smoking history descriptors of a sample of Former and Never Smokers identified in the Smoking Induced Epithelial Gene Expression database (SIEGE)*

| | Smoking Status | | | |
| | Former | Never | Test | p-value |
Description of sample	(n = 22)	(n = 26)		
Age				
Average (years)	57.2**	33.7	t = 5.3	3.06E-06
Standard deviation	16.7	13.8		
Coeffecient of variation (cv)	29.2	41.0		
Race (%)				
African American	54.5	23.1	χ² = 7.7	0.05
Caucasian	45.5	57.7		
Hispanic	0.0	15.4		
Other	0.0	3.8		
Gender (%)				
Female	31.8	26.9	χ² = 0.1	0.71
Male	68.2	73.1		
Cessation interval				
Average (years)	11.5			
Median (years)	8			
Range (years)	0-46			
Pack-years				
Average	37.6			

* The SIEGE database links a patient's clinical and biological sample data with individual gene expression values (Spira *et al.,* 2004; Shah *et al.,* 2005)

** Values reported in this table are the results of a *de novo* query and are shown in italics

and their cytogenetic location is provided (1p13.3, 1p22.1, 1p36.33, 1q21, 2p16.1, 3p21.1, 4p16, 9p22, 16q12, 17q22 and 19q13.2). Of these 11 genes, three were upregulated and 8 were downregulated, as follows:

Overexpressed in bronchial epithelial cells of former smokers compared to never smokers

CEACAM6: Carcinoembryonic antigen-related cell adhesion molecule 6 is a member of the glycosylphosphatidylinositol (GPI)-linked immunoglobulin super-family found to be an important determinant of malignant phenotype in a variety of gastrointestinal malignancies. Upregulation of CEACAM6 expression in hyperplastic polyps and early adenomas represents one of the earliest observable molecular events leading to colorectal tumours (Jantscheff *et al.,* 2003); upregulation of CEACAM6 in former smokers might have analogous results. CEACAM6 and its downstream targets have been recently described as determining pancreatic adenocarcinoma cellular invasiveness (Duxbury *et al.,* 2004).

GAK: Cyclin G Associated Kinase is a serine/threonine kinase that exhibits high homology outside its kinase domain with auxilin (Lee *et al.,* 2005). Like auxilin, GAK mediates binding of clathrin and adaptors to the plasma membrane (and the trans-Golgi network). GAK modulates internalization of both transferrin and epidermal growth factor receptors (EGFR) (Lee *et al.,* 2005), suggesting an influence on signaling. EGFR- mediated signaling results in cell proliferation or differentiation associated with increased propensity for cell transformation and tumour formation (Schlessinger, 2000). Upon ligand stimulation, EGFRs are activated by autophosphorylation and internalized, at least in part through clathrin-mediated endocytosis (Schlessinger *et al.,* 1983). Internalized receptors then are delivered to the lysosome and degraded or recycled to the cell surface. As the receptor transits through the cell's interior, various EGF-mediated signaling molecules are activated, including extra-cellular signal-regulated kinases 1/2 (ERK1/2) via the Ras/raf pathway (Robinson & Cobb, 1997; Schlessinger, 2000), and Akt via the phosphatidylinositol 3-kinase pathway (Cantley, 2002). Down-regulation of GAK resulted in out-growth of cells in soft agar, raising the possibility that loss of GAK function may promote tumorigenesis (Zhang *et al.,* 2004). The consequence of over-expression of GAK (as seen in former smokers) is not yet determined.

UBAP1: Ubiquitin associated protein 1 is a member of the UBA domain family, whose members confer target specificity to multiple enzymes of the ubiquitination system. (Qian *et al.,* 2001). An increased degradation of suppressor proteins, such as p53 or p27, by the ubiquitin system could be oncogenic; conversely, a lack of degradation of cell cycle-promoting proteins, such as the v-fos and v-jun products, could be oncogenic (Pallares-Trujillo *et al.,* 1997). Taking into account its cytogenetic location (9p22-21),

Table 2A. SIEGE*-identified 50 genes differentially expressed by Former Smokers (FS) compared to Never Smokers (NS) ordered by FS/NS expression ratio

AFFX_ID[a]	F N PVAL[b]	FS/NS Ratio	GENBANK ID[c]	GENBANK description	Location	SNP[d]
202620_s_at	0.00033308	1.8814212	NM_000935	"procollagen-lysine, 2-oxoglutarate 5-dioxygenase (lysine hydroxylase) 2 "	3q23-q24	SNP_5352
218610_s_at	0.00072537	1.78843887	NM_018340	hypothetical protein FLJ11151	16p13.13	SNP_55313
201431_s_at	0.00006062	1.75648426	NM_001387	dihydropyrimidinase-like 3	5q32	SNP_1809
217755_at	0.00004385	1.7412881	NM_016185	hematological and neurological expressed 1	17q25.2	SNP_51155
211657_at	0.0004723	1.59085804	M18728	carcinoembryonic antigen-related cell adhesion molecule 6 (non-specific cross reacting antigen)	19q13.2	SNP_4680
214106_s_at	0.00033354	1.51393292	AI762113	"GDP-mannose 4,6-dehydratase"	6p25	SNP_2762
218503_at	0.0001274	1.45972167	NM_017794	KIAA1797	9p21	SNP_54914
202281_at	0.00025561	1.43178932	NM_005255	cyclin G associated kinase	4p16	SNP_2580
200967_at	0.00065002	1.43098509	NM_000942	peptidylprolyl isomerase B (cyclophilin B)	15q21-q22	SNP_5479
208898_at	0.00067413	1.38985512	AF077614	"ATPase, H+ transporting, lysosomal 34kDa, V1 subunit D "	14q23-q24.2	SNP_51382
220964_s_at	0.00064422	1.36054263	NM_030981	"RAB1B, member RAS oncogene family "	11q12	SNP_81876
221507_at	0.00079181	1.32741003	BG258639	"transportin 2 (importin 3, karyopherin beta 2b)"	19p13.2	SNP_30000
219299_at	0.00080772	1.32174034	NM_017956	hypothetical protein FLJ20772	8q24.13	SNP_55039
200599_s_at	0.00049698	1.29153066	NM_003299	tumor rejection antigen (gp96) 1	12q24.2-q24.3	SNP_7184
46270_at	0.00082068	1.2493878	AL039447	ubiquitin associated protein 1	9p22-p21	SNP_51271
200757_s_at	0.00057839	1.19889932	NM_001219	calumenin	7q32	SNP_813
203445_s_at	0.00088085	0.87466922	NM_005730	"CTD (carboxy-terminal domain, RNA polymerase II, polypeptide A) small phosphatase 2 "	12q13-q15	SNP_10106
201064_s_at	0.00040051	0.80796488	NM_003819	"poly(A) binding protein, cytoplasmic 4 (inducible form) "	1p32-p36	SNP_8761
202360_at	0.00041074	0.79717116	NM_014757	mastermind-like 1 (Drosophila)	5q35	SNP_9794
48612_at	0.00073978	0.7935941	AA225490	hypothetical protein FLJ31821	16q12.1	SNP_146268

Table 2A. (contd)

AFFX ID[a]	F N PVAL[b]	FS/NS Ratio	GENBANK ID[c]	GENBANK description	Location	SNP[d]
218306_s_at	0.00053994	0.77697076	NM_003922	hect (homologous to the E6-AP (UBE3A) carboxyl terminus) domain and RCC1 (CHC1)-like domain (RLD) 1	15q22	SNP_8925
219940_s_at	0.00094399	0.76189006	NM_018386	hypothetical protein FLJ11305	13q34	SNP_55795
201997_s_at	0.00003772	0.74712113	NM_015001	SMART/HDAC1 associated repressor protein	1p36.33-p36.11	SNP_23013
203740_at	0.00061719	0.73946929	NM_005792	M-phase phosphoprotein 6	16q23.3	SNP_10200
213295_at	0.00013467	0.73527999	AA555096	cylindromatosis (turban tumor syndrome)	16q12-q13	SNP_1540
200937_s_at	0.00045695	0.72570523	NM_000969	ribosomal protein L5	1p22.1	SNP_6125
205489_at	0.00018136	0.72061577	NM_001888	"crystallin, mu "	16p13.11-p12.3	SNP_1428
203378_at	0.00022184	0.70261664	AB020631	pre-mRNA cleavage complex II protein Pcf11	11q13	SNP_51585
220755_s_at	0.00043697	0.69454732	NM_016947	chromosome 6 open reading frame 48	6p21.3	SNP_50854
208798_x_at	0.00086306	0.67875023	AF204231	golgin-67	15q11.2	SNP_23015
204382_at	0.00051709	0.6736213	NM_015654	DKFZP564C103 protein	17q25.2	SNP_26151
203638_s_at	0.00013277	0.67138275	NM_022969	"fibroblast growth factor receptor 2 (bacteria-expressed kinase, keratinocyte growth factor receptor, craniofacial dysostosis 1, Crouzon syndrome, Pfeiffer syndrome, Jackson-Weiss syndrome)"	10q26	SNP_2263
210347_s_at	0.00007791	0.66514071	AF080216	B-cell CLL/lymphoma 11A (zinc finger protein)	2p16.1	SNP_53335
211004_s_at	0.00080829	0.65604347	BC002553	"aldehyde dehydrogenase 3 family, member B1 "	11q13	SNP_221
207547_s_at	0.00058863	0.65046545	NM_007177	TU3A protein	3p21.1	SNP_11170
201562_s_at	0.00004862	0.64839184	NM_003104	sorbitol dehydrogenase	15q15.3	SNP_6652
205752_s_at	0.00012478	0.64093046	NM_000851	glutathione S-transferase M5	1p13.3	SNP_2949
212230_at	0.00015284	0.63258006	AV725664	phosphatidic acid phosphatase type 2B	1pter-p22.1	SNP_8613

Table 2A. (contd)

AFFX ID[a]	F N PVAL[b]	FS/NS Ratio	GENBANK ID[c]	GENBANK description	Location	SNP[d]
207913_at	0.00026546	0.62450786	NM_000774	"cytochrome P450, family 2, subfamily F, polypeptide 1 "	19q13.2	SNP_1572
205405_at	0.00051687	0.61887887	NM_003966	"sema domain, seven thrombospondin repeats (type 1 and type 1-like), transmembrane domain (TM) and short cytoplasmic domain, (semaphorin) 5A "	5p15.2	SNP_9037
218576_s_at	0.00080193	0.60851745	NM_007240	dual specificity phosphatase 12	1q21-q22	SNP_11266
213228_at	0.00002634	0.60039769	AK023913	phosphodiesterase 8B	5q14.1	SNP_8622
204754_at	0.00037455	0.59244992	W60800	hepatic leukemia factor	17q22	SNP_3131
215190_at	0.00087568	0.58734254	AV717062	dendritic cell protein	11p13	SNP_10480
217629_at	0.00007568	0.55651177	AA365670	Transcribed sequence with strong similarity to protein sp: P00722 (E. coli) BGAL_ECOLI Beta-galactosidase	---	---
200878_at	0.00000139	0.54652474	AF052094	endothelial PAS domain protein 1	2p21-p16	SNP_2034
216557_x_at	0.00002723	0.53152499	U92706	immunoglobulin heavy constant gamma 1 (G1m marker)	14q32.33	SNP_3500
209821_at	0.00076114	0.52773746	AB024518	chromosome 9 open reading frame 26 (NF-HEV)	9p24.1	SNP_90865
211734_s_at	0.00008407	0.51216168	BC005912	"Fc fragment of IgE, high affinity I, receptor for; alpha polypeptide "	1q23	SNP_2205
204734_at	0.00014456	0.47458065	NM_002275	keratin 15	17q21.2	SNP_3866

*Smoking Induced Epithelial Gene Expression (SIEGE). The SIEGE database links a patient's clinical and biological sample data with individual gene expression values (Spira *et al.*, 2004; Shah *et al.*, 2005).
a = gene annotation identity number (for each probe) in the October 2003 NᴇᴛAffx HG-U133A Annotation files
b = p-value for the comparison former versus never smokers
c = NIH genetic sequence database identity number
d = single nucleotide polymorphisms
Values reported in this table are the results of a *de novo* query.

Table 2B. SIEGE*-identified genes differentially expressed by Former Smokers (FS) compared to Never Smokers (NS) according to biological process and relative expression. In red are those genes whose annotated functions might contribute to airway carcinogenesis

Biological Process	Expression Upregulated in FS	Expression Downregulated in FS
Alcohol metabolism		ALDH3B1; SORD
Amino acid phosphorylation	FLJ11151	
ATP biosynthesis	ATP6V1D	
Carbohydrate metabolism	GMDS	SORD
Cell adhesion	GMDS	CYP2F1
Cell communication	DPYSL3; GMDS; RAB1B	FGFR2; SEMA5A; PDE8B
Cell growth/maintenance	GAK; RAB1B; TNPO2; ATP6V1D	HERC1; RPL5; TU3A; PPAP2B; DUSP12; HLF
Cell motility		PPAP2B
Cell proliferation	GAK	MPHOSPH6
Coenzyme metabolism	ATP6V1D	
Cytoplasm organization		RPL5
Dephosphorylation		DUSP12
Development		MAML1; FGFR2; SEMA5A; HLF; KRT15
DNA Recombination		FLJ31821
Gametogenesis/reproduction		PPAP2B
Hemostasis/Blood Coagulation		PABPC4
Intracelluar transport	RAB1B	
Intracellular signaling	RAB1B	
Ligase Activity		HERC1
Lipid metabolism		
Macromolecule biosynthesis		PABPC4; RPL5; GSTM5
Macromolecule catabolism	UBAP1	PABPC4
mRNA cleavage		PCF11
Neurogenesis		MAML1; SEMA5A
Nucleic acid metabolism	DPYSL3; GMDS; ATP6V1D	PABPC4; FLJ31821; SHARP; BCL11A; PDE8B
Nucleocytoplasmic transport	TNPO2	
Phosphorus metabolism	FLJ11151; GAK	FGFR2; DUSP12
Protein biosynthesis		PABPC4; RPL5
Protein catabolism	UBAP1	
Protein folding	PPIB; TRA1	
Protein metabolism	CEACAM6, FLJ11151; GAK; PLOD2; PPIB; TBPO2; TRA1; UBAP1	HERC1; RPL5 FGFR2; HLF
Protein nucleus transport	TNPO2	
Protein phosphorylation		FGFR2
Protein transport	RAB1B	
Proton transport	ATP6V1D	
Regulation of cell cycle	GAK	MPHOSPH6
Regulation of transcription		SHARP; PCF11; BCL11A; HLF
Ribosome biogenesis		RPL5
RNA catabolism		PABPOC4
Signal transduction	DPYSL3; RAB1B	PDE8B
Ubiquitin-dependent protein catabolism	UBAP1	
Vesicle-mediated transport		HERC1

*Smoking Induced Epithelial Gene Expression. The SIEGE database links a patients clinical and biological sample data with individual gene expression values (Spira *et al.*, 2004; Shah *et al.*, 2005).
The table lists the genes for which a functional annotation was obtained from Entrez Gene, EASE and GO (Ashburner *et al.*, 2000).
Values reported in this Table are the results of a *de novo* query.

Table 3. SIEGE*-identified genes differentially expressed by Former Smokers (FS) compared to Never Smokers (NS) selected for functional contribution to carcinogenesis, ordered by FS/NS expression ratio

Gene Name	F_NPVAL[a]	F/N ratio**	GENBANK ID[b]	GENBANK description	Location	SNP[c]
CEACAM6	0.0004723	1.59085804	M18728	carcinoembryonic antigen-related cell adhesion molecule 6 (non-specific cross reacting antigen)	19q13.2	SNP_468
GAK	0.00025561	1.43178932	NM_005255	cyclin G associated kinase	4p16	SNP_2580
UBAP1	0.00082068	1.2493878	AL039447	ubiquitin associated protein 1	9p22-p21	SNP_51271
SHARP	0.00003772	0.74712113	NM_015001	SMART/HDAC1 associated repressor protein	1p36.33-p36.11	SNP_23013
CYLD	0.00013467	0.73527999	AA555096	cylindromatosis (turban tumor syndrome)	16q12-q13	SNP_1540
RPL5	0.00045695	0.72570523	NM_000969	ribosomal protein L5	1p22.1	SNP_6125
BCL11A	0.00007791	0.66514071	AF080216	B-cell CLL/lymphoma 11A (zinc finger protein)	2p16.1	SNP_53335
TU3A	0.00058863	0.65046545	NM_007177	TU3A protein	3p21.1	SNP_11170
GSTM5	0.00012478	0.64093046	NM_000851	glutathione S-transferase M5	1p13.3	SNP_2949
DUSP12	0.00080193	0.60851745	NM_007240	dual specificity phosphatase 12	1q21-q22	SNP_11266
HLF	0.00037455	0.59244992	W60800	hepatic leukemia factor	17q22	SNP_3131

*Smoking Induced Epithelial Gene Expression. The SIEGE database links a patients' clinical and biological sample data with individual gene expression values (Spira *et al.*, 2004; Shah *et al.*, 2005).
** First three genes listed are upregulated while remaining genes are downregulated.
[a] p-value for the comparison former versus never smokers
[b] NIH genetic sequence database identity number
[c] single nucleotide polymorphisms
Values reported in this Table are the results of a *de novo* query.

this UBA domain family member is being studied as a putative target for silencing in many epithelial cancers, including lung cancer (Wistuba *et al.*, 1999).

Underexpressed in bronchial epithelial cells of former smokers compared with never smokers

SHARP: Notch transmembrane receptors cleave after ligand binding, leaving the Notch intracellular domain to trans-locate to the nuclear compartment, interact with transcription factor RBP-Jκ, and activate transcription of Notch target genes (Vadlamudi *et al.*, 2005). SHARP is a novel component of the HDAC co-repressor complex, recruited by RBP-J to repress transcription of target genes in the absence of activated Notch (Oswald *et al.*, 2002). SHARP interacts with the p21-activated kinase 1 (Pak1), enhancing the corepressor functions of SHARP, thereby modulating Notch sig-naling in human cancer cells (Vadlamudi *et al.*, 2005). Underexpression of SHARP in former smokers might reduce trans-criptional repression of Notch tar-get (growth) genes in transformed cells.

CYLD: This tumour suppressor gene is mutated in familial cylindromatosis, an autosomal dominant that confers a predisposition to multiple tumours of the skin. Recent studies suggest that trans-fected CYLD has deubiquitinating enzyme activity, inhibits the activation of transcription factor NF-κB and is a major regulator of the JNK signaling pathway (Reiley *et al.*, 2004). Under-expression of CYLD in former smokers could reduce the inhibition of NF-κB and JNK stimulated (growth) gene transcription.

RPL5: Ribosomal protein L5 (along with ribosomal proteins L11, and L23) activates *TP53* by inhibiting oncoprotein MDM2-mediated *TP53* suppression (Dai & Lu, 2004). The MDM2-L5-L11-L23 complex functions to inhibit MDM2-mediated p53 ubiquitination and thus activates p53. L5 enhances *TP53* transcriptional activity and induces p53-dependent G_1 cell cycle arrest (Dai & Lu, 2004). Underexpression of RPL5 in former smokers might reduce p53 half-life (through ubiquinated destruction) reducing the ability of cells with damaged DNA to arrest in G1 and halt replication.

BCL11A: The B cell leukemia 11A protein is a transcriptional repressor that binds directly to a GC-rich motif and results in deacetylation of histones H3 and/or H4 that were associated with the promoter region of a reporter gene (Senawong *et al.*, 2005). The human locus of BCL11A has been shown to be involved in a translocation event, t(2; 14)(p13; q32.3), that may underlie some forms of chronic lymphocytic leukemia (CLL), suggesting that BCL11A may be involved in human lymphoid malignancies through either chromosomal translocation or amplification (Satter-white *et al.*, 2001). The histone deacetylase SIRT1 probably underlies the mechanism of BCL11A-mediated transcriptional repression in mammalian cells (Senawong *et al.*, 2005). The reduced expression of BCL11A in former smokers may remove the transcriptional repression by inhibiting euchromatin deacetylation.

TU3A: (DRR 1) The short arm of human chromosome 3 in the region of 3p14-p25 is believed to harbor tumour suppressor genes based on the observation of frequent deletions in this region in several types of tumours, including lung, kidney, breast, and ovarian carcinomas (Killary *et al.*, 1992). Wang and coworkers have cloned a gene they named DRR 1 (downregulated in renal cell carcinoma) and mapped it to 3p21.1 by fluorescence *in situ* hybridization analysis (Wang *et al.*, 2000). The gene showed loss of expression in eight of eight renal cell carcinoma cell lines, one of seven ovarian cancer cell lines, one of one cervical cancer cell line, one of one gastric cancer cell line, and one of one non-small cell lung cancer cell line. Although its function is not yet described, transfection of the gene into *DRR 1*-negative cell lines led to clear growth retardation, suggesting a role in cell growth and maintenance (Wang *et al.*, 2000). In former smokers, reduced expression of this putative tumour suppressor gene could therefore result in enhanced growth.

GSTM5: This gene encodes a glutathione S-transferase that belongs to the *mu* class. The *mu* class of enzymes detoxifies electrophilic compounds, including carcinogens, therapeutic drugs, environmental toxins and products of oxidative stress by conjugation with glutathione to produce a water-soluble (excretable) product. The genes encoding the *mu* class of enzymes are organized in a gene cluster on chromosome 1p13.3 and are known to be highly polymorphic. These genetic variations can change an individual's susceptibility to carcinogens and toxins as well as affect the toxicity and efficacy of certain drugs (Takahashi *et al.*, 1993). Reduced GSTM5 expression in former smokers would reduce the ability of the epithelium to detoxify electrophilic carcinogens.

DUSP12: Also called YVH1, dual specificity phosphatase 12 inactivates its target kinases by dephosphorylating both the phosphoserine/threonine and phosphotyrosine residues. Although the specific function of the protein is not yet described, it negatively regulates members of the mitogen-activated protein (MAP) kinase superfamily (MAPK/ERK, SAPK/JNK, p38), which is associated with cellular proliferation and differentiation (Muda *et al.*, 1999). Loss of negative MAP kinase regulation in former smokers with reduced DUSP12 expression might lead to enhanced cellular growth.

HLF: Hepatic Leukemia Factor is normally expressed in liver and kidney, and has been found to be closely related to the leucine zipper-containing transcription factors DBP (albumin D-box binding protein) and TEF (thyrotroph embryonic factor) which regulate developmental stage-specific gene expression (Inaba *et al.*, 1992). Although HLF (on chromosome 17) is not normally expressed in lymphoid cells, translocation 17;19 fuses an equivalent portion of *E2A* (chromosome 19) to the gene *HLF*, leading to expression of the protein E2A-HLF (Inaba *et al.*, 1992). This translocation is associated with pediatric acute lymphoblastic leukemia (ALL), the most common form of childhood cancer. The oncogenic fusion protein contributes to leukemia development by causing abnormal transcriptional regulation of key target genes. Since the E2A portion of the fusion proteins contains transcriptional activation domains, and the HLF portion contains DNA binding domains, leukemogenesis may be due, at least in part, to excessive transcriptional induction of target genes defined by HLF (LeBrun, 2003).

It is therefore apparent that the airway epithelial cells in the sample of former smokers analyzed in SIEGE over-express at least three genes and underexpress eight genes that have been shown to contribute to lung cancer in human or model systems. This altered gene expression has persisted in these study participants for an average of 12.5 years (median 8 years) after cessation of smoking.

Alteration of bronchial epithelial cell gene expression of current smokers

As reported by Spira and collaborators (2004), the airway epithelial cell expression of ninety-seven genes was altered in smokers compared with never smokers (differentially expressed by Student's t test $p < 1.06 \times 10^{-5}$). Of the 97 genes that passed the permutation analysis, 68 (73%) represented increased gene expression among current smokers. The greatest increases were in genes that coded for xenobiotic functions such as CYP1B1 (30-fold) and DBDD (5-fold), antioxidants such as GPX2 (3-fold) and ALDH3A1 (6-fold), and genes involved in electron transport such as NADPH (4-fold). In general, genes that were increased in smokers tended to be involved in regulation of oxidant stress and glutathione metabolism, xenobiotic metabolism, and secretion. Expression of several putative oncogenes (pirin, CA12, and CEACAM6) was also increased. Genes that decreased in smokers tended to be involved in regulation of inflammation, although expression of several putative tumour suppressor genes (TU3A, SLIT1, and -2, and GAS6) was decreased. Changes in the expression of select genes were confirmed by real-time reverse transcription polymerase chain reaction (RT-PCR).

Comparison of bronchial epithelial cell gene expression of former with never and with current smokers

Figure 2A, reproduced from Spira (2004), shows a multidimensional scaling plot of never and current smokers according to the expression of the 97 genes that distinguish current smokers from never smokers. Also reproduced from Spira (2004), Figure 2B shows that former smokers who discontinued smoking < 2 years before this study tend to cluster with current smokers, whereas former smokers who discontinued smoking for > 2 years group clustered more closely with never smokers.

Tobacco-associated molecular lesions in developing lung cancer

The genes that showed persistent deregulated expression in healthy former smokers (without cancer) are shown to be similar to many of the genes found mutated (or lost) in lung cancer.

The cytogenetic location of genes altered in former smokers (Table 3) corresponds to the cytogenetic changes reported in the development of lung cancer. Following the morphological progression from hyperplasia, to metaplasia, to dysplasia, carcinoma-in-situ and finally invasive cancer, there seems to be a corresponding increase in the prevalence of 3p and 9p deletions along with an increase in the total number of chromosomal alterations, showing evidence of accumulation of genetic damage (Thiberville *et al.*, 1995). Early genetic changes in squamous cell lung carcinogenesis include LOH on 3p at 3p12, 3p14.2 (FHIT locus) (Fong *et al.*, 1997; Sozzi *et al.*, 1998) and at 3p14.1-21.2, 3p21, 3p22-24, 3p25 (Sundaresan *et al.*, 1992) on 9p21 (Wistuba *et al.*, 1999). Morphologically more advanced lesions were characterized by LOH of other chromosome regions, particularly 17p13 (*TP53* gene), but also including 13q (RB gene), and 5q (APC-MCC region) as well as K-ras mutations (Chung *et al.*, 1995; Wistuba *et al.*, 1999). Table 4, reproduced from Sozzi (2006), summarizes the frequency of the molecular changes in established lung cancer.

This review now will focus upon the lesions found in the epithelial cells of former smokers that correspond to the molecular lesions that lead to positive and negative alterations in signals for growth and apoptosis identified in established lung cancer. Particular attention will be paid to 3p loss/*FHIT* inactivation (TU3A), 9p loss/p16[INK4A] inactivation (UBAP1) and 17p loss/*TP53* inactivation (GAK, RPL5, UBAP1).

3p loss/FHIT inactivation

Chromosome arm 3p is one of the earliest and most frequent sites of genetic loss in lung cancer. To define potential tumour suppressor gene regions on 3p, Wistuba *et al.* (2000) performed high-resolution LOH allelotyping using 54 microsatellite markers, including 19 markers in the 600-kb 3p21.3 region with specimens from 31 lung cancer cell lines and a panel of 28 3p markers on 97 lung cancer and 54 preneoplastic/preinvasive microdissected respiratory epithelial samples. Allelic losses of 3p were detected in 96% of the lung cancers and in 78% of the preneoplastic/preinvasive lesions. These investigators concluded that 3p allelic loss is nearly universal in lung cancer pathogenesis and involves multiple, discrete, LOH sites that often show areas of LOH interspersed with areas of retention of heterozygosity. They report a progressive increase in the frequency and size of 3p allele loss regions with increasing severity of histopathological preneo-plastic/preinvasive changes, and observed that 3p LOH was not randomly distributed. Preneoplastic lesions and frank tumour from the same patient often lose the same parental allele by a currently unknown mechanism. In their series, lung cancer appears to have allele loss and breakpoints first occurring in the 600-kb 3p21.3 region (Wistuba

A

B

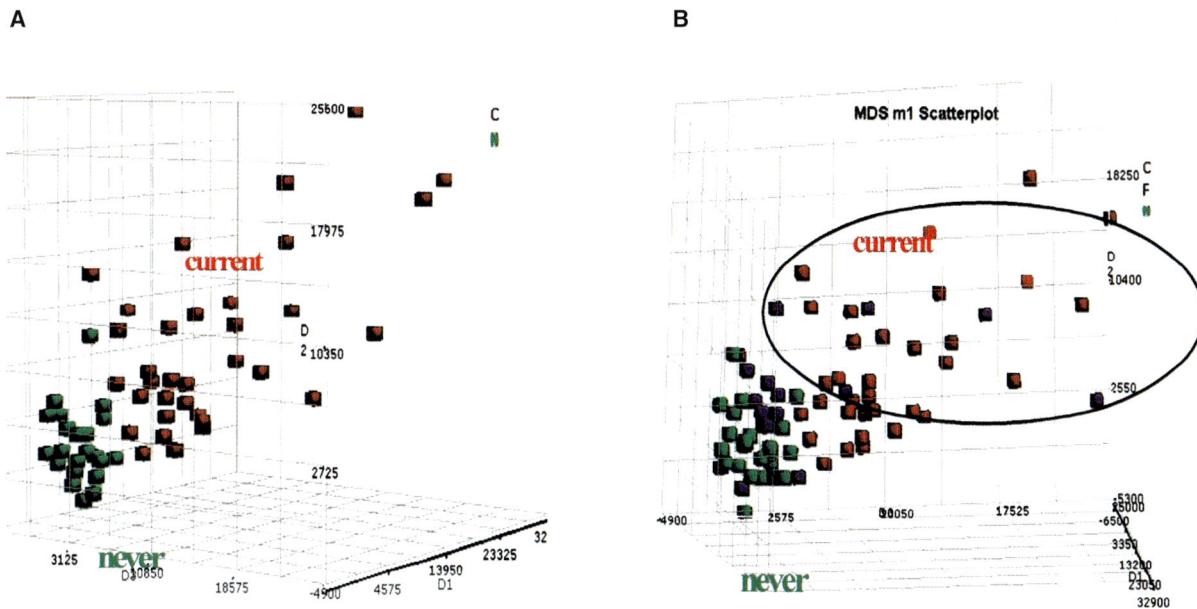

Figure 2. Multidimensional scaling plot of samples from Current, Never and Former Smokers according to 97 genes differentially expressed between Current and Never Smokers

Reproduced from Spira et al., PNAS 2004; 101: 10143–10148. Copyright 2004 National Academy of Sciences, USA
(A) Samples of current (red boxes) and never (green boxes) smokers plotted according to the expression of these genes. The axes of the figures have no units.

(B) The majority of former smokers (blue boxes) group closely to never smokers. However, a number of samples from former smokers are positioned in the grid closer to current smokers (in black circle).

et al., 2000) that contains the tumour suppressor genes RASS1A (Dammann et al., 2000) and Semaphorin 3B (SEMA3B) (Tomizawa et al., 2001).

This region is nearby, but not identical to, the TU3A gene at 3p21.1 that showed reduced expression by former smokers' airway epithelial cells. The 54 microsatellite markers used by Wistuba (2000) did not include D3S1289, the marker directed at the 3p21.1 region affected in former smokers. While inclusion of this region might not have changed the Wistuba conclusions, other investigators who interrogated this region found 70% LOH for D3S1289 in lung cancer specimens resected from 26 lung cancer

patients (without occupational exposure) (Hirose et al., 2002).

Multiple genes residing on chromosome 3p are important in the development of lung cancer. Sozzi and collaborators (2006) refer to the complexity of this region and nicely summarize how the biologic complexity of 3p silencing mechanisms (point mutation, LOH, epigenetic silencing, haploinsufficiency), compounded by variability and accuracy of investigator methods (LOH, comparative genomic hybridization (CGH), single nucleotide polymorphism (SNP)), has made this region so difficult to map for tumour suppressor genes (Sozzi et al., 2006).

Zabarovsky et al. (2002) reaffirm that loss of expression of DRR1 (TU3A) may play an important role in the development of epithelial tumours; thus this gene needs to be studied in lung cancer. Perhaps the observation that this gene is down regulated in the airway epithelium of former smokers and is adjacent to the region almost always silenced in lung cancer will lead to further research at this locus.

9p loss/p16INK4A inactivation

One of the most frequently silenced genes in lung cancer, p16, (Cairns et al., 1994, 1995) is frequently inactivated through multiple mechanisms in NSCLC

Table 4. Frequency of molecular changes in lung cancer histotypes as summarized in Sozzi et al. (2006)

Alteration	Small-cell lung cancer	Non-small cell lung cancer
Receptor tyrosine kinases	c-kit 70%	EGFR overexpression: 90% (SCC); 50% (ADC) Her2/neu: 30% (ADC)
	MET point mutations (rare)	MET overexpression: 25%
Ras point mutations	-	10–30% (ADC)
MYC family amplification	65% high level	50% low level
p53 inactivation	75–100%	50%
Rb inactivation	90%	15–30%
p16^{INK4A} inactivation	0–10%	30–40%
FHIT inactivation	80%	50–70%
3p, 9p, 13q, 17p allelic loss	90%	70%
Bcl2 overexpression	75–90%	30%

SCC = squamous cell carcinoma; ADC = adenocarcinoma; EGFR = epidermal growth factor receptor; Rb = retinoblastoma gene; FHIT = Fragile histidine triad; HER2/neu = human epidermal growth factor receptor; MET = c-MET protein also known as hepatocyte growth factor; BC12 = B-cell CLL/lymphoma 2; MYC = myelocytomatosis viral oncogene

Reproduced from Table 6.1, Frequency of molecular changes in lung cancer, page 90 in Sozzi et al., (2006) Thompson Publishing Services

(Herman et al., 1995; Merlo et al., 1995; Shapiro et al., 1995). The p14^{ARF} gene at the same 9p21 locus has emerged as a new tumour suppressor gene (Mao et al., 1995). The INK4a gene encodes both p14^{ARF} and p16 proteins that initiate in different first exons and continue in alternative reading frames through a common exon 2. The p16 protein (Figure 3) blocks the interaction of cyclin dependent kinase 4 (CDK4) with cyclin D (and CDK2 with cycline E), preventing phosphorylation of the retinoblastoma (Rb) protein which sequesters E2F and halts the cell cycle, resulting in growth arrest (Chin et al., 1998). The p14ARF protein leads to growth arrest by blocking MDM2 inhibition of p53 (Figure 3), resulting in increased TP53 levels which activate transcription of p21 and blockade of CDK4/cyclinD

(Chin et al., 1998).

Within this same 9p21 locus, KIAA1797 (a gene of unknown function, Table 2A) and UBAP1 (discussed above, Tables 2A, 2B, 3) found to be overexpressed in former smokers, are 13.3M apart and straddle p16^{INK4A} (NCBI MapViewer). As stated earlier, UBAP1 protein may confer target specificity to enzymes of the ubiquitination system (Qian et al., 2001). An increased degradation of suppressor proteins, such as p53 or p27, by the ubiquitin system could be oncogenic early in the course of neoplastic transformation of former smoker airway epithelium. Conversely, a lack of degradation of cell cycle-promoting proteins, such as the v-fos and v-jun products, could be oncogenic if this locus were lost with that of p16INK4A

(Pallares-Trujillo et al., 1997). While overexpression of UBAP1 may be important in initiation of carcinogenesis, given the frequent deletion of this locus in lung cancer, it is more likely that its loss of function is more significant for tumour growth and development.

17p loss/TP53 inactivation

The last defensive barrier before cellular transformation (Figure 1, Figure 3), TP53 is the cellular gatekeeper for growth and division (Levine, 1997). The p53 protein enhances the rate of transcription of seven known genes that direct a cell with damaged DNA to a viable growth arrest or to apoptosis (Table 5) allowing the injured cell an opportunity for DNA repair (Levine, 1997). The native protein is a tetramer of alpha helices and loops that bind to DNA and two non-parallel beta sheets that provide scaffold structure (Cho et al., 1994). The protein requires C-terminal activation to bind to DNA and become a transcription factor. The C-terminal binds to DNA ends and internal deletion loops in DNA as generated by replication errors that are then detected and fixed by mismatch-repair processes (Levine, 1997).

More than 60% of human lung cancers contain mutations in this gene (Greenblatt et al., 1994), and its epigenetic inactivation has been recently proposed (Baylin & Ohm, 2006). The majority of TP53 mutations are found in sequences that encode amino acids in the DNA binding domain (exons 5, 7 and 8). Mutations in amino acid residues such as R248 and R273, the two most frequently altered residues in the protein, result in defective contacts with DNA and loss of ability of p53 to act as a transcription factor. The IARC TP53 mutation database (http://www-p53.iarc.fr/index.html) has been developed to identify and compare

P53-Rb Pathway

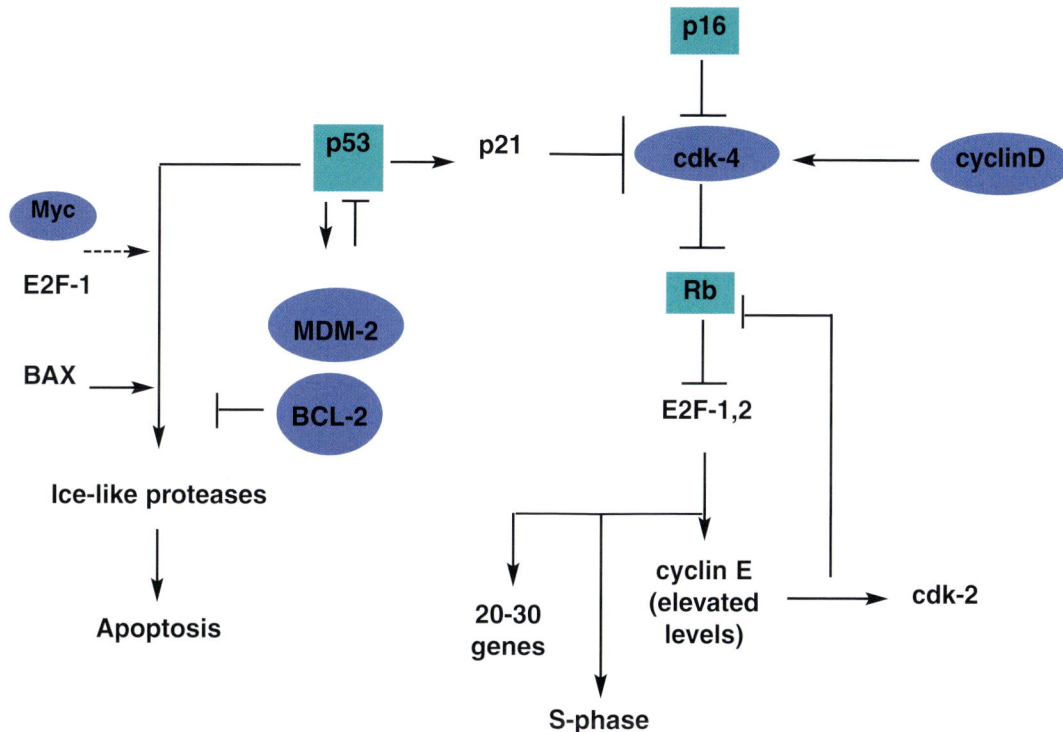

Figure 3. The p53–Rb Pathway

The p53-Rb pathway permits one to postulate the interrelationships among a number of oncogenes (purple circles) and tumor suppressor genes (green squares) that regulate the G1–S phase restriction point, its relation to a DNA damage checkpoint mediated by p53, and the choice by p53 whether to initiate a G1 arrest (via p21) or apoptosis. The available evidence suggests an important role for Rb and its two related gene products, p107 and p130 (along with E2F-4 and -5), in p53-mediated G1–S phase regulation. Shown are the p53–MDM2 autoregulatory loop that reverses this checkpoint control and the gene products that positively or negatively act on the probability of entering apoptosis.

Reprinted from Cell, Vol. 88, Levine A, p 53 the Cellular Gatekeeper for Growth and Division, pages 323-331 (1997) with permission from Elsevier

the mutation patterns in this gene (Olivier *et al.,* 2002).

The G:C to T:A transversions observed at selected ^{Me}CG sites in lung cancer are thought to represent a hypermutability of these guanine nucleobases to the tobacco-smoke carcinogen PAH-diolepoxides ("PAH hotspot" codons 157, 158, 245, 248, and 273) (Denissenko *et al.,* 1996; Denissenko *et al.,* 1997; Smith *et al.,* 2000). Thus, smoking affects the mechanism in addition to the frequency of lung carcinogenesis (Le Calvez *et al.,* 2005). This particular mutation pattern of transversions at G bases (G to T, 30%) seen in lung cancers of smokers, is uncommon in never smokers (13%) and in cancers not directly related to tobacco (9%) (Pfeifer *et al.,* 2002), but the majority of lung cancer mutations are a heterogeneous mix of transversions and transitions (Le Calvez *et al.,* 2005). These mutations lead to a missense p53 protein with impaired function in lung cancers from smokers (73%), former smokers (47%) and never smokers (48%)(supplemental data Tables 5–7 in http://www.cancerresearchjournals.org) (Le Calvez *et al.,* 2005). The RR of

Table 5. Products of genes transcriptionally activated by p53

p21, WAF1, Cip1	Inhibits several cyclin-cyclin-dependent kinases; bind cdk's cyclins, and PCNA; arrest the cell cycle
MDM2	Product of an oncogene; inactivates p53-mediated transcription and so forms an autoregulatory loop with p53 activity
GADD45	Induced upon DNA damage; binds to PCNA and can arrest the cell cycle; involved directly in DNA nucleotide excision repair
Cyclin G	A novel cyclin (it does not cycle with cell division) of unknown function and no known cyclin dependent kinase
Bax	A member of the BC12 family that promotes apoptosis; not induced by p53 in all cells
IGF-BP3	The insulin-like growth factor binding protein-3; blocks signalling of a mitogenic growth factor

cdk's: cyclin-dependent kinases
Reprinted from Cell, Vol. 88, Levine A, p53 the Cellular Gatekeeper for Growth and Division, pages 323–331 (1997) with permission from Elsevier

having a cancer with a *TP53* mutation (and abnormal p53 protein) increases with tobacco use (current smokers: RR 5.2; with a linear dose-response; former smokers: RR 1.7) (Le Calvez *et al.,* 2005). Recently, Schabath *et al.* documented that in lung cancer, TP53 polymorphism was another mechanism of functional injury (Schabath *et al.,* 2006). Polymorphisms of *TP53* and *p73*, a family member with structural and functional homology, were associated with the development of lung cancer among current smokers, and the risk persisted in those with *TP53* polymorphisms after smoking cessation (Schabath *et al.,* 2006).

In airway epithelial cells of current, former and never smokers who have not (yet) developed cancer, there is no evidence of a smoking-related change in *TP53* expression (supplemental data Table 9 at http://www-pnas.org/cgi/content/full/0401422101/DC1, Spira *et al.,* 2004). However, as discussed earlier, the airway epithelial cells from former smokers (compared to never smokers) show reduced expression of ribosomal protein L5 (RPL5) which may lead to loss of MDM2 suppression and ubiquinated destruction of p53 protein (Dai & Lu, 2004). Thus, former smokers might inhibit their "gatekeeper" by under-expression of *RPL5*, reducing the ability of cells with damaged DNA to arrest in G_1 and halt replication.

Relevance to Early Cessation of Smoking

Hanahan and Weinberg (2000) have suggested that cells acquire a malignant growth advantage in 4–7 rate-limiting events. The epidemiologic data suggest that on average, after 20 years of smoking the acquisition of these changes in gene regulation begins to manifest as clinical disease. Further, the epidemiologic data reviewed elsewhere in this volume suggest that early breaking of the cigarette addiction prevents the carcinogenic exposures that leads to cell transformation and death from lung malignancy. The understanding that genes deregulated by cigarette smoking can continue to stimulate indolent neoplasia long after smoking has stopped should encourage the earliest possible attempts to quit smoking.

Summary and Conclusions

This section documents a biologic plausibility for the reduction of persistent lung cancer risk observed among former smokers compared to current smokers, although remaining elevated compared to never smokers. This documentation includes evidence, in former smokers compared with never smokers, of altered expression of 11 genes known (or suspected) to show similar alterations in lung cancer. Finally, this altered gene expression has been shown to persist in the airway epithelial cells of former smokers for a decade after smoking cessation. Data suggesting that risk for lung cancer may be elevated among former smokers with residual molecular lesions and among those with polymorphisms in gatekeeper and DNA repair genes are consistent with epidemiologic and clinical studies.

Effects of Smoking on Atherogenesis and Clotting and Changes in Cardiovascular Diseases with Smoking Cessation

Introduction

This section describes the effects of tobacco smoking on the process of plaque formation and thrombosis, and the effects of smoking cessation on these processes. Cardiovascular disease (CVD) includes coronary heart disease (CHD), cerebrovascular disease, peripheral arterial disease (PAD) and abdominal aortic aneurysm (AAA). There are common and distinct features to CVD, but atherosclerosis and thrombosis play important roles in each form of disease. Multiple risk factors contribute to the risk of atherosclerosis and thrombosis, including blood lipids, diabetes, hypertension, genetic predisposition, physical inactivity and smoking. The most common form of CVD is coronary heart disease (CHD). Manifestations of CHD—e.g., angina, myocardial infarction, sudden cardiac death, and arrhythmia—are precipitated by tissue hypoxia caused by vessel occlusion from a combination of plaque and thrombosis. Cerebrovascular disease also affects small arteries and therefore involves similar mechanisms, but additional mechanisms likely also contribute to PAD and AAA. For example, inflammation and other biomechanical factors are noted to affect the expansion of AAA.

The atherosclerotic and thrombotic process

Atherosclerosis is the result of a process involving oxidation and inflammation in the artery wall. Low-density lipoprotein (LDL) is transported through endothelial cells into the vascular intima of the artery. Here LDL is retained and oxidised by reactive oxygen species. Oxidized LDL is taken up by macrophages, which as a consequence become 'foam' cells, named so for their appearance after engorging LDL. The accumulated foam cells form 'fatty streaks'. The activated macrophages trigger a state of chronic inflammation involving numerous inflammatory mediators, including neutrophil leukocytes and T-lymphocytes. As this inflammation process evolves, smooth muscle cells are recruited and induced to proliferate and produce collagen, causing fatty streaks to be transformed to fibrous plaques. This process also involves microvascularisation with formation of fragile new micro-vessels within the plaque, which contribute to plaque instability.

Fibrous plaques can become unstable with the risk of rupture. Rupture can occur if the endothelial layer covering the plaque is thin and as a consequence is denuded or if bleeding occurs in the fragile new microvessels in the plaque. Plaque rupture then exposes blood components to tissue factor, which initiates coagulation and the formation of thrombus. In most cases this will be sub-clinical, but if flow in the vessel is compromised it leads to cardiovascular events. The coronary vessels are particularly prone to this process. Plaques that reach a size that reduces the diameter of the coronary vessels and thus the blood flow in the vessels cause disease manifestations such as angina pectoris and claudication, whereas rupture of unstable plaques with formation of thrombus causes disease manifestations such as myocardial infarction and stroke when occurring in coronary or cerebral arteries.

These lesions, whether fatty streaks or fibrous plaques, are not static but rather undergo continuous remodelling from stable to unstable plaques. Stable plaques contain mainly smooth muscle cells in a matrix of collagen, and are low in inflammatory activators. A solid cap of endothelial cells covers stable plaques. Unstable plaques contain more inflammatory activity; a core of dead cells, cholesterol and debris. This type of plaque is often fragile and denuded, causing the lesions to be exposed to blood flow resulting in thrombus formation.

Acute coronary events are usually caused by the development of platelet-rich thrombus associated with atheromatous plaque rupture or erosion. Healthy endothelium inhibits thrombosis within the vessel. Coagulation is initiated after exposure of blood to tissue factor present in atheromatous plaques. Platelet responses cannot distinguish between traumatic and pathologic vessel damage. Levels of systemic biomarkers of haemostasis may reflect the presence of atherosclerosis and predisposition to thrombosis.

The haemostatic system is comprised of two inextricably linked components: cellular, principally platelets, and plasma protein-based coagulation cascade (Hemker & Beguin, 2000; Falati *et al.,* 2002; Monroe & Hoffman, 2002; MacCallum, 2005). Coagulation is initiated by contact of blood containing activated clotting factor VIIa (FVIIa) with tissue factor (TF). Subsequent activation of both FIX and FX by FVIIa leads to generation of thrombin, the key enzyme product of coagulation system activation (Mann *et al.,* 2003; Ichinose, 2001). The extrinsic or TF pathway is switched off by a specific inhibitor, tissue factor inhibitor, and continuing generation of thrombin is then dependent upon recruitment of the intrinsic pathway through activation of FXI and the cofactors VIII and V by thrombin (Mann *et al.,* 2003). Thrombin converts fibrinogen to fibrin, and the resulting fibrin polymers are cross-linked, and thereby stabilized by FXIIIa. Several endogenous inhibitors of coagulation regulate the clotting process further. Fibrin is lysed by plasmin, which is cleaved from its precursor, plasminogen, by the enzyme tissue-type plasminogen activator (tPA). Fibrinolysis is inhibited by plasminogen activator inhibitor type 1 (PAI-1), which inhibits binding of plasminogen to fibrin.

Exposure of vessel wall subendothelium leads to a series of steps in which platelets initially adhere to underlying subendothelial collagen and von Willebrand factor. Platelets become activated and aggregation takes place whereby adjacent platelets link to each other by fibrinogen, von Willebrand factor, and possibly by fibronectin bridges, and thereby forming the initial haemostatic plug (Jackson *et al.,* 2003; Ruggeri, 2003). Platelet activation is accompanied by a series of intracellular reactions, such as generation of thromboxane A2, the release of which leads to further activation.

The progression of cardiovascular disease to clinical events depends on this balance between atherosclerotic plaque stability and instability. The endothelium is central to regulation of this homeostatic process, and endothelial functions are important in the development of cardiovascular disease. These functions include control over thrombosis and thrombolysis, regulation of vessel tone, regulation of platelet and leukocyte interactions with the vessel wall, adhesion of monocytes and growth of vessel wall (Libby, 2002; Puranik & Celermajer, 2003; Scott, 2004).

The effects of cigarette smoking and smoking cessation on the atherosclerotic and haemostatic process

Tobacco smoke has numerous constituents, and the resulting effect of cigarette smoking on the atherosclerotic process is complex, involving metabolic, neurohumoral, hematological and hemodynamic effects (Figure 4). The time courses of these are both acute and chronic in nature. Through observational and experimental studies the resulting dose-response-dependent effect of cigarette smoking on atherosclerosis in both central and peripheral arteries has been established. Accumulated smoking exposure is strongly associated with degree of atherosclerosis determined by coronary angiography both cross-sectional (Herbert, 1975; Ramsdale *et al.,* 1985; Wang *et al.,* 1994; Ambrose & Barua, 2004), prospectively in the formation of new lesions (Waters *et al.,* 1996), and in echocardiography studies of intimae-media thickness of carotid arteries and thickness of the proximal aorta (Inoue *et al.,* 1995).

Studies of the mechanism of the effect of cigarette smoking on the atherosclerotic process have concentrated on endothelial function, oxidative processes, platelet function, fibrinolysis, inflammation, modification of lipids and vasomotor function. There are common pathways to these effects and overlap in the mechanisms responsible. Their effects have been elucidated through observational cohort studies, experimental observations and laboratory studies in humans and animals; an overview of each will be offered below. The intent is to describe potential mechanisms by which cigarette smoking may result in CVD and which may change with smoking cessation. The factors are described in the context of how they are altered by cigarette smoking and cessation and not in context of how they may play a role in CVD independent of cessation.

Constituents of cigarette smoke that contribute to cardiovascular disease

Nicotine

The role of nicotine alone on atherosclerosis is debated. Nicotine acts in the central nervous system (CNS) leading to release of noradrenaline, adrenocorticotrophic hormone, endorphin, prolactin and cortisol (Taylor *et al.,* 1998). There is no doubt that nicotine acutely increases heart rate, cardiac output, and blood pressure, but whether these effects translate to increased atherosclerosis and cardiac risk is not established. Nicotine also causes arterial constriction, which has been shown to impair regional cardiac perfusion in patients with ischemic heart disease (Benowitz & Gourlay, 1997). Regarding endothelial function, nicotine exposure alone has led to increased, decreased or no effect on flow mediated vasodilation (FMD) and availability of nitric oxide (NO) (Li *et al.,* 1994; Mayhan & Sharpe, 1999; Clouse *et al.,* 2000). Nicotine infusion has limited effect on platelet function (Whiss *et al.,* 2000). Through increased nicotine effects and increased adrenergic drive, smoking may increase shear stress, which may cause unstable plaques to disrupt.

Despite these effects, a recent comprehensive review concluded that the majority of current evidence suggests that nicotine exposure from cigarette smoking has at most minor effects on the atherosclerotic process (Ambrose & Barua, 2004). This is corroborated by studies comparing the relative effects of cigarette smoking and smokeless tobacco, i.e. oral snuff, with a similar amount of nicotine-exposure. There is a higher incidence of vascular disease in cigarette smoking than in smokeless

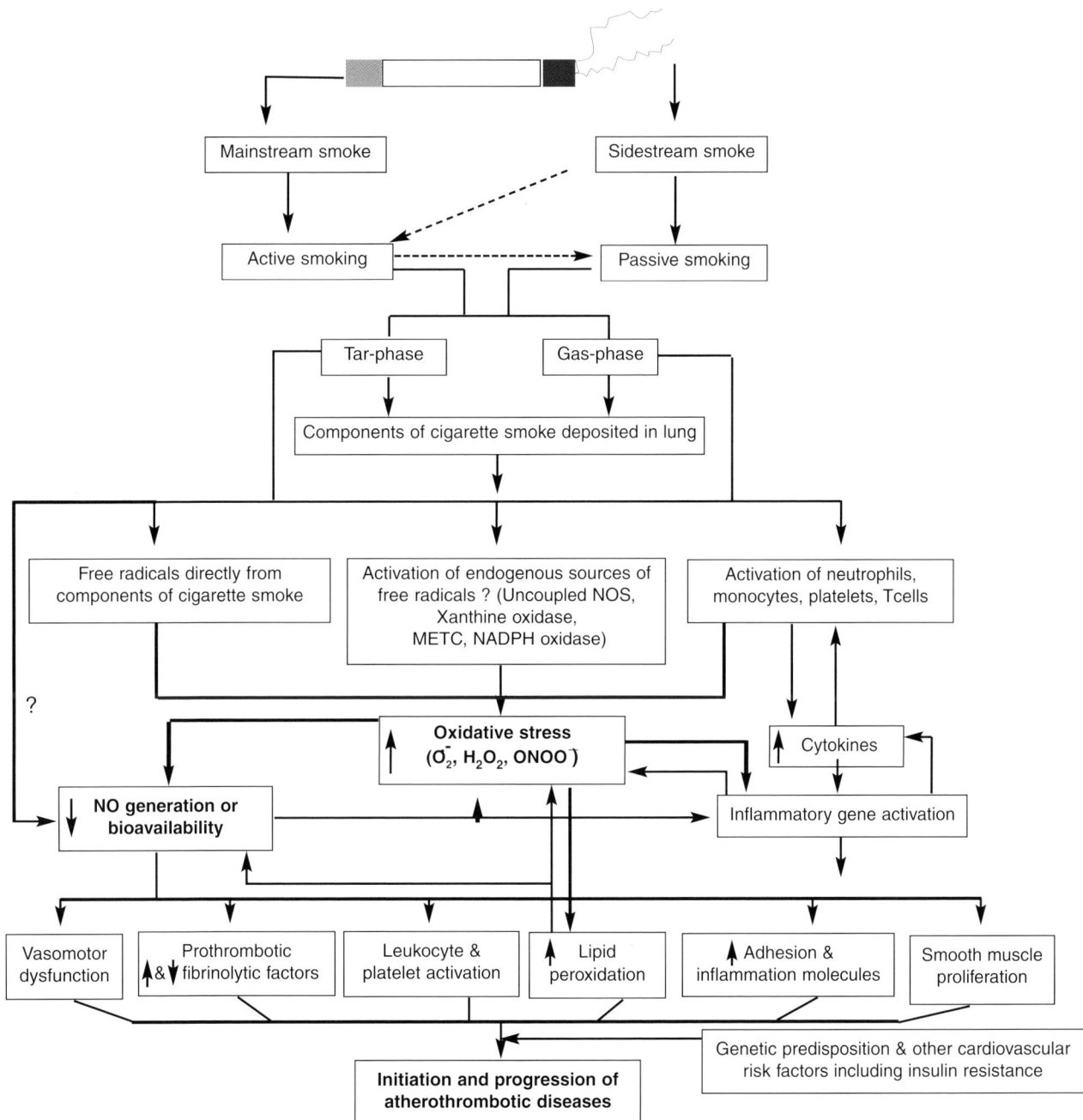

Figure 4. Potential pathways and mechanisms for cigarette smoking-mediated cardiovascular dysfunction

The bold boxes and arrows in the flow diagram represent the probable central mechanisms in the complex pathophysiology of cigarette-smoking-mediated athero-thrombotic disease. H_2O_2 hydrogen peroxide; METC = mitochondrial electron transport chain; NADPH = nicotinamide adenine dinucleotide phosphate reduced form; NOS = nitric oxide synthase; ONOO peroxinitrate; $O_2^{\cdot -}$ superoxide.
Reprinted from J. Am. Coll. Cardiol., Vol. 43(10), Ambrose & Barua, The pathophysiology of cigarette smoking and cardiovascular disease: an update, pages 1731–1737, copyright (2004), with permission from the American College of Cardiology Foundation.

tobacco users (Asplund, 2003). White blood cell count, levels of C-reactive protein (CRP) and fibrinogen, antioxidant vitamin levels, and thromboxane A2 metabolite excretion (reflecting platelet activation) are similar in snuff-users and non-smokers (Asplund, 2003). Cigarette smoking but not snuff use was associated with increased carotid and femoral intimae-media thickness and increased levels of CRP, adding strength to the argument that components of tobacco combustion and not nicotine are responsible for the effects on the atherosclerotic process (Wallenfeldt *et al.,* 2001).

Free Radicals

Cigarette smoking contains numerous free radicals in both the gas phase and the tar phase. The radicals in the tar phase are long-lived (up to months) and in the gas phase are short-lived (seconds). The effects of free radicals— or reactive oxygen species—on NO availability will be mentioned below. Cigarette smoking enhances the process of superoxide-anion-mediated degradation of endothelium-derived relaxing factor (EDRF) via increased oxidative stress. Smoking increases oxidized LDL (Flavahan, 1992) and decreases availability of the dietary antioxidants beta-carotene and vitamins C and E (Chow *et al.,* 1986; Schectman *et al.,* 1989; Duthie & Wahle, 1990).

Carbon monoxide (CO)

CO has strong affinity to haemoglobin and lowers the capacity of blood to carry oxygen to target organs. Although this can be critical in a situation with reduced blood flow relative to oxygen demand, studies of the independent effect of CO are sparse. At present CO is not thought to independently acceler-ate the atherosclerotic process (Zevin *et*

al., 2001; Ambrose & Barua, 2004). CO-exposure reduces ventricular fibrillation threshold in animals (DeBias *et al.,* 1976). It is possible that CO at the levels at which smokers are exposed may increase electrical instability (Turino, 1981; Taylor *et al.,* 1998), which can increase the risk of cardiac death but does not affect the atherosclerotic process. This is also true for the increased catecholamine drive induced by smoking.

Endothelial function

The term endothelial function is a poorly-defined entity which usually covers a broad spectrum of functions important for development of cardiovascular disease. In experimental studies cigarette smoking impairs endothelial function. This has been demonstrated through impaired endothelium dependent flow mediated vasodilatation in various vascular beds in several studies (Celermajer *et al.,* 1993; Adams *et al.,* 1998). The mechanism has been demonstrated to be through reduced nitrous oxide (NO) availability. NO is a free radical responsible for the vasodilator function of the endothelium, but NO also influences platelet aggregation, leukocyte activity, monocyte adhesion, fibrinolysis, and inflammation. NO is formed locally by endothelial NO synthase enzyme (eNOS), is chemically unstable, and has a short half-life, which means that it acts only locally.

The expression and activation of eNOS is altered by exposure to cigarette smoking, resulting in decreased availability of NO (Ambrose & Barua, 2004). In addition, tobacco smoke contains numerous free radicals that react with NO and reduce the level of NO available locally (Ohara *et al.,* 1993; Puranik & Celermajer, 2003). The combined effect of reduced availability of NO can be measured as reduced flow mediated vasodilatation (FMD). Acute

exposure to smoking in non-smokers causes impaired FMD (Lekakis *et al,* 1998). The effect of smoking on expression of eNOS may be modified by diet or genetic predisposition. This was suggested after subjects who were homozygous for a gene polymorphism coding for eNOS (Glu298 Asp) did not demonstrate the same impairment of FMD when exposed to cigarette smoking (Leeson *et al,* 2002). In a study in rural China there was no difference in FMD between smokers and non-smokers (Woo *et al.,* 1997) although differences were later demonstrated in urbanized Chinese (Woo *et al.,* 2000). Endothelial dysfunction is probably only partially reversible upon smoking cessation: flow-mediated vasodilatation was better in former smokers than in continued smokers but poorer than in never-smokers, indicating some reversibility of the effect of smoking on endothelial function (Celermajer *et al.,* 1993; Raitakari *et al.,* 1999). Another study, however, has indicated complete and rapid restoration of endothelial func-tion shortly after smoking cessation (Moreno *et al,* 1998).

Through its effect on availability of NO, cigarette smoking has a more widespread effect on the atherosclerotic process. NO is not only a mediator of vasodilatation, it is also involved in endothelial regulation of inflammatory mechanisms in the intima of the vessels, in adhesion of monocytes to the endothelium, in platelet activation, formation of thrombus and fibrinolytic activity (Ambrose & Barua, 2004). The effect of cigarette smoking on these factors has been shown in a number of studies. Cigarette smokers have higher levels of adhesion molecules (sICAM, sVCAM, sE-selectin and sP-selectin) (Blann *et al.,* 1997; Ridker *et al.,* 1998; Takeuchi *et al.,* 2002). sE-selectin (but not the remaining adhesion molecules) was higher in former smokers than in never smokers.

Endothelial function is also regulated by endothelin (ET-1). ET-1 has opposite effects of NO: Like NO it is unstable with a short half-life indicating that it acts locally. In humans there is a constant level of both NO and ET1 in the vascular bed which regulates vessel tonus. Like NO, ET-1 is also involved in thrombosis, vascular growth, monocyte adhesion and inflammatory regulation (Puranik & Celermajer, 2003). When NO expression is suppressed, the balance tips in favour of endothelin effects. Smoking has been shown to increase levels of ET-1 both acutely and chronically (Borissova et al., 2004; Hirai et al., 2004).

Endothelial progenitor cells (EPC) are produced in response to ischemia and vascular injury from bone marrow. They are mobilized to repair endothelial injury and are inversely correlated to risk of CVD. Smoking inhibits eNOS, which has been shown to be important for EPC mobilization from bone marrow (Aicher et al., 2003). The level of EPC is lower in smokers than in non-smokers. After smoking cessation the EPC-count increases rapidly, particularly in light smokers, and decreased again when smoking is resumed after 4 weeks (Kondo et al., 2004). Notably, the increase in EPC after smoking cessation was significantly higher in light smokers. This suggests that light smokers may have a better chance of recovery than heavy smokers and that bone marrow or endothelium in heavy smokers is to some extent irreversibly damaged.

Oxidative process

Oxidative stress refers to a situation when the amounts of reactive oxygen species overcome the antioxidant defence system's capacity. This results in oxidation of molecules such as lipids and DNA. A central mechanism of cigarette smoking in causing atherosclerosis is its net oxidative effect. Free-radical-mediated oxidative stress is central in the development of atherosclerosis and is largely mediated through endothelial function. Free radicals can arise from the cigarette smoke itself; both the tar and the gas phase of the smoke contain numerous free radicals. Free radicals also arise from the activation of macrophages and neutrophils. The reactive oxygen species, which initiate the atherosclerotic process, are principally inactivated by the enzyme glutathione peroxidase. Cigarette smoke inhibits glutathione peroxidase and other enzymes, which inhibit oxidation of LDL, resulting in a net increase in oxidative activity and in oxidized LDL (Mukherjee et al., 1993; Nishio & Watanabe, 1997; Blankenberg et al., 2003). In vitro studies have shown that exposure to cigarette smoke causes an oxidation of plasma LDL (Frei et al., 1991; Pech-Amsellem et al., 1996) and an increased uptake of LDL in macrophages in the intima (Yokode et al., 1988). A direct link from cigarette smoking through increased LDL oxidization to increased atherosclerosis has been shown in hyperlipidemic rabbits (Yamaguchi et al., 2001).

A mere two weeks of smoking cessation can ameliorate the enhanced platelet aggregability and intraplatelet redox imbalance in long-term smokers, possibly by decreasing oxidative stress (Morita et al., 2005). Cigarette smoking cessation was followed by a marked increase in plasma antioxidant concentrations within four weeks of abstinence in the study by Polidori and colleagues (2003) on healthy smokers who subsequently quit.

Haemostatic factors

Platelet function

Although platelets play an important role in the development of an acute coronary event, it has been difficult to prove the associations between platelet properties and coronary heart disease risk in epidemiological studies. Problems in handling platelets in vivo and uncertainty about relevant markers of platelet function represent some of those difficulties. Increased platelet volume and spontaneous platelet aggregation have been suggested to predict the risk of recurrent myocardial infarction (Trip et al., 1990; Martin et al., 1991; MacCallum, 2005).

The effects of cigarette smoking on platelet function are at least partially controlled through endothelial function. Several studies have shown that smoking increases platelet aggregation. In one study, inhalation of only 2 cigarettes increases platelet adhesion 100-fold (Taylor et al., 1998). Law and colleagues suggest that smoking has maximal effect on platelet aggregation at low doses, and that other mechanisms come into play in higher doses (Law & Wald, 2003). Therefore, coronary heart disease risk may rise quickly on exposure to small amounts of tobacco smoke and then more slowly as the number of cigarettes per day increases. Cigarette smoking inhibits effects of cyclo-oxygenase, which leads to prostacyclin (PGI2) inhibition and increased thromboxane synthesis in platelets. These act synergistically in thrombus (Fitzgerald et al., 1988; Taylor et al., 1998). After stimulation from smoking, platelets release platelet-derived growth factors, which stimulate smooth muscle cells to migrate into intimae of blood vessels and proliferate, an important process in the formation of plaques (Nowak et al., 1987). P-selectin expression, a marker of platelet activation, is increased in smokers compared with non-smokers (Pernerstorfer et al., 1998). Baseline platelet-dependent thrombin generation appears to be significantly greater in smokers than in non-smokers and appears to rise further immediately after smoking (Hioki *et al.,* 2001). Platelet thrombus size has also been shown to increase after smoking (Hung *et al.,* 1995).

In one study, hematological characteristics (including number of platelets) increased with increasing pack-years and daily number of cigarettes, but were similar to those in never smokers within two years of abstinence (Van Tiel *et al.,* 2002). Clotting time has been shown to increase with daily cigarette consumption in smokers and to approach the level of never smokers with increasing years of abstinence (Yarnell *et al.,* 1987). Similar results were found for haematocrit. In general, values had not quite reached the level of never smokers after 10 years of abstinence.

Fibrinogen

Plasma fibrinogen is the most widely reported haemostatic variable associated with cardiovascular disease risk (Meade *et al.,* 1986). A recent large meta-analysis comprising data from 31 prospective studies including 154 211 participants who were followed up for a total of 1.38 million person-years demonstrated a moderately strong association between plasma fibrinogen level and the risk of coronary heart disease, stroke and other vascular mortality (Fibrinogen Studies Collaboration, 2004). The potential mechanisms whereby fibrinogen could contribute to cardiovascular disease risk include increased fibrin formation, platelet aggregation, plasma viscosity and through binding of leucocytes to endothelial cells (Kamath & Lip, 2003). Fibrinogen is elevated in smokers (Kannel *et al.,* 1987), and fibrinogen levels increase with the number of cigarettes smoked and quickly fall after smoking cessation (Kannel, 2005), although in some studies levels have

remained elevated up to 10 years after smoking cessation (Yarnell *et al.,*1987; Wannamethee, 2005)

D-dimer

D-dimer is a product of lysis of cross-linked fibrin. Increased D-dimer levels indicate increased fibrin turnover. As for fibrinogen, several prospective studies have shown an association of D-dimer level with coronary heart disease risk (Danesh *et al.,* 2001). Cross-sectional studies show increased levels of D-dimer in smokers compared to non-smokers (Lee *et al.,* 1995) and reduced levels in former smokers, although levels remained significantly raised even after two decades of abstinence (Wannamethee *et al.,* 2005).

Exposure of TF to blood containing FVIIa is thought to produce strong thrombogenic stimulus that is critical to the development of coronary thrombosis after plaque rupture. Among 56 endarterectomy patients, smokers had increased TF expression and activity compared with non-smokers (Matetzky *et al.,* 2000). In a study comparing 10 smokers and 15 non-smokers, the former had significantly higher plasma TF activity, with levels rising further 2 hours after smoking (Sambola *et al.,* 2003).

Fibrinolysis

Studies show lower levels of tissue plasminogen activator (tPA) in smokers (Barua *et al.,* 2002). Levels of thromboxane A2, which is released by activated platelets, are higher in smokers (Benowitz *et al.,* 1993; Ludvig *et al.,* 2005). Impairment of plasma fibrinolytic activity has been associated with coronary heart disease risk in several prospective observational studies. Reduced release of tPA antigen levels and decreased activity, which indicates impaired fibrinolytic activity, have been

reported by Newby *et al.,* (1999, 2001). The level of its inhibitor, plasminogen activator inhibitor type 1 (PAI-1), which forms a complex with tPA, is associated with tPA level. Newby (2001) reported higher PAI-1 levels in smokers compared to former and neversmokers although differences were not statistically significant in the small size study (n=22). Impaired fibrinolytic activity, caused both by increased circulating PAI-1 and impaired endothelial tPA release, could be a factor linking smoking to the coronary heart disease risk. Impaired plasma fibrinolysis (PAI-1 and tPA) in smokers and restored fibrinolysis in former smokers have been reported (Simpson *et al.,* 1997).

Inflammation

Most inflammatory markers are correlated with haemostatic factors, and interaction between these is complex. Observational studies have associated cigarette smoking with increased levels of a number of inflammatory markers, namely: leukocytes, hs-CRP, fibrinogen, and IL6, and markers of leucocyte recruitment, namely: VCAM-1, ICAM-1, E- and P-selectin, with intermediary values in former smokers (Bermudez *et al.,* 2002). Inflammation is triggered by effects on endothelial function with activation of neutrophils and macrophages and secretion of a number of chemotactic factors (Taylor *et al.,* 1998; Ambrose & Barua, 2004). In experimental studies, exposure to cigarette smoking causes increased levels of pro-inflammatory cytokines IL-6, TNF-α and IL-1β in addition to increased lipid per oxidation (Zhang *et al.,* 2002).

Several studies have shown increased concentrations of inflammatory and haemostatic markers in smokers with a dose-dependent relationship (Bakhru & Erlinger, 2005; Wannamethee *et al.,* 2005). The time-course of decline in these markers after smoking cessation differs; some studies have shown rapid normalisation in haemostatic and inflammatory markers whereas others have not. In a Scottish study of 22 920 men aged 60–79 free of CVD examined at baseline and after 20 years, former smokers had levels of CRP, leukocyte count, fibrinogen, plasma viscosity, tPA and D-dimer that were much lower than in continued smokers but did not reach the level of never smokers until after >20 years of not smoking (Wannamethee et al., 2005). For most of these inflammatory and haemostatic markers, the time course after smoking cessation did not differ between light and heavy smokers. In contrast, in cross-sectional analyses of the NHANES III study comprising 15 489 men and women, although both CRP, WBC and fibrinogen were higher in smokers than in never smokers in a dose-dependent manner, inflammatory response subsided within 5 years of giving up smoking, and as a group former smokers did not have significantly higher levels than never smokers after adjustment (Bakhru & Erlinger, 2005). The MONICA study also found higher levels of inflammatory markers with increasing daily consumption and pack-years of smoking and decreased levels with time since smoking cessation in men, but the risk did not quite reach the level of neversmokers, even with >30 years of tobacco abstinence. In women, associations between levels of inflammation markers and smoking were not present, perhaps due to lack of control for inhalation habits, reported to differ from those in men, and to a reduced number of former and current smokers in participant women, decreasing the power of the study to detect associations if present (Frohlich et al., 2003). Similar results were reported from a United Kingdom study

with rapid decline in white blood cell count, granulocytes and monocytes following smoking cessation but still slightly elevated levels after a decade of abstinence in comparison with never smokers (Smith et al., 2003). The Scottish study only comprised men, and in the NHANES study results were not presented by gender. A Swedish study showed complementary results on the associations between amount of cigarettes smoked and inflammatory markers by showing that within smoking strata the risk of CVD increased with higher measures of Carboxyhemoglobin (COHb%) and that levels of COHb% were correlated with markers of inflammation (Lind et al., 2004).

Also, in experimental studies smoking reduction and cessation have been accompanied by a decrease in WBC, fibrinogen, lipids, BP and heart rate (Eliasson et al., 2001; Bolliger et al., 2002; Hatsukami et al., 2005).

Associations between cigarette smoking and smoking cessation and the levels of haemostatic factors were assessed among 7735 men aged 40–59 years participating in the British Regional Heart Study (Wannamethee et al., 2005). Current smokers had markedly higher plasma fibrinogen, D-dimer, von Willebrand factor and t-PA levels and higher plasma and blood viscosity compared to lifelong never smokers. Former smokers tended to have slightly higher levels than lifelong smokers (Table 6). Duration of cessation of smoking was also associated with the levels of haemostatic factors. Compared to current smokers, plasma fibrinogen level was substantially lower among those who had quit less than five years earlier, but the lowest levels were found among those who had quit smoking more than 20 years earlier. In other haemostatic factors the effect of time since quitting was less clear.

Modification of lipids

Smokers have a more atherogenic lipid profile than neversmokers: they have higher total cholesterol, LDL-cholesterol, VLDL-cholesterol and triglycerides and lower HDL-cholesterol. Cigarette smoking affects activity of lipoprotein lipase and through nicotine effects on catecholamine increases lipolysis and release of free fatty acids which increase VLDL. The role of diet in lipid profile between smokers and non-smokers is not clear. Reactive oxygen species—free radicals—present in inhaled smoke cause plasma LDL oxidation directly or indirectly through activation of macrophages (Yamaguchi et al., 2005). This is confirmed by higher rates of lipid per oxidation in studies of smokers and in experimental studies (Yamaguchi et al., 2004). Experimental studies with isolated oxidants in inhaled smoke have shown increased oxidisation of LDL resulting in increased atherosclerosis in hyper-lipidemic rabbits (Yamaguchi et al., 2001). Cigarette smoking also decreased the activity of paraoxonase, an enzyme that protects against LDL oxidization (Nishio & Watanabe, 1997).

As noted above, cigarette smoking causes increased oxidization of LDL, a trigger of the inflammatory process in the intimae of the arteries through stimulation of monocyte adhesion to the vessel wall (Weber et al., 1995). Increased adhesion to vessel wall of monocytes in smokers compared to never smokers has been shown in experimental settings (Weber et al., 1996). Unfortunately, dietary supplementation of antioxidant vitamins (vitamins C and E), expected to inhibit the oxidative process, has not proven successful in preventing CVD (Lonn & Yusuf, 1997). This apparent contradiction has been termed the 'oxidative paradox'.

Table 6. Smoking status and adjusted mean levels (95% CI) of haemostatic and inflammatory markers for CVD

	Never (n = 873)	Ex-smokers (n = 1503)	Primary pipe cigar smokers (n = 44)	Secondary pipe cigar smokers (n = 109)	Current smokers (n = 391)	P-value[a]	P-value[b]
CRP (mg/L)[c]	1.35 (1.26, 1.46)	1.58 (1.49, 1.66)	1.22 (0.91, 1.68)	1.72 (1.42, 2.10)	2.53 (2.27, 2.80)	< 0.0001	< 0.0001
White cell count (x 10^9/L)[c]	6.42 (6.30,6.49)	6.62 (6.48, 6.69)	6.48 (5.99,7.03)	7.24 (6.96, 7.61)	7.92 (7.69, 8.08)	< 0.0001	< 0.0001
Fibrinogen (g/L)	3.13 (3.08, 3.18)	3.20 (3.17, 3.24)	3.16 (2.96, 3.37)	3.26 (3.13, 3.39)	3.51 (3.44, 3.54)	< 0.0001	< 0.0001
Albumin (g/L)	44.4 (44.2, 44.6)	44.2 (44.0, 44.3)	44.0 (43.2, 44.8)	44.0 (43.5, 44.5)	43.9 (43.6, 44.2)	0.002	0.02
HCT (%)	45.1 (44.9, 45.3)	45.0 (44.9, 45.2)	45.2 (44.2, 46.2)	45.7 (45.1, 46.3)	46.0 (45.7, 46.4)	< 0.0001	< 0.0001
Blood viscosity (mPa s)	3.39 (3.36, 3.40)	3.38 (3.37, 3.40)	3.36 (3.28, 3.45)	3.43 (3.38, 3.49)	3.48 (3.45, 3.51)	< 0.0001	< 0.0001
Plasma viscosity (mPa s)	1.275 (1.270, 1.280)	1.281 (1.278, 1.286)	1.263 (1.241, 1.285)	1.277 (1.263, 1.292)	1.289 (1.282, 1.297)	0.003	0.02
Factor VIII (iu/dL)	129.9 (127.7, 131.9)	132.1 (130.5, 133.7)	131.2 (122.0, 140.5)	124.5 (118.7, 130.3)	124.5 (121.3, 127.7)	0.007	0.0003
VWF (iu/dL)	134.9 (131.6, 137.7)	136.3 (134.1, 138.6)	140.3 (137.1, 153.4)	132.8 (123.5, 140.3)	138.8 (134.3, 143.4)	0.14	0.45
t-PA (ng/mL)	10.2 (9.9, 10.5)	10.8 (10.6, 11.0)	10.7 (9.5, 11.9)	10.8 (10.3, 11.6)	11.6 (11.2, 12.0)	< 0.0001	< 0.0001
d-dimer (ng/mL)	75.6 (71.5, 79.4)	79.8 (76.7, 83.1)	78.3 (62.2, 98.5)	81.1 (70.1, 93.7)	94.4 (88.2, 102.5)	< 0.0001	0.0002

95% CI = 95% confidence interval

Adjusted for age, social class, physical activity, alcohol intake, BMI, systolic blood pressure, and HDL-cholesterol.

CRP, C-reactive protein; HCT, haematocrit mpAs

a Comparisons between current smokers and never smokers

b Differences between groups

c Geometric mean used

Reproduced from Wannamethee et al., Associations between cigarette smoking, pipe/cigar smoking, and smoking cessation and haemostatic and inflammatory markers for cardiovascular disease, Eur. Heart J., 2005, Vol. 26(17), pages 1765–1773, by permission of Oxford University Press.

Vasomotor function

In addition to the vasomotor effects regulated by endothelial function, smoking may have a direct effect on the tonus of coronary arteries through adrenergic stimulation, at least partially due to the effects of nicotine, causing reduced blood flow. Smoking has been shown to have an acute vasoconstrictor effect during angiography. This reaction is paradoxical because smoking exposure, with its accompanying reduced oxygen availability and increased demand due to increased heart rate and cardiac output, requires increased blood flow (Quillen et al., 1993).

Should the timing of risk reduction be different for those with and without clinically significant cardiovascular disease at the time of cessation?

Based on the described mechanisms, it would be expected that effects on haemostatis and plaque instability would be partly reversible whereas the accumulated effects on plaque formation would not be reversible. However, smoking cessation would have the effect of reducing the rate of progression of the atherosclerotic process in comparison with continued smoking. Cardiovascular events that involve occlusion of vessels, e.g. myocardial infarction and stroke, are relatively more dependent on plaque stability, whereas events determined by insufficient delivery of oxygen due to reduced blood flow in vessels, e.g. angina and intermittent claudication, are expected to be more dependent on plaque size and thus less affected by smoking cessation.

A biphasic response to smoking cessation in CVD risk is compatible with the dual effects of smoking—acute and reversible effects on haemostasis and plaque stability and more prolonged effect on plaque formation. Furthermore, as noted, evolution of risk would be expected to differ according to pathogenetic mechanisms of the corresponding disease. Plaque formation is not expected to be fully reversible, thus smokers would not be expected to ever reach risk level of never smokers concerning CVD.

Mechanisms of Pathophysiology in Chronic Obstructive Pulmonary Disease (COPD)

Introduction

The Global Initiative for Chronic Obstructive Lung Disease (GOLD) has recently formulated a "Global Strategy for the Diagnosis, Management and Prevention of COPD" (www.gold copd.org) (NIH, 2003; Pauwels et al., 2001; Hansel & Barnes, 2004). A working definition of COPD is given within the GOLD Global Strategy as: "A disease state characterised by airflow limitation that is not fully reversible. The airflow limitation is usually progressive and associated with an abnormal inflammatory response of the lungs to noxious particles or gases." This is the first time that a definition of COPD has highlighted the fact that it is an inflammatory disease, or has made an attempt to emphasise its etiology.

However, this brief definition does not detail risk factors such as cigarette smoke, does not describe the symptoms of COPD, and does not describe the range of pathological processes and diseases encompassed within COPD (Snider, 2003). In practice, the main source of "noxious particles or gases" referred to in the GOLD definition is cigarette smoking, constituting the main risk factor for COPD (Anto et al., 2001). COPD may also be caused by exposure to mineral dusts, fumes from indoor biomass fuels, and outdoor air pollution (Dennis et al., 1996; Anto et al., 2001; Jones et al., 2003). Spirometry is fundamental to the diagnosis and staging of COPD, and the GOLD stages of severity of COPD are arbitrarily defined by the post-bronchodilator forced expiratory volume in 1 second (FEV_1) (Table 7). Bronchodilatory reversibility in COPD is a poorly reproducible variable (Calverley et al., 2003).

The large amounts of oxidants contained in cigarette smoke cause an exaggerated host leukocyte inflammatory response involving macrophages, neutrophils, and T cells in patients with COPD (Barnes, 2000; Cosio et al., 2002; Barnes et al., 2003; Di Stefano et al., 2004; Shapiro & Ingenito, 2005). In response to long-term cigarette exposure, cycles of inflammation, repair and regeneration fibrosis, proteolysis and tissue destruction occur within the lungs.

The Pathology of COPD

At separate anatomical sites different pathological events occur in COPD, with distinct physiological sequelae that result in varying clinical manifestations: chronic bronchitis, obstructive bronchiolitis, and emphysema occur in the respiratory tree (Figure 5). Pulmonary vascular disease and cor pulmonale, systemic disease with cachexia, and respiratory and peripheral muscle weakness are also important features of more severe COPD.

Chronic bronchitis

Chronic bronchitis is an inflammatory disease of the large airways that generally causes little ventilatory limitation. Mucus-producing goblet cell hyperplasia occurs in the epithelium, and there is hypertrophy of mucous glands in the submucosa. Chronic bronchitis develops in approximately half of all heavy smokers and involves excess mucus production and expectoration (Willemse et al., 2004). Chronic bronchitis was originally described for clinical and epidemiology purposes by the United Kingdom Medical Research Council (MRC) as productive cough on most days for at least three months for at least two consecutive years that cannot be attributed to other pulmonary or cardiac causes (Medical Research Council, 1965).

In addition, the term "chronic bronchitis" can also be used to describe histopathological features. Chronic stimulation leads to up-regulation of mucin (MUC) genes, especially MUC5B in the bronchiolar lumen and MUC5AC in the bronchiolar epithelium (Caramori et al., 2004). A 15-year study has found that patients at GOLD Stage 0 with chronic bronchitis are not vulnerable to developing subsequent airways obstruction (Vestbo & Lange, 2002).

Obstructive bronchiolitis

Obstructive bronchiolitis involves the small or peripheral airways, and is an inflammatory and fibrotic condition of small airways < 3mm in diameter. Hogg and colleagues (2004) have studied the histopathology of the small airways in lungs from patients with different severities of COPD (GOLD I–IV). They have identified a prominent infiltration with macrophages and neutrophils in all stages of COPD, with more prominent wall thickening in more severe disease, and identified prominent lymphoid follicles only in COPD of stages III and IV (Figure 6).

Emphysema

Emphysema is defined by permanent, destructive enlargement of the air-spaces distal to the terminal bronchioli, with destruction of the interstitium, affecting the respiratory bronchioles and sometimes the alveoli (Figure 5).

Centrilobular emphysema occurs more frequently in the upper lung fields in mild disease. A fundamental defect is ventilation/perfusion (Va/Q) imbalance that becomes reflected in abnormalities in gas transfer, which eventually manifests as respiratory failure. Loss of alveolar attachments from small airways alters elastic recoil of the lung and contributes to airflow obstruction.

Pulmonary vascular disease

Pulmonary vascular disease begins early in the course of COPD as intimal thickening, followed by smooth muscle hypertrophy and inflammatory infiltration.

Systemic COPD

Systemic cachectic COPD involves disturbances in metabolism with cachexia, as well as increased respiratory and skeletal muscle fatigue with wasting. This is a predictor of increased mortality even when level of abnormal lung function is controlled in the analysis (Schols et al., 1998; Celli et al., 2004).

Table 7. Global initiative for chronic obstructive lung diseaase (GOLD) stages of severity

Severity stage	Symptoms	Post-bronchodilator FEV$_1$ (% predicted)	FEV$_1$/FVC (%)
0: At risk	chronic bronchitis	normal	normal
I: Mild	+/- symptoms +/- cough/sputum	> 80	< 70
II: Moderate	+/- symptoms	50–80	< 70
III: Severe	+/- cough/sputum/dyspnoea	30–50	< 70
IV: Very severe	cough/sputum/dyspnoea +/- respiratory failure +/- right heart failure	< 30 or respiratory failure or right heart failure	< 70

From NIH/NHLBI/WHO (2003). GOLD guidelines were revised in November 2006 and are available at www.goldcopd.org.

Chronic bronchitis
Mucous: sputum

Obstructive bronchiolitis
Obstruction: FEV_1

Centrilobular emphysema
Destruction: hypoxia

Goblet cell hyperplasia
and squamous
metaplasia

Increased mucous

Smooth muscle
hypertrophy

Collapsed
lumen

Increased
mucous

Loss of
attachments

Inflammation
with fibrosis

Goblet cells
metaplasia

Inflammation
with fibrosis

Submucosal bronchial
gland hypertrophy

Degeneration of
cartilage

Smooth muscle
hypertrophy

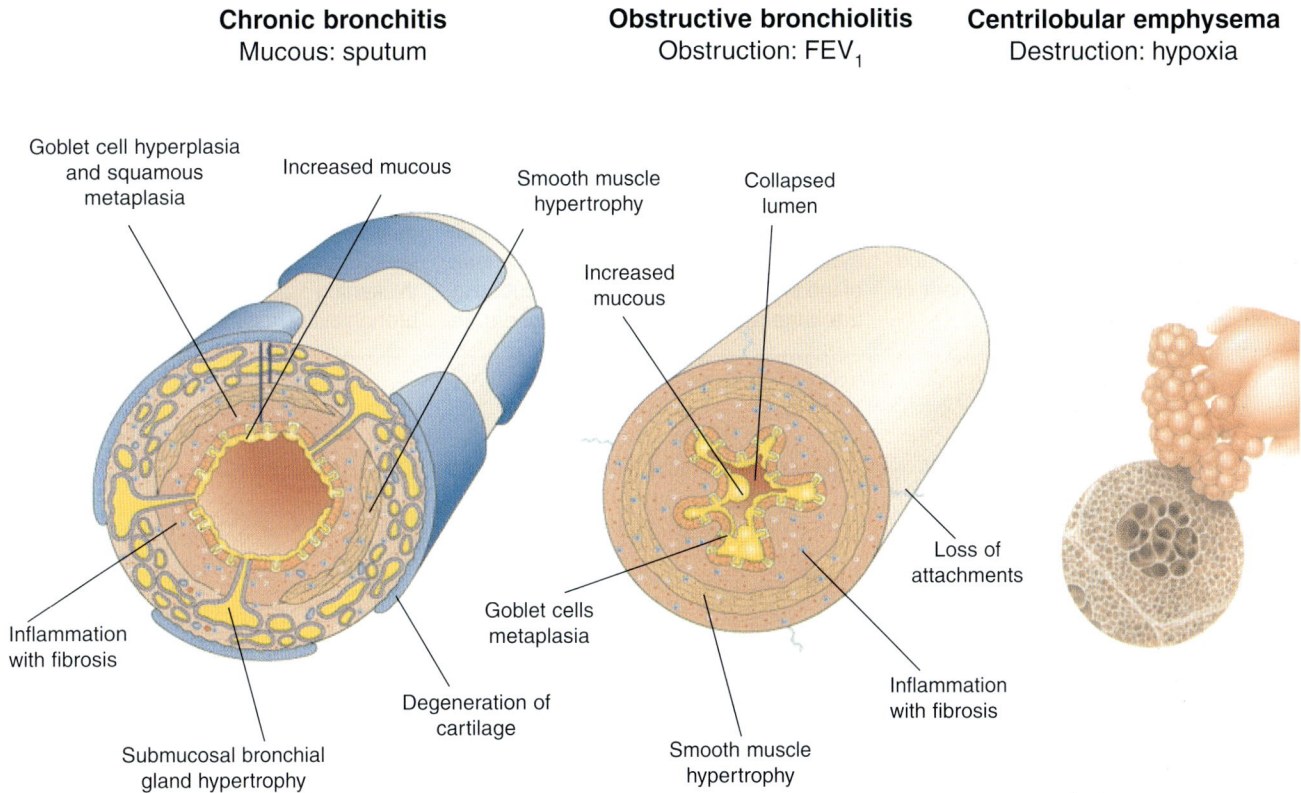

Figure 5. Lung Pathology of COPD

From An Atlas of COPD by Trevor Hansel & Peter J. Barnes. Copyright (2004) Parthenon Publishing Group. Reproduced by permission of Taylor & Francis Books UK.

The skeletal muscle weakness may exacerbate dyspnoea, and skeletal and respiratory muscle training is an important aspect of pulmonary rehabilitation (Salman *et al.*, 2003). In addition, there are features of inflammation in the peripheral blood, and hypogonadism and other endocrine problems are commonly noted (Creutzberg & Casaburi, 2003; Sin & Man, 2003; Gan *et al.*, 2005; Laghi *et al.*, 2005).

Smoking Cessation Study Limitations

There is a shortage of data on the effects of smoking cessation on parameters of inflammation: in particular there is a need for longitudinal studies in well-controlled groups of smoking patients that are asymptomatic, symptomatic with chronic bronchitis, and with COPD of different grades of severity. Unfortunately, much of the available data is cross-sectional, so the differences

between smokers and former smokers are assessed without consideration of the kinetics of the processes in individual subjects that would be documented in longitudinal determinations.

Specimens to Assess Mechanisms

The ultimate standard for assessment of inflammation is to perform histopathological analysis of resected lung tissue at surgery for lung volume reduction or lung malignancy, or lung tissue obtained at post mortem (Hogg *et al.,* 2004). Invasive bronchoscopic techniques enable assessment of inflammation in endobronchial mucosal biopsy or bronchoalveolar lavage (BAL). Non-invasive assessment of biomarkers may be performed in blood, urine, exhaled breath and sputum, though there are considerable methodological and technical issues in the measurement of breath and sputum biomarkers.

Hogg and colleagues have published a series of important observations on the histopathology of the lungs in cigarette smokers, studying both asymptomatic smokers and individuals with COPD of varying severity (Hogg *et al.,* 2004). These data are cross-sectional due to the requirement for resected or autopsy lung. Goblet cell hyperplasia, as opposed to the thickness of the bronchial gland layer, is reduced in the large airways of former smokers. In

more severe COPD the small airways develop the particular pathological features of an intense lymphocytic infiltrate and prominent lymphoid follicles containing helper T (Th) and cytotoxic T (Tc) cells and B cells (Hogg *et al.,* 2004). These changes may represent chronic bacterial colonisation. Severe COPD may not be reversible due to prominent structural remodelling: small airway thickening and fibrosis (obstructive bronchiolitis) associated with interstitial

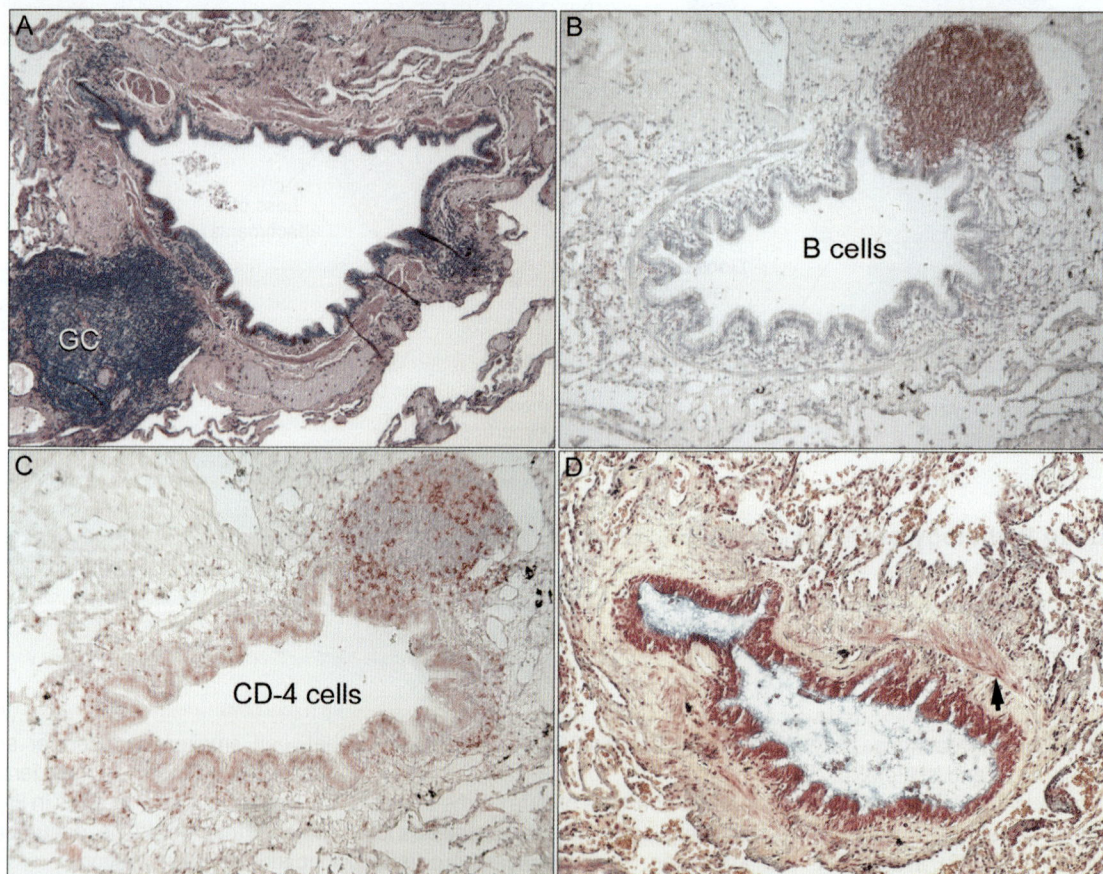

Figure 6. Pathological findings in patients with COPD

Panel A shows a collection of bronchial lymphoid tissue with a lymphoid follicle containing a germinal center (GC) surrounded by a rim of darker-staining lymphocytes that extend to the epithelium of both the small airway and alveolar surface (Movat's stain x 6). Panel B shows another follicle, in which the germinal center stains strongly for B cells (x6) and Panel C shows a serial section of the same airway stained for CD4 cells, which are scattered around the edge of the follicle and in the airway wall (x6.5). Panel D, shows an airway that has been extensively remodeled by connective-tissue deposition in the subep-ithelial and advential compartments ofr the airway wall. The arrow points to the smooth muscle that separates the subepithelial from the adventitial compart-ments (Movat's stain, x6).

From Hogg *et al.* (2004). Copyright (2004) Massachusetts Medical Society. All rights reserved.

alveolar destruction (emphysema). In histopathological studies inflammation may persist many years after smoking cessation, despite reversal of the accelerated decline in lung function produced by smoking; therefore it is likely that not all features of inflammation cause impaired lung function.

Skold and coworkers undertook longitudinal bronchoscopic studies in the 1990s assessing changes after smoking cessation in non-symptomatic individuals: macroscopic signs of chronic bronchitis disappeared with 12 months, with decreased blood leukocytes and decreased numbers of neutrophils and activated macrophages in BAL and sputum specimens by 6 months (Skold et al., 1992, 1993, 1996). Other smoking cessation studies have documented changes in Clara cell secretory protein in BAL and other measures of lower respiratory tract inflammation (Andersson et al., 2000). A recent longitudinal study of bronchial mucosal biopsies obtained after smoking cessation in COPD patients showed persistence of inflammation (Hogg, 2006; Lapperre et al., 2006).

In peripheral blood there are increased levels of leukocytes in smokers, and these levels do not always return to normal after smoking cessation (Skold et al., 1996; Willemse et al., 2004). Leukocytosis together with elevated C-reactive protein (CRP), fibrinogen, and IL-6 were found to be elevated in a large meta-analysis of patients with COPD (Gan et al., 2004). A series of studies have monitored the acute effects of smoking cessation on blood parameters (Jensen et al., 1992; Meliska et al., 1995; Skold et al., 1996; Jensen et al., 1998).

Breath levels of nitric oxide (NO) are lower in smokers (Montuschi et al, 2001), but alveolar NO is elevated in COPD (Brindicci et al., 2005), while parameters of oxidant stress are elevated in breath condensate (iso-prostane, hydrogen peroxide) (Montuschi et al, 2000). Smoking cessation is associated with an increase in exhaled NO (Robbins et al., 1997). However, there are considerable technical problems with breath condensate analysis, including interpretation of data that is not specific as to the source of condensate solutes and a fluctuating dilution of respiratory droplets from condensed water vapor, which represents the overwhelming majority of condensate volumes (Effros et al., 2005; Horvath et al., 2005).

Sputum levels of TNF-α, soluble-TNFR, IL-8, GRO-α and MIP-1α are elevated in COPD patients (Vernooy et al., 2002), but levels are also higher in former smokers (Keatings et al., 1996, 1997; Stockley et al., 2001). In addition, there are increased levels of myelo-peroxidase (MPO) (Hill et al., 1999; Crooks et al., 2000). In an important recent study on the effects of smoking cessation, there was a consistent but paradoxical increase in inflammation 1 year after quitting attributed to repair of tissue damage in the airways (Willemse et al., 2005).

Processes

Oxidative Stress

Cigarette smoke has been estimated to contain some 1017 oxidant molecules per inhalation, and there is considerable evidence that oxidative stress is increased in patients with COPD (Repine et al., 1997; MacNee, 2000; van der Vliet & Cross, 2000; MacNee & Rahman, 2001; Boots et al., 2003). The lungs have a large epithelial surface area that is exposed to reactive oxygen and nitrogen species within cigarette smoke, further oxidants are generated during inflammatory processes, and an oxidant/antioxidant balance is thought to be important in the pathogenesis of COPD (Comhair & Erzurum, 2002).

Inflammation

Cigarette smoke and other inhaled irritants initiate an inflammatory response in the peripheral airways and lung parenchyma (Barnes et al., 2003) (Figure 7). Following chronic exposure to oxidants, epithelial cell injury and macrophage activation cause release of chemotactic factors that recruit neutrophils from the circulation. Macrophages and neutrophils release proteases that break down connective tissue. Both serine proteases such as neutrophil elastase (NE) and matrix metalloproteinases (MMPs) are implicated in this process. Cytotoxic CD8+ T cells may also be involved in the inflammatory cascade. Over many years of injury, cycles of inflammation and repair occur that may result in resolution, but can be associated with excess mucus production, proteolysis, fibrosis, and both airway and parenchymal remodelling.

Inflammation, when present in "healthy" smokers, is very similar to that in COPD, in terms of inflammatory cells, mediators and proteases, but is less pronounced. This suggests that the inflammation in COPD represents an exaggeration of the normal inflammatory response to noxious agents (Barnes, 2000). The mechanisms for this amplification are not yet certain, but may be determined by genetic factors (Barnes, 1999), latent virus (such as adenovirus) (Gilmour et al., 2001; Meshi et al., 2002) and impaired histone deacetylase (HDAC) activity (Barnes et al., 2004). Histone acetylation causes the activation of nuclear core histones, resulting in the transcription of genes that cause inflammation. The reversal of this process by HDAC is impaired in alveolar macrophages from patients with COPD (Ito et al., 2000, 2001). COPD causes a particular type of inflammation especially associated with mononuclear cells (macrophages and CD8+ T cells) as well as neutrophils. This inflammation may resolve or may become associated with fibrosis, proteolysis and remodelling. The nature of the inflammatory infiltrate is broadly similar in large and small airways as well as within the alveoli and pulmonary artery wall.

Proteases

The key to the pathogenesis of emphysema is believed to be an imbalance of proteases and antiproteases in the lung (Stockley, 1994). Excess extracellular matrix deposition in the small airways may be due to a protease-antiprotease imbalance favouring fibrosis (Vignola et al., 1998). Proteases are also involved in the third component of COPD, excess mucus production, being potent stimulators of mucus secretion. Two of the cell types implicated as key effectors in the pathogenesis of COPD, namely the neutrophil and the macrophage, are together able of secreting proteases capable of digesting all the components of the extracellular matrix. Serine proteases (neutrophil elastase (NE), cathepsin G and protease 3 and cysteine proteases (cathepsins)) are produced by neutrophils. Matrix metalloproteinases (MMPs) are a group of over 20 closely related endopeptidases, also involved in emphysema pathology, produced by neutrophils, alveolar macrophages and airway epithelial cells (Shapiro, 1994).

Fibrosis

MMP-9 may play a role in the activation of transforming growth factor-β (TGF-β) (Dallas et al., 2002; Kranenburg et al., 2002), as well as in the release of chemotactic peptides and activation of

α1-anti-trypsin; thus being involved closely with both proteolysis and fibrosis. Protease activated receptor 2 (PAR-2) is a transmembrane receptor preferentially activated by trypsin and tryptase, and PARs play an important role in matrix remodelling, cell migration and proliferation and inflammation. PAR-2 has increased expression on the smooth muscle of bronchial vessels in patients with chronic bronchitis when compared to patients with COPD (Miotto et al., 2002). PAR-2 induces the proliferation of human airway smooth muscle cells (Berger et al., 2001) and human lung fibroblast proliferation (Akers et al., 2000), as well as MMP-9 release from airway epithelial cells (Vliagoftis et al., 2000). Transforming growth factor-β1 has increased expression in small airway and alveolar epithelial cells in COPD, and participates in the fibrotic processes that take place in the small airways (de Boer et al., 1998; Takizawa et al., 2001). Cigarette smoke extract has been shown to induce COX-2 with concurrent synthesis of prostaglandin E2 by normal human lung fibroblasts producing a pro-inflammatory environment (Martey et al., 2004). Hence MMP-9, PAR-2 and TGF-β may be interrelated in causing fibrosis in COPD.

Reversibility and structural remodelling

Some features of inflammation may be more reversible than others, and as COPD progresses there is likely to be less and less reversibility in the pulmonary inflammatory processes with the advent of structural remodeling that includes fibrosis, tissue reorganisation and destruction.

Issues for Assessment of the Mechanisms of COPD

The diagnosis of emphysema can be made accurately using high resolution CT scans (Goldin, 2004; Newell et al., 2004; Stockley, 2004; de Jong et al., 2005; Shaker et al., 2005). There is, however, the need for new improved imaging modalities to study the small airways (Hill & van Beek, 2004).

There is a paradigm that oxidants in cigarette smoke cause inflammation that is the basis of the pathology of COPD. However, there is a lack of information in longitudinal studies on the effects of smoking cessation on parameters of inflammation. Inflammation persists in histopathology of surgically resected and post mortem lung tissue many years after smoking cessation. Mucosal bronchial biopsies obtained on bronchoscopy are from larger airways, and may be poorly representative of small airways pathology (Lapperre et al., 2006). Inflammation increases in sputum samples taken at up to 12 months after smoking cessation, and this corresponds to improved lung function. Hence, paradoxically, inflammation may be beneficial in some instances. Non-invasively obtained specimens, such as breath and sputum, could be used to study inflammatory biomarkers after smoking cessation.

Understanding the molecular, cellular and pathophysiological basis of the events that occur after smoking cessation can give insight into potentially reversible molecular mechanisms, and will assist in the definition of targets for pharmacotherapy (Barnes & Hansel, 2004).

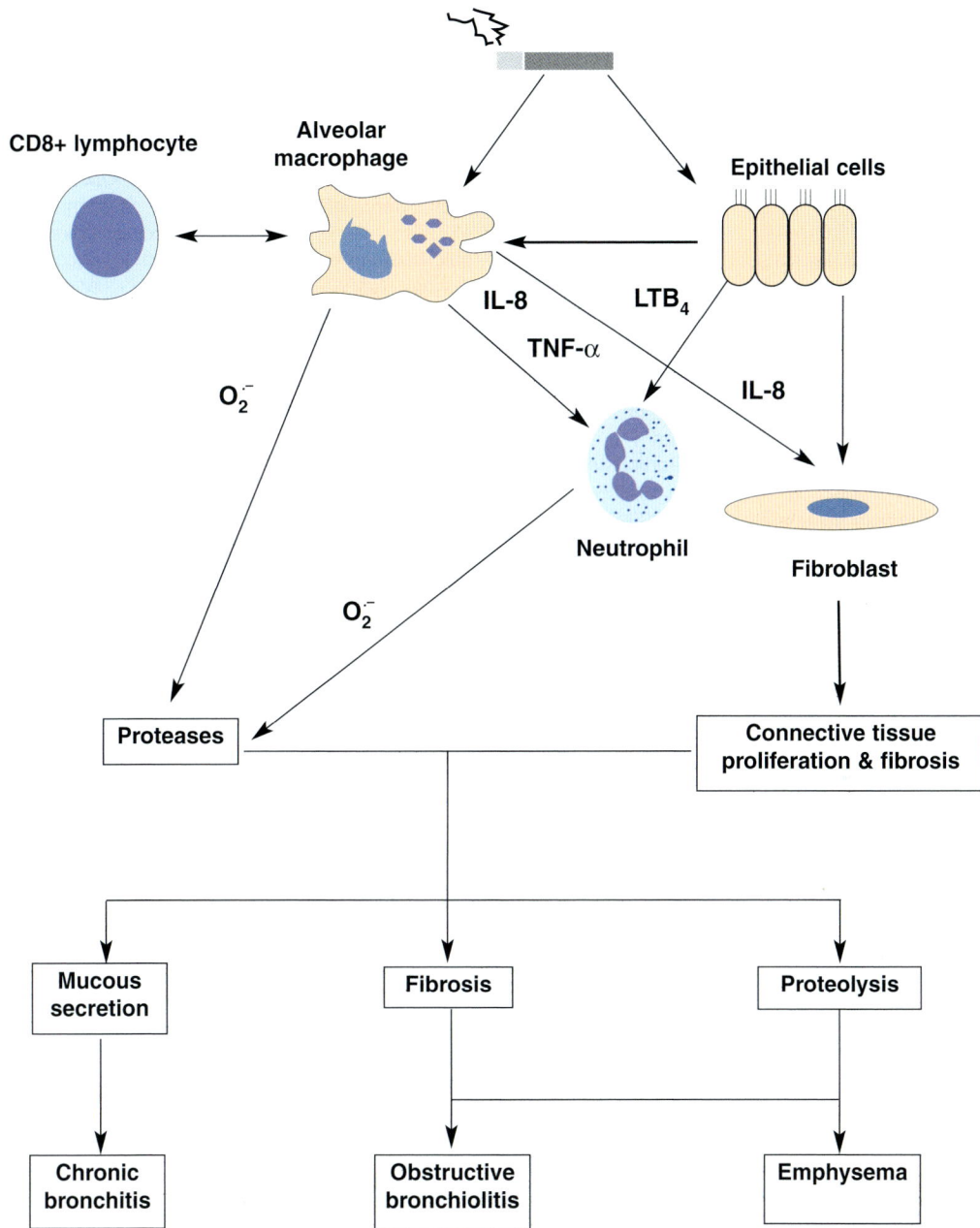

Figure 7. Cells in the pathology of COPD

Initiation of the inflammatory response in the peripheral airways and lung parenchyma following cigarette smoke and inhalation of irritant components ($O_2^{.-}$ = oxygen radicals)

From an Atlas of COPD by Trevor Hensel & Peter J. Barnes. Copyright (2004) Parthenon Publishing Group. Reprodced by permission of Taylor Francis Books UK.

References

Adams MR, Robinson J, McCredie R, et al. (1998). Smooth muscle dysfunction occurs independently of impaired endothelium-dependent dilation in adults at risk of atherosclerosis. *J Am Coll Cardiol,* 32(1):123-127.

Ahrendt SA, Decker PA, Alawi EA, et al. (2001). Cigarette smoking is strongly associated with mutation of the K-ras gene in patients with primary adeno-carcinoma of the lung. *Cancer,* 92(6):1525-1530.

Aicher A, Heeschen C, Mildner-Rihm C, et al. (2003). Essential role of endothelial nitric oxide synthase for mobilization of stem and progenitor cells. *Nat Med,* 9(11):1370-1376.

Akers IA, Parsons M, Hill MR, et al. (2000). Mast cell tryptase stimulates human lung fibroblast proliferation via protease-activated receptor-2. *Am J Physiol Lung Cell Mol Physiol,* 278(1):L193-L201.

Ambrose JA, Barua RS (2004). The pathophysiology of cigarette smoking and cardiovascular disease: an update. *J Am Coll Cardiol,* 43(10):1731-1737.

Andersson O, Cassel TN, Skold CM, et al. (2000). Clara cell secretory protein. Levels in BAL fluid after smoking cessation. Chest, 118(1):180-182.

Anto JM, Vermeire P, Vestbo J, et al. (2001). Epidemiology of chronic obstructive pulmonary disease. *Eur Respir J,* 17(5):982-994.

Ashburner M, Ball CA, Blake JA, et al. (2000). Gene ontology: tool for the unification of biology. The Gene Ontology Consortium. *Nat Genet,* 25(1):25-29.

Asplund K (2003). Smokeless tobacco and cardiovascular disease. *Prog Cardiovasc Dis,* 45(5):383-394.

Auerbach O, Stout AP, Hammond EC, et al. (1961). Changes in bronchial epithelium in relation to cigarette smoking and in relation to lung cancer. *N Engl J Med,* 265:253-267.

Bain C, Feskanich D, Speizer FE, et al. (2004). Lung cancer rates in men and women with comparable histories of smoking. *J Natl Cancer Inst,* 96(11):826-834.

Bakhru A, Erlinger TP (2005). Smoking cessation and cardiovascular disease risk factors: results from the Third National Health and Nutrition Examination Survey. *PLoS Med,* 2(6):e160.

Barnes PJ (1999). Genetics and pulmonary medicine. 9. Molecular genetics of chronic obstructive pulmonary disease. *Thorax,* 54(3):245-252.

Barnes PJ (2000). Chronic obstructive pulmonary disease. *N Engl J Med,* 343(4):269-280.

Barnes PJ, Shapiro SD, Pauwels RA (2003). Chronic obstructive pulmonary disease: molecular and cellular mechanisms. *Eur Respir J,* 22(4):672-688.

Barnes PJ, Ito K, Adcock IM (2004). Corticosteroid resistance in chronic obstructive pulmonary disease: inactivation of histone deacetylase. *Lancet,* 363(9410):731-733.

Barnes PJ, Hansel TT (2004). Prospects for new drugs for chronic obstructive pulmonary disease. *Lancet,* 364(9438):985-996.

Bartkova J, Horejsi Z, Koed K, et al. (2005). DNA damage response as a candidate anti-cancer barrier in early human tumorigenesis. *Nature,* 434(7035):864-870.

Barua RS, Ambrose JA, Saha DC, et al. (2002). Smoking is associated with altered endothelial-derived fibrinolytic and antithrombotic factors: an in vitro demonstration. *Circulation,* 106(8):905-908.

Baylin SB, Ohm JE (2006). Epigenetic gene silencing in cancer - a mechanism for early oncogenic pathway addiction? *Nat Rev Cancer,* 6(2):107-116.

Beland FA, Kadlubar FF (1985). Formation and persistence of arylamine DNA adducts in vivo. *Environ Health Perspect,* 62:19-30.

Belinsky SA, Nikula KJ, Palmisano WA, et al. (1998). Aberrant methylation of p16(INK4a) is an early event in lung cancer and a potential biomarker for early diagnosis. *Proc Natl Acad Sci USA,* 95(20):11891-11896.

Belinsky SA (2005). Silencing of genes by promoter hypermethylation: key event in rodent and human lung cancer. *Carcinogenesis,* 26(9):1481-1487.

Benowitz NL, FitzGerald GA, Wilson M, et al. (1993). Nicotine effects on eicosanoid formation and hemostatic function: comparison of transdermal nicotine and cigarette smoking. *J Am Coll Cardiol,* 22(4):1159-1167.

Benowitz NL, Gourlay SG (1997). Cardiovascular toxicity of nicotine: implications for nicotine replacement therapy. *J Am Coll Cardiol,* 29(7):1422-1431.

Berger P, Perng DW, Thabrew H, et al. (2001). Tryptase and agonists of PAR-2 induce the proliferation of human airway smooth muscle cells. *J Appl Physiol,* 91(3):1372-1379.

Bermudez EA, Rifai N, Buring JE, et al. (2002). Relation between markers of systemic vascular inflammation and smoking in women. *Am J Cardiol,* 89(9):1117-1119.

Black WC (2000). Overdiagnosis: An underrecognized cause of confusion and harm in cancer screening. *J Natl Cancer Inst,* 92(16):1280-1282.

Blankenberg S, Rupprecht HJ, Bickel C, et al. (2003). Glutathione peroxidase 1 activity and cardiovascular events in patients with coronary artery disease. *N Engl J Med,* 349(17):1605-1613.

Blann AD, Steele C, McCollum CN (1997). The influence of smoking on soluble adhesion molecules and endothelial cell markers. *Thromb Res,* 85(5):433-438.

Bolliger CT, Zellweger JP, Danielsson T, et al. (2002). Influence of long-term smoking reduction on health risk markers and quality of life. *Nicotine Tob Res,* 4(4):433-439.

Boots AW, Haenen GR, Bast A (2003). Oxidant metabolism in chronic obstructive pulmonary disease. *Eur Respir J,* 22 Suppl. 46:14s-27s.

Borissova AM, Tankova T, Kirilov G, et al. (2004). The effect of smoking on peripheral insulin sensitivity and plasma endothelin level. *Diabetes Metab,* 30(2):147-152.

Brazma A, Hingamp P, Quackenbush J, et al. (2001). Minimum information about a microarray experiment (MIAME)-toward standards for microarray data. *Nat Genet*, 29(4):365-371.

Brindicci C, Ito K, Resta O, et al. (2005). Exhaled nitric oxide from lung periphery is increased in COPD. *Eur Respir J*, 26(1):52-59.

Caballero OL, Cohen D, Liu Q, et al. (2001). Loss of chromosome arms 3p and 9p and inactivation of P16 (INK4a) in normal epithelium of patients with primary lung cancer. *Genes Chromosomes Cancer*, 32(2):119-125.

Cairns P, Mao L, Merlo A, et al. (1994). Rates of p16 (MTS1) mutations in primary tumors with 9p loss. *Science*, 265(5170):415-417.

Cairns P, Polascik TJ, Eby Y, et al. (1995). Frequency of homozygous deletion at p16/CDKN2 in primary human tumours. *Nat Genet*, 11(2):210-212.

Calverley PM, Burge PS, Spencer S, et al. (2003). Bronchodilator reversibility testing in chronic obstructive pulmonary disease. *Thorax*, 58(8):659-664.

Cantley LC (2002). The phosphoinositide 3-kinase pathway. *Science*, 296(5573):1655-1657.

Caramori G, Di Gregorio C, Carlstedt I, et al. (2004). Mucin expression in peripheral airways of patients with chronic obstructive pulmonary disease. *Histopathology*, 45(5):477-484.

Celermajer DS, Sorensen KE, Georgakopoulos D, et al. (1993). Cigarette smoking is associated with dose-related and potentially reversible impairment of endothelium-dependent dilation in healthy young adults. *Circulation*, 88(5 Pt 1):2149-2155.

Celli BR, Cote CG, Marin JM, et al. (2004). The body-mass index, airflow obstruction, dyspnea, and exercise capacity index in chronic obstructive pulmonary disease. *N Engl J Med*, 350(10):1005-1012.

Chan CK, Wells CK, McFarlane MJ, et al. (1989). More lung cancer but better survival. Implications of secular trends in ìnecropsy surpriseî rates. *Chest*, 96(2):291-296.

Chin L, Pomerantz J, DePinho RA (1998). The INK4a/ARF tumor suppressor: one geneótwo productsótwo pathways. *Trends Biochem Sci*, 23(8):291-296.

Cho Y, Gorina S, Jeffrey PD, et al. (1994). Crystal structure of a p53 tumor suppressor-DNA complex: understanding tumorigenic mutations. *Science*, 265(5170):346-355.

Chow CK, Thacker RR, Changchit C, et al. (1986). Lower levels of vitamin C and carotenes in plasma of cigarette smokers. *J Am Coll Nutr*, 5(3):305-312.

Chung GT, Sundaresan V, Hasleton P, et al. (1995). Sequential molecular genetic changes in lung cancer development. *Oncogene*, 11(12):2591-2598.

Church DF, Pryor WA (1985). Free-radical chemistry of cigarette smoke and its toxicological implications. *Environ Health Perspect*, 64:111-126.

Clouse WD, Yamaguchi H, Phillips MR, et al. (2000). Effects of transdermal nicotine treatment on structure and function of coronary artery bypass grafts. *J Appl Physiol*, 89(3):1213-1223.

Comhair SA, Erzurum SC (2002). Antioxidant responses to oxidant-mediated lung diseases. *Am J Physiol Lung Cell Mol Physiol*, 283(2):L246-L255.

Cosio MG, Majo J, Cosio MG (2002). Inflammation of the airways and lung parenchyma in COPD: role of T cells. *Chest*, 121(5 Suppl):160S-165S.

Creutzberg EC, Casaburi R (2003). Endocrinological disturbances in chronic obstructive pulmonary disease. *Eur Respir J*, 46:76s-80s.

Crooks SW, Bayley DL, Hill SL, et al. (2000). Bronchial inflammation in acute bacterial exacerbations of chronic bronchitis: the role of leukotriene B4. *Eur Respir J*, 15(2):274-280.

Dai MS, Lu H (2004). Inhibition of MDM2-mediated p53 ubiquitination and degradation by ribosomal protein L5. *J Biol Chem*, 279(43):44475-44482.

Dallas SL, Rosser JL, Mundy GR, et al. (2002). Proteolysis of latent transforming growth factor-beta (TGF-beta)-binding protein-1 by osteoclasts. A cellular mechanism for release of TGF-beta from bone matrix. *J Biol Chem*, 277(24):21352-21360.

Dammann R, Li C, Yoon JH, et al. (2000). Epigenetic inactivation of a RAS association domain family protein from the lung tumour suppressor locus 3p21.3. *Nat Genet*, 25(3):315-319.

Danesh J, Whincup P, Walker M, et al. (2001). Fibrin D-dimer and coronary heart disease: prospective study and meta-analysis. *Circulation*, 103(19):2323-2327.

David-Beabes GL, London SJ (2001). Genetic polymorphism of XRCC1 and lung cancer risk among African-Americans and Caucasians. *Lung Cancer*, 34(3):333-339.

de Boer WI, van Schadewijk A, Sont JK, et al. (1998). Transforming growth factor beta1 and recruitment of macrophages and mast cells in airways in chronic obstructive pulmonary disease. *Am J Respir Crit Care Med*, 158(6):1951-1957.

de Jong PA, Muller NL, Pare PD, et al. (2005). Computed tomographic imaging of the airways: relationship to structure and function. *Eur Respir J*, 26(1):140-152.

DeBias DA, Banerjee CM, Birkhead NC, et al. (1976). Effects of carbon monoxide inhalation on ventricular fibrillation. *Arch Environ Health*, 31(1):42-46.

Denissenko MF, Pao A, Tang M, et al. (1996). Preferential formation of benzo[a]pyrene adducts at lung cancer mutational hotspots in P53. *Science*, 274(5286):430-432.

Denissenko MF, Chen JX, Tang MS, et al. (1997). Cytosine methylation determines hot spots of DNA damage in the human P53 gene. *Proc Natl Acad Sci USA*, 94(8):3893-3898.

Dennis RJ, Maldonado D, Norman S, et al. (1996). Wood smoke exposure and risk for obstructive airways disease among women. *Chest*, 109(3 Suppl):55S-56S.

Di Stefano A, Caramori G, Ricciardolo FL, et al. (2004). Cellular and molecular mechanisms in chronic obstructive pulmonary disease: an overview. *Clin Exp Allergy*, 34(8):1156-1167.

Duthie GG, Wahle KJ (1990). Smoking, antioxidants, essential fatty acids and coronary heart disease. *Biochem Soc Trans*, 18(6):1051-1054.

Duxbury MS, Ito H, Benoit E, et al. (2004). CEACAM6 is a determinant of pancreatic adenocarcinoma cellular invasiveness. *Br J Cancer*, 91(7): 1384-1390.

Effros RM, Su J, Casaburi R, et al. (2005). Utility of exhaled breath condensates in chronic obstructive pulmonary disease: a critical review. *Curr Opin Pulm Med*, 11(2):135-139.

Eliasson B, Hjalmarson A, Kruse E, et al. (2001). Effect of smoking reduction and cessation on cardiovascular risk factors. *Nicotine Tob Res*, 3(3):249-255.

Ezzati M, Henley SJ, Lopez AD, et al. (2005). Role of smoking in global and regional cancer epidemiology: current patterns and data needs. *Int J Cancer*, 116(6):963-971.

Falati S, Gross P, Merrill-Skoloff G, et al. (2002). Real-time in vivo imaging of platelets, tissue factor and fibrin during arterial thrombus formation in the mouse. *Nat Med*, 8(10):1175-1181.

Fibrinogen Studies Collaboration (2004). Collaborative meta-analysis of prospective studies of plasma fibrinogen and cardiovascular disease. *Eur J Cardiovasc Prev Rehabil*, 11(1):9-17.

FitzGerald GA, Oates JA, Nowak J (1988). Cigarette smoking and hemostatic function. *Am Heart J*, 115(1 Pt 2):267-271.

Flavahan NA (1992). Atherosclerosis or lipoprotein-induced endothelial dysfunction. Potential mechanisms underlying reduction in EDRF/nitric oxide activity. *Circulation*, 85(5):1927-1938.

Fong KM, Biesterveld EJ, Virmani A, et al. (1997). FHIT and FRA3B 3p14.2 allele loss are common in lung cancer and preneoplastic bronchial lesions and are associated with cancer-related FHIT cDNA splicing aberrations. *Cancer Res*, 57(11):2256-2267.

Fontana RS, Sanderson DR, Woolner LB, et al. (1991). Screening for lung cancer. A critique of the Mayo Lung Project. *Cancer*, 67(4 Suppl.):1155-1164.

Foulds L (1954). The experimental study of tumor progression: a review. *Cancer Res*, 14(5):327-339.

Frei B, Forte TM, Ames BN, et al. (1991). Gas phase oxidants of cigarette smoke induce lipid peroxidation and changes in lipoprotein properties in human blood plasma. Protective effects of ascorbic acid. *Biochem J*, 277 (Pt 1):133-138.

Frohlich M, Sund M, Lowel H, et al. (2003). Independent association of various smoking characteristics with markers of systemic inflammation in men. Results from a representative sample of the general population (MONICA Augsburg Survey 1994/95). *Eur Heart J*, 24(14):1365-1372.

Gan WQ, Man SF, Senthilselvan A, et al. (2004). Association between chronic obstructive pulmonary disease and systemic inflammation: a systematic review and a meta-analysis. *Thorax*, 59(7):574-580.

Gan WQ, Man SF, Sin DD (2005). The interactions between cigarette smoking and reduced lung function on systemic inflammation. *Chest*, 127(2): 558-564.

Gealy R, Zhang L, Siegfried JM, et al. (1999). Comparison of mutations in the p53 and K-ras genes in lung carcinomas from smoking and nonsmoking women. *Cancer Epidemiol Biomarkers Prev*, 8(4 Pt 1):297-302.

Gilmour PS, Rahman I, Hayashi S, et al. (2001). Adenoviral E1A primes alveolar epithelial cells to PM(10)-induced transcription of interleukin-8. *Am J Physiol Lung Cell Mol Physiol*, 281(3):L598-L606.

Goldin JG (2004). Quantitative CT of emphysema and the airways. *J Thorac Imaging*, 19(4):235-240.

Gorgoulis VG, Vassiliou LV, Karakaidos P, et al. (2005). Activation of the DNA damage checkpoint and genomic instability in human precancerous lesions. *Nature*, 434(7035):907-913.

Greenblatt MS, Bennett WP, Hollstein M, et al. (1994). Mutations in the p53 tumor suppressor gene: clues to cancer etiology and molecular pathogenesis. *Cancer Res*, 54(18):4855-4878.

Guengerich FP, Johnson WW (1997). Kinetics of ferric cytochrome P450 reduction by NADPH-cytochrome P450 reductase: rapid reduction in the absence of substrate and variations among cytochrome P450 systems. *Biochemistry*, 36(48):14741-14750.

Hainaut P, Pfeifer GP (2001). Patterns of p53 G̀ó>T transversions in lung cancers reflect the primary mutagenic signature of DNA-damage by tobacco smoke. *Carcinogenesis*, 22(3):367-374.

Hanahan D, Weinberg RA (2000). The hallmarks of cancer. *Cell*, 100(1):57-70.

Hanawalt PC (2001). Controlling the efficiency of excision repair. *Mutat Res*, 485(1):3-13.

Hansel TT, Barnes PJ (2004). *An Atlas of Chronic Obstructive Pulmonary Disease*. London, The Parthenon Publishing Group Inc.

Hatsukami DK, Kotlyar M, Allen S, et al. (2005). Effects of cigarette reduction on cardiovascular risk factors and subjective measures. *Chest*, 128(4): 2528-2537.

Hecht SS, Peterson LA, Spratt TE (1994). Tobacco-specific nitrosamines. In: Hemminki K, Dipple A, Shuker DEG, et al., eds., *DNA Adducts: Identification and Biological Significance*. IARC Scientific Publications No. 125: 91-106.

Hecht SS (1999a). DNA adduct formation from tobacco-specific N-nitrosamines. *Mutat Res*, 424(1-2):127-142.

Hecht SS (1999b). Tobacco smoke carcinogens and lung cancer. *J Natl Cancer Inst*, 91(14):1194-1210.

Hemker HC, Beguin S (2000). Phenotyping the clotting system. *Thromb Haemost*, 84(5):747-751.

Henschke CI, McCauley DI, Yankelevitz DF, et al. (1999). Early Lung Cancer Action Project: overall design and findings from baseline screening. *Lancet*, 354(9173):99-105.

Herbert WH (1975). Cigarette smoking and arteriographically demonstrable coronary artery disease. *Chest*, 67(1):49-52.

Herman JG, Merlo A, Mao L, et al. (1995). Inactivation of the CDKN2/p16/MTS1 gene is frequently associated with aberrant DNA methylation in all common human cancers. *Cancer Res*, 55(20):4525-4530.

Hernandez-Boussard TM, Hainaut P (1998). A specific spectrum of p53 mutations in lung cancer from smokers: review of mutations compiled in the IARC p53 database. *Environ Health Perspect*, 106(7):385-391.

Hill AT, Bayley D, Stockley RA (1999). The interrelationship of sputum inflammatory markers in patients with chronic bronchitis. *Am J Respir Crit Care Med*, 160(3):893-898.

Hill C, Van Beek E.J.R. (2004). MRI of the chest: present and future. *Imaging*, 16:61-70.

Hioki H, Aoki N, Kawano K, et al. (2001). Acute effects of cigarette smoking on platelet-dependent thrombin generation. *Eur Heart J*, 22(1):56-61.

Hirai Y, Adachi H, Fujiura Y, et al. (2004). Plasma endothelin-1 level is related to renal function and smoking status but not to blood pressure: an epidemiological study. *J Hypertens*, 22(4):713-718.

Hoffmann D, Hecht SS (1985). Nicotine-derived N-nitrosamines and tobacco-related cancer: current status and future directions. *Cancer Res*, 45(3):935-944.

Hoffmann D, Hecht SS (1990). Advances in Tobacco Carcinogenesis. In: Cooper CS, Grover PL, eds., *Chemical Carcinogenesis and Mutagenesis I. Handbook of experimental pharmacology; v.94.* Berlin, 63-102.

Hoffmann D, Hoffmann I, El Bayoumy K (2001). The less harmful cigarette: a controversial issue. a tribute to Ernst L. Wynder. *Chem Res Toxicol*, 14(7):767-790.

Hogg JC, Chu F, Utokaparch S, et al. (2004). The nature of small-airway obstruction in chronic obstructive pulmonary disease. *N Engl J Med*, 350(26):2645-2653.

Hogg JC (2006). Why does airway inflammation persist after the smoking stops? *Thorax*, 61(2):96-97.

Horvath I, Hunt J, Barnes PJ, et al. (2005). Exhaled breath condensate: methodological recommendations and unresolved questions. *Eur Respir J*, 26(3):523-548.

Hung J, Lam JY, Lacoste L, et al. (1995). Cigarette smoking acutely increases platelet thrombus formation in patients with coronary artery disease taking aspirin. *Circulation*, 92(9):2432-2436.

Husgafvel-Pursiainen K, Hackman P, Ridanpaa M, et al. (1993). K-ras mutations in human adenocarcinoma of the lung: association with smoking and occupational exposure to asbestos. *Int J Cancer*, 53(2):250-256.

Hussain SP, Amstad P, Raja K, et al. (2001). Mutability of p53 hotspot codons to benzo(a)pyrene diol epoxide (BPDE) and the frequency of p53 mutations in nontumorous human lung. *Cancer Res*, 61(17):6350-6355.

IARC (1972). *IARC Monographs on the Evaluation of Carcinogenic Risk of Chemicals to Man, Vol. 1, Some Inorganic Substances , Chlorinated Hydrocarbons, Aromatic Amines, N-Nitroso Compounds, and Natural Products.* Lyon, IARCPress

IARC (1978). *IARC Monographs on the Evaluation of the Carcinogenic Risk of Chemicals to Humans, Vol. 17, Some N-Nitroso Compounds.* Lyon, IARC Press.

IARC (1983). *IARC Monographs on the Evaluation of the Carcinogenic Risk of Chemicals to Humans, Vol.32, Polynuclear Aromatic Compounds, Part 1: Chemical, Environmental and Experimental Data.* Lyon, IARCPress.

IARC (1985). *IARC Monographs on the Evaluation of the Carcinogenic Risk of Chemicals to Humans, Vol. 37, Tobacco Habits Other than Smoking; Betel-Quid and Areca-Nut Chewing; and Some Related Nitrosamines.* Lyon, IARCPress.

IARC (1986). *IARC Monographs on the Evaluation of the Carcinogenic Risk of Chemicals to Humans, Vol. 38, Tobacco smoking.* Lyon, IARCPress.

IARC (1987). *IARC Monographs on the Evaluation of Carcinogenic Risks to Humans, Suppl. 7, Overall Evaluations of Carcinogenicity: An Updating of IARC Monographs Volumes 1 to 42.* Lyon, IARCPress.

IARC (1994). *IARC Monographs on the Evaluation of Carcinogenic Risks to Humans, Vol. 60, Some Industrial Chemicals.* Lyon, IARCPress.

IARC (2004). *IARC Monographs on the Evaluation of Carcinogenic Risks to Humans, Vol. 83, Tobacco Smoke and Involuntary Smoking.* Lyon, IARCPress.

Ichinose A (2001). Physiopathology and regulation of factor XIII. *Thromb Haemost*, 86(1):57-65.

Inaba T, Roberts WM, Shapiro LH, et al. (1992). Fusion of the leucine zipper gene HLF to the E2A gene in human acute B-lineage leukemia. *Science*, 257(5069):531-534.

Inoue T, Oku K, Kimoto K, et al. (1995). Relationship of cigarette smoking to the severity of coronary and thoracic aortic atherosclerosis. *Cardiology*, 86(5):374-379.

Ito H, Matsuo K, Hamajima N, et al. (2004). Gene-environment interactions between the smoking habit and polymorphisms in the DNA repair genes, APE1 Asp148Glu and XRCC1 Arg399Gln, in Japanese lung cancer risk. *Carcinogenesis*, 25(8):1395-1401.

Ito K, Barnes PJ, Adcock IM (2000). Glucocorticoid receptor recruitment of histone deacetylase 2 inhibits interleukin-1beta-induced histone H4 acetylation on lysines 8 and 12. *Mol Cell Biol*, 20(18):6891-6903.

Ito K, Lim S, Caramori G, et al. (2001). Cigarette smoking reduces histone deacetylase 2 expression, enhances cytokine expression, and inhibits glucocorticoid actions in alveolar macrophages. *FASEB J*, 15(6):1110-1112.

Jackson SP, Nesbitt WS, Kulkarni S (2003). Signaling events underlying thrombus formation. *J Thromb Haemost*, 1(7):1602-1612.

Jantscheff P, Terracciano L, Lowy A, et al. (2003). Expression of CEACAM6 in resectable colorectal cancer: a factor of independent prognostic significance. *J Clin Oncol*, 21(19):3638-3646.

Jensen EJ, Pedersen B, Schmidt E, et al. (1992). Serum IgE in nonatopic smokers, nonsmokers, and recent exsmokers: relation to lung function, airway symptoms, and atopic predisposition. *J Allergy Clin Immunol*, 90(2):224-229.

Jensen EJ, Pedersen B, Frederiksen R, et al. (1998). Prospective study on the effect of smoking and nicotine substitution on leucocyte blood counts and relation between blood leucocytes and lung function. *Thorax*, 53(9):784-789.

Jones HA, Marino PS, Shakur BH, et al. (2003). In vivo assessment of lung inflammatory cell activity in patients with COPD and asthma. *Eur Respir J*, 21(4):567-573.

Jones PA, Laird PW (1999). Cancer epigenetics comes of age. *Nat Genet*, 21(2):163-167.

Kadlubar FF (1994). DNA Adducts of carcinogenic aromatic amines. In: Hemminki K, Dipple A, Shuker DEG, et al., eds., *DNA Adducts, identification and Biological Significance.* IARC Scientific Publications No. 125: 199-216.

Kamath S, Lip GY (2003). Fibrinogen: biochemistry, epidemiology and determinants. *QJM*, 96(10):711-729.

Kannel WB, DiAgostino RB, Belanger AJ (1987). Fibrinogen, cigarette smoking, and risk of cardiovascular disease: insights from the Framingham Study. *Am Heart J*, 113(4):1006-1010.

Kannel WB (2005). Overview of hemostatic factors involved in atherosclerotic cardiovascular disease. *Lipids*, 40(12): 1215-1220.

Keatings VM, Collins PD, Scott DM, et al. (1996). Differences in interleukin-8 and tumor necrosis factor-alpha in induced sputum from patients with chronic obstructive pulmonary disease or asthma. *Am J Respir Crit Care Med*, 153(2):530-534.

Keatings VM, Barnes PJ (1997). Granulocyte activation markers in induced sputum: comparison between chronic obstructive pulmonary disease, asthma, and normal subjects. *Am J Respir Crit Care Med*, 155(2):449-453.

Killary AM, Wolf ME, Giambernardi TA, et al. (1992). Definition of a tumor suppressor locus within human chromosome 3p21-p22. *Proc Natl Acad Sci USA*, 89(22):10877-10881.

Kondo T, Hayashi M, Takeshita K, et al. (2004). Smoking cessation rapidly increases circulating progenitor cells in peripheral blood in chronic smokers. *Arterioscler Thromb Vasc Biol*, 24(8):1442-1447.

Kranenburg AR, de Boer WI, van Krieken JH, et al. (2002). Enhanced expression of fibroblast growth factors and receptor FGFR-1 during vascular remodeling in chronic obstructive pulmonary disease. *Am J Respir Cell Mol Biol*, 27(5):517-525.

Laghi F, Antonescu-Turcu A, Collins E, et al. (2005). Hypogonadism in men with chronic obstructive pulmonary disease: prevalence and quality of life. *Am J Respir Crit Care Med*, 171(7):728-733.

Laird PW, Jaenisch R (1996). The role of DNA methylation in cancer genetic and epigenetics. *Annu Rev Genet*, 30:441-464.

Lange P, Nyboe J, Appleyard M, et al. (1992). Relationship of the type of tobacco and inhalation pattern to pulmonary and total mortality. *Eur Respir J*, 5(9):1111-1117.

Lapperre TS, Postma DS, Gosman MM, et al. (2006). Relation between duration of smoking cessation and bronchial inflammation in COPD. *Thorax*, 61: 115-121.

Law MR (1990). Genetic predisposition to lung cancer. *Br J Cancer*, 61(2):195-206.

Law MR, Wald NJ (2003). Environmental tobacco smoke and ischemic heart disease. *Prog Cardiovasc Dis*, 46(1):31-38.

Le Calvez F, Mukeria A, Hunt JD, et al. (2005). TP53 and KRAS mutation load and types in lung cancers in relation to tobacco smoke: distinct patterns in never, former, and current smokers. *Cancer Res*, 65(12):5076-5083.

LeBrun DP (2003). E2A basic helix-loop-helix transcription factors in human leukemia. *Front Biosci*, 8:s206-s222.

Lee AJ, Fowkes FG, Lowe GD, et al. (1995). Fibrin D-dimer, haemostatic factors and peripheral arterial disease. *Thromb Haemost*, 74(3):828-832.

Lee DW, Zhao X, Zhang F, et al. (2005). Depletion of GAK/auxilin 2 inhibits receptor-mediated endocytosis and recruitment of both clathrin and clathrin adaptors. *J Cell Sci*, 118(Pt 18):4311-4321.

Leeson CP, Hingorani AD, Mullen MJ, et al. (2002). Glu298Asp endothelial nitric oxide synthase gene polymorphism interacts with environmental and dietary factors to influence endothelial function. *Circ Res*, 90(11):1153-1158.

Lekakis J, Papamichael C, Vemmos C, et al. (1998). Effects of acute cigarette smoking on endothelium-dependent arterial dilatation in normal subjects. *Am J Cardiol*, 81(10):1225-1228.

Levine AJ (1997). p53, the cellular gatekeeper for growth and division. *Cell*, 88(3):323-331.

Li Z, Barrios V, Buchholz JN, et al. (1994). Chronic nicotine administration does not affect peripheral vascular reactivity in the rat. *J Pharmacol Exp Ther*, 271(3):1135-1142.

Liang G, Xing D, Miao X, et al. (2003). Sequence variations in the DNA repair gene XPD and risk of lung cancer in a Chinese population. *Int J Cancer*, 105(5):669-673.

Libby P (2002). Inflammation in atherosclerosis. *Nature*, 420(6917):868-874.

Lind P, Engstrom G, Stavenow L, et al. (2004). Risk of myocardial infarction and stroke in smokers is related to plasma levels of inflammation-sensitive proteins. *Arterioscler Thromb Vasc Biol*, 24(3):577-582.

Lonn EM, Yusuf S (1997). Is there a role for antioxidant vitamins in the prevention of cardiovascular diseases? An update on epidemiological and clinical trials data. *Can J Cardiol*, 13(10):957-965.

Ludvig J, Miner B, Eisenberg MJ (2005). Smoking cessation in patients with coronary artery disease. *Am Heart J*, 149(4):565-572.

MacCallum PK (2005). Markers of hemostasis and systemic inflammation in heart disease and atherosclerosis in smokers. *Proc Am Thorac Soc*, 2(1):34-43.

MacNee W (2000). Oxidants/antioxidants and COPD. *Chest*, 117(5 Suppl 1): 303S-317S.

MacNee W, Rahman I (2001). Is oxidative stress central to the pathogenesis of chronic obstructive pulmonary disease? *Trends Mol Med*, 7(2):55-62.

Malarcher AM, Schulman J, Epstein LA, et al. (2000). Methodological issues in estimating smoking-attributable mortality in the United States. *Am J Epidemiol*, 152(6):573-584.

Mann KG, Brummel K, Butenas S (2003). What is all that thrombin for? *J Thromb Haemost*, 1(7):1504-1514.

Mao L, Merlo A, Bedi G, et al. (1995). A novel p16INK4A transcript. *Cancer Res*, 55(14):2995-2997.

Marcus PM, Bergstralh EJ, Fagerstrom RM, et al. (2000). Lung cancer mortality in the Mayo Lung Project: impact of extended follow-up. *J Natl Cancer Inst*, 92(16):1308-1316.

Marshall CJ, Vousden KH, Phillips DH (1984). Activation of c-Ha-ras-1 proto-oncogene by in vitro modification with a chemical carcinogen, benzo(a)-pyrene diol-epoxide. *Nature*, 310 (5978): 586-589.

Martey CA, Pollock SJ, Turner CK, et al. (2004). Cigarette smoke induces cyclooxygenase-2 and microsomal prostaglandin E2 synthase in human lung fibroblasts: implications for lung inflammation and cancer. *Am J Physiol Lung Cell Mol Physiol*, 287(5):L981-L991.

Martin JF, Bath PM, Burr ML (1991). Influence of platelet size on outcome after myocardial infarction. *Lancet*, 338(8780):1409-1411.

Matetzky S, Tani S, Kangavari S, et al. (2000). Smoking increases tissue factor expression in atherosclerotic plaques: implications for plaque thrombogenicity. *Circulation*, 102(6): 602-604.

Mayhan WG, Sharpe GM (1999). Chronic exposure to nicotine alters endothelium-dependent arteriolar dilatation: effect of superoxide dismutase. *J Appl Physiol*, 86(4):1126-1134.

Meade TW, Mellows S, Brozovic M, et al. (1986). Haemostatic function and ischaemic heart disease: principal results of the Northwick Park Heart Study. *Lancet*, 2(8506):533-537.

Medical Research Council (1965). Definition and classification of chronic bronchitis for clinical and epidemiological purposes. A report to the Medical Research Council by their Committee on the Aetiology of Chronic Bronchitis. *Lancet*, 1(7389):775-779.

Meliska CJ, Stunkard ME, Gilbert DG, et al. (1995). Immune function in cigarette smokers who quit smoking for 31 days. *J Allergy Clin Immunol*, 95(4):901-910.

Memisoglu A, Samson L (2000). Base excision repair in yeast and mammals. *Mutat Res*, 451(1-2):39-51.

Merlo A, Herman JG, Mao L, et al. (1995). 5í CpG island methylation is associated with transcriptional silencing of the tumour suppressor p16/CDKN2/MTS1 in human cancers. *Nat Med*, 1(7):686-692.

Meshi B, Vitalis TZ, Ionescu D, et al. (2002). Emphysematous lung destruction by cigarette smoke. The effects of latent adenoviral infection on the lung inflammatory response. *Am J Respir Cell Mol Biol*, 26(1):52-57.

Miotto D, Hollenberg MD, Bunnett NW, et al. (2002). Expression of protease activated receptor-2 (PAR-2) in central airways of smokers and non-smokers. *Thorax*, 57(2):146-151.

Monroe DM, Hoffman M (2002). Coagulation factor interaction with platelets. *Thromb Haemost*, 88(2): 179.

Montuschi P, Collins JV, Ciabattoni G, et al. (2000). Exhaled 8-isoprostane as an in vivo biomarker of lung oxidative stress in patients with COPD and healthy smokers. *Am J Respir Crit Care Med*, 162(3 Pt 1):1175-1177.

Montuschi P, Kharitonov SA, Barnes PJ (2001). Exhaled carbon monoxide and nitric oxide in COPD. *Chest*, 120(2):496-501.

Mooney LA, Santella RM, Covey L, et al. (1995). Decline of DNA damage and other biomarkers in peripheral blood following smoking cessation. *Cancer Epidemiol Biomarkers Prev*, 4(6):627-634.

Moreno H, Jr., Chalon S, Urae A, et al. (1998). Endothelial dysfunction in human hand veins is rapidly reversible after smoking cessation. *Am J Physiol*, 275(3 Pt 2):H1040-H1045.

Morita H, Ikeda H, Haramaki N, et al. (2005). Only two-week smoking cessation improves platelet aggregability and intraplatelet redox imbalance of long-term smokers. *J Am Coll Cardiol*, 45(4):589-594.

Muda M, Manning ER, Orth K, et al. (1999). Identification of the human YVH1 protein-tyrosine phosphatase orthologue reveals a novel zinc binding domain essential for in vivo function. *J Biol Chem*, 274(34):23991-23995.

Mukherjee S, Woods L, Weston Z, et al. (1993). The effect of mainstream and sidestream cigarette smoke exposure on oxygen defense mechanisms of guinea pig erythrocytes. *J Biochem Toxicol*, 8(3):119-125.

Newby DE, Wright RA, Labinjoh C, et al. (1999). Endothelial dysfunction, impaired endogenous fibrinolysis, and cigarette smoking: a mechanism for arterial thrombosis and myocardial infarction. *Circulation*, 99(11):1411-1415.

Newby DE, McLeod AL, Uren NG, et al. (2001). Impaired coronary tissue plasminogen activator release is associated with coronary atherosclerosis and cigarette smoking: direct link between endothelial dysfunction and athero-thrombosis. *Circulation*, 103(15): 1936-1941.

Newell JD, Jr., Hogg JC, Snider GL (2004). Report of a workshop: quantitative computed tomography scanning in longitudinal studies of emphysema. *Eur Respir J*, 23(5):769-775.

NIH/NHLBI/WHO (2003). Global Initiative for Chronic Obstructive Lung Disease (GOLD): Global Strategy for the Diagnosis, Management, and Prevention of Chronic Obstructive Pulmonary Disease. p. 1-111.

Nishio E, Watanabe Y (1997). Cigarette smoke extract inhibits plasma paraoxonase activity by modification of the enzymeís free thiols. *Biochem Biophys Res Commun*, 236(2):289-293.

Norbury CJ, Hickson ID (2001). Cellular responses to DNA damage. *Annu Rev Pharmacol Toxicol*, 41:367-401.

Nowak J, Murray JJ, Oates JA, et al. (1987). Biochemical evidence of a chronic abnormality in platelet and vascular function in healthy individuals who smoke cigarettes. *Circulation*, 76(1):6-14.

Ohara Y, Peterson TE, Harrison DG (1993). Hypercholesterolemia increases endothelial superoxide anion production. *J Clin Invest*, 91(6):2546-2551.

Olivier M, Eeles R, Hollstein M, et al. (2002). The IARC TP53 database: new online mutation analysis and recommendations to users. *Hum Mutat*, 19(6):607-614.

Oswald F, Kostezka U, Astrahantseff K, et al. (2002). SHARP is a novel component of the Notch/RBP-Jkappa signalling pathway. *EMBO J*, 21(20):5417-5426.

Pallares-Trujillo J, Agell N, Garcia-Martinez C, et al. (1997). The ubiquitin system: a role in disease? *Med Res Rev*, 17(2):139-161.

Pastorino U, Bellomi M, Landoni C, et al. (2003). Early lung-cancer detection with spiral CT and positron emission tomography in heavy smokers: 2-year results. *Lancet*, 362(9384):593-597.

Pauwels RA, Buist AS, Calverley PM, et al. (2001). Global strategy for the diagnosis, management, and prevention of chronic obstructive pulmonary disease. NHLBI/WHO Global Initiative for Chronic Obstructive Lung Disease (GOLD) Workshop summary. *Am J Respir Crit Care Med*, 163(5):1256-1276.

Pech-Amsellem MA, Myara I, Storogenko M, et al. (1996). Enhanced modifications of low-density lipoproteins (LDL) by endothelial cells from smokers: a possible mechanism of smoking-related atherosclerosis. *Cardiovasc Res*, 31(6):975-983.

Pegg AE (2000). Repair of O(6)-alkylguanine by alkyltransferases. *Mutat Res*, 462(2-3):83-100.

Pelkonen M, Notkola IL, Tukiainen H, et al. (2001). Smoking cessation, decline in pulmonary function and total mortality: a 30 year follow up study among the Finnish cohorts of the Seven Countries Study. *Thorax*, 56(9):703-707.

Pernerstorfer T, Stohlawetz P, Stummvoll G, et al. (1998). Low-dose aspirin does not lower in vivo platelet activation in healthy smokers. *Br J Haematol*, 102(5):1229-1231.

Peto R, Darby S, Deo H, et al. (2000). Smoking, smoking cessation, and lung cancer in the UK since 1950: combination of national statistics with two case-control studies. *BMJ*, 321(7257): 323-329.

Pfeifer GP, Denissenko MF, Olivier M, et al. (2002). Tobacco smoke carcinogens, DNA damage and p53 mutations in smoking-associated cancers. *Oncogene*, 21(48):7435-7451.

Pigula FA, Keenan RJ, Ferson PF, et al. (1996). Unsuspected lung cancer found in work-up for lung reduction operation. *Ann Thorac Surg*, 61(1):174-176.

Polidori MC, Mecocci P, Stahl W, et al. (2003). Cigarette smoking cessation increases plasma levels of several antioxidant micronutrients and improves resistance towards oxidative challenge. *Br J Nutr*, 90(1):147-150.

Puranik R, Celermajer DS (2003). Smoking and endothelial function. *Prog Cardiovasc Dis*, 45(6):443-458.

Qian J, Yang J, Zhang X, et al. (2001). Isolation and characterization of a novel cDNA, UBAP1, derived from the tumor suppressor locus in human chromosome 9p21-22. *J Cancer Res Clin Oncol*, 127(10):613-618.

Quillen JE, Rossen JD, Oskarsson HJ, et al. (1993). Acute effect of cigarette smoking on the coronary circulation: constriction of epicardial and resistance vessels. *J Am Coll Cardiol*, 22(3):642-647.

Raitakari OT, Adams MR, McCredie RJ, et al. (1999). Arterial endothelial dysfunction related to passive smoking is potentially reversible in healthy young adults. *Ann Intern Med*, 130(7):578-581.

Ramsdale DR, Faragher EB, Bray CL, et al. (1985). Smoking and coronary artery disease assessed by routine coronary arteriography. *Br Med J*, 290(6463):197-200.

Reik W, Dean W, Walter J (2001). Epigenetic reprogramming in mammalian development. *Science*, 293(5532):1089-1093.

Reiley W, Zhang M, Sun SC (2004). Negative regulation of JNK signaling by the tumor suppressor CYLD. *J Biol Chem*, 279(53):55161-55167.

Renan MJ (1993). How many mutations are required for tumorigenesis? Implications from human cancer data. *Mol Carcinog*, 7(3):139-146.

Repine JE, Bast A, Lankhorst I (1997). Oxidative stress in chronic obstructive pulmonary disease. Oxidative Stress Study Group. *Am J Respir Crit Care Med*, 156(2 Pt 1):341-357.

Ridker PM, Hennekens CH, Roitman-Johnson B, et al. (1998). Plasma concentration of soluble intercellular adhesion molecule 1 and risks of future myocardial infarction in apparently healthy men. *Lancet*, 351(9096):88-92.

Robbins RA, Millatmal T, Lassi K, et al. (1997). Smoking cessation is associated with an increase in exhaled nitric oxide. *Chest*, 112(2):313-318.

Robinson MJ, Cobb MH (1997). Mitogen-activated protein kinase pathways. *Curr Opin Cell Biol*, 9(2):180-186.

Ruggeri ZM (2003). Von Willebrand factor, platelets and endothelial cell interactions. *J Thromb Haemost*, 1(7): 1335-1342.

Saccomanno G, Archer VE, Auerbach O, et al. (1974). Development of carcinoma of the lung as reflected in exfoliated cells. *Cancer*, 33(1):256-270.

Salman GF, Mosier MC, Beasley BW, et al. (2003). Rehabilitation for patients with chronic obstructive pulmonary disease: meta-analysis of randomized controlled trials. *J Gen Intern Med*, 18(3):213-221.

Sambola A, Osende J, Hathcock J, et al. (2003). Role of risk factors in the modulation of tissue factor activity and blood thrombogenicity. *Circulation*, 107(7):973-977.

Satterwhite E, Sonoki T, Willis TG, et al. (2001). The BCL11 gene family: involvement of BCL11A in lymphoid malignancies. *Blood*, 98(12):3413-3420.

Schabath MB, Wu X, Wei Q, et al. (2006). Combined effects of the p53 and p73 polymorphisms on lung cancer risk. *Cancer Epidemiol Biomarkers Prev*, 15(1):158-161.

Schectman G, Byrd JC, Gruchow HW (1989). The influence of smoking on vitamin C status in adults. *Am J Public Health*, 79(2):158-162.

Schlessinger J, Schreiber AB, Levi A, et al. (1983). Regulation of cell proliferation by epidermal growth factor. *CRC Crit Rev Biochem*, 14(2):93-111.

Schlessinger J (2000). Cell signaling by receptor tyrosine kinases. *Cell*, 103(2):211-225.

Schols AM, Slangen J, Volovics L, et al. (1998). Weight loss is a reversible factor in the prognosis of chronic obstructive pulmonary disease. *Am J Respir Crit Care Med*, 157(6 Pt 1):1791-1797.

Scott J (2004). Pathophysiology and biochemistry of cardiovascular disease. *Curr Opin Genet Dev*, 14(3):271-279.

Senawong T, Peterson VJ, Leid M (2005). BCL11A-dependent recruitment of SIRT1 to a promoter template in mammalian cells results in histone deacetylation and transcriptional repression. *Arch Biochem Biophys* , 434(2):316-325.

Shah V, Sridhar S, Beane J, et al. (2005). SIEGE: Smoking Induced Epithelial Gene Expression Database. *Nucleic Acids Res*, 33(Database issue):D573-D579.

Shaker SB, Maltbaek N, Brand P, et al. (2005). Quantitative computed tomography and aerosol morphometry in COPD and alpha1-antitrypsin deficiency. *Eur Respir J*, 25(1):23-30.

Shapiro GI, Park JE, Edwards CD, et al. (1995). Multiple mechanisms of p16INK4A inactivation in non-small cell lung cancer cell lines. *Cancer Res*, 55(24):6200-6209.

Shapiro SD (1994). Elastolytic metalloproteinases produced by human mononuclear phagocytes. Potential roles in destructive lung disease. *Am J Respir Crit Care Med*, 150(6 Pt 2):S160-S164.

Shapiro SD, Ingenito EP (2005). The pathogenesis of chronic obstructive pulmonary disease: advances in the past 100 years. *Am J Respir Cell Mol Biol*, 32(5):367-372.

Shields PG (1999). Molecular epidemiology of lung cancer. *Ann Oncol*, 10 Suppl 5:S7-11.

Shuker DE, Bartsch H (1994). DNA adducts of nitrosamines. In: Hemminki K, Dipple A, Shuker DE, et al., eds., *DNA Adducts: Identification and Biological Significance*. IARC Scientific Publications No. 125: 73-89.

Simmons MS, Connett JE, Nides MA, et al. (2005). Smoking reduction and the rate of decline in FEV(1): results from the Lung Health Study. *Eur Respir J*, 25(6):1011-1017.

Simpson AJ, Gray RS, Moore NR, et al. (1997). The effects of chronic smoking on the fibrinolytic potential of plasma and platelets. *Br J Haematol*, 97(1):208-213.

Sin DD, Man SF (2003). Why are patients with chronic obstructive pulmonary disease at increased risk of cardiovascular diseases? The potential role of systemic inflammation in chronic obstructive pulmonary disease. *Circulation*, 107(11):1514-1519.

Skold CM, Hed J, Eklund A (1992). Smoking cessation rapidly reduces cell recovery in bronchoalveolar lavage fluid, while alveolar macrophage fluorescence remains high. *Chest*, 101(4):989-995.

Skold CM, Forslid J, Eklund A, et al. (1993). Metabolic activity in human alveolar macrophages increases after cessation of smoking. *Inflammation*, 17(3):345-352.

Skold CM, Blaschke E, Eklund A (1996). Transient increases in albumin and hyaluronan in bronchoalveolar lavage fluid after quitting smoking: possible signs of reparative mechanisms. *Respir Med*, 90(9):523-529.

Slaughter DP, Southwick HW, Smejkal W (1953). Field cancerization in oral stratified squamous epithelium; clinical implications of multicentric origin. *Cancer*, 6(5):963-968.

Slebos RJ, Hruban RH, Dalesio O, et al. (1991). Relationship between K-ras oncogene activation and smoking in adenocarcinoma of the human lung. *J Natl Cancer Inst*, 83(14):1024-1027.

Smith LE, Denissenko MF, Bennett WP, et al. (2000). Targeting of lung cancer mutational hotspots by polycyclic aromatic hydrocarbons. *J Natl Cancer Inst*, 92(10):803-811.

Smith MR, Kinmonth AL, Luben RN, et al. (2003). Smoking status and differential white cell count in men and women in the EPIC-Norfolk population. *Atherosclerosis*, 169(2):331-337.

Snider GL (2003). Nosology for our day: its application to chronic obstructive pulmonary disease. *Am J Respir Crit Care Med*, 167(5):678-683.

Sozzi G, Pastorino U, Moiraghi L, et al. (1998). Loss of FHIT function in lung cancer and preinvasive bronchial lesions. *Cancer Res*, 58(22):5032-5037.

Sozzi G, Andriani F, Roz L, et al. (2006). Lung carcinogenesis: biology. In: Hirsch FR, Bunn PA, Jr., Kato H, et al., eds., *Textbook of Prevention and Detection of Early Lung Cancer*. Taylor & Francis: 91-116.

Spira A, Beane J, Shah V, et al. (2004). Effects of cigarette smoke on the human airway epithelial cell transcriptome. *Proc Natl Acad Sci USA*, 101(27):10143-10148.

Spitz MR, Wu X, Wang Y, et al. (2001). Modulation of nucleotide excision repair capacity by XPD polymorphisms in lung cancer patients. *Cancer Res*, 61(4):1354-1357.

Stockley RA (1994). The role of proteinases in the pathogenesis of chronic bronchitis. *Am J Respir Crit Care Med*, 150(6 Pt 2):S109-S113.

Stockley RA, Bayley D, Hill SL, et al. (2001). Assessment of airway neutrophils by sputum colour: correlation with airways inflammation. *Thorax*, 56(5):366-372.

Stockley RA (2004). The HRCT scan pursuing real life pathology. *Thorax*, 59(10):822-823.

Strong MS, Incze J, Vaughan CW (1984). Field cancerization in the aerodigestive tractóits etiology , manifestation, and significance. *J Otolaryngol*, 13(1):1-6.

Sundaresan V, Ganly P, Hasleton P, et al. (1992). p53 and chromosome 3 abnormalities, characteristic of malignant lung tumours, are detectable in preinvasive lesions of the bronchus. *Oncogene*, 7(10):1989-1997.

Swensen SJ, Jett JR, Sloan JA, et al. (2002). Screening for lung cancer with low-dose spiral computed tomography. *Am J Respir Crit Care Med*, 165(4):508-513.

Takahashi Y, Campbell EA, Hirata Y, et al. (1993). A basis for differentiating among the multiple human Mu-glutathione S-transferases and molecular cloning of brain GSTM5. *J Biol Chem*, 268(12):8893-8898.

Takeuchi N, Kawamura T, Kanai A, et al. (2002). The effect of cigarette smoking on soluble adhesion molecules in middle-aged patients with Type 2 diabetes mellitus. *Diabet Med*, 19(1):57-64.

Takizawa H, Tanaka M, Takami K, et al. (2001). Increased expression of transforming growth factor-beta1 in small airway epithelium from tobacco smokers and patients with chronic obstructive pulmonary disease (COPD). *Am J Respir Crit Care Med*, 163(6):1476-1483.

Tang D, Phillips DH, Stampfer M, et al. (2001). Association between carcinogen-DNA adducts in white blood cells and lung cancer risk in the physicians health study. *Cancer Res*, 61(18):6708-6712.

Taylor BV, Oudit GY, Kalman PG, et al. (1998). Clinical and pathophysiological effects of active and passive smoking on the cardiovascular system. *Can J Cardiol*, 14(9):1129-1139.

Thiberville L, Payne P, Vielkinds J, et al. (1995). Evidence of cumulative gene losses with progression of premalignant epithelial lesions to carcinoma of the bronchus. *Cancer Res*, 55(22):5133-5139.

Tomizawa Y, Sekido Y, Kondo M, et al. (2001). Inhibition of lung cancer cell growth and induction of apoptosis after reexpression of 3p21.3 candidate tumor suppressor gene SEMA3B. *Proc Natl Acad Sci USA*, 98(24):13954-13959.

Trip MD, Cats VM, van Capelle FJ, et al. (1990). Platelet hyperreactivity and prognosis in survivors of myocardial infarction. *N Engl J Med*, 322(22):1549-1554.

Turino GM (1981). Effect of carbon monoxide on the cardiorespiratory system. Carbon monoxide toxicity: physiology and biochemistry. *Circulation*, 63(1):253A-259A.

van der Vliet A, Cross CE (2000). Oxidants, nitrosants, and the lung. *Am J Med*, 109(5):398-421.

Van Tiel E, Peeters PH, Smit HA, et al. (2002). Quitting smoking may restore hematological characteristics within five years. *Ann Epidemiol*, 12(6):378-388.

Vernooy JH, Kucukaycan M, Jacobs JA, et al. (2002). Local and systemic inflammation in patients with chronic obstructive pulmonary disease: soluble tumor necrosis factor receptors are increased in sputum. *Am J Respir Crit Care Med*, 166(9):1218-1224.

Vestbo J, Lange P (2002). Can GOLD Stage 0 provide information of prognostic value in chronic obstructive pulmonary disease? *Am J Respir Crit Care Med*, 166(3):329-332.

Vignola AM, Riccobono L, Mirabella A, et al. (1998). Sputum metalloproteinase-9/tissue inhibitor of metalloproteinase-1 ratio correlates with airflow obstruction in asthma and chronic bronchitis. *Am J Respir Crit Care Med*, 158(6):1945-1950.

Vliagoftis H, Schwingshackl A, Milne CD, et al. (2000). Proteinase-activated receptor-2-mediated matrix metalloproteinase-9 release from airway epithelial cells. *J Allergy Clin Immunol*, 106(3):537-545.

Vousden KH, Bos JL, Marshall CJ, et al. (1986). Mutations activating human c-Ha-ras1 protooncogene (HRAS1) induced by chemical carcinogens and depurination. *Proc Natl Acad Sci USA*, 83(5):1222-1226.

Wallenfeldt K, Hulthe J, Bokemark L, et al. (2001). Carotid and femoral atherosclerosis, cardiovascular risk factors and C-reactive protein in relation to smokeless tobacco use or smoking in 58-year-old men. *J Intern Med*, 250(6):492-501.

Wang L, Darling J, Zhang JS, et al. (2000). Loss of expression of the DRR 1 gene at chromosomal segment 3p21.1 in renal cell carcinoma. *Genes Chromosomes Cancer*, 27(1):1-10.

Wang XL, Tam C, McCredie RM, et al. (1994). Determinants of severity of coronary artery disease in Australian men and women. *Circulation*, 89(5):1974-1981.

Wannamethee SG, Lowe GD, Shaper AG, et al. (2005). Associations between cigarette smoking, pipe/cigar smoking, and smoking cessation, and haemostatic and inflammatory markers for cardiovascular disease. *Eur Heart J*, 26(17):1765-1773.

Waters D, Lesperance J, Gladstone P, et al. (1996). Effects of cigarette smoking on the angiographic evolution of coronary atherosclerosis. A Canadian Coronary Atherosclerosis Intervention Trial (CCAIT) Substudy. CCAIT Study Group. *Circulation*, 94(4):614-621.

Weber C, Erl W, Weber PC (1995). Enhancement of monocyte adhesion to endothelial cells by oxidatively modified low-density lipoprotein is mediated by activation of CD11b. *Biochem Biophys Res Commun*, 206(2):621-628.

Weber C, Erl W, Weber K, et al. (1996). Increased adhesiveness of isolated monocytes to endothelium is prevented by vitamin C intake in smokers. *Circulation*, 93(8):1488-1492.

Westra WH, Slebos RJ, Offerhaus GJ, et al. (1993). K-ras oncogene activation in lung adenocarcinomas from former smokers. Evidence that K-ras mutations are an early and irreversible event in the development of adenocarcinoma of the lung. *Cancer*, 72(2):432-438.

Whiss PA, Lundahl TH, Bengtsson T, et al. (2000). Acute effects of nicotine infusion on platelets in nicotine users with normal and impaired renal function. *Toxicol Appl Pharmacol*, 163(2):95-104.

Willemse BW, Postma DS, Timens W, et al. (2004). The impact of smoking cessation on respiratory symptoms, lung function, airway hyperresponsiveness and inflammation. *Eur Respir J*, 23(3):464-476.

Willemse BW, Ten Hacken NH, Rutgers B, et al. (2005). Effect of 1-year smoking cessation on airway inflammation in COPD and asymptomatic smokers. *Eur Respir J*, 26(5):835-845.

Wistuba II, Lam S, Behrens C, et al. (1997). Molecular damage in the bronchial epithelium of current and former smokers. *J Natl Cancer Inst*, 89(18):1366-1373.

Wistuba II, Behrens C, Milchgrub S, et al. (1999). Sequential molecular abnormalities are involved in the multistage development of squamous cell lung carcinoma. *Oncogene*, 18(3):643-650.

Wistuba II, Behrens C, Virmani AK, et al. (2000). High resolution chromosome 3p allelotyping of human lung cancer and preneoplastic/preinvasive bronchial epithelium reveals multiple, discontinuous sites of 3p allele loss and three regions of frequent breakpoints. *Cancer Res*, 60(7):1949-1960.

Wolffe AP, Matzke MA (1999). Epigenetics: regulation through repression. *Science*, 286(5439):481-486.

Woo KS, Robinson JT, Chook P, et al. (1997). Differences in the effect of cigarette smoking on endothelial function in chinese and white adults. *Ann Intern Med*, 127(5):372-375.

Woo KS, Chook P, Leong HC, et al. (2000). The impact of heavy passive smoking on arterial endothelial function in modernized Chinese. *J Am Coll Cardiol*, 36(4):1228-1232.

Yamaguchi Y, Matsuno S, Kagota S, et al. (2001). Oxidants in cigarette smoke extract modify low-density lipoprotein in the plasma and facilitate atherogenesis in the aorta of Watanabe heritable hyperlipidemic rabbits. *Atherosclerosis*, 156(1):109-117.

Yamaguchi Y, Matsuno S, Kagota S, et al. (2004). Peroxynitrite-mediated oxidative modification of low-density lipoprotein by aqueous extracts of cigarette smoke and the preventive effect of fluvastatin. *Atherosclerosis*, 172(2):259-265.

Yamaguchi Y, Haginaka J, Morimoto S, et al. (2005). Facilitated nitration and oxidation of LDL in cigarette smokers. *Eur J Clin Invest*, 35(3):186-193.

Yarnell JW, Sweetnam PM, Rogers S, et al. (1987). Some long term effects of smoking on the haemostatic system: a report from the Caerphilly and Speedwell Collaborative Surveys. *J Clin Pathol*, 40(8):909-913.

Yokode M, Kita T, Arai H, et al. (1988). Cholesteryl ester accumulation in macrophages incubated with low density lipoprotein pretreated with cigarette smoke extract. *Proc Natl Acad Sci USA*, 85(7):2344-2348.

Zabarovsky ER, Lerman MI, Minna JD (2002). Tumor suppressor genes on chromosome 3p involved in the pathogenesis of lung and other cancers. *Oncogene*, 21(45):6915-6935.

Zevin S, Saunders S, Gourlay SG, et al. (2001). Cardiovascular effects of carbon monoxide and cigarette smoking. *J Am Coll Cardiol*, 38(6):1633-1638.

Zhang J, Liu Y, Shi J, et al. (2002). Sidestream cigarette smoke induces dose-response in systemic inflammatory cytokine production and oxidative stress. *Exp Biol Med (Maywood)*, 227(9):823-829.

Zhang L, Gjoerup O, Roberts TM (2004). The serine/threonine kinase cyclin G-associated kinase regulates epidermal growth factor receptor signaling. *Proc Natl Acad Sci USA*, 101(28):10296-10301.

Zhou W, Liu G, Miller DP, et al. (2003). Polymorphisms in the DNA repair genes XRCC1 and ERCC2, smoking, and lung cancer risk. *Cancer Epidemiol Biomarkers Prev*, 12(4):359-365.

Websites

http://www.pnas.org/cgi/content/full/0401422101/DC1

http://pulm.bumc.bu.edu/siegeDB

http://www-p53.iarc.fr/index.html

http://www.cancerresearchjournals.org

http://www.goldcopd.org

Epidemiological Considerations in Evaluating the Effects of Cessation

A number of methodological issues in the design, analysis, and interpretation of epidemiological studies and randomised trials need careful attention to assess the effects on health of smoking cessation. The majority of these methodological problems, shown in Table 1, cause the true magnitude of the health benefits of smoking cessation to be underestimated. Problems due to misclassification and confounding by other aspects of lifestyle can be minimised by careful attention to measures at baseline and follow up and by analyses that control for lifestyle variables. Many of the problems are most acute in studies with short follow-up in populations in which the risks of smoking are not yet mature. Large observational studies with long-term follow-up over several decades have proved exceptionally useful for characterising the full magnitude of the benefits of smoking cessation.

Study designs used to examine the health effects of smoking cessation

A number of different study designs have been used to evaluate the health consequences of smoking cessation. Observational cohort studies, which follow large numbers of participants over time, can be used to derive estimates of the absolute risk of various disease outcomes in continuing smokers, former smokers and never smokers. Observational case–control studies focus on a single disease and assess detailed smoking histories retrospectively in cases and controls; they then use this information to derive estimates of the relative risk of the disease in question according to smoking history. Intervention trials randomise smokers to smoking cessation interventions and examine effects on morbidity and mortality at follow up. Each type of study has its particular methodological strengths and weaknesses. Observational studies need to be large and to have long follow-up in order to provide estimates that are sufficiently precise to be useful. Studies meeting these descriptions have been particularly informative, and have provided convincing evidence of major reductions in disease risk following long-term smoking cessation relative to the risk in individuals who continue to smoke.

Classifying smoking behaviour

Proper classification of smoking behaviour is critically important for evaluating the health consequences of smoking cessation. Misclassification of smoking status can derive from inaccurate reporting of smoking habit at enrolment of study subjects (e.g. current smokers classified as non-smokers or former smokers), and from changes in smoking habits in prospective studies which are not captured by repeated measurements (e.g. former smokers who relapse and current smokers who give up). These sources of misclassification will result in underestimation of the extent of the health gains that stem from successful quitting.

Cigarette smoking is notoriously a chronic relapsing condition. In countries such as the USA and the United Kingdom about 40% of smokers make a serious quit attempt each year, but the long-term success rate of such attempts is only about 3% (Jarvis et al., 1997; Royal College of Physicians, 2000). This means that a snapshot of smoking status at a point in time provides an imperfect guide to long-term smoking status. Because of the dynamic nature of change in smoking behaviour, any categorization of smoking status at a point in time becomes a simplification (USDHHS, 1990). At one extreme, many smokers make no efforts to change, and about 30% report not going for longer than a single day without smoking in the past five years (Jarvis et al., 2003); former smokers of long duration (two to five years or longer) are unlikely to return to smoking; and uptake of smoking by adult non-smokers above the age of twenty-five is rare in many populations. At the other extreme, however, there are also many smokers who make repeated efforts to quit, and transitions in and out of smoking are frequent.

Table 1. Potential methodological problems in investigating the health consequences of smoking cessation

Problem	Effect	Relevance		
		Cohort studies	Case-control studies	Randomised interventions
Carrying out study in population where smoking epidemic is not mature	Under-estimation of risks of smoking and hence, of the benefits of quitting	Considerably important	Considerably important	Considerably important
Carrying out study in population with few long-term former smokers	Under-estimation of the benefits of quitting	Considerably important	Considerably important	Depends on endpoint
Current smokers quitting in response to disease onset	Apparent benefits of cessation are reduced	Considerably important	Problem can be avoided with careful study design	Not applicable
Smoking habits changing during follow-up (baseline smokers quitting, and former smokers relapsing repeatedly)	Apparent benefits of cessation are reduced	Problem can be be reduced by repeat surveys of population	Not applicable	Problem can be reduced by repeat surveys of population
Self-reported former smokers are actually smoking	Apparent benefits of cessation are reduced	Problem relatively small in individuals who report quitting more than 2 years previously	Problem relatively small in individuals who report quitting more than 2 years previously	Biochemical validation advisable
Former smokers tend to have smoked less than persistent smokers	Failure to account for the difference may exaggerate the apparent benefits of cessation	Problem can be minimised with appropriate data collection and analysis	Problem can be minimised with appropriate data collection and analysis	Not applicable
Former smokers tend to have a healthier lifestyle than persistent smokers	Failure to account for the difference may exaggerate the apparent benefits of cessation	Effect probably small	Effect probably small	Not applicable

Modified from USDHHS (1990)

The subgroup of particular concern for studies of smoking cessation are those who report having quit at one time, but then resume smoking. The Lung Health Study, a randomised trial of smoking cessation in adult smokers with evidence of early chronic obstructive lung disease, provides an example (Anthonisen *et al.*, 1994). Three patterns of response were identified: sustained quitters were defined as carbon-monoxide (CO) verified former smokers at the first and all subsequent annual follow-ups, who additionally reported no significant intervening lapses. Continuing smokers reported smoking at all annual follow-ups. Intermittent smokers were verified former smokers at at least one follow-up and who were smoking at a minimum of one annual follow-up (Murray *et al.*, 1998). At eleven years after initial enrolment, 19% of participants were sustained quitters, 52% continuing smokers, and 29% intermittent smokers (Anthonisen *et al.*, 2002). Observational studies which require participants to have been abstinent for at least two years at baseline in order to be categorized as former smokers will reduce the problem of relapse to smoking influencing the estimation of the health effects of quitting, as relatively few former smokers are likely to go back to smoking after this duration of abstinence (see Table 2).

Definition of smoking and of ex-smoking

In the great majority of studies, smoking is ascertained by self-report. Questions used to determine current smoking and former smoking vary across studies and countries. In the United Kingdom national statistics, a current cigarette smoker is someone who responds yes to "Do you smoke cigarettes at all nowadays?" (Rickards *et al.*, 2004); while in several countries a distinction is drawn between daily and non-daily smoking, and national cigarette smoking prevalence may be defined as daily smoking (as in Sweden, Australia, and Canada). Ex-cigarette or former smokers may be defined as those who report having smoked at least 100 cigarettes in their life, but no current cigarette use (National Health and Nutritional Examination Survey (NHANES); National Health Interview Survey (NHIS), United States); or, in the United Kingdom, as those who do not currently smoke cigarettes but who respond yes to "Have you ever smoked cigarettes regularly?" (Rickards *et al.*, 2004) These variations in the approach to defining smoking status are likely to be of considerable importance for ecological comparisons of smoking prevalence across countries, but may be of less relevance for establishing baseline smoking in observational cohorts, as the questions used to ascertain smoking history in observational studies are more detailed than those in national surveys.

Misclassification of exposure can also result from the treatment of individuals who smoke cigars or pipes, or, in populations where this is common, who use smokeless tobacco. Estimates of former smoking may or may not take account of ex-cigarette smokers who continue to smoke pipes or cigars. In the Multiple Risk Factor Intervention Trial (MRFIT) there was a focus on cigarette smoking, and men who smoked pipes or cigars, but not cigarettes, at baseline were counted as non-smokers. Those who switched from cigarettes to pipes/cigars during the course of the study could be counted as former smokers, despite evidence of continued smoke inhalation (Neaton *et al.*, 1981). Similarly, in the Whitehall Study, ex-smoking was defined solely in terms of cigarettes and took no account of pipe/cigar smoking (Rose & Hamilton, 1978).

Factors affecting the accuracy of self-reported smoking status

Smoking status can be determined objectively by biochemical markers of smoke inhalation (Jarvis *et al.*, 1987; USDHHS, 1990). While many observational and cohort studies have relied exclusively on self-report, a number of major studies have incorporated biochemical markers of smoking. The Lung Health Study used CO and saliva cotinine to validate claims of cessation (Murray *et al.*, 2002), while measures of thiocyanate and CO were taken in MRFIT (Neaton *et al.*, 1981). Population surveys such as NHANES in the US and the Health Survey for England (HSE) (Prior et al., 2003) collect serum or saliva samples for cotinine assay. Cotinine is widely accepted as the most sensitive

Table 2. Number of self-reported former smokers and never smokers categorized as smoking by cotinine in the Health Survey for England

	N (%)	% smoking by cotinine	Mean cotinine in confirmed non-smokers (ng/ml)	Mean cotinine in misreported non-smokers (ng/ml)
Never smokers	9278	2.0	0.8	147
Former smokers	4907	4.9	0.9	160
Reported time since quitting				
< 6 months	89 (1.8)	15.7	1.6	136
6–12 months	150 (3.1)	24.7	2.3	172
1–2 years	152 (3.1)	17.8	1.3	204
2–5 years	465 (9.5)	7.7	1.1	11
5–9 years	662 (13.5)	7.1	1.0	162
10–19 years	1316 (26.8)	3.8	0.8	183
20+ years	2073 (42.2)	1.5	0.7	135

Data from the Health Survey for England 1998 and 2001 combined. Self-reported smoking status based on initial interview responses confirmed by no reported smoking and no use of nicotine replacement products at nurse visit when saliva specimen for cotinine was collected. A cotinine concentration ≥ 15 ng/ml was taken to indicate current smoking.

and specific of available tests (SRNT Subcommittee on Biochemical Verification, 2002).

Observational studies in which no intervention occurs, or intervention studies in which there is minimal intervention or interaction with smokers, are less likely to prompt false reports of smoking cessation than studies in which intensive intervention does occur (USDHHS, 1990). Perceived social pressure to report non-smoking is likely to be minimal in population surveys in which smoking is one of many health behaviours covered, and probably also in observational studies where no intervention is applied. Observational studies have in general not employed biomarkers of smoking to confirm self-reported smoking status at baseline. However, such data are available from general population surveys of smoking. Table 2 gives percentages of respondents with misreported smoking status observed in the Health Survey for England, a large continuing survey on representative samples of the adult population. Among self-reported never smokers, 2% had cotinine levels indicative of smoking. Among former smokers, the corresponding percentage was considerably higher (4.9%). The extent of misreport showed a strong relationship to time since quitting, being similar to never smokers in those who reported quitting more than twenty years previously (1.5%), but ranging between 15–25% in those who reported quitting for less than two years (Table 2). The cotinine levels observed in these discrepant never and former smokers were not marginally raised, but were well into the smoking range, indicating substantial amounts of inhaled smoke.

It is important to emphasize that the great majority of former smokers (70%) had quit for ten years or longer, and that substantial levels of misreport were observed mostly in the minority (15%) who had quit within the previous two

years. This indicates that observational studies that require former smokers to have quit for a minimum of one to two years at baseline to be included in the ex-smoking category may avoid much of this problem. It is also reassuring that self-reports of never smoking appear in general to be highly reliable (only 2% giving evidence of current smoking, see also Riboli *et al.*, 1995; Hackshaw *et al.*, 1997), suggesting that contamination of the reference group of never smokers by smokers in observational studies is likely to be of minimal significance.

The extent of misreport of smoking status may be greater in studies which enrol smokers in interventions to promote cessation in order to investigate the effects on health outcomes. In MRFIT, which incorporated an intensive special intervention condition to promote cigarette cessation, thiocyanate-validated cessation rates differed substantially from self-reported cessation. The reported cessation at one year of 43% in the special intervention group was reduced to 31% using biochemical validation by thiocyanate according to the complex formula adopted by MRFIT researchers which allowed continued pipe/cigar smoking (Neaton *et al.*, 1981), while the best estimate of complete smoking cessation, derived from the overall reduction in smoking-attributable thiocyanate, was estimated at no more than 19% (Jarvis *et al.*, 1984). In the usual care group, by contrast, the corresponding figures were 13.5%, 11.7% and 2.9%, indicating markedly less misreport among those participants assigned to the arm that did not involve as much pressure to quit. Differences in misreport between intervention and control participants, albeit of smaller magnitude, were also observed in the Lung Health Study: at one year 17% of participants assigned to the smoking intervention had saliva cotinines discrepant with their self-report of non-smoking, compared with 10% in those

assigned to usual care. The discrepancy between self-report and cotinine-assessed smoking reduced across years in those who received the smoking intervention (falling from 17% at year one to 12% by year five). There was a tendency for the same individuals to give cotinine-discrepant self-reports across years. The high rates of misreport of smoking status observed in these intervention trials may be attributable to perceived pressure to stop smoking and a desire to give socially approved responses. Social and cultural norms in some countries may give rise to pressures on some groups (e.g. women in Asian countries) to deny their smoking under some circumstances.

Biases caused by quitting in response to disease development

Within a population it is likely that a proportion of the former smokers gave up smoking after developing a smoking-related disease, and that signs and symptoms related to the early stages of the disease, or receipt of a diagnosis, played a part in motivating them to give up.

The consequences of this phenomenon are illustrated in Figure 1, in which the observed mortality rate from lung cancer among former smokers in the baseline American Cancer Society Cancer Prevention Study I (CPS-I) is plotted against years since quitting, and the lung cancer mortality rate predicted if smoking had continued is also shown. The predicted rate is based on a model that takes into account age, duration of smoking and number of cigarettes per day, and the parameters of the model were estimated from the lung cancer mortality rates observed in the individuals in the study who continued to smoke. In the first year after quitting smoking, the observed rate among the quitters is more than double the predicted rate in continuing smokers. Therefore, if such individuals are counted as former smokers when estimating the benefits of giving up smoking, disease risks in former smokers will be over-estimated and the benefits of quitting will be under-estimated. It should be noted that the bias illustrated in Figure 1 cannot be avoided by considering the first ten years after quitting as a single category: such an approach will only dilute any true reduction in risk.

In case–control studies where detailed information is collected from all those taking part, including the reasons for quitting among former smokers, it is possible — at least in principle — to avoid this bias by asking the cases to describe their smoking habits at the time of the initial symptoms of their disease and by asking the controls to describe their smoking habits at a comparable

index date. This approach has been used by Peto *et al.* (2000) and also in a number of other case–control studies. Of course, such studies are limited by the accuracy of the smoking histories obtained, especially where they have not been derived from the case in person, but from his or her spouse or another relative. The approach cannot generally be used in cohort studies, as detailed information on the reasons for quitting will not generally be available for all those who develop disease throughout the period of follow-up.

In a cohort study, elimination of all cases of prevalent disease at the start of the study will result in under-estimation of subsequent mortality rates in those who have given up smoking, resulting in over-estimation of the benefits of quitting smoking.

Few patients with lung cancer survive for more than five years after diagnosis. Therefore, for mortality from lung cancer, the bias illustrated in Figure 1 will be largely confined to the initial five years after quitting. Hence, approximately unbiased estimates of the risk in former smokers of more than five years' duration can be derived, enabling unbiased estimates of the benefits of giving up smoking on lung cancer mortality in case-control studies and, where the length of follow-up permits, also in cohort studies. For other cancers with poor survival rates, the situation will be similar to that for lung cancer.

For cancers with higher survival rates than lung cancer, and also for chronic obstructive pulmonary disease (COPD) and many other important smoking-related diseases, a considerable proportion of the individuals who develop the disease are likely to survive for many years. This reduces the extent to which unbiased estimates of the benefits of stopping smoking can be estimated, even at substantial periods of time after quitting.

There is evidence that, among patients with lung cancer, average survival is several months longer among those who have given up smoking than among those who continue to smoke (Gritz *et al.*, 2005). However, even for patients who do not smoke after a diagnosis of lung cancer, only a small proportion will survive for longer than five years. In contrast, for COPD, for symptoms indicating early-stage cardio-vascular disease, and for many other smoking-related diseases, an apprecia-ble number of those affected are likely to survive for several years. In these diseases the severity of the disease may well be reduced substantially by quitting smoking and its time-course may also be prolonged substantially. Therefore, for studies of mortality it is impossible to derive unbiased estimates of the

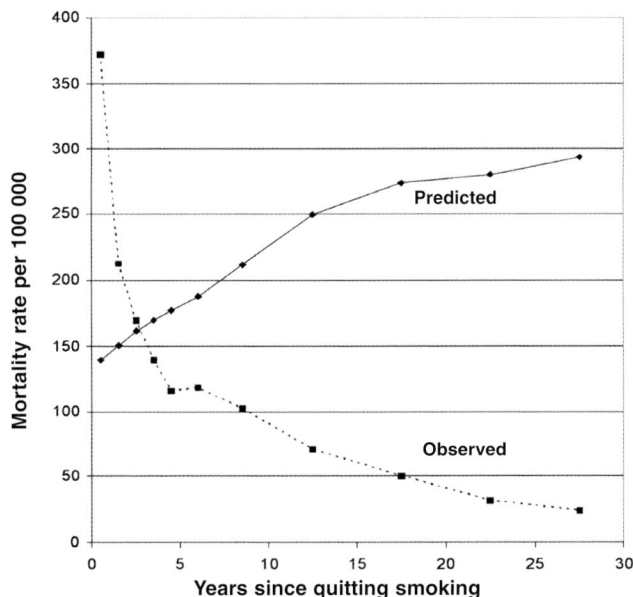

Figure 1. Observed lung cancer mortality among former smokers versus time since quitting in the baseline CSP-1; also the predicted lung cancer mortality rate that would have occurred if smoking had continued

Source: D. Burns unpublished analyses

benefits of giving up smoking for these diseases, even in the period more than ten years after quitting.

Bias due to differences in smoking history between smokers who quit and those who continue to smoke

Most of the information on the health benefits of giving up smoking has come from observational studies. In these studies, former smokers are those participants who have self-selected to give up smoking. This raises the question of whether those who stop smoking and those who continue differ in other respects in ways which affect disease risk. It cannot be assumed that those who become former smokers are, while smoking, similar to continuing smokers in terms of their risk of developing smoking-related disease. For example, smokers who quit may have lower smoke intakes and be less nicotine-dependent than continuing smokers. There is evidence from a prospective study of cohorts of smokers in the general population that this is indeed the case (Jarvis *et al.*, 1997). The effects of any such tendency for lighter smokers to be more likely than heavy smokers to quit will be to overestimate the apparent benefits of cessation, as former smokers may not have been as likely to have developed smoking-related disease if they had not quit. Analyses that stratify by intensity of smoking can control for this potential bias. However, it should be emphasized that any such effects are likely to be of marginal importance only, as the magnitude of changes in death rates following cessation in observational studies far exceeds anything that could reflect residual confounding. The results of the Lung Health Study, which found a significant benefit of smoking cessation on mortality in an intention-to-treat comparison between the smoking intervention and controls, also confirm that the benefits of cessation cannot be due in any significant way to self-selection (Anthonisen *et al.*, 2005).

Are apparent health gains from quitting smoking partly attributable to changes in other aspects of lifestyle?

Smokers tend to differ from non-smokers on a number of other health-relevant behaviours in addition to smoking (Thun *et al.*, 2000). As a group, they have unhealthier diets and lower vitamin intakes, take less physical activity and drink more alcohol. For some of these behaviours, there is evidence that former smokers move toward the healthier pattern displayed by never smokers. In particular, their diets (Morabia & Wynder, 1990; Cade & Margetts, 1991; Whichelow *et al.*, 1991; Dallongeville *et al.*, 1998; Dyer *et al.*, 2003) are much closer to those of never smokers than those of continuing cigarette smokers. Some of the observed reduction in disease risk in former smokers by comparison with continuing smokers could in principle be due to confounding by a shift to a generally healthier lifestyle that occurs following smoking cessation. However, analyses of the CPS II cohort to examine this issue found that adjustment for potential confounders (diet, physical activity, alcohol consumption) made little difference to estimates of risk in comparison with never smokers, even for cardiovascular outcomes (Thun *et al.*, 2000). There is also genuine uncertainty as to whether it is appropriate to treat some behaviours associated with smoking and which change with cessation as confounders. It can be argued that these behaviours should not be controlled for, because they represent adverse effects of smoking and/or intermediates in the causal pathway. For example, both physical inactivity and low body mass index can be caused by smoking or smoking-related diseases (Perkins *et al.*, 1993; Thun *et al.*, 2000).

Table 1 summarises the main issues that relate to accurate classification of smoking status: reverse causality due to smokers quitting after disease onset, confounding when smokers' characteristics are related both to giving up smoking and to disease risk, and the problems of interpretation raised by studies in populations in which the full detrimental effects of smoking on health are not yet apparent.

References

Anthonisen NR, Connett JE, Kiley JP, et al. (1994). Effects of smoking intervention and the use of an inhaled anticholinergic bronchodilator on the rate of decline of FEV$_1$. The Lung Health Study. *JAMA*, 272(19):1497-1505.

Anthonisen NR, Connett JE, Murray RP (2002). Smoking and lung function of Lung Health Study participants after 11 years. *Am J Respir Crit Care Med*, 166(5):675-679.

Anthonisen NR, Skeans MA, Wise RA, et al. (2005). The effects of a smoking cessation intervention on 14.5-year mortality: a randomized clinical trial. *Ann Intern Med*, 142(4):233-239.

Cade JE, Margetts BM (1991). Relationship between diet and smoking--is the diet of smokers different? *J Epidemiol Community Health*, 45(4):270-272.

Dallongeville J, Marecaux N, Fruchart JC, et al. (1998). Cigarette smoking is associated with unhealthy patterns of nutrient intake: a meta-analysis. *J Nutr*, 128(9):1450-1457.

Dyer AR, Elliott P, Stamler J, et al. (2003). Dietary intake in male and female smokers, ex-smokers, and never smokers: the INTERMAP study. *J Hum Hypertens*, 17(9):641-654.

Gritz ER, Dresler C, Sarna L (2005). Smoking, the missing drug interaction in clinical trials: ignoring the obvious. Cancer *Epidemiol Biomarkers Prev,* 14(10):2287-2293.

Hackshaw AK, Law MR, Wald NJ (1997). The accumulated evidence on lung cancer and environmental tobacco smoke. *BMJ,* 315(7114):980-988.

Jarvis M, West R, Tunstall-Pedoe H, et al. (1984). An evaluation of the intervention against smoking in the multiple risk factor intervention trial. *Prev Med,* 13(5):501-509.

Jarvis MJ, Tunstall-Pedoe H, Feyerabend C, et al. (1987). Comparison of tests used to distinguish smokers from nonsmokers. *Am J Public Health,* 77(11):1435-1438.

Jarvis MJ (1997). Patterns and predictors of unaided smoking cessation in the general population. In: Bolliger CT, Fagerström KO, eds., *The Tobacco Epidemic.* 151-164.

Jarvis MJ, Wardle J, Waller J, et al. (2003). Prevalence of hardcore smoking in England, and associated attitudes and beliefs: cross sectional study. *BMJ,* 326(7398):1061.

Morabia A, Wynder EL (1990). Dietary habits of smokers, people who never smoked, and exsmokers. *Am J Clin Nutr,* 52(5):933-937.

Murray RP, Anthonisen NR, Connett JE, et al. (1998). Effects of multiple attempts to quit smoking and relapses to smoking on pulmonary function. Lung Health Study Research Group. *J Clin Epidemiol,* 51(12):1317-1326.

Murray RP, Connett JE, Istvan JA, et al. (2002). Relations of cotinine and carbon monoxide to self-reported smoking in a cohort of smokers and ex-smokers followed over 5 years. *Nicotine Tob Res,* 4(3):287-294.

Neaton JD, Broste S, Cohen L, et al. (1981). The multiple risk factor intervention trial (MRFIT). VII. A comparison of risk factor changes between the two study groups. *Prev Med,* 10(4):519-543.

Perkins KA, Rohay J, Meilahn EN, et al. (1993). Diet, alcohol, and physical activity as a function of smoking status in middle-aged women. *Health Psychol,* 12(5):410-415.

Peto R, Darby S, Deo H, et al. (2000). Smoking, smoking cessation, and lung cancer in the UK since 1950: combination of national statistics with two case-control studies. *BMJ,* 321(7257):323-329.

Prior G, Deverill C, Malbut K, et al. (2003). Health Survey for England. Methodology and documentation. London, The Stationery Office.

Riboli E, Haley NJ, Tredaniel J, et al. (1995). Misclassification of smoking status among women in relation to exposure to environmental tobacco smoke. *Eur Respir J,* 8(2):285-290.

Rickards L, Fox K, Roberts C, et al. (2004). Living in Britain. Results from the 2002 General Household Survey. London, The Stationery Office.

Rose G, Hamilton PJ (1978). A randomised controlled trial of the effect on middle-aged men of advice to stop smoking. *J Epidemiol Community Health,* 32(4):275-281.

Royal College of Physicians (2000). *Nicotine Addiction in Britain.* London, Royal College of Physicians.

SRNT Subcommittee on Biochemical Verification (2002). Biochemical verification of tobacco use and cessation. *Nicotine Tob Res,* 4:149-159.

Thun MJ, Apicella LF, Henley SJ (2000). Smoking vs other risk factors as the cause of smoking-attributable deaths: confounding in the courtroom. *JAMA,* 284(6):706-712.

United States Department of Health and Human Service (USDHHS) (1990). *The Health Benefits of Smoking Cessation. A Report of the Surgeon General.* Rockville, MD, Centers for Disease Control, Office on Smoking and Health.

Whichelow MJ, Erzinclioglu SW, Cox BD (1991). A comparison of the diets of non-smokers and smokers. *Br J Addict,* 86(1):71-81.

Lung Cancer Risk After Smoking Cessation

Introduction

More is known about the impact of smoking cessation on the risk of lung cancer than on any other cancer. Comprehensive reviews by IARC (1986, 2004) and the U.S. Surgeon General (USDHHS, 1990, 2004) cite more than 50 published and unpublished epidemiologic studies on this topic (Best, 1966; Hammond, 1966; Kahn, 1966; Graham & Levin, 1971; Cederlof *et al.*, 1975; Doll *et al.*, 1976; Doll *et al.*, 1980; Rogot & Murray, 1980; Wigle *et al.*, 1980; Joly *et al.*, 1983; Correa *et al.*, 1984; Lubin *et al.*, 1984; Alderson *et al.*, 1985; Wu *et al.*, 1985; Gao *et al.*, 1988; Higgins & Wynder, 1988; Pathak *et al.*, 1986; Damber & Larsson, 1986; Carstensen *et al.*, 1987; Garfinkel & Stellman, 1988; Benhamou *et al.*, 1989; Jedrychowski *et al.*, 1990; Becher *et al.*, 1991; Jockel *et al.*, 1992 ; Morabia & Wynder, 1992; Chyou *et al.*, 1993; Gao *et al.*, 1993; De Stefani *et al.*, 1994; Suzuki *et al.*, 1994; De Stefani *et al.*, 1996; Barbone *et al.*, 1997; Muscat *et al.*, 1997; Pohlabeln *et al.*, 1997; Khuder *et al.*, 1998; Matos *et al.*, 1998; Jacobs *et al.*, 1999; Speizer *et al.*, 1999; Agudo *et al.*, 2000; Kreuzer *et al.*, 2000 ; Osann *et al.*, 2000; Peto *et al.*, 2000; Mao *et al.*, 2001; Simonato *et al.*, 2001; Stellman *et al.*, 2001; Bhurgri *et al.*, 2002; Petrauskaite *et al.*, 2002; Stellman *et al.*, 2003). Another 17 studies (Sobue *et al.*, 1993; Friedman *et al.*, 1997; Hrubec & McLaughlin, 1997; Wakai *et al.*, 2001; Godtfredsen *et al.*, 2002; Lam *et al.*, 2002; Sobue *et al.*, 2002; Thun *et al.*, 2002; Andó *et al.*, 2003; Gajalakshmi *et al.*, 2003; Doll *et al.*, 2004; Jee *et al.*, 2004; Miller *et al.*, 2004; Ebbert *et al.*, 2005; Godtfredsen *et al.*, 2005; Wen *et al.*, 2005; Zhang *et al.*, 2005) were identified by the Working Group that were not included in the earlier reviews. Based on the extensive epidemiologic evidence, IARC (2004) has concluded that "Stopping smoking at any age avoids the further increase in risk of lung cancer incurred by continued smoking," and that "The younger the age at cessation, the greater the benefit."

While the benefits of smoking cessation for lung cancer are well established qualitatively, there is still uncertainty about the size and timing of these benefits and the extent to which they may vary according to age at cessation, antecedent smoking history, histologic type of lung cancer, and the presence or absence of other diseases caused by smoking. Most studies were conducted in time periods and countries where the full effect of prolonged cigarette smoking had not yet reached its peak; thus these studies underestimate the impact of lifetime smoking on lung cancer risk and do not fully capture the benefits of prolonged cessation (Peto *et al.*, 2000). Furthermore, almost all studies have examined the change in lung cancer risk after smoking cessation in terms of relative rather than absolute risk. There are now large numbers of former smokers who are concerned about their residual risk in terms of the probability that they may develop lung cancer because of past smoking. While it is obvious that absolute risk varies according to age, gender, and past smoking practices, it is not clear whether the absolute risk of developing lung cancer actually decreases after smoking cessation, as is the case with relative risk, or whether it continues to increase but at a slower rate than would result from continued smoking.

Relative risk by time since cessation

A total of 34 studies including results in men, 21 in women, and 6 in both sexes combined have examined the risk of developing or dying from lung cancer among former smokers compared with either people who continue to smoke or those who have never smoked (Tables 1 and 2). Most of these studies express the comparison as a ratio (relative risk or odds ratio) comparing the incidence or death rate from lung cancer in former smokers to that of never smokers. Fewer studies have compared the lung cancer risk in former smokers to that of current smokers. The comparison with continuing smokers is more relevant to a smoker who is contemplating cessation than is the contrast with never smokers. People who smoke have the option of

Table 1. Cohort studies: relative risk of lung cancer by smoking status and/or years since quitting smoking

Reference Country and years of follow-up	Subjects	Number of cases	Smoking cessation/status categories	Relative risk vs. never-smokers	95% CI	Relative risk vs. current smokers	95% CI	Comments
Asia								
Wakai et al. (2001) Japan 1988–1997	Japanese Collaborative Cohort Study (JACC) 33 654 males	228	Current smoker	5.2	(3.6, 7.5)	1.0		Outcome=mortality
			Former smoker					Adjusted for age
			Years since quitting					
		36	0–4	4.8	(3.0, 7.8)	0.9	(0.7, 1.3)	Individuals with history of lung cancer were excluded from analysis
		21	5–9	3.2	(1.8, 5.5)	0.6	(0.4, 1.0)	
		11	10–14	2.0	(1.0, 4.0)	0.4	(0.2, 0.7)	
		4	15–19	1.3	(0.5, 3.6)	0.3	(0.1, 0.7)	
		9	≥20	1.0	(0.5, 2.1)	0.2	(0.1, 0.4)	Exposure assessed at baseline only
		32	Non-smoker	1.0		0.2	(0.1, 0.3)	
								Subjects limited to former/current smokers who started smoking at ages 18-22
Sobue et al. (2002) Japan 1990–1999	Japan Public Health Center Study 91 738 participants		MEN *All incident*					Outcome=incidence
		231	Current smoker	4.5	(3.0, 6.8)	1.0		Adjusted for age and area
		67	Former smoker	2.2	(1.4, 3.4)	0.5	(0.4, 0.7)	
		26	Non-smoker	1.0		0.2	(0.1, 0.3)	
			Squamous cell, small cell carcinoma					Individuals with history of any cancer excluded from analysis
		104	Current smoker	12.7	(4.7, 34.7)	1.0		
		25	Former smoker	5.1	(1.8, 14.6)	0.4	(0.3, 0.6)	
		4	Non-smoker	1.0		0.1	(0.04, 0.3)	Exposure assessed at baseline only
			Adenocarcinoma					
		81	Current smoker	2.8	(1.6, 4.9)	1.0		
		23	Former smoker	1.3	(0.7, 2.5)	0.5	(0.3, 0.8)	
		15	Non-smoker	1.0		0.4	(0.2, 0.7)	

Table 1 (cont). Cohort studies in lung cancer

Reference Country and years of follow-up	Subjects	Number of cases	Smoking cessation/status categories	Relative risk vs. never-smokers	95% CI	Relative risk vs. current smokers	95% CI	Comments
Asia								
Sobue (contd)			*WOMEN*					
			All incident					
		16	Current smoker	4.2	(2.4, 7.2)	1.0		
		4	Former smoker	3.7	(1.4, 10.2)	0.9	(0.3, 2.7)	
		78	Non-smoker	1.0		0.2	(0.1, 0.3)	
			Squamous cell, small cell carcinoma					
		5	Current smoker	17.5	(4.9, 62.1)	1.0		
		1	Former smoker	10.8	(1.2, 94.4)	0.6	(0.1, 5.1)	
		5	Non-smoker	1.0		0.1	(0.03, 0.3)	
			Adenocarcinoma					
		5	Current smoker	2.0	(0.8, 5.0)	1.0		
		3	Former smoker	4.3	(1.3, 13.8)	2.2	(0.5, 9.2)	
		54	Non-smoker	1.0		0.5	(0.2, 1.2)	
Lam et al. (2002) China 1987–1999	1268 retired military men, 60 or older	15	Current smoker	2.4	(0.9, 6.2)	1.0		Outcome= mortality
		19	Former smoker	2.3	(0.9, 5.8)	1.0	(0.5, 2.0)	Adjusted for age, systolic blood pressure, BMI, total cholesterol, triglycerides, alcohol consumption, exercise, existing disease at baseline
		6	Never smoker	1.0		0.4	(0.2, 1.0)	
			No disease at baseline					
		6	Current smoker	5.2	(0.6, 45.0)	1.0		Current smoker= still smoking at baseline Former smoker= stopped for at least 2 yrs
		4	Former smoker	2.7	(0.3, 25.6)	0.5	(0.1, 1.8)	Exposure assessed at baseline only
		1	Never smoker	1.0		0.2	(0.02, 1.7)	

Table 1 (cont). Cohort studies in lung cancer

Reference Country and years of follow-up	Subjects	Number of cases	Smoking cessation/status categories	Relative risk vs. never-smokers	95% CI	Relative risk vs. current smokers	95% CI	Comments
Ando et al. (2003) Japan 1988–1997	Japan Collaborative Cohort Study 45 010 men 55 724 women		MEN					Outcome= mortality
		317	Current smoker	4.5	(3.1, 6.4)	1.0		Adjusted for age
		120	Former smoker	2.4	(1.6, 3.5)	0.5	(0.4, 0.6)	Excluded individuals with previous history of lung cancer
			Years since quitting					
		38	<5	4.3	(2.7, 6.9)	1.0	(0.7, 1.3)	Exposure assessed at baseline only
		17	5–9	2.2	(1.2, 4.0)	0.5	(0.3, 0.8)	
		12	10–14	1.9	(1.0, 3.6)	0.4	(0.2, 0.8)	
		11	≥15	0.8	(0.4, 1.7)	0.2	(0.1, 0.3)	
		32	Never smoker	1.0		0.2	(0.1, 0.3)	
			WOMEN					
		21	Current smoker	3.6	(2.2, 5.7)	1.0		
		6	Former smoker	2.6	(1.1, 5.8)	0.7	(0.3, 1.7)	
		101	Never smoker	1.0		0.3	(0.2, 0.5)	
Jee et al. (2004) Korea 1993–2001	Korean Cancer Prevention Study 1 212 906 participants		MEN					Outcome= mortality
		2733	Current smoker	4.6	(4.0, 5.3)	1.0		Adjusted for age
		708	Former smoker	2.2	(1.9, 2.6)	0.5	(0.46, 0.54)	Excluded participants with history of cancer
		212	Never smoker	1.0		0.2	(0.17, 0.23)	
			WOMEN					
		136	Current smoker	2.5	(2.0, 3.1)	1.0		
		50	Former smoker	1.7	(1.2, 2.3)	0.7	(0.5, 1.0)	
		399	Never smoker	1.0		0.4	(0.3, 0.5)	
			MEN					Outcome= incidence
		3258	Current smoker	4.0	(3.5, 4.4)	1.0		Adjusted for age
		879	Former smoker	2.0	(1.7, 2.3)	0.5	(0.46, 0.54)	
		308	Never smoker	1.0		0.3	(0.27, 0.34)	

Table 1 (cont). Cohort studies in lung cancer

Reference Country and years of follow-up	Subjects	Number of cases	Smoking cessation/status categories	Relative risk vs. never-smokers	95% CI	Relative risk vs. current smokers	95% CI	Comments
Wen et al. (2005) Taipei 1989–2001	Underwent annual medical screening at Taipei Outpatient Service Center 30 244 male government employees and teachers		Current smoker Former smoker Years since quitting 0–5 0–16 17+ Never smoker	4.3 3.3 1.0	(2.7, 6.7) (1.9, 5.8)	1.0 0.6 0.4 0.7 0.3	(0.4, 1.0) (0.2, 1.0) (0.4, 1.1) (0.1, 0.9)	Outcome= mortality Adjusted for age Current smokers= smoking at time of recruitment; former smokers= quit for at least 6 months Exposure assessed at baseline only
Europe Tverdal et al. (1993)[b] Norway 1972–88	Norwegian Men Screening Study 44 290 men, 24 535 women	144 1 1 5 4 4	MEN Current smoker Former smoker Years since quitting < 3 months 3–12 months 1–5 years > 5 years Never smoker	16.1 3.4 2.3 2.8 1.3 1.0	(6.1, 44.8) (0.4, 30.4) (0.3, 30.0) (0.8, 10.5) (0.3, 5.4)	1.0 0.2 0.1 0.2 0.1 0.1	(0.03, 1.4) (0.02, 1.0) (0.1, 0.4) (0.03, 0.2) (0.04, 0.3)	Outcome=mortality Relative risks calculated from annual mortality rate per 100 000 persons; adjusted for age and area Exposure assessed at baseline only
Ben-Shlomo et al. (1994)[b] UK 1967–87	Whitehall Study 19 018 men	365 14 23 15 6 10	Current smoker Former smoker Years since quitting 1–9 10–19 20–29 ≥ 30 per 10 years Never smoker	11.9[†] 8.7 4.1 2.6 1.0 0.5 1.0	(6.61, 21.4) (4.0, 18.9) (2.0, 8.2) (1.2, 5.5) (0.3, 3.1) (0.4, 0.7)	1.0 0.7 0.3 0.2 0.1 0.04 0.1	(0.4, 1.2) (0.2, 0.5) (0.1, 0.3) (0.04, 0.2) (0.05, 0.2)	Outcome=mortality Adjusted for age and civil service employment grade †Adjusted for age Included individuals with pre-existing disease Exposure assessed at baseline only

Table 1 (cont). Cohort studies in lung cancer

Reference Country and years of follow-up	Subjects	Number of cases	Smoking cessation/status categories	Relative risk vs. never-smokers	95% CI	Relative risk vs. current smokers	95% CI	Comments
Doll et al. (2004) UK 1951–2001	British Doctor's cohort 34 439 British male doctors		AGE RANGE=35–44					Outcome= mortality
			Continuing cigarette smoker	3.0		1.0		
			Never smoker	1.0		0.3		
			AGE RANGE=45–54					
			Continuing cigarette smoker	11.0		1.0		
			Stopped smoking by 35–44	0.3		0.03		
			Never smoker	1.0		0.1		
			AGE RANGE=55–64					
			Continuing cigarette smoker	19.3		1.0		
			Stopped smoking by 35–44	0.3		0.01		
			Stopped smoking by 45–54	0.3		0.01		
			Never smoker	1.0		0.1		
			AGE RANGE=65–74					
			Continuing cigarette smoker	17.8		1.0		
			Stopped smoking by 35–44	0.8		0.04		
			Stopped smoking by 45–54	2.2		0.1		
			Stopped smoking by 55–64	2.8		0.2		
			Never smoker	1.0		0.1		
			AGE RANGE=75–84					
			Continuing cigarette smoker	5.8		1.0		
			Stopped smoking by 35–44	1.7		0.3		
			Stopped smoking by 45–54	1.0		0.2		
			Stopped smoking by 55–64	1.7		0.3		
			Never smoker	1.0		0.2		
			ALL AGES					
			Continuing cigarette smoker	12.11		1.0		
			Stopped smoking by 35–44	0.9		0.1		
			Stopped smoking by 45–54	1.3		0.1		
			Stopped smoking by 55–64	1.3		0.1		
			Never smoker	1.0		0.1		

Table 1 (cont). Cohort studies in lung cancer

Reference Country and years of follow-up	Subjects	Number of cases	Smoking cessation/status categories	Relative risk vs. never-smokers	95% CI	Relative risk vs. current smokers	95% CI	Comments
Miller et al. (2004) Europe 1992–2002	EPIC study 478 021 participants		**MEN**					Outcome= incidence
			Current smoker					[†] The current smokers referent group is defined as 15–24 cig/day
		63	<15 cig/day	10.0	(5.2, 19.0)	1.0		
		123	15–24 cig/day	22.5	(12.1, 42.0)			
		78	25+ cig/day	40.7	(21.2, 78.0)			Stratified by center
			Former smoker					
			Years since quitting					Participants excluded if had personal history of cancer at another site
		73	0–10	6.0	(3.0, 11.9)	0.3	(0.2, 0.4)	
		32	11–20	2.4	(1.1, 5.1)	0.1	(0.07, 0.16)	
		27	>20	1.3	(0.6, 2.9)	0.1	(0.04, 0.1)	
		13	Never smoker	1.0		0.04[†]	(0.02, 0.1)	
			WOMEN					
			Current smoker					
		74	<15 cig/day	3.5	(2.2, 5.6)	1.0		
		103	15–24 cig/day	9.6	(6.2, 14.8)			
		42	25+ cig/day	18.3	(10.8, 30.9)			
			Former smoker					
			Years since quitting					
		44	0–10	2.6	(1.5, 4.7)	0.3	(0.2, 0.4)	
		13	11–20	1.1	(0.5, 2.4)	0.1	(0.06, 0.2)	
		18	>20	1.3	(0.6, 2.9)	0.1	(0.08, 0.2)	
		61	Never smoker	1.0		0.1	(0.07, 0.14)	
Godtfredsen et al. (2005) Denmark 1964–2003	3 longitudinal studies 11 151 men 8 563 women	576	Heavy smoker	10.0	(6.8, 14.6)	1.0	(0.5, 1.0)	Outcome= incidence
		52	Reducer	7.0	(4.4, 11.1)	0.7	(0.4, 0.6)	Adjusted for sex, cohort of origin, inhalation habits, tobacco type, years smoked
		104	Light smoker	4.0	(2.6, 6.1)	0.4	(0.4, 0.7)	
		52	Quitter	5.0	(3.2, 7.9)	0.5	(0.1, 0.2)	
		52	Former smoker	2.0	(1.3, 3.2)	0.2	(0.1, 0.1)	
		28	Never smoker	1.0		0.1		

Table 1 (cont). Cohort studies in lung cancer

Reference Country and years of follow-up	Subjects	Number of cases	Smoking cessation/status categories	Relative risk vs. never-smokers	95% CI	Relative risk vs. current smokers	95% CI	Comments
North America								
Garfinkel & Stellman (1988)[b] USA 1982–86	Cancer Prevention Study II 619 925 women		**1-20 cigarettes/day** *With history of heart disease, stroke or cancer*					Outcome=mortality Standardized mortality ratios based on age-specific rates in nonsmokers within cohort. Exposure assessed at baseline only
		335	Current smoker	10.3	(8.6, 12.4)	1.0		
			Years since quitting					
		52	< 2	13.6	(10.0, 18.5)	1.3	(1.0, 1.7)	
		33	3–5	8.4	(5.8, 12.2)	0.8	(0.6, 1.1)	
		20	6–10	3.3	(2.1, 5.2)	0.3	(0.2, 0.5)	
		21	11–15	3.0	(1.9, 4.7)	0.3	(0.2, 0.5)	
		41	≥ 16	1.6	(1.1, 2.2)	0.2	(0.1, 0.3)	
		174	Never smoker	1.0		0.1	(0.08, 0.12)	
			No history of heart disease, stroke, or cancer					
		258	Current smoker	14.5	(12.0, 17.6)	1.0		
			Years since quitting					
		17	< 2	8.9	(5.4, 14.6)	0.6	(0.4, 1.0)	
		15	3–5	7.8	(4.6, 13.2)	0.5	(0.3, 0.8)	
		12	6–10	3.9	(2.2, 7.0)	0.3	(0.2, 0.5)	
		7	11–15	1.9	(0.9, 4.0)	0.1	(0.05, 0.2)	
		19	≥ 16	1.4	(0.9, 2.2)	0.1	(0.06, 0.2)	
		88	Never smoker	1.0		0.1	(0.08, 0.13)	
			≥ 21 cigarettes/day *With history of heart disease, stroke or cancer*					
		195	Current smoker	21.2	(17.3, 26.0)	1.0		
			Years since quitting					
		39	< 2	32.4	(22.9, 45.9)	1.6	(1.1, 2.3)	
		23	3–5	20.3	(13.1, 31.4)	1.0	(0.7, 1.6)	
		17	6–10	11.4	(6.9, 18.8)	0.5	(0.3, 0.9)	
		6	11–15	4.1	(1.8, 9.3)	0.2	(0.1, 0.5)	
		9	≥ 16	4.0	(2.0, 7.8)	0.2	(0.1, 0.4)	
		174	Never smoker	1.0		0.05	(0.08, 0.12)	

Table 1 (cont). Cohort studies in lung cancer

Reference Country and years of follow-up	Subjects	Number of cases	Smoking cessation/status categories	Relative risk vs. never-smokers	95% CI	Relative risk vs. current smokers	95% CI	Comments
Garfinkel & Stellman (1988)[b] USA 1982–86 (contd)			*No history of heart disease, stroke, or cancer*					
		146	Current smoker	27.5	(22.1, 34.3)	1.0		
			Years since quitting					
		14	< 2	24.0	(13.9, 41.4)	0.9	(0.5, 1.6)	
		7	3–5	13.0	(6.1, 27.7)	0.5	(0.2, 1.1)	
		9	6–10	12.4	(6.3, 24.2)	0.5	(0.3, 1.0)	
		2	11–15	2.7	(0.7, 10.9)	0.1	(0.02, 0.4)	
		4	≥ 16	3.6	(1.3, 9.7)	0.1	(0.01, 0.1)	
		88	Never smoker	1.0		0.04	(0.03, 0.5)	
Chyou et al. (1993)[b] USA 1965–90	American Men of Japanese Ancestry Study 7961 men	181	Current smoker	11.4	(6.5, 20.1)	1.0		Outcome= incidence
			Former smoker (pack–years)					Adjusted for age
		14	< 25	2.2	(1.1, 4.8)	0.2	(0.1, 0.3)	*p* for trend = 0.0002
		10	25–49.9	3.1	(1.4, 7.1)	0.3	(0.2, 0.6)	Prevalent cases excluded
		8	≥ 50	6.3	(2.6, 15.3)	0.6	(0.3, 1.2)	Exposure assessed at baseline only
		13	Never smoker	1.0		0.1	(0.06, 0.2)	

Table 1 (cont). Cohort studies in lung cancer

Reference Country and years of follow-up	Subjects	Number of cases	Smoking cessation/status categories	Relative risk vs. never-smokers	95% CI	Relative risk vs. current smokers	95% CI	Comments
Friedman et al. (1997) USA 1979–1987	Kaiser Permanente Medical Care Program cohort study 60 838 participants		WOMEN Years since quitting					Outcome= mortality
			Age 35-49					Current smoker= answered 'yes' to question about still smoking cigarettes regularly or occasionally
		0	2–10	0				
		0	11–20	0				
		0	>20	0				
		1	Never	1.0				
			Age 50-64					
		3	2–10	8.0	(1.9, 33.5)			
		1	11–20	1.8	(0.2, 15.4)			Former smoker= quit smoking cigarettes at least 2 years before completing questionnaire
		0	>20	0				
		5	Never	1.0				
			Age 65-74					
		2	2–10	15.4	(2.2, 109.3)			
		2	11–20	9.6	(1.4, 68.2)			
		3	>20	13.7	(2.3, 82.0)			
		2	Never	1.0				
			Age 75+					
		1	2–10	10.4	(1.1, 100.0)			
		1	11–20	5.7	(0.6, 54.8)			
		1	>20	4.8	(0.5, 46.1)			
		3	Never	1.0				
			All ages					Adjusted by age
		6	2–10	8.4	(3.1, 22.7)			
		4	11–20	3.8	(1.2, 11.9)			
		4	>20	4.4	(1.4, 13.8)			
		11	Never	1.0				

Table 1 (cont). Cohort studies in lung cancer

Reference Country and years of follow-up	Subjects	Number of cases	Smoking cessation/status categories	Relative risk vs. never-smokers	95% CI	Relative risk vs. current smokers	95% CI	Comments
Friedman et al. (1997) USA 1979–1987 (contd)			MEN					Adjusted by age
			Age 35–49					
		1	2–10	–				
		0	11–20	–				
		0	>20	–				
		0	Never	1.0				
			Age 50–64					
		6	2–10	8.0	(2.4, 26.2)			
		2	11–20	1.6	(0.3, 8.2)			
		1	>20	1.0	(0.1, 8.6)			
		5	Never	1.0				
			Age 65–74					
		2	2–10	4.7	(0.9, 24.2)			
		6	11–20	5.4	(1.6, 17.7)			
		1	>20	0.7	(0.1, 6.0)			
		5	Never	1.0				
			Age 75+					
		3	2–10	13.3	(3.0, 59.4)			
		0	11–20	0				
		4	>20	3.1	(0.8, 12.4)			
		4	Never	1.0				
			All ages					
		12	2–10	8.5	(3.9, 18.4)			
		8	11–20	2.7	(1.1, 6.4)			
		6	>20	1.6	(0.6, 4.2)			
		14	Never	1.0				
Hrubec et al. (1997) USA 1954–1980	U.S. veterans (Dorn study) approximately 300 000 subjects (< 0.5% women)		Former smoker (age started)					Outcome=mortality Exposure assessed at baseline only
		91	<15	5.2	(4.1, 6.6)			
		388	15–19	4.4	(3.8, 5.1)			
		213	20–24	3.2	(2.7, 3.8)			
		86	25+	2.0	(1.6, 2.6)			
			Years since quitting					
		56	<5	16.1	(10.4, 24.8)			
		87	5–9	7.8	(5.7, 10.5)			
		261	10–19	5.1	(4.2, 6.1)			
		215	20–29	3.3	(2.8, 4.0)			
		82	30–39	2.0	(1.6, 2.6)			
		49	40+	1.5	(1.1, 2.0)			

Table 1 (cont). Cohort studies in lung cancer

Reference Country and years of follow-up	Subjects	Number of cases	Smoking cessation/status categories	Relative risk vs. never-smokers	95% CI	Relative risk vs. current smokers	95% CI	Comments
Hrubec et al. (1997) USA 1954–1980 (contd)			Former smoker					
			Entire follow-up	2.8	(2.1,3.6)			
			1970–1974 follow-up	3.6	(2.6,4.8)			
			1965–1969 follow-up	3.0	(2.3,3.9)			
			1954–1964	4.8	(3.8,4.0)			
		325	Never smoker	1.0				
Speizer et al. (1999)[b] USA 1976–92	Nurses' Health Study 121 700 women	391	Current smoker	10.0	(7.6, 13.2)	1.0		Outcome=incidence
			Former smoker					Adjusted for age, 2-year follow-up interval and age started smoking
			Years since quitting					
		24	< 2	4.0	(2.5, 6.4)	0.4	(0.2, 0.7)	Excluded women with personal history of cancer at baseline except for non-melanoma skin cancer
		34	2–4.9	6.0	(3.9, 9.2)	0.6	(0.4, 1.0)	
		41	5–9.9	6.0	(4.0, 9.0)	0.6	(0.4, 0.9)	
		17	10–14.9	1.0	(0.6, 1.7)	0.1	(0.1, 0.3)	
		28	≥ 15	1.0	(0.6, 1.6)	0.1	(0.1, 0.2)	
		58	Never smoker	1.0		0.1	(0.1, 0.1)	
Ebbert et al. (2003) USA 1986–1999	Iowa Women's Health Study 41 836 women	387	**1–19 pack-years of smoking**			1.0		Outcome=incidence
			Current smoker					Adjusted for age, physical activity, education, BMI, waist circumference, alcohol use, fruit consumption
			Former Smoker					
			Years since quitting					
		1	0–5	0.7	(0.1, 4.9)	0.04	(0.01, 0.3)	Excluded women with personal history of cancer at baseline
		6	6–10	4.2	(1.7, 10.5)	0.2	(0.1, 0.6)	
		7	11–20	2.1	(1.0, 4.6)	0.1	(0.1, 0.3)	
		11	21–30	2.8	(1.5, 5.5)	0.2	(0.1, 0.3)	
		5	>30	1.1	(0.4, 2.9)	0.1	(0.02, 0.2)	
		30	All	2.0	(1.3, 3.2)	0.1	(0.1, 0.2)	
		94	Never smoker	1.0				

Table 1 (cont). Cohort studies in lung cancer

Reference Country and years of follow-up	Subjects	Number of cases	Smoking cessation/status categories	Relative risk vs. never-smokers	95% CI	Relative risk vs. current smokers	95% CI	Comments
Ebbert et al. (2003) USA 1986–1999 (contd)			**≥20 pack-years**					
		387	Current smokers			1.0		
			Former Smoker					
			Years since quitting					
		74	0–5	15.3	(11.1, 21.3)	0.9	(0.7, 1.1)	
		22	6–10	9.4	(5.7, 15.3)	0.5	(0.3, 0.8)	
		11	11–20	4.3	(2.3, 8.0)	0.2	(0.1, 0.4)	
		7	21–30	7.3	(3.2, 16.7)	0.4	(0.2, 0.9)	
		0	>30	0		0		
		114	All	10.4	(7.8, 14.0)	0.6	(0.5, 0.7)	
		94	Never smokers	1.0				
Anthonisen et al. (2005) USA, Canada 1986–2001	Lung Health Study 5 887 35 to 60 year-old patients with asympto-matic airway obstruction		Continued smoker	~ 2.4		1.0		Outcome=mortality Study is a randomized trial examining smoking cessation programs and use of bronchodilator and their impact on total disease specific mortality Relative risks computed from death rates Participants all had evidence of airway obstruction, but no evidence of other disease
			Intermittent quitter	~ 1.9	p=0.001	~0.8		
			Sustained quitter	1.0		~0.4		

Table 1 (cont). Cohort studies in lung cancer

Reference Country and years of follow-up	Subjects	Number of cases	Smoking cessation/status categories	Relative risk vs. never-smokers	95% CI	Relative risk vs. current smokers	95% CI	Comments
Ebbert et al. (2005) USA 1998–2003	Mayo Clinic patients 5 229 patients with NSCLC and SCLC		**WOMEN**					Outcome=post-diagnosis mortality
			NSCLC					
			Per 10 years of quitting	0.9	(0.8, 1.0)			Adjusted for age at diagnosis, packs per day smoked, years smoked, histology, tumor grade, stage, treatment
			Never smoker	1.0				
			SCLC					
			Per 5 years of quitting	1.0	(0.8, 1.3)			
			Never smoker	1.0				
			MEN					
			NSCLC					
			Per 10 years of quitting	1.0	(0.9, 1.1)			
			Never smoker	1.0				
			SCLC					
			Per 5 years of quitting	1.0	(0.9, 1.2)			
			Never smoker	1.0				
			ALL					
			NSCLC					
			Per 10 years of quitting	1.0	(0.9, 1.0)			
			Never smoker	1.0				
			SCLC					
			Per 10 years of quitting	1.0	(0.8, 1.3)			
			Never smoker	1.0				

Table 1 (cont). Cohort studies in lung cancer

Reference Country and years of follow-up	Subjects	Number of cases	Smoking cessation/status categories	Relative risk vs. never-smokers	95% CI	Relative risk vs. current smokers	95% CI	Comments
Zhang et al. (2005) Canada 1980–1993	Canadian National Breast Screening Study 49 165 women	73	Current smoker	14.0	(7. 6, 26.1)	1.0		Outcome= mortality
			Former smoker					Adjusted for age, education, BMI, moderate physical activity, alcohol consumption, HRT use, total fat, cereal fiber, β-carotene, vitamin A, vitamin C, vitamin E
			Years since quitting					
		14	1–9 yrs	5.5	(2.5, 11.9)	0.4	(0.2, 0.7)	
		6	10–19 yrs	2.7	(1.0, 7.1)	0.2	(0.1, 0.4)	
		1	≥20 yrs	0.6	(0.1, 4.2)	0.04	(0.01, 0.3)	
			Age at quitting					
		1	<30 yrs	0.8	(0.1, 6.1)	0.1	(0.01, 0.4)	
		3	30–39	1.5	(0.4, 5.2)	0.1	(0.03, 0.3)	
		8	40–49	3.7	(1.5, 9.1)	0.3	(0.1, 0.6)	Current smokers defined as those who currently smoke and those who quit smoking for less than 1 year at baseline Exposure assessed at baseline only
		9	50–59	7.8	(3.2, 18.7)	0.6	(0.3, 1.1)	
		12	Never smoker	1.0		0.07	(0.04, 0.13)	
U.S. Surgeon General's Report (1990)[a]	CPS-II (unpublished tabulation)	608	MEN 1–20 cig/day Current smoker	18.8	(14.9, 23.7)	1.0		Outcome=mortality Analyses include prevalent cancers, heart disease, and "sick" at enrollment
			Former smoker					
		33	<1	26.7	(17.8, 40.0)	1.4	(1.0, 2.0)	
		71	1–2	22.4	(16.3, 30.8)	1.2	(0.9, 1.5)	
		82	3–5	16.5	(12.1, 22.4)	0.9	(0.7, 1.1)	Exposure assessed at baseline only
		80	6–10	8.7	(6.4, 11.8)	0.5	(0.4, 0.6)	
		69	11–15	6.0	(4.4, 8.3)	0.3	(0.2, 0.4)	
		144	≥16	3.1	(2.4, 4.1)	0.16	(0.1, 0.19)	
		81	Never smoker	1.0		0.05	(0.04, 0.07)	

Table 1 (cont). Cohort studies in lung cancer

Reference Country and years of follow-up	Subjects	Number of cases	Smoking cessation/status categories	Relative risk vs. never-smokers	95% CI	Relative risk vs. current smokers	95% CI	Comments
U.S. Surgeon General's Report (1990)[a] (contd)			**≥21 cig/day**					
		551	Current smoker	26.9	(20.2, 35.8)	1.0		
			Former smoker					
		64	<1	50.7	(40.2, 64.0)	1.9	(1.5, 2.3)	
		117	1–2	33.2	(23.9, 46.1)	1.2	(0.9, 1.7)	
		96	3–5	20.9	(15.7, 27.7)	0.8	(0.6, 1.0)	
		106	6–10	15.0	(11.2, 20.2)	0.6	(0.4, 0.7)	
		95	11–15	12.6	(9.4, 16.8)	0.5	(0.4, 0.6)	
		112	≥16	5.5	(4.1, 7.4)	0.2	(0.16, 0.3)	
		81	Never smoker	1.0		0.04	(0.03, 0.05)	
			WOMEN					
			1–19 cig/day					
		145	Current smoker	7.3	(5.9, 9.1)	1.0		
			Former smoker					
		5	<1	7.9	(3.2, 19.2)	1.1	(0.4, 2.63)	
		13	1–2	9.1	(5.2, 16.0)	1.3	(0.7, 2.2)	
		7	3–5	2.9	(1.4, 6.2)	0.4	(0.2, 0.8)	
		4	6–10	1.0	(0.4, 2.7)	0.1	(0.05, 0.4)	
		6	11–15	1.5	(0.7, 3.4)	0.2	(0.1, 0.5)	
		23	≥16	1.4	(0.9, 2.2)	0.2	(0.1, 0.3)	
		181	Never smoker	1.0		0.14	(0.11, 0.2)	
			≥20 cig/day					
		434	Current smoker	16.3	(13.7, 19.4)	1.0		
			Former smoker					
		31	<1	34.3	(23.4, 50.2)	2.1	(1.4, 3.1)	
		42	1–2	19.5	(13.9, 27.3)	1.2	(0.9, 1.7)	
		42	3–5	14.6	(10.4, 20.4)	0.9	(0.6, 1.3)	
		32	6–10	9.1	(6.3, 13.3)	0.6	(0.4, 0.8)	
		20	11–15	5.9	(3.7, 9.4)	0.4	(0.2, 0.6)	
		18	≥16	2.6	(1.6, 4.2)	0.2	(0.10, 0.26)	
		181	Never smoker	1.0		0.06	(0.05, 0.08)	

Table 1 (cont). Cohort studies in lung cancer

Reference Country and years of follow-up	Subjects	Number of cases	Smoking cessation/status categories	Relative risk vs. never-smokers	95% CI	Relative risk vs. current smokers	95% CI	Comments
International								
Jacobs et al. (1999)[b] 25 years Baseline examination 1957–1964	Seven-Country Study 12 763 men		Years since quitting					Outcome=mortality
		11	< 1	3.1	1.5–6.3			Relative risks calculated from 25-year mortality rate per 1000 men; adjusted for age and cohort
		19	1–9	1.5	0.8–2.7			
		5	> 10	0.2	0.1–0.5			
		24	Never smoker	1.0				Exposure assessed at baseline only

BMI, body mass index; CI, confidence interval; HC, hospital controls; PC, population controls; CC, cancer controls; HRT, hormone replacement therapy; NCC, non-cancer controls; NSCLC, non-small cell lung cancer; SCLC, small cell lung cancer

*p < 0.05

[a]Study is listed in 1990 Surgeon General's Report "The Health Benefits of Smoking Cessation"

[b]Study is listed in 2004 IARC monograph Vol. 83 "Tobacco Smoke and Involuntary Smoking"

Italicized relative risks and 95% CIs indicate that the results were calculated by the Working Group

The necessary relative risks were calculated by the following principle: $RR_{former\ vs.\ current} = RR_{former\ vs.\ never} / RR_{current\ vs.\ never}$

If results for both former smokers vs. nonsmokers and former smokers vs. current smokers are italicized (e.g. Tverdal (1993), Doll (2004)), relative risks were computed from given mortality rates

$$Standard\ error = \sqrt{\frac{1}{a} + \frac{1}{b}}$$, where a = number of events in the reference category and b=number of events in the former smokers category

$$95\%\ CI = (e^{\ln RR - 1.96 * se}, e^{\ln RR + 1.96 * se})$$

Table 2. Case–control studies: relative risk of lung cancer by years since quitting smoking

Reference	Subjects	Smoking cessation/status categories	Cases	Odds ratio relative to never smokers	95% CI	Odds ratios relative to current smokers	95% CI	Comments
Asia								
Gao et al. (1993)[b] Japan	Men	Current smoker	184	6.6	(3.5, 12.6)	1.0		Outcome=incidence
		Former smoker:						Adjusted for age
		Years since quitting						Participants with
		1–4	31	5.1	(2.3, 11.4)	0.8	(0.5, 1.1)	respiratory diseases were
		5–9	21	3.5	(1.2, 8.0)	0.5	(0.3, 0.8)	excluded from control
		10–14	16	3.8	(1.6, 9.5)	0.6	(0.3, 1.0)	group
		15–19	7	3.3	(1.1, 10.7)	0.5	(0.2, 1.1)	
		≥ 20	8	1.4	(0.5, 3.7)	0.2	(0.1, 0.4)	Ex-smokers= quit 1 year
		Never smoker	13	1.0		0.2	(0.1, 0.4)	or more prior to visiting hospital
								Current smokers= current smokers + quit <1 year prior to visiting hospital
Sobue et al. (1993) Japan	Men	Age at enrolment 55–64						Outcome=incidence
		Current smoker	169			1.0		Ex-smokers=quit 1 year or more prior to enrolment
		Former smoker:						
		Years since quitting						Individuals with smoking-related diseases were
		1–4	30			0.9	(0.5, 1.5)	excluded from controls
		5–9	14			0.5	(0.3, 0.9)	
		10+	14			0.3	(0.2, 0.6)	All individuals started
		60–64						smoking at ages 18–22
		Current smoker	197			1.0		
		Former smoker:						
		Years since quitting						
		1–4	35			0.9	(0.5, 1.5)	
		5–9	24			0.6	(0.3, 1.1)	
		10+	22			0.4	(0.2, 0.6)	
		65–74						
		Current smoker	183			1.0		
		Former smoker:						
		Years since quitting						
		1–4	32			1.0	(0.5, 1.8)	
		5–9	26			0.7	(0.4, 1.3)	
		10+	27			0.4	(0.2, 0.7)	

Table 2 (cont). Case–control studies lung cancer

Reference	Subjects	Smoking cessation/status categories	Cases	Odds ratio relative to never smokers	95% CI	Odds ratios relative to current smokers	95% CI	Comments
Sobue et al. (1993) Japan (contd)	Men	70–79						
		Current smoker	140					
		Former smoker: Years since quitting						
		1–4	31			0.9	(0.4, 1.7)	
		5–9	15			0.5	(0.2, 1.1)	
		10+	25			0.5	(0.3, 0.9)	
Stellman et al. (2001) [b] USA Japan	Men USA (Hospital Controls)	Current smoker	148	40.4	(21.8, 79.6)	1.0		Outcome=incidence
		Former smoker: Years since quitting	207					Adjusted for age, education and hospital
		1–4		20.2		0.5	(0.3, 1.0)	
		5–9		20.2		0.5	(0.2, 0.9)	p for trend < 0.001
		10–15		16.2		0.4	(0.2, 0.8)	
		≥ 16		4.0		0.1	(0.1, 0.2)	
		Never smoker	16	1.0		0.02		
	Japan (Hospital Controls)	Current smoker	107	3.5	(1.6, 7.5)	1.0		Adjusted for age, education and hospital
		Former smoker: Years since quitting	284					
		1–4		3.0		0.9	(0.3, 2.9)	p for trend < 0.001
		5–9		2.7		0.8	(0.3, 1.8)	
		10–15		0.7		0.2	(0.1, 0.5)	
		≥ 16		0.7		0.2	(0.1, 0.4)	
		Never smoker	19	1.0		0.3		
	Japan (Community Controls)	Current smoker	107	6.3	(3.7, 10.9)	1.0		Adjusted for age and education
		Former smoker: Years since quitting	284					
		1–4		3.0		0.9	(0.5, 1.7)	p for trend < 0.001
		5–9		2.7		0.8	(0.5, 1.4)	Excluded cases with other tobacco related cancer
		10–15		0.7		0.2	(0.1, 0.4)	Controls were free of tobacco-related diseases
		≥ 16		0.7		0.2	(0.1, 0.3)	Current smokers included those who had smoked within the past year
		Never smoker	19	1.0		0.2		

Table 2 (cont). Case–control studies lung cancer

Reference	Subjects	Smoking cessation/status categories	Cases	Odds ratio relative to never smokers	95% CI	Odds ratios relative to current smokers	95% CI	Comments
Bhurgri et al. (2002)[b] Pakistan	Men and women	Current smoker	183	33.3	(24.0, 46.1)	1.0		Outcome=incidence
		Former smoker: Years since quitting						Adjusted for age, sex and hospital
		2–4	36	56.7	(36.6, 87.9)	1.7	(0.9, 3.4)	
		5–9	25	30.0	(18.4, 48.9)	0.9	(0.4, 1.8)	Current smoker includes ex-smokers for less than 2 years
		10–14	13	10.0	(5.4, 18.5)	0.3	(0.1, 0.7)	
		15–19	5	6.7	(2.7, 16.9)	0.2	(0.1, 0.5)	
		≥ 20	13	6.7	(3.6, 12.4)	0.2	(0.1, 0.3)	
		Never smoker	45	1.0		0.03	(0.02, 0.05)	
Gajalakshmi et al. (2003) India	Men	Current smoker	113	3.9	(2.9, 5.1)	1.0		Outcome=incidence
		Former smoker: Years since quitting						Adjusted for age, educational level, chewing tobacco, alcohol consumption, and center
		≤3	7	2.2	(1.0, 4.7)	0.6	(0.2, 1.3)	
		3.1–10	9	1.4	(0.7, 2.8)	0.4	(0.2, 0.8)	Controls included both healthy individuals and individuals with non-tobacco-related cancers
		10.1–15	4	1.8	(0.7, 4.9)	0.5	(0.2, 1.5)	
		>15	4	1.0	(0.4, 2.6)	0.3	(0.1, 0.7)	Former smokers were defined as those who stopped smoking at least 1 year prior to enrolment
		Never smoker	87	1.0		0.3	(0.2, 0.4)	The odds ratios presented are from cigarette smokers only

Table 2 (cont). Case–control studies lung cancer

Reference	Subjects	Smoking cessation/status categories	Cases		Odds ratio relative to never smokers	95% CI	Odds ratios relative to current smokers	95% CI	Comments
Europe									
Jedrychowski et al. (1990)[b] Poland	Men	Current smoker	715						Outcome=mortality
		Former smoker: Years since quitting:							Adjusted for age
		>5–10	64		0.7	(0.4, 1.0)			Current smokers
		>10	73		0.4	(0.3, 0.6)			includes those who
		Never smoker	49		1.0				quit <5 years
	Women	Current smoker	107						
		Former smoker Years since quitting							
		>5	13		0.5	(0.2, 1.5)			
		Never smoker	78		1.0				
Becher et al. (1991)[b] Germany	Men and Women	Former smoker: Years since quitting	M	W					Outcome=incidence
		0–1	101	33			1.0		Risks for both sexes and both groups of
		2–4	10	2			1.0	(0.4, 2.2)	controls combined
		5–9	16	2			0.8	(0.3, 1.3)	(Hospital and
		≥10	16	1			0.3	(0.1, 0.5)	population)
		Nonsmoking interval (years)	M	W					Hospital controls had diseases unrelated to
		0–<1	127	34			1.0		smoking
		1–2	11	3			0.7	(0.3, 1.7)	Adjusted for lifetime- cumulative cigarette
		≥3	5	1			0.2	(0.1, 0.5)	consumption
									Smokers who quit <1 year prior to interview were considered current smokers
Jöckel et al. (1992)[b] Germany	Men	Former smoker: Years since quitting							Outcome=incidence
		0–5	111				1.0		Hospital controls and population controls
		> 5–10	16				0.9	(0.4, 1.9)	combined
		> 10	16				0.4	(0.2, 0.7)	
	Women	Former smoker: Years since quitting							Smokers who quit <5 years prior to interview where considered
		0–5	35				1.0		current smokers
		> 5	3				0.2	(0.03, 1.1)	

Table 2 (cont). Case–control studies lung cancer

Reference	Subjects	Smoking cessation/status categories	Cases	Odds ratio relative to never smokers	95% CI	Odds ratios relative to current smokers	95% CI	Comments
Barbone et al. (1997)[b] Italy	Men	Current smoker	562	13.8	(8.7, 21.9)	1.0		Outcome=mortality
		Former smoker:						Cases and controls were deceased men who underwent autopsy
		Years since quitting						
		1–4	32	13.9	(6.8, 28.5)	1.0	(0.7, 1.4)	
		5–14	89	9.1	(5.3, 15.5)	0.7	(0.5, 0.8)	Adjusted for age
		15–24	33	6.8	(3.6, 12.8)	0.5	(0.3, 0.7)	
		≥ 25	15	2.1	(1.0, 4.3)	0.2	(0.1, 0.3)	
		Never smoker	22	1.0		0.1	(0.07, 0.2)	
Pohlabeln et al. (1997)[b] Germany	Men	Current smoker	269	5.0	(3.1, 8.1)	1.0		Outcome=incidence
		Former smoker: Years since quitting						Adjusted for age, region of residence and cumulative cigarette consumption (pack–years)
		< 1	166	101.5	(62.4, 165.1)	20.3	(9.8, 42.3)	
		1	60	34.5	(20.4, 58.4)	6.9	(3.3, 14.2)	
		2–5	77	8.0	(4.8, 13.4)	1.6	(1.0, 2.4)	
		6–10	59	5.0	(3.0, 8.5)	1.0	(0.6, 1.5)	
		11–20	64	3.0	(1.5, 4.2)	0.6	(0.4, 0.8)	
		> 20	29	1.5	(0.6, 1.8)	0.3	(0.2, 0.4)	
		Never/occasional smoker	18	1.0		0.2	(0.1, 0.4)	
Agudo et al. (2000)[b] Europe	Women	Current smoker	880	8.9	(7.5, 10.6)	1.0		Outcome=incidence
		Former smoker: Years since quitting						Adjusted for age and center
		< 9	116	3.8	(2.9, 5.1)	0.4	(0.3, 0.5)	
		10–19	62	1.7	(1.2, 2.4)	0.2	(0.15, 0.25)	Never smokers include smokers who had smoked less than 400 cigarettes in their lifetime.
		20–29	16	0.7	(0.4, 1.2)	0.1	(0.04, 0.1)	
		≥ 30	22	1.1	(0.7, 1.8)	0.1	(0.07, 0.2)	
		Never smoker	460	1.0		0.1	(0.09, 0.11)	Smokers who quit <2 years prior to interview were considered current smokers

Table 2 (cont). Case–control studies lung cancer

Reference	Subjects	Smoking cessation/status categories	Cases	Odds ratio relative to never smokers	95% CI	Odds ratios relative to current smokers	95% CI	Comments
Kreuzer et al. (2000)[b] Germany, Italy	Men	Current smoker	2525			1.0		Outcome=incidence
		Former smoker:	1117					Adjusted for age, center and average amount of smoking
		Years since quitting						
		2–9				0.7	(0.6, 0.8)	Smokers who quit <2 years prior to interview were considered current smokers
		10–19				0.2	(0.2, 0.3)	
		≥ 20				0.1	(0.1, 0.1)	
	Women	Current smoker	501			1.0		
		Former smoker:	172					Hospital controls did not include individuals with smoking-related disease
		Years since quitting						
		2–9				0.5	(0.3, 0.7)	
		10–19				0.2	(0.1, 0.3)	
		≥ 20				0.2	(0.1, 0.3)	
Simonato et al. (2001)[b] Europe	Men	Current smoker	4077	25.0	(20.9, 30)	1.0		Outcome=incidence
		Former smoker:						Adjusted for age, education and center
		Years since quitting						
		2–9	974	17.5	(14.5, 21.2)	0.7	(0.6, 0.7)	Smokers who quit <2 years prior to interview were considered current smokers
		10–19	546	7.5	(6.2, 9.1)	0.3	(0.2, 0.3)	
		20–29	229	5.0	(4.0, 6.2)	0.2	(0.1, 0.2)	
		≥30	89	2.5	(1.9, 3.3)	0.1	(0.06, 0.1)	
		Never smoker	120	1.0		0.04	(0.03, 0.05)	
	Women	Current smoker	891	10.0	(8.9, 11.2)	1.0		Hospital controls did not include individuals with smoking-related disease
		Former smoker:						
		Years since quitting						
		2–9	116	4.0	(3.3, 4.9)	0.4	(0.3, 0.6)	
		10–19	62	2.0	(1.5, 2.6)	0.2	(0.1, 0.3)	
		20–29	16	0.8	(0.6, 1.6)	0.08	(0.05, 0.1)	
		≥30	22	1.0	(0.7, 1.5)	0.1	(0.08, 0.2)	
		Never smoker	467	1.0		0.1	(0.10, 0.14)	
Petrauskaite et al. (2002)[b] Lithuania	Men	Current smoker	148	10.0	(3.7, 27.0)	1.0		Outcome=mortality
		Former smoker:						Adjusted for age and year of death
		Years since quitting						
		2–4	31	11.0	(4.2, 34.0)	1.1	(0.6, 2.0)	Smokers who quit <2 years prior to interview were considered current smokers
		5–9	14	6.0	(2.0, 18.2)	0.6	(0.3, 1.3)	
		10–19	11	4.0	(1.3, 12.6)	0.4	(0.2, 0.9)	
		≥ 20	14	4.0	(1.3, 12.2)	0.4	(0.2, 0.9)	
		Never smoker	4	1.0		0.1	(0.04, 0.3)	

Table 2 (cont). Case–control studies lung cancer

Reference	Subjects	Smoking cessation/status categories	Cases	Odds ratio relative to never smokers NCC CC	95% CI NCC CC	Odds ratios relative to current smokers NCC CC	95% CI CC	Comments
North America								
Morabia & Wynder (1992)[b] USA	Men and Women	Current smoker	36	3.7* 2.3	(1.0, 5.2)	1.0 1.0		Outcome = incidence
		Former smoker:						Bronchioloalveolar carcinoma only
		Years since quitting:						
		1–9	14	2.9* 3.8*	(2.1, 7.1)	0.8 1.7	(0.9, 3.2)	Adjusted for age and sex
		10–19	13	2.6* 2.1	(0.9, 4.9)	0.7 0.9	(0.5, 1.7)	Hospital controls did not
		20–52	9	1.5 1.5	(0.6, 4.0)	0.4 0.7	(0.3, 1.5)	have condition known to
		Never smoker	15	1.0 1.0		0.3 0.4	(0.2, 0.7)	be related to tobacco use *p<0.05
Muscat et al. (1997)[b] USA	Men	Current smoker	120	18.0	(8.3, 39.0)	1.0		Outcome=incidence
		Former smoker:						Adjusted for age and education
		Years since quitting:						
		1–5	23	12.4	(5.2, 29.6)	0.7	(0.4, 1.1)	Hospital controls were
		6–10	20	12.9	(5.3, 31.1)	0.7	(0.5, 1.2)	admitted for conditions
		> 10	56	6.1	(2.8, 13.6)	0.3	(0.2, 0.4)	unrelated to tobacco exposure
		Never smoker	7	1.0		0.1	(0.05, 0.2)	
	Women	Current smoker	100	20.2	(11.1, 36.7)	1.0		
		Former smoker:						
		Years since quitting:						
		1–5	14	15.9	(7.1, 35.4)	0.8	(0.4, 1.4)	
		6–10	11	11.5	(5.0, 26.7)	0.6	(0.3, 1.1)	
		> 10	16	4.2	(2.0, 9.0)	0.2	(0.1, 0.4)	
		Never smoker	13	1.0		0.1	(0.06, 0.2)	
Khuder et al. (1998)[b] USA	Men	Current smoker	245	10.4	(6.6, 16.4)	1.0		Outcome=incidence
		Former smoker:						
		Years since quitting:						
		1–4	88	9.6	(5.8, 15.9)	0.9	(0.7, 1.1)	
		5–14	63	6.4	(3.8, 10.7)	0.6	(0.5, 0.8)	
		≥ 15	63	4.0	(2.4, 6.6)	0.4	(0.3, 0.5)	
		Never smoker	23	1.0		0.04	(0.03, 0.1)	

Table 2 (cont). Case–control studies lung cancer

Reference	Subjects	Smoking cessation/status categories	Cases	Odds ratio relative to never smokers	95% CI	Odds ratios relative to current smokers	95% CI	Comments
Osann et al. (2000)[b] USA	Women	Current smoker	77	14.8	(4.3, 51.4)	1.0		Outcome=incidence
		Former smoker: Years since quitting						Small-cell carcinoma only
		<12	17	8.6	(2.1, 34.9)	0.6	(0.3, 1.0)	Adjusted for age, education and pack–years
		>12 or nonsmoker (Former smokers with long duration of abstinence grouped with never smokers)	4	1.0		0.1	(0.02, 0.2)	
Mao et al. (2001)[b] Canada	Men	Current smoker	869	17.3	(12.4, 24.2)	1.0		Outcome=incidence
		Former smoker: Years since quitting						Adjusted for age group, province, years of exposure to passive smoking, total consumption of vegetables, vegetable juices and meat
		≤ 10	403	14.5	(10.2, 20.6)	0.8	(0.7, 0.9)	
		11–19	214	7.3	(5.0, 10.5)	0.4	(0.3, 0.5)	
		20–28	106	3.5	(2.4, 5.2)	0.2	(0.17, 0.2)	
		≥ 29	55	1.5	(1.0, 2.4)	0.1	(0.07, 0.11)	
		Never smoker	45	1.0		0.1	(0.07, 0.13)	Population controls did not have cancer at any site
	Women	Current smoker	894	13.2	(10.6, 16.4)	1.0		
		Former smoker: Years since quitting						
		≤ 10	327	11.8	(9.0, 15.4)	0.9	(0.9, 1.1)	
		11–19	88	3.3	(2.4, 4.6)	0.3	(0.2, 0.4)	
		20–28	39	1.6	(1.0, 2.3)	0.1	(0.09, 0.18)	
		≥ 29	36	1.5	(1.0, 2.3)	0.1	(0.08, 0.12)	
		Never smoker	161	1.0		0.1	(0.08, 0.12)	

Table 2 (cont). Case–control studies lung cancer

Reference	Subjects	Smoking cessation/status categories	Cases	Odds ratio relative to never smokers	95% CI	Odds ratios relative to current smokers	95% CI	Comments
Stellman et al. (2003)[b] USA	Men White	Current smoker	798	21.0	(15.8, 27.8)	1.0		Outcome=incidence
		Former smoker:						Adjusted for age at diagnosis, BMI, education
		Years since quitting						
		1–10	434	14.5	(10.9, 19.5)	0.7	(0.6, 0.8)	Hospital controls were patients without diagnosis of tobacco-related illness
		11–20	234	7.8	(5.8, 10.6)	0.4	(0.35, 0.5)	
		≥ 21	184	3.7	(2.8, 5.1)	0.2	(0.17, 0.2)	
		Never smoker	60	1.0		0.04	(0.03, 0.1)	
	Black	Current smoker	164	18.2	(7.6, 43.4)	1.0		
		Former smoker:						
		Years since quitting						
		1–10	57	13.7	(5.9, 37.5)	0.8	(0.6, 1.1)	
		11–20	14	4.2	(1.6, 12.7)	0.2	(0.13, 0.4)	
		≥ 21	13	3.9	(1.4, 12.3)	0.2	(0.1, 0.4)	
		Never smoker	6	1.0		0.1	(0.04, 0.2)	
	Women White	Current smoker	702	19.3	(15.4, 24.2)	1.0		
		Former smoker:						
		Years since quitting						
		1–5	167	10.1	(7.9, 13.0)	0.5	(0.4, 0.6)	
		6–15	192	6.7	(4.8, 9.4)	0.35	(0.30, 0.4)	
		≥ 16	138	3.4	(2.6, 4.4)	0.2	(0.15, 0.24)	
		Never smoker	122	1.0		0.1	(0.04, 0.2)	
	Black	Current smoker	102	17.2	(8.7, 33.7)	1.0		
		Former smoker:						
		Years since quitting						
		1–5	24	11.0	(5.0, 24.2)	0.6	(0.4, 1.0)	
		6–15	11	6.5	(2.0, 20.7)	0.4	(0.2, 0.7)	
		≥ 16	15	7.2	(2.9, 17.5)	0.4	(0.2, 0.7)	
		Never smoker	11	1.0		0.1	(0.05, 0.19)	

Table 2 (cont). Case–control studies lung cancer

Reference	Subjects	Smoking cessation/status categories	Cases	Odds ratio relative to never smokers	95% CI	Odds ratios relative to current smokers	95% CI	Comments
South America								
De Stefani et al. (1994)[b] Uruguay	Men	*Manufactured* Current smoker	78			1.0		Outcome=incidence
		Former smoker: Years since quitting						Adjusted for age, residence, education and amount of smoking
		1–4	10			0.5	(0.2, 1.4)	
		5–9	9			0.7	(0.2, 1.9)	
		≥ 10	10			0.5	(0.2, 1.5)	
		Hand-rolled Current smoker	275			1.0		
		Former smoker: Years since quitting						
		1–4	50			0.9	(0.5, 1.4)	
		5–9	17			0.5	(0.3, 1.0)	
		≥ 10	27			0.2	(0.1, 0.3)	
Suzuki et al. (1994)[b] Brazil	Men and Women	Current smoker	78	22.0	(6.5, 76.0)	1.0		Outcome=incidence
		Former smoker: Years since quitting						Adjusted for age, sex, race and smoking in pack-years
		1–5	15	*11.0*	*(5.1, 23.9)*	0.5	*(0.2–1.4)*	
		5–10	10	*11.0*	*(4.7, 25.9)*	0.5	*(0.2–1.5)*	Hospital controls were without cancer and respiratory diseases
		> 10	9	*4.4*	*(1.8, 10.6)*	0.2	*(0.1–0.6)*	
		Never smoker	11	*1.0*		*0.045*	*(0.05-2.0)*	
De Stefani et al. (1996)[b] Uruguay	Men	Current smoker	362	10.9	(6.9, 17.1)	*1.0*		Outcome=incidence
		Former smoker: Years since quitting						Adjusted for age, residence, urban/rural status and education
		1–4	64	*9.0*	*(5.2, 15.9)*	*0.8*	*(0.5, 1.5)*	
		5–9	27	*6.2*	*(3.2, 12.2)*	*0.6*	*(0.3, 1.0)*	
		≥ 10	17	*2.8*	*(1.4, 5.7)*	*0.3*	*(0.2, 0.4)*	
		Never smoker	27	*1.0*		*0.1*	*(0.05, 0.18)*	

Table 2 (cont). Case–control studies lung cancer

Reference	Subjects	Smoking cessation/status categories	Cases	Odds ratio relative to never smokers	95% CI	Odds ratios relative to current smokers	95% CI	Comments
Matos et al. (1998)[b] Argentina	Men	Current smoker	112	*10.0*	*(5.4, 18.6)*	1.0		Outcome=incidence
		Former smoker: Years since quitting						Adjusted for age and hospital
		1–5	28	14.0	(7.0, 28.1)	1.4	(0.8, 2.6)	
		6–10	21	9.0	(4.3, 18.7)	0.9	(0.4, 1.6)	Smokers who quit <1 year before the interview where considered current smokers
		≥ 11	27	3.0	(1.5, 6.0)	0.3	(0.2, 0.6)	
		Never smoker	11	1.0		0.1	(0.06, 0.2)	

BMI – body mass index; CI – confidence interval; HC – hospital controls; PC – population controls; CC – cancer controls; NCC – non-cancer controls
*p < 0.05
[a]Study is listed in 1990 Surgeon General's Report "The Health Benefits of Smoking Cessation"
[b]Study is listed in 2004 IARC monograph Vol. 83 "Tobacco Smoke and Involuntary Smoking"
Italicized relative risks and 95% CIs indicate that the results were calculated by the Working Group
The necessary relative risks were calculated by the following principle: $RR_{former\ vs.\ current} = RR_{former\ vs.\ never} / RR_{current\ vs.\ never}$
If results for both former smokers vs. nonsmokers and former smokers vs. current smokers are italicized (e.g. Tverdal (1993), Doll (2004)), relative risks were computed from given mortality rates

$Standard\ error = \sqrt{\dfrac{1}{a} + \dfrac{1}{b}}$, where a = number of events in the reference category and b=number of events in the former smokers category

$95\%\ CI = (e^{\ln RR - 1.96 * se}, e^{\ln RR + 1.96 * se})$

stopping smoking, but cannot return to the status of never having smoked in the past.

Tables 1 and 2 summarize the results of 22 cohort and 24 case–control studies, respectively, that measure the relative risk of lung cancer in former smokers compared to either continuing or never smokers. Figures 1–4 present these results graphically. Table 3 provides some additional information about the criteria used in these studies to define cessation, exclude subjects with prevalent disease, and account for exposure from pipe and/or tobacco smoking. With the exception of the study by Garfinkel & Stellman (1988), that followed a large cohort in a country with relatively early and high uptake of smoking in women, the tables and figures are restricted to studies published since 1990, since these provide the best indication of the current impact of cigarette smoking and benefits of smoking cessation in the 20 countries represented. For the studies that presented relative risk estimates comparing former smokers with never or current smokers but not both, the Working Group calculated relative risk and 95 percent confidence interval estimates using the following equations:

$$RR_{former\ vs.\ current} = RR_{former\ vs.\ never} / RR_{current\ vs\ never}$$

$$95\%\ CI = (e^{\ln RR - 1.96*se}, e^{\ln RR + 1.96*se}).$$

Standard error(se) = $\sqrt{\frac{1}{a} + \frac{1}{b}}$, where a = number of events in the reference category and b = number of events in the former smokers category;

In the case of two studies (Tverdal *et al.*, 1993; Doll *et al.*, 2004), the Working Group calculated the relative risk and 95% confidence intervals based on the published incidence or death rates. Estimates calculated by the Working Group are shown in italics in Tables 1 and 2 and as open circles with dashed lines for the confidence intervals in

Figures 1-4.

All of the published studies show that the risk of developing or dying from lung cancer is lower among former smokers than in those who continue to smoke, and that the relative risk decreases with time since cessation. The pattern is qualitatively similar when former smokers are compared with never smokers (Figures 1 and 2) or to current smokers (Figures 3 and 4). However, as time since cessation increases, the relative risk estimates decrease towards 1.0 when former smokers are compared to never smokers (shown on an arithmetic scale in Figures 1 and 2) and below 1.0 in the comparison with current smokers (shown on a logarithmic scale in Figures 3 and 4). Several studies report that the relative risk estimates comparing former with never smokers actually reach 1.0, implying that no residual increase in lung cancer risk from past smoking persists among smokers who have quit many years before. However, the interpretation of this finding is complex, because former smokers who have abstained from smoking for twenty or more years usually quit at an early age and have a short duration of smoking. [The Working Group noted that the residual excess risk in former smokers cannot be determined at any particular age except in analyses that stratify simultaneously on age at cessation plus time since cessation or attained age.]

Conceptually, the question of whether lung cancer risk among former smokers ever returns to that of never smokers is important to cancer biologists, even though it has only hypothetical relevance

to smokers contemplating cessation. While smokers cannot return to the status of lifelong nonsmokers, as noted above, the comparison between lung cancer risk in current and former smokers helps to separate the consequences of initiation and residual genetic damage from the promoting effect of continued smoking. As discussed elsewhere, the higher lung cancer risk in a former smoker, compared with a never smoker, exists because of residual genetic damage that persists despite cessation of smoking. Continued smoking accelerates the rate at which clones of abnormal cells accumulate further genetic or epigenetic damage, increasing the likelihood that one or more cells will be transformed into an invasive malignancy. The duration of smoking is more strongly related to lung cancer risk than is any other parameter of smoking (Doll & Peto, 1978; Flanders *et al.*, 2003). However, even in the absence of continued smoking, former smokers have a somewhat higher risk than never smokers of developing lung cancer. The multistage nature of carcinogenesis provides a conceptual framework for understanding why lung cancer risk increases rapidly with continued smoking, but much more gradually after cessation and prolonged abstinence.

The size of the reduction in lung cancer risk observed after smoking cessation is strongly influenced by the risk observed in current smokers in the study populations (Figures 1–4). Therefore, the benefit of smoking cessation appears largest in countries and populations where the full effects of long-term smoking are already manifest, particularly among men in the United States, United Kingdom, and Eastern European countries. In these countries, the relative risk of lung cancer among all male current cigarette smokers compared with that of never smokers now exceeds 20 in many studies, and exceeds 50 among those who have

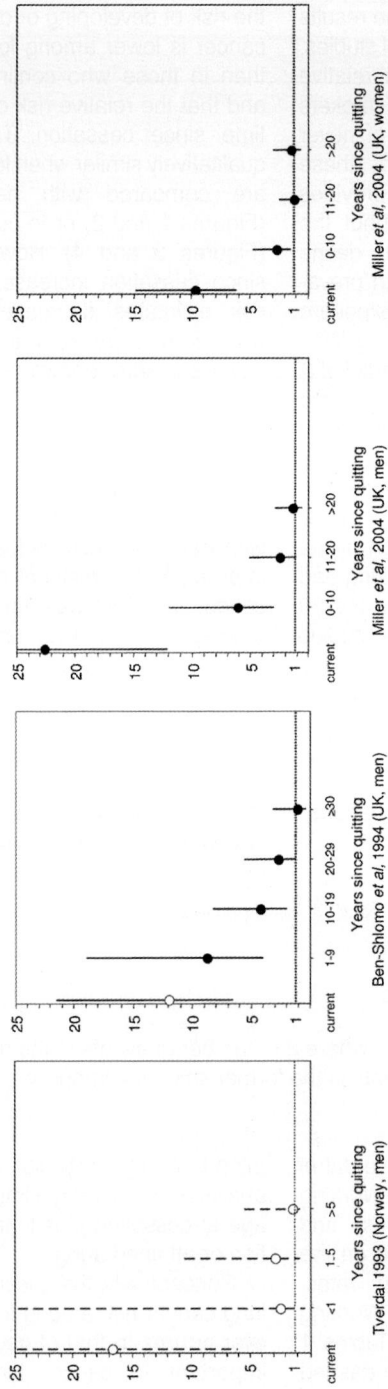

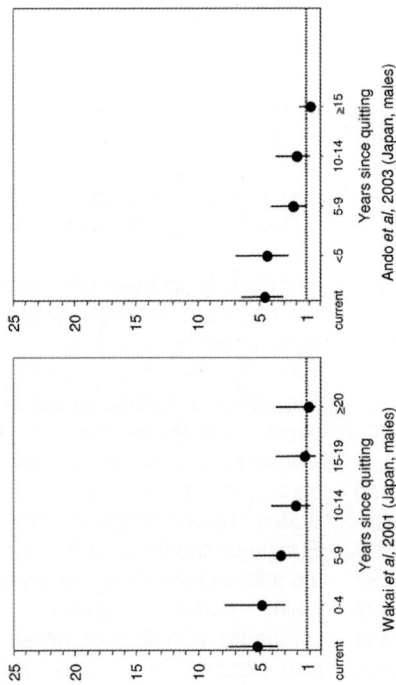

Asia

Europe

Figure 1. Cohort studies comparing the relative risk of lung cancer in former to never smokers by years since quitting

North America

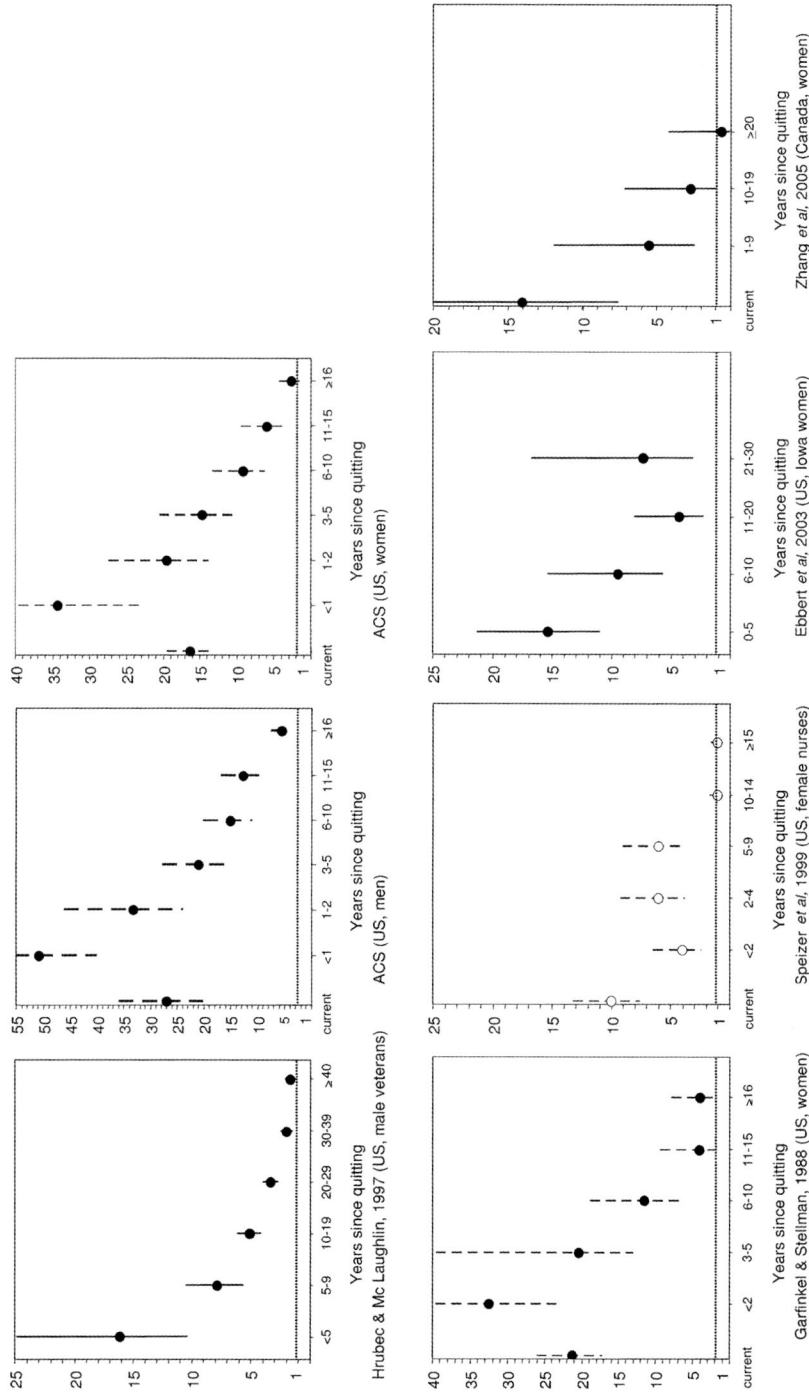

Relative risk estimates as reported in respective studies

Relatived risk estimates calculated by the Working Group

Reported and calculated 95% confidence intervals respectively

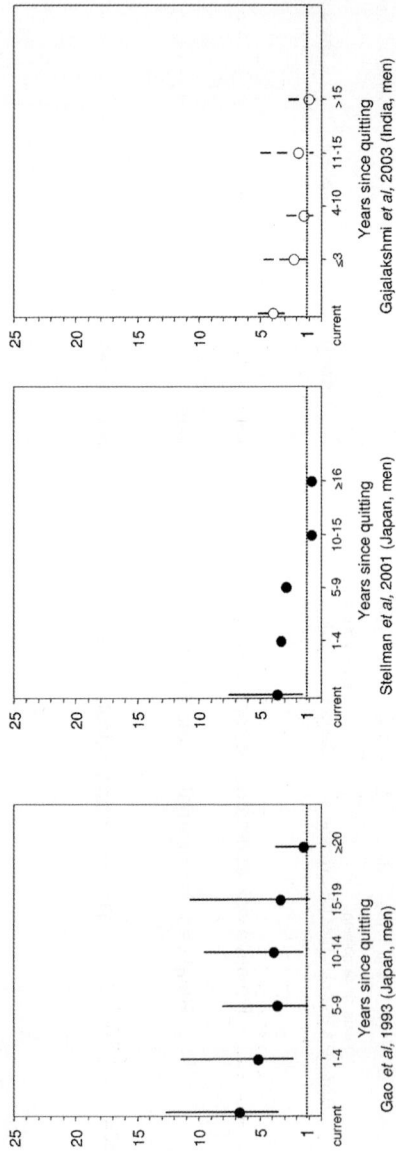

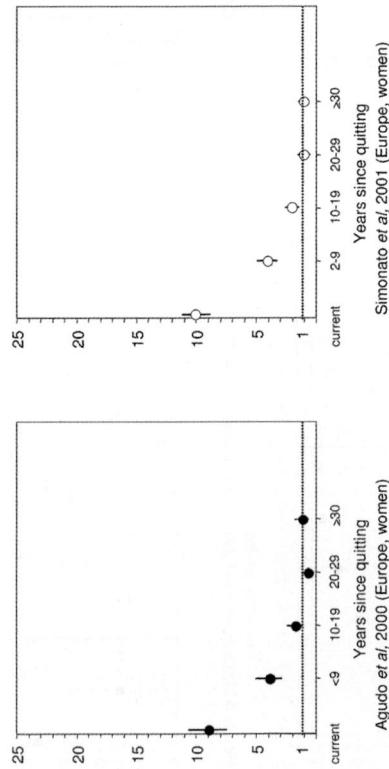

Figure 2. Case–control studies comparing the relative odds of lung cancer in former to never smokers by years since quitting

Europe

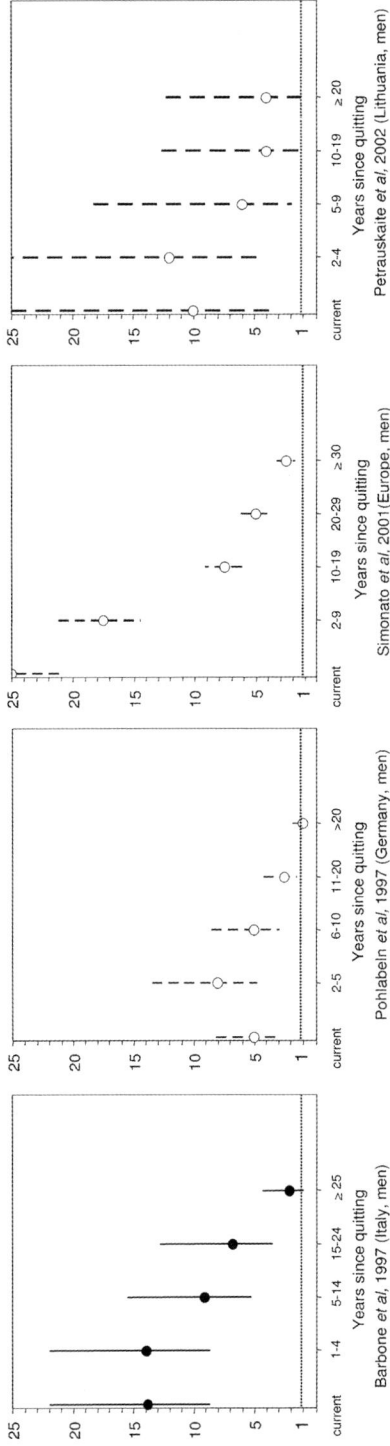

North America

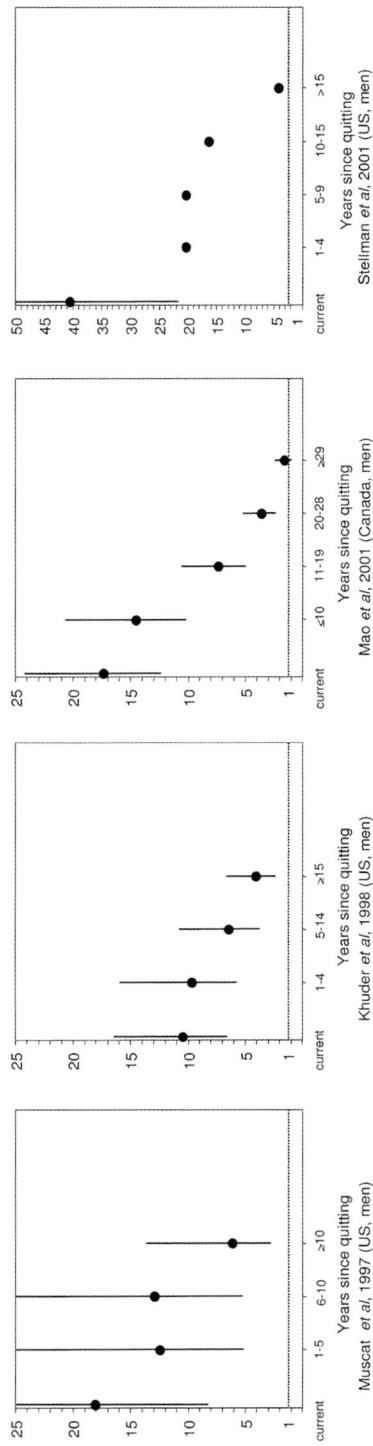

Figure 2. (contd)

North America

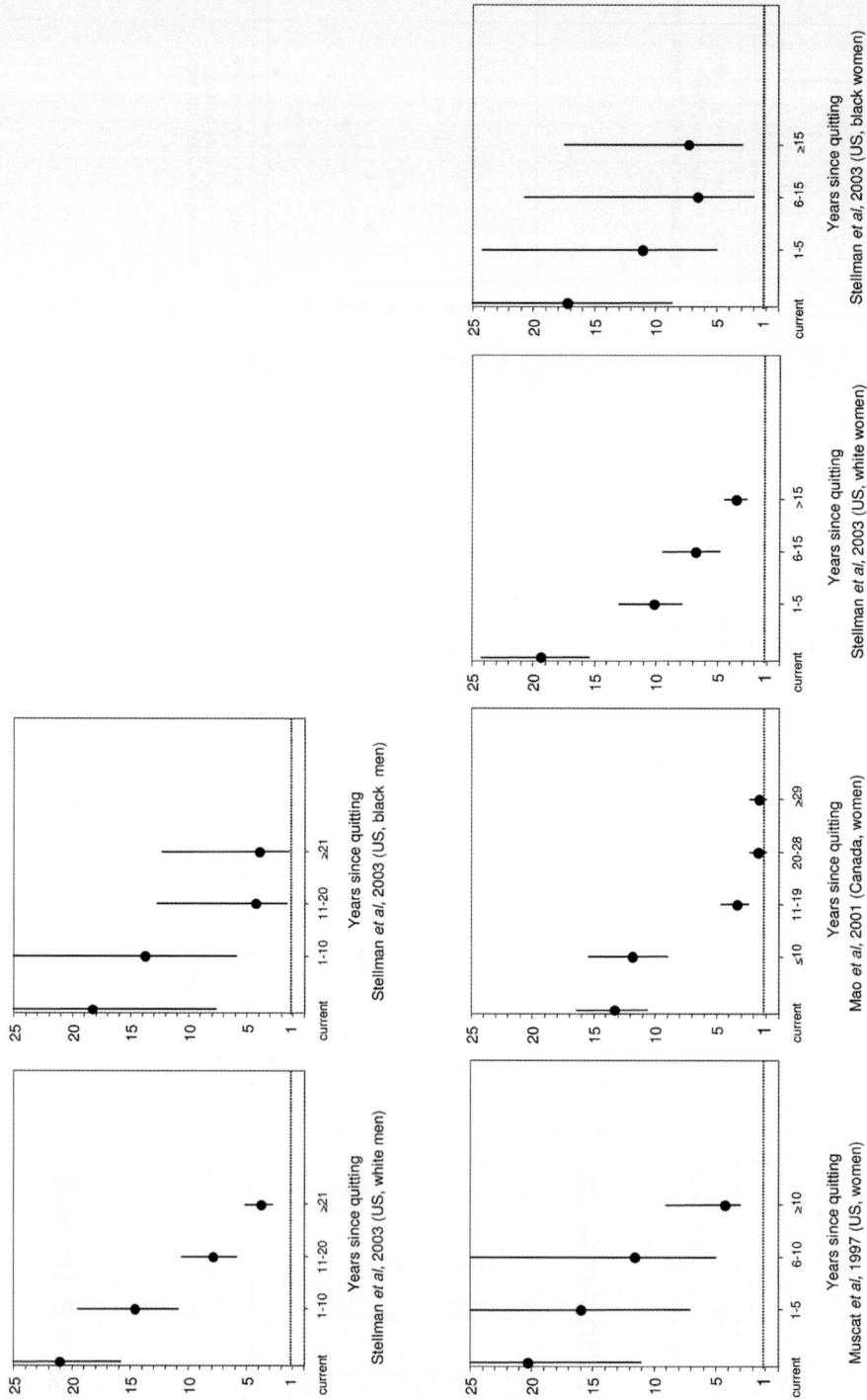

Figure 2. (contd)

South America

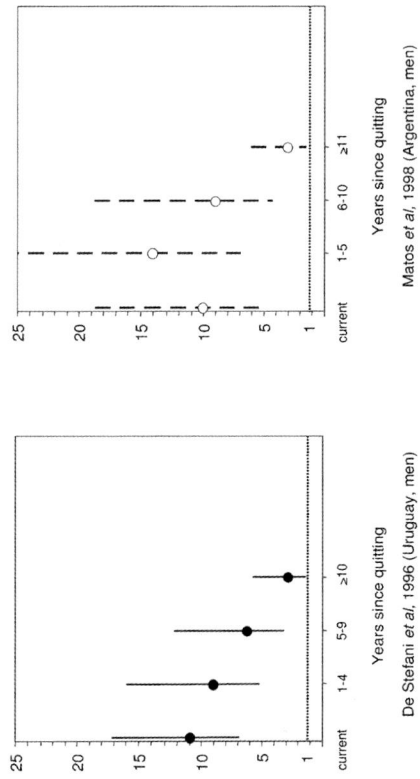

De Stefani *et al*, 1996 (Uruguay, men)

Years since quitting

Matos *et al*, 1998 (Argentina, men)

Years since quitting

- ● Odds ratio estimates as reported in respective studies

- ○ Odds ratio estimates calculated by the Working Group

- ┊┊ Reported and calculated 95% confidence intervals respectively

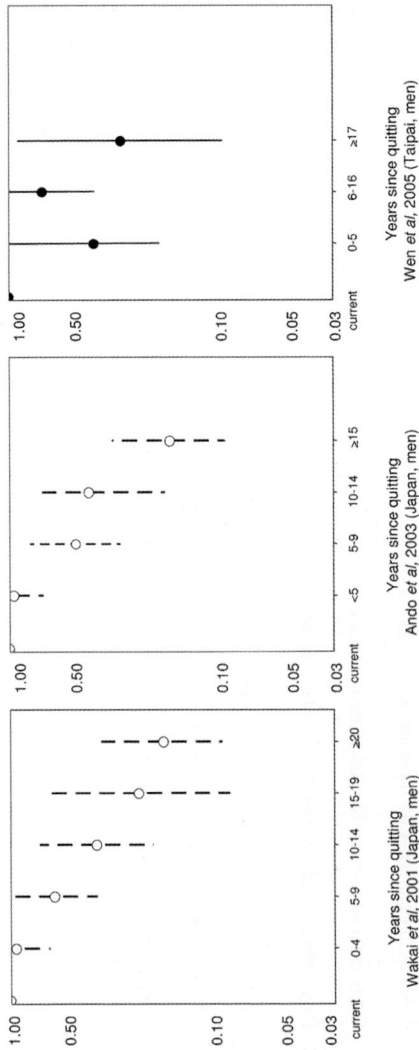

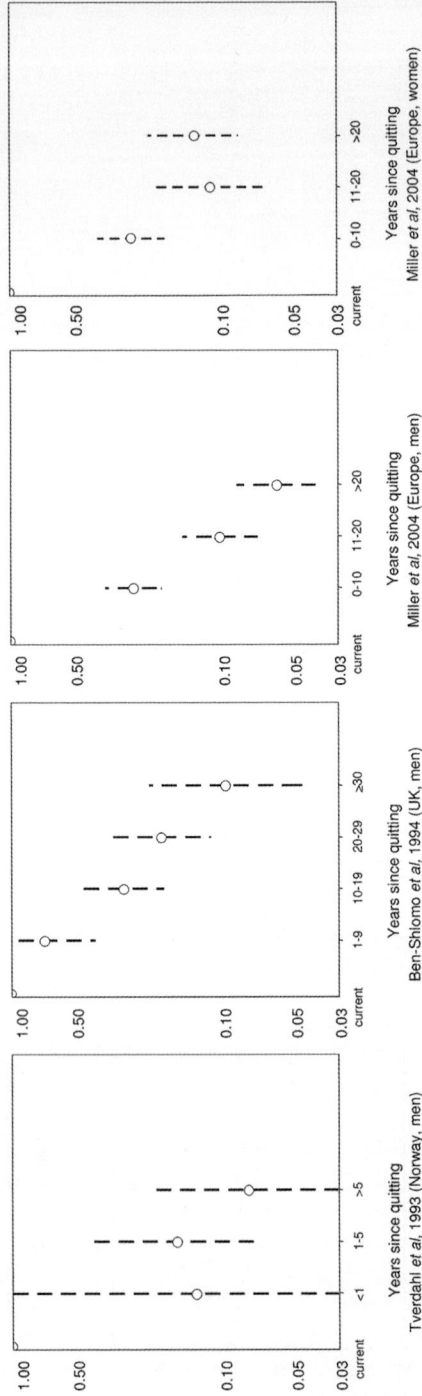

Figure 3. Cohort studies comparing the relative risk in former to current smokers by years since quitting in logarithmic scale

North America

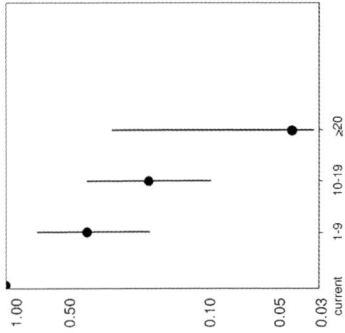

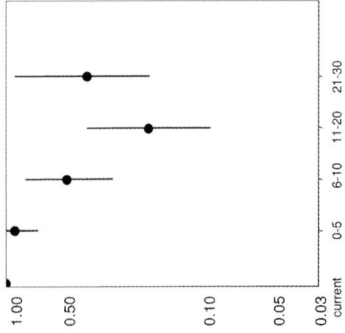

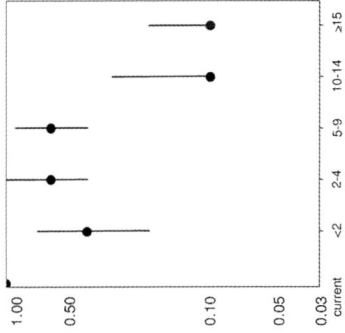

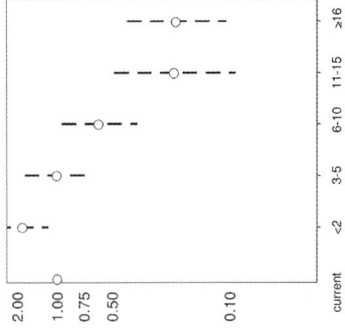

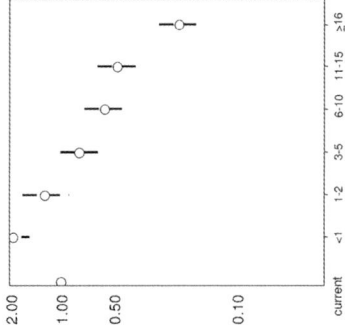

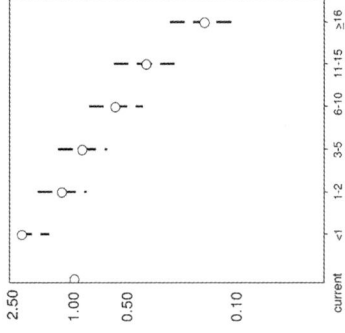

Relative risks estimates as reported in respective studies

Relative risks estimates calculated by the Working Group

Reported and calculated 95% confidence intervals respectively

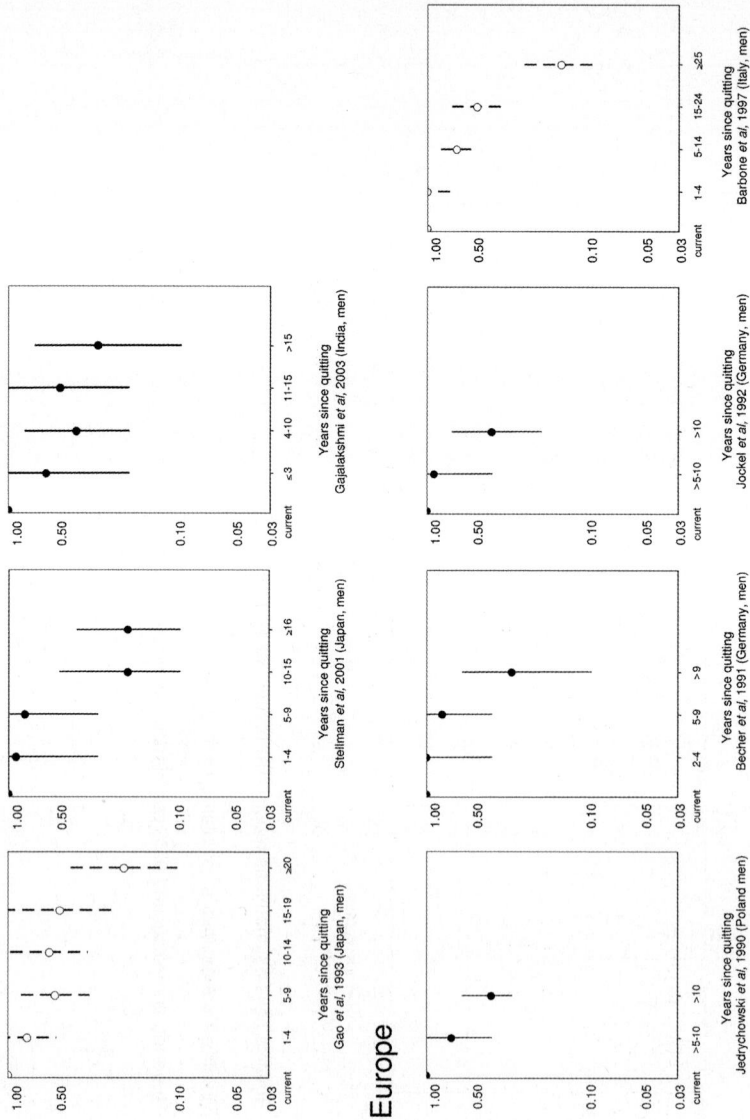

Figure 4. Case–control studies comparing the relative odds of lung cancer in former to current smokers by years since quitting in logarithmic scale

● Odds ratio estimates as reported in respective studies

○ Odds ratio estimates calculated by the Working Group

- - - Reported and calculated 95% confidence intervals respectively

Europe

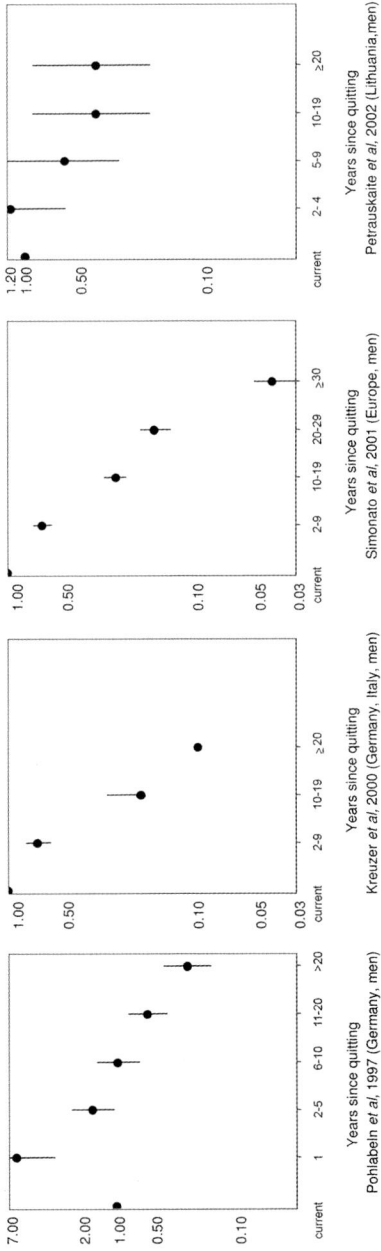

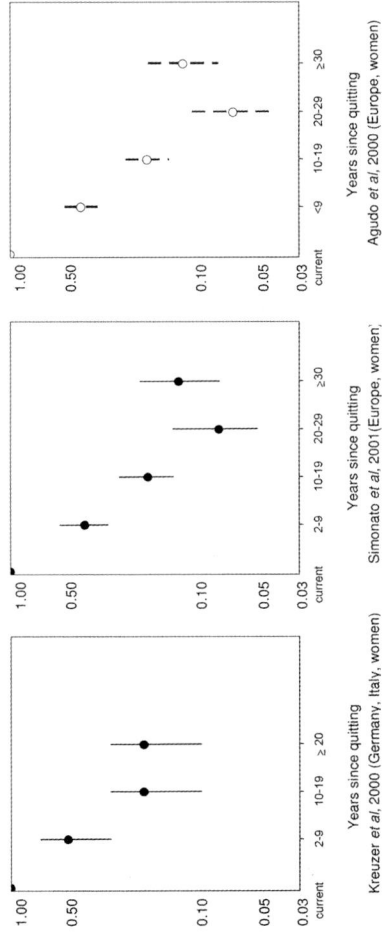

Figure 4 (contd)

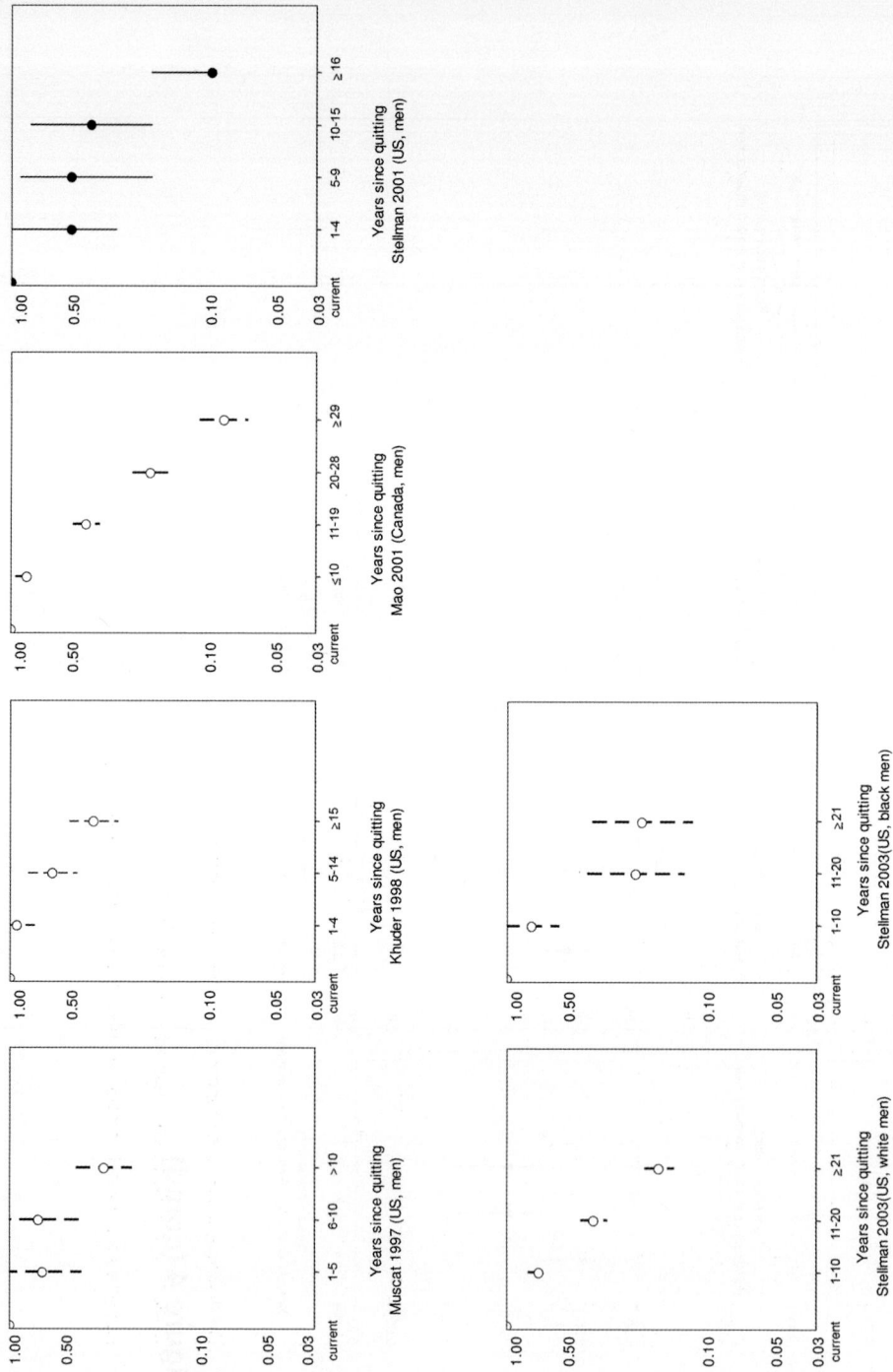

Figure 4 (contd)

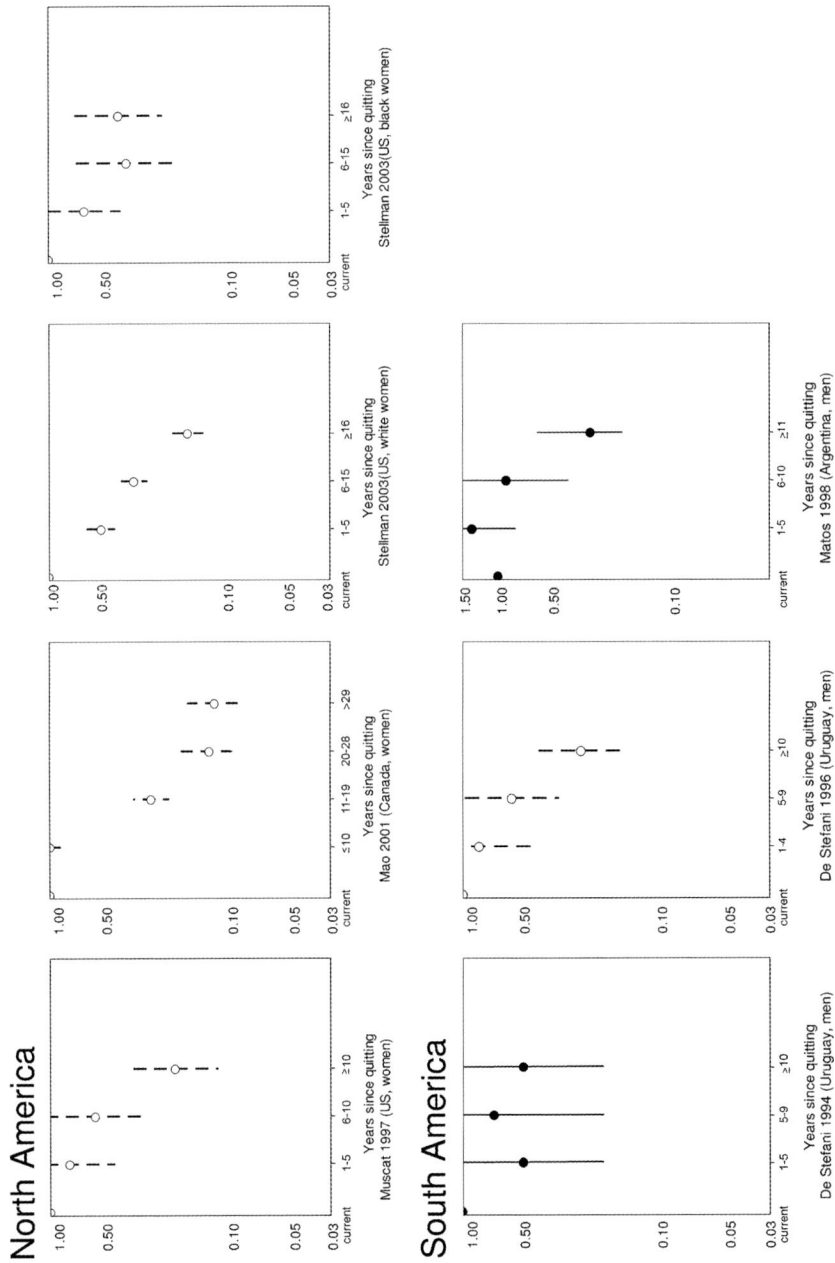

North America

Muscat 1997 (US, women)
Years since quitting
current · 1-5 · 6-10 · ≥10

Mao 2001 (Canada, women)
Years since quitting
current · ≤10 · 11-19 · 20-28 · >29

Stellman 2003(US, white women)
Years since quitting
current · 1-5 · 6-15 · ≥16

Stellman 2003(US, black women)
Years since quitting
current · 1-5 · 6-15 · ≥16

South America

De Stefani 1994 (Uruguay, men)
Years since quitting
current · 1-5 · 5-9 · ≥10

De Stefani 1996 (Uruguay, men)
Years since quitting
current · 1-4 · 5-9 · ≥10

Matos 1998 (Argentina, men)
Years since quitting
current · 1-5 · 6-10 · ≥11

● Odds ratio estimates as reported in respective studies

○ Odds ratio estimates calculated by the Working Group

╎╎ Reported and calculated 95% confidence intervals respectively

Table 3. Criteria used to define cessation, exclude prevalent disease, and account for exposure to smoke from pipe or cigar smoking in studies measuring relative risk of lung cancer in former smokers

Study	Cessation definition	Exclusions	Pipes/cigars
Cohort Studies			
Asia			
Ando et al. (2003)	Those who stopped smoking prior to participation in the study	Prevalent cases of lung cancer	Did not ask about cigars or pipes because almost all tobacco products in Japan are cigarettes
Jee et al. (2004)	Those who smoked, but then quit	Participants with personal history of any type of cancer	Not discussed
Wen et al. (2005)	Those who quit for at least 6 months prior to interview. Current, smoking at time of interview	Not discussed	Not discussed
Europe			
Tverdal et al. (1993)	Those who quit prior to interview	Not discussed	The category for current daily smokers has separate categories for cigarettes only, pipe only; but there is only one category for former smokers: "ex-cigarettes". It is not specified if it excludes former pipe or cigar smokers (it does exclude current pipe and cigar smokers)
BenSchlomo et al. (1994)	Ex-cigarette smokers: ever smoked cigarettes, but did not smoke any tobacco product at baseline	Not discussed	Current cigarette smoker=currently smoking cigarettes, irrespective of whether also smoked pipe or cigar.
Doll et al. (2004)	Those who either were ex-smokers in 1951 whose last habit involved only cigarettes or current cigarette smokers who had stopped. Years of cessation not defined; only category is "ex-smoker"	Not discussed	Cigarettes only; former cigarette smokers who were current pipe/cigar smokers considered secondary pipe or cigar smokers. Those who had never smoked cigarettes but were current cigar or pipe smokers were referred to as primary smokers.
Miller et al. (2004)	Those who quit prior to baseline	Participants with personal history of any type of cancer	Not discussed
Godtfredsen et al. (2005)	Continued ex-smokers, those who were ex-smoker at base-line and at follow-up. Quitters, those who quit during follow-up	Not discussed	This study reports exclusive cigarette use and use of other products (cigars, cheroots, pipes, or mixed).
North America			
Garfinkel & Stellman (1988)	Those who quit prior to baseline	Looked at results among all women and then among those with no history of heart disease, stroke or cancer	Not discussed
Chyou et al. (1993)	Years of cessation not defined; only category is "past"	Excluded prevalent cases of lung cancer	Not discussed

Table 3. Cessation definitions, exclusions and pipe/cigar smoking (contd)

Study	Cessation definition	Exclusions	Pipes/cigars
Friedman et al. (1997)	Ex-smokers, those who quit smoking cigarettes at least 2 years prior to completing questionnaire. Current, those who admitted to ever smoking cigarettes and to still smoke cigarettes regularly or ocassionally	Not discussed	Cigarettes only
Hrubec & McLaughlin (1997)	Those who quit prior to baseline questionnaire	Not discussed	Former cigarette smokers smoked cigarettes regularly in the past but did not smoke cigars or pipes on a regular basis at baseline
Speizer et al. (1999)	Those who quit prior to baseline questionnaire	Participants with personal history of any type of cancer	Not discussed
Ebbert et al. (2003)	Those who quit prior to baseline questionnaire	Participants with personal history of any type of cancer	Not discussed
Anthonisen et al. (2005)	Sustained quitters, those who stopped smoking in the first year after randomisation and maintained biochemically validated abstinence	Participants had evidence of airway obstruction, but little evidence of other diseases	Not discussed
Ebbert et al. (2005)	Those reporting at least 6 months of abstinence at the time of diagnosis	All participants had NSCLC or SCLC (study looked at post-diagnosis mortality)	History of use of other tobacco products obtained during interview, but otherwise not discussed
Zhang et al. (2005)	Ex-smokers, those who quit at least 1 year prior to enrolment. Current, those who were smoking at or quit less than 1 year prior to enrolment	Not discussed	Not discussed
US Surgeon General's Report (1990)	Those who quit prior to baseline	CPS-II lung cancer analyses made no exclusions for prevalent cancer, heart disease, stroke or "sick" at enrolment	Not discussed
Jacobs et al. (1999)	Those who quit prior to baseline	Men who had quit smoking within 1 year before baseline were excluded from analysis	Information on pipe and cigar smoking obtained during interview, but otherwise not discussed

Case-control studies

Asia

Gao et al. (1993)	Ex-smokers, those who quit at least 1 year prior to visiting hospital	Individuals with respiratory diseases or cancer were excluded from the control group	Not discussed

Table 3. Cessation definitions, exclusions and pipe/cigar smoking (contd)

Study	Cessation definition	Exclusions	Pipes/cigars
Stellman *et al.* (2001)	Ex-smokers, those who quit at least 1 year prior to enrolment. Current, those who quit less than 1 year prior to enrolment	Cases-excluded people with history of other tobacco-related cancer. Controls-excluded subjects with history of tobacco related illnesses	Individuals who smoked cigars or pipes exclusively were excluded from analyses; suggests that cigarette smokers (current and ex) who smoke(d) cigars or pipes are not excluded from analysis
Europe			
Jedrychowski *et al.* (1990)	Ex-smokers, those who quit at least 5 years prior to enrolment. Current, those smoking or those who quit than 5 years prior to enrollment	Individuals with diseases of the respiratory tract were excluded from controls	Not discussed
Becher *et al.* (1991)	Ex-smokers, those who quit at least 1 year prior to enrolment. Current smoker, currently smoking or those who quit less than 1 year prior to enrolment	Individuals with diseases related to smoking were excluded from control group	Smokers of pipes and/or cigars were grouped separately for analysis
Jockel *et al.* (1992)	Ex-smokers, those who quit at least 5 years prior to enrolment. Current, those smoking or who quit less than than 5 years prior to enrolment enrolment	Controls excluded if had condition related to smoking	Use of other tobacco products obtained during interview, but otherwise not discussed
Barbone *et al.* (1997)	Those who quit prior to enrolment	Controls excluded if had chronic lung disease or smoking-related cancer	One cigar/pipe=3 cigarettes for exclusive smokers of pipes/cigars; otherwise not discussed
Pohlabeln *et al.* (1997)	Those who quit prior to enrolment	Cases with lung metastases from a different primary tumour were excluded	Not discussed
Agudo *et al.* (2000)	Ex-smokers, those who quit at least 2 years prior to enrolment. Current, those smoking or those who quit less than 2 years ago	Controls excluded if admitted for tobacco related conditions	Excluded participants if smoked tobacco products other than cigarettes
Kreuzer *et al.* (2000)	Ex-smokers, those who quit at least 2 years prior to enrolment. Current, those smoking or who quit less than 2 years ago	Controls excluded if had smoking related disease	Excluded participants if smoked other tobacco products
Simonato *et al.* (2001)	Ex-smokers, those who quit at least 2 years prior to enrolment. Current, those smoking or who quit less than 2 years ago	Controls excluded if had smoking related disease	Excluded participants if smoked other tobacco products
Petrauskaite *et al.* (2002)	Ex-smokers, those who quit at least 2 years prior to enrolment. Current, those smoking or who quit less than 2 years ago	Controls excluded if had cancer of the respiratory tract	Not discussed

Table 3. Cessation definitions, exclusions and pipe/cigar smoking (contd)

Study	Cessation definition	Exclusions	Pipes/cigars
North America			
Morabia & Wynder (1992)	Those who quit prior to baseline	Controls excluded if had tobacco-related cancers, myocardial infarction, emphysema, and chronic bronchitis	Not discussed
Muscat *et al.* (1997)	Those who quit prior to baseline	Controls excluded if had tobacco-related condition	Not discussed
Khuder *et al.* (1998)	Those who quit prior to baseline	Not discussed	Not discussed
Osann *et al.* (2000)	Those who quit prior to baseline; because of small numbers, if quit > 12 years ago, then grouped with non-smokers	Not discussed	Not discussed
Mao *et al.* (2001)	Those who quit prior to baseline	Controls excluded if had cancer at any site	Information on pipe, cigar and chewing tobacco collected but not reported. Not clear if excluded from cigarette analysis
Stellman *et al.* (2003)	Those who quit prior to baseline	Controls excluded if had tobacco-related condition	Not discussed
South America			
De Stefani *et al.* (1994)	Those who quit prior to baseline	Controls excluded if had tobacco-related condition	Not discussed
Suzuki *et al.* (1994)	Those who quit prior to baseline	Controls excluded if had cancer or respiratory disease	20 cigarettes=4 cigars=5 smokes of a pipe; suggests pipe/cigar smokers not excluded
De Stefani *et al.* (1996)	Those who quit prior to baseline	Controls were cancer patients but were excluded if had oral cancer or cancer of pharynx, oesophagus, stomach, bladder	Not discussed
Matos *et al.* (1998)	Ex-smokers, those who quit at least 1 year prior to enrolment. Current, those smoking or who quit less than 1 year prior to enrolment	Controls excluded if had tobacco-related condition	'pipe/cigar only' is excluded from analyses

SCLC: small cell lung cancer
NSCLC: non-small cell lung cancer

smoked 40 cigarettes per day for forty or more years (Thun *et al.,* 2002; Doll *et al.,* 2004). For example, the fifty-year follow-up of male British Doctors illustrates the strength of the association at older ages in lifelong smokers (Table 4) (Doll *et al.,* 2004). The number of lung cancer deaths observed among male doctors who continued to smoke into the age intervals 65-74 or 75-84 years, was 26 and 21 times higher, respectively, than would be expected from the death rate in never-smokers, but was less among former smokers who quit at progressively earlier ages (Table 4). In contrast, the relative risk associated with current smoking is currently much smaller in populations and countries where the maximal impact of tobacco smoking on lung cancer has not yet emerged (Figures 1- 4). The wide range of relative risk estimates associated with time since cessation by smoking intensity is shown in Table 5 and depicted graphically in Figure 5. Contributing to this variation is the wide range in the duration of smok-

ing across these populations. [The Working Group noted that the benefits of smoking cessation are seriously underestimated in countries and populations where the impact of long-term smoking is still increasing].

In order to summarize the information on the long-term benefits of smoking cessation for lung cancer with greater statistic stability, the Working Group elected to combine the results for men and women separately within each geographic region (Asia, Europe, North America, South America). The results were separated by gender, study region and referent group (either current or never smokers). A weighted average of the relative risk was computed for studies within each category (Table 6) (Greenland, 1998). In analyses of categories and duration intervals with no evidence of heterogeneity, weighting was based on the inverse of each study's variance, and the analysis was based on a fixed effects model (Greenland, 1998). When heterogeneity

was present, studies were weighted according to the within and between study variance and analyzed using a random effects model. The analyses combined cohort and case-control studies because of the small number of studies within each category. Only studies that provided 95% confidence intervals were included in this analysis.

The aggregated data show notable differences in the trends across gender and geographic region (Table 6). The highest relative risks in comparisons between former and never smokers are seen among men and women in North America, where six of the seven studies were conducted in the United States. The relative risk estimates are somewhat lower in the studies from Europe, because they represent an average of studies from Southern Europe, where the full effects of smoking are not yet manifest, and those conducted in Northern and Eastern Europe, where lifetime cigarette smoking began much earlier. The magnitude and slope

Table 4. Mortality from lung cancer among never smokers, former smokers, and continuing cigarette smokers, in relation to stopping smoking at ages 35-64 (men born 1900-1930 and observed 1951–2001), compared with that expected at death rates for US male never smokers

	Observed (expected US rate)*					Mortality ratio (UK continuing cigarette smoker versus US lifelong non-smoker)
Age range (years)	Lifelong never smokers	Former cigarette smokers, by age stopped			Continuing cigarette smokers	
		35–44	45–54	55–64		
35–44	1 (0.8)	-	-	-	3 (1.3)	2
45–54	3 (2.2)	1 (1.0	-	-	33 (3.3)	10
55–64	3 (4.3)	1 (1.8)	7 (1.7)	-	58 (4.1)	14
65–74	5 (6.7)	4 (2.7)	11 (2.5)	14 (1.6)	89 (3.4)	26
75–84	6 (5.5)	10 (2.5)	6 (2.2)	10 (1.6)	35 (1.7)	21
Total**	18 (19.5)	16 (8.1)	24 (6.4)	24 (3.2)	218 (13.7)	16
Mortality ratio	0.9	2.0	3.8	7.5	15.9	

*Among US male non-smokers in the five-year range starting at a given age, the annual lung cancer death rate is taken to be 11.2 times the fourth power of (age/1000). This is based on a large US prospective study in the 1980s, but similar results were seen in a large US prospective study in the 1960s, indicating that US never smoker lung cancer death certification rates have been approximately constant over the past few decades.

**Total for former cigarette smokers who stopped at ages 25-34 is observed 7, expected 4.7; mortality ratio is 1.5

Reproduced with permission from Doll et al., BMJ 2004; 328: 1519–1527.

Table 5. Relative risk in former smokers vs. never smokers by duration of abstinence and intensity of smoking

Study	Sex	Years since quitting	Cases	Cig/day	RR (95% CI)	Outcome
Hrubec & McLaughlin (1997) USA	Men	<5	3	1–9	7.6 (2.3, 24.9)	Mortality
			20	10–20	12.5 (7.1, 21.7)	
			22	21–39	20.6 (11.9, 35.6)	
			11	40+	26.9 (13.6, 53.4)	
		5–9	5	1–9	3.6 (1.5, 9.0)	
			27	10–20	5.1 (3.3, 8.0)	
			38	21–39	11.5 (7.8, 17.0)	
			17	40+	13.6 (8.0, 22.9)	
		10–19	15	1–9	2.2 (1.3, 3.6)	
			104	10–20	4.3 (3.4, 5.4)	
			100	21–39	6.8 (5.4, 8.7)	
			42	40+	7.8 (5.6, 10.9)	
		20–39	16	1–9	1.7 (1.0, 2.8)	
			102	10–20	3.3 (2.6, 4.1)	
			61	21–39	3.4 (2.6, 4.5)	
			36	40+	5.9 (4.2, 8.3)	
		30–39	5	1–9	0.5 (0.2, 1.3)	
			39	10-20	2.1 (1.5, 2.9)	
			25	21-39	2.8 (1.9, 4.3)	
			13	40+	4.5 (2.6, 7.9)	
		40+	12	1–9	1.1 (0.6, 1.9)	
			23	10–20	1.6 (1.0, 2.4)	
			10	21–39	1.8 (0.9, 3.3)	
			4	40+	2.3 (0.9, 6.2)	
Simonato et al. (2001) Europe	Men	Current smokers	105	<5	8.3 (6.4, 10.8)	Incidence
			1041	5–14	16.7 (13.8, 20.1)	
			1954	15–24	33.3 (27.7, 40.1)	
			708	25–34	50.0 (41.2, 60.7)	
			269	35+	50.0 (40.3, 62.0)	
		2-9	22	<5	6.7 (4.2, 10.5)	
			246	5–14	10.8 (8.7, 13.5)	
			473	15–24	22.7 (18.6, 27.7)	
			157	25–34	33.0 (26.0, 41.9)	
			76	35+	22.5 (16.9, 30.0)	
		10-19	12	<5	2.3 (1.2, 4.1)	
			175	5–14	5.7 (4.5, 7.1)	
			232	15–24	8.7 (7.0, 10.8)	
			67	25–34	9.5 (7.1, 12.8)	
			60	35+	17.0 (12.5, 23.2)	

Table 5. Relative risk in former vs. never smokers (contd)

Study	Sex	Years since quitting	Cases	Cig/day	RR (95% CI)	Outcome
Simonato et al. (2001) (contd)		20–29	8	<5	2.1 (1.0, 4.3)	
			98	5–14	3.8 (2.8, 5.0)	
			82	15–24	5.3 (4.0, 7.1)	
			29	25–34	8.5 (5.7, 12.8)	
			12	35+	4.5 (2.5, 8.1)	
		30+	8	<5	1.1 (0.5, 2.2)	
			50	5–14	2.0 (1.4, 2.8)	
			22	15–24	2.7 (1.7, 4.2)	
			5	25–34	3.0 (1.2, 7.3)	
			4	35+	3.5 (1.3, 9.5)	
	Women	Current smokers	44	<5	2.5 (1.8, 3.4)	
			330	5–14	6.7 (5.8, 7.7)	
			354	15–24	14.3 (12.4, 16.4)	
			101	25–34	25.0 (20.2, 31.0)	
			62	35+	50.0 (38.4, 65.2)	
		2–9	11	<5	1.7 (0.9, 3.1)	
			48	5–14	3.7 (2.8, 5.1)	
			42	15–24	4.1 (3.0, 5.7)	
			8	25–34	6.8 (3.4, 13.6)	
			9	35+	35.0 (18.1, 67.7)	
		10–19	6	<5	0.5 (0.2, 1.2)	
			24	5–14	1.5 (1.0, 2.2)	
			21	15–24	3.7 (2.4, 5.8)	
			9	25–34	11.0 (5.7, 21.3)	
			2	35+	1.5 (0.4, 6.0)	
		20–29	3	<5	0.4 (0.1, 1.1)	
			8	5–14	0.7 (0.4, 1.5)	
			3	15–24	1.4 (0.5, 4.4)	
			2	25–34	4.0 (1.0, 16.0)	
			0	35+	-	
		30+	9	<5	0.9 (0.5, 1.8)	
			12	5–14	1.9 (1.1, 3.4)	
			1	15–24	0.6 (0.1, 4.1)	
			0	25–34	-	
			0	35+	-	
Garfinkel & Stellman (1988) USA	Women	Current smokers	335	1–20	10.3 (8.6, 12.4)	Mortality
			195	≥ 21	21.2 (17.3, 26.0)	
		<2	52	1-20	13.6 (10.0, 18.5)	
			39	≥ 21	32.4 (22.9, 45.9)	
		3-5	33	1–20	8.4 (5.8, 12.2)	
			23	≥21	20.3 (13.1, 31.4)	

Table 5. Relative risk in former vs. never smokers (contd)

Study	Sex	Years since quitting	Cases	Cig/day	RR (95% CI)	Outcome
Garfinkel & Stellman (contd)		6–10	20	1–20	3.3 (2.1, 5.2)	
			17	≥ 21	11.4 (6.9, 18.8)	
		11–15	21	1–20	3.0 (1.9, 4.7)	
			6	≥ 21	4.1 (1.8, 9.3)	
		≥ 16	41	1–20	1.6 (1.1, 2.2)	
			9	≥ 21	4.0 (2.0, 7.8)	
Surgeon General (1990) USA*	Men	Current smokers	608	1–20	18.8 (14.9, 23.7)	Mortality
			551	≥ 21	26.9 (20.2, 35.8)	
		<1	33	1–20	26.7 (17.8, 40.0)	
			64	≥ 21	50.7 (40.2, 64.0)	
		1–2	71	1–20	22.4 (16.3, 30.8)	
			117	≥ 21	33.2 (23.9, 46.1)	
		3–5	82	1–20	16.5 (12.1, 22.4)	
			96	≥ 21	20.9 (15.7, 27.7)	
		6–10	80	1–20	8.7 (6.4, 11.8)	
			106	≥ 21	15.0 (11.2, 20.2)	
		11–15	69	1–20	6.0 (4.4, 8.3)	
			95	≥ 21	12.6 (9.4, 16.8)	
		≥ 16	144	1–20	3.1 (2.4, 4.1)	
			112	≥ 21	5.5 (4.1, 7.4)	
	Women	Current smokers	145	1–20	7.3 (5.9, 9.1)	
			434	≥ 21	16.3 (13.7, 19.4)	
		<1	5	1–20	7.9 (3.2, 19.2)	
			31	≥ 21	34.3 (23.4, 50.2)	
		1–2	13	1–20	9.1 (5.2, 16.0)	
			42	≥ 21	19.5 (13.9, 27.3)	
		3–5	7	1–20	2.9 (1.4, 6.2)	
			42	≥ 21	14.6 (10.4, 20.4)	
		6–10	4	1–20	1.0 (0.4, 2.7)	
			32	≥ 21	9.1 (6.3, 13.3)	
		11–15	6	1–20	1.5 (0.7, 3.4)	
			20	≥ 21	5.9 (3.7, 9.4)	
		≥16	23	1–20	1.4 (0.9, 2.2)	
			18	≥ 21	2.6 (1.6, 4.2)	

* Data from ACS CPS II
Estimates calculated by the Working Group are shown in italics

By cigarettes per day

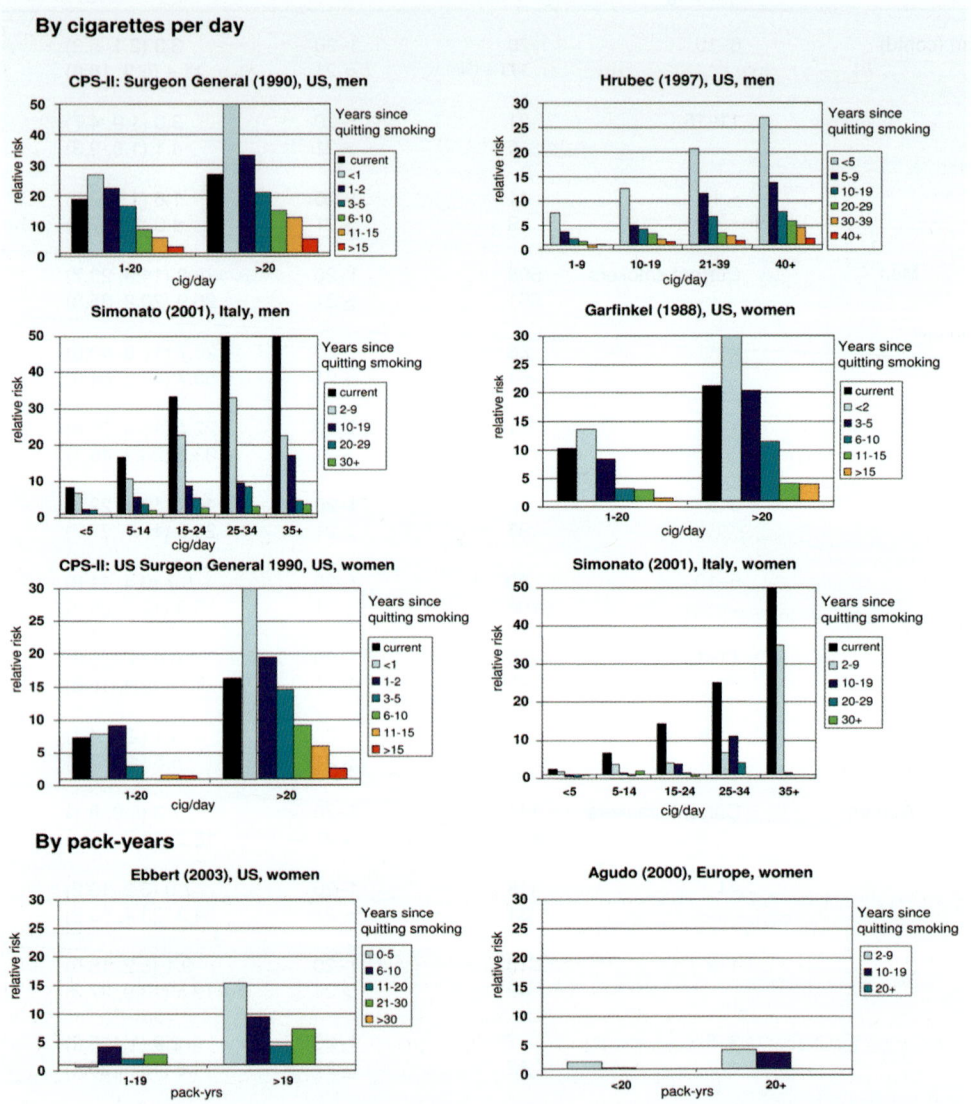

CPS-II: Surgeon General (1990), US, men

Hrubec (1997), US, men

Simonato (2001), Italy, men

Garfinkel (1988), US, women

CPS-II: US Surgeon General 1990, US, women

Simonato (2001), Italy, women

By pack-years

Ebbert (2003), US, women

Agudo (2000), Europe, women

Figure 5. Decline in relative risk among former smokers with increasing time since cessation

Table 6. Aggregated sex- and region-specific relative risk estimates for lung cancer comparing former with never and former with current smokers by years since quitting

	<10		10-19		20-29		30-39	
	RR	95% CI	RR	95% CI	RR	95% CI	RR	95% CI
MEN								
Former vs. never smokers								
N America (7)*	14.29	9.58–21.30	6.36	4.96–8.14	3.42	2.97–3.94	1.88	1.54–2.30
Europe (7)	11.60	6.91–19.5	4.30	2.62–7.06	2.28	1.16–4.49	2.38	1.82–3.12
S America (2)	9.30	5.87–14.72	2.90	1.77–4.75				
Asia (4)	3.42	2.51–4.67	1.75	1.15–2.66	1.12	0.63–2.01		
Former vs. current smokers								
S America (3)	0.83	0.55–1.25	0.31	0.24–0.41				
Asia (6)	0.79	0.66–0.95	0.36	0.26–0.51	0.24	0.14–0.40		
N America (7)	0.78	0.67–0.92	0.28	0.15–0.51	0.20	0.18–0.22	0.10	0.08--0.13
Europe (11)	0.75	0.56–0.99	0.30	0.23–0.41	0.18	0.12–0.29	0.06	0.02–0.14
WOMEN								
Former vs. never smokers								
N America (9)	11.78	8.75–15.87	3.48	2.47-4.89	2.24	0.64–7.84	1.50	0.99–2.27
Europe (3)	3.81	3.27–4.45	1.81	1.47-2.23	0.87	0.62–1.21	1.04	0.77–1.40
Former vs. current smokers								
N America (9)	0.73	0.58–0.92	0.23	0.13-0.40	0.14	0.04–0.42	0.10	0.08–0.12
Europe (4)	0.39	0.32–0.47	0.17	0.12-0.24	0.11	0.07–0.17	0.11	0.08–0.16

RR = Relative Risk
95% CI = 95% confidence interval on the relative risk estimates
*In parentheses: number of studies included per region
Values shown in this table were calculated by the Working Group and are shown in italics

(not shown) of the estimates were similar between men and women in North America, but was more than twice as high in men as in women in Europe, and cannot yet be compared between men and women in Asia or South America. In contrast, analyses that compared former smokers with current smokers found the lowest relative risk estimates among men in Europe and North America and the highest relative risk estimates among men in South America. These regional differences reflect historical differences in tobacco use among men and women in different countries. As stated above, these data underestimate the benefit of

long-term cessation in populations where the full effects of smoking on lung cancer risk are not yet manifest.

The short-term benefits of smoking cessation on lung cancer risk are more difficult to measure than are the long-term benefits. This is because of biases introduced during the early years of follow-up by smokers who quit smoking because of preexisting lung cancer or other health problems from smoking. Even studies that exclude persons with previously diagnosed lung cancer or other smoking-related diseases from analysis of cohort studies, or that exclude the first several years of

follow-up from consideration, are not completely free of this bias. Table 7 presents the results from 14 studies in men and 6 studies of women that suggest, but do not conclusively establish, some benefit in reducing lung cancer risk within the first five years after smoking cessation. None of the RR estimates for men and only two for women are significantly below 1.0.

Absolute risk by age at cessation

Five studies have examined patterns in the absolute risk of lung cancer in relation to age at smoking cessation

(Halpern *et al.,* 1993; Peto *et al.,* 2000; Thun *et al.,* 2002; Doll *et al.,* 2004; Crispo *et al.,* 2004). Peto *et al.* (2000) estimated the cumulative probability of death from lung cancer at various ages among men in the United Kingdom, based on relative risk estimates derived from two case–control studies of current and former smokers who quit at various ages (Doll & Hill, 1950, 1952; Darby *et al.,* 1998). This study combined the relative risk estimates from these case–control studies with age-specific lung cancer death rates among male never smokers in the Cancer Prevention Study (CPS)-II cohort, and with nation-ally representative data on the prevalence of never, current, and former smoking and age-specific lung cancer death rates among men in the United Kingdom. The estimated cumulative incidence of dying from lung cancer at 5-year age intervals between ages 45 and 75 years is shown in Figure 6, and the actual estimates in Table 8.

The results of this analysis provide powerful evidence that: (a) stopping smoking by age 30 avoids more than 90% of the lung cancer risk that would other-wise result from continued smoking and (b) that even people who have smoked for many years but who stop smoking by age 50 avoid much of the lung cancer risk that would result from continuing to smoke (Peto *et al.,* 2000).

Similar results were reported by Thun *et al.* (2002), based on an analysis of the cumulative probability of death from lung cancer among men and women in CPS-II during follow-up from 1984 to 1991 (Figure 7). The cumulative probability is highest in men and women who continue to smoke, becomes progres-sively lower in those who quit at earlier ages, and is lowest in those who never smoked. The actual values from CPS-II, shown both in Figure 7 and Table 8, are somewhat lower than in the previous example, because the analyses exclude prevalent cases and represent the actual values in the study rather than extrapolating to the general population. Nevertheless, the pattern in the two studies (Peto *et al.,* 2000; Thun *et al.,* 2002) is virtually identical.

In a previous report from CPS-II, Halpern *et al.* used logistic regression to model the annual death rate (per 100 000) from lung cancer among men and women who were current smokers, never smokers, or who had stopped smoking at various ages, based on the first six years of follow-up (Figure 8; Halpern *et al.,* 1993). This analysis pro-vides the only published report on the change in absolute lung cancer death rates (per 100 000 per year) following smoking cessation. However, it is limited in that it is based on statistical modeling of the death rates, rather than simple graphical representation of the empirical data, and it does not exclude the first 2–4 years after cessation. Consequently, the model predicts that the annual death rate from lung cancer will increase in the first 2-5 years after cessation, then level off for the next 10–15 years, and then increase again after age 70 or 75 years, although even then the absolute lung cancer risk in former smokers remained substantially less than that of continuing smokers. Despite its limitations, the

Table 7. Short-term benefits of smoking cessation on lung cancer: Relative risk in former smokers with ≤ 5 years since quitting as compared to continuous smokers

Country	Study	RR	95% CI
	Males		
India	Gajalakshmi *et al.* (2003)	0.6	(0.2, 1.3)
Japan	Gao *et al.* (1993)	*0.8*	*(0.5, 1.1)*
Japan	Stellman *et al.* (2001)	0.9	(0.3, 2.9)
Japan	Wakai *et al.* (2001)	*0.9*	*(0.7, 1.0)*
Japan	Ando *et al.* (2003)	*1.0*	*(0.7, 1.3)*
Germany	Becher *et al.* (1991)	1.0	(0.4, 2.6)
Italy	Barbone *et al.* (1997)	*1.0*	*(0.7, 1.4)*
Lithuania	Petrauskaite *et al.* (2002)	1.1	(0.6, 2.0)
United States	Muscat *et al.* (1997)	*0.7*	*(0.4, 1.1)*
United States	Khuder *et al.* (1998)	*0.9*	*(0.7, 1.1)*
United States	Stellman *et al.* (2001)	0.5	(0.3, 1.0)
Uruguay	DeStefani *et al.* (1994)	0.5	(0.2, 1.4)
Uruguay	DeStefani *et al.* (1996)	*0.8*	*(0.5, 1.5)*
Argentina	Matos *et al.* (1998)	1.4	(0.8, 2.6)
	Weighted analysis	*0.9*	*(0.8, 1.0)*
	Females		
United States	Garfinkel & Stellman (1988)	*0.8*	*(0.6, 1.1)*
United States	Muscat *et al.* (1997)	*0.8*	*(0.4, 1.4)*
United States	Speizer *et al.* (1999)	*0.6*	*(0.4, 1.0)*
United States	Ebbert *et al.* (2003)	0.9	(0.7, 1.1)
United States	Stellman *et al.* (2003) (white)	*0.5*	*(0.4, 0.6)*
United States	Stellman *et al.* (2003) (black)	*0.6*	*(0.4, 1.0)*
	Weighted analysis	*0.7*	*(0.5, 0.9)*

95% CI = 95% confidence interval on the relative risk estimates
Estimates calculated by the Working Group are shown in italics

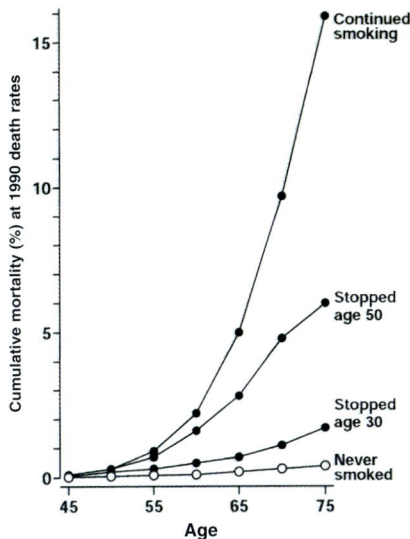

Figure 6. Cumulative risk (%) of death from lung cancer (in the absence of other causes of death) in men at ages 45–75 years; in continuing cigarette smokers, former smokers who stopped at age 50 or at age 30 and lifelong nonsmokers. The estimates are extrapolated to men in the general population of the United Kingdom in 1990.

Reproduced with permission from Peto *et al.*, BMJ 2000; 321: 323–329

model illustrates that the absolute death rate from lung cancer does not decrease after smoking cessation. Rather, the principal benefit of cessation comes from avoiding the much larger increase that would occur with continued smoking.

Other studies (Crispo *et al.*, 2004; Brennan *et al.*, 2006), have measured the cumulative incidence of lung cancer in relation to smoking status among men in selected European countries by combining relative risk estimates from a multicenter case-control study with national lung cancer incidence rates (Figure 9) (Brennan *et al.*, 2006). As in other studies (Halpern *et al.*, 1993;

Peto *et al.*, 2000; Thun *et al.*, 2002; Doll *et al.*, 2004; Crispo *et al.*, 2004), the cumulative probability is highest in men who continue to smoke, progressively lower in those who quit at earlier ages, and lowest in those who never smoked.

Change in risk after cessation by histologic type of lung cancer

Several studies have examined whether the change in risk after lung cancer cessation are similar for adenocarcinoma and squamous cell carcinoma, the two most common histologic types of lung cancer (Barbone *et al.*, 1997; Pohlabeln *et al.*, 1997; Matos *et al.*, 1998; Ebbert *et al.*, 2003). Results from these studies are presented in Table 9 and are shown graphically in Figure 10. The relative risk appears to decrease more rapidly with increasing length of

abstinence for squamous cell carcinoma than for adenocarcinoma.

Synthesis

A large number of epidemiologic studies have compared lung cancer risk in persons who stop smoking with the risk of those who continue. The major published studies show lower lung cancer risk in former than in current smokers. The absolute annual risk of developing or dying from lung cancer does not decrease after stopping smoking. Rather, the principal benefit from cessation derives from avoiding the much steeper increase in risk that would result from continuing to smoke. Stopping smoking before middle age avoids much of the lifetime risk incurred by continuing to smoke. Stopping smoking in middle or old age confers

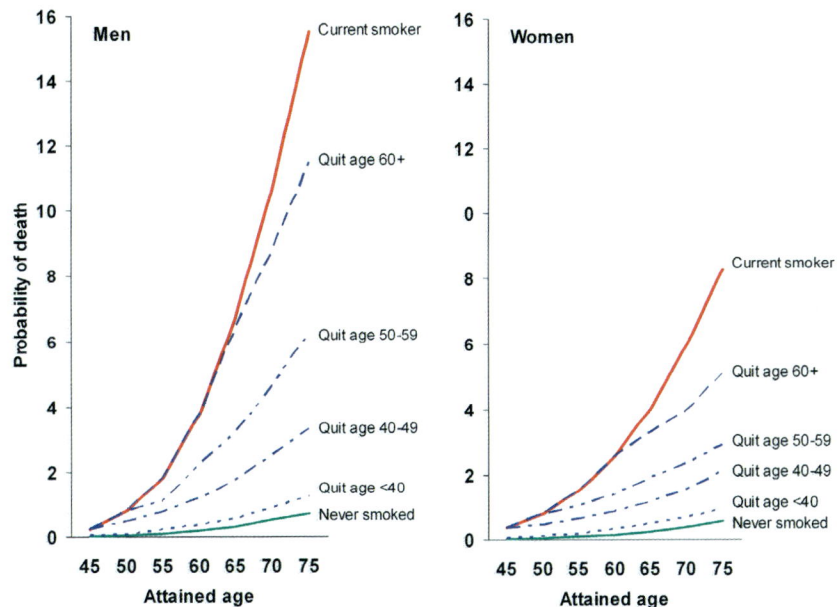

Figure 7. Cumulative probability of death from lung cancer in current smokers, never smokers, and men and women who quit smoking at various ages (CPS-II)

Reprinted by permission by MacMillan Publishers Ltd: Oncogene, Thun *et al.* (2002)

Table 8. Cumulative risk of death from lung cancer by age, smoking status, and age at cessation

UK men 1990[1]

Risk by age	Never[1] Smoker	Current Smoker	Former Smokers (age at cessation in years)			
			<40	40-49	50-59	60+
45	0.0	0.1	0.1	0.1	0.1	0.1
50	0.1	0.3	0.2	0.2	0.3	0.3
55	0.1	0.9	0.3	0.5	0.7	0.9
60	0.1	2.2	0.5	1.0	1.6	2.2
65	0.2	5.0	0.7	1.5	2.8	4.1
70	0.3	9.7	1.1	2.4	4.8	7.2
75	0.4	15.9	1.7	3.0	6.0	9.9

CPS-II men, 1984-1991 (excluding prevalent disease)[2]

Risk by age	Never Smoker	Current Smoker	<40	40-49	50-59	60+
45	0.0	0.1	0.0	0.1	0.1	0.1
50	0.0	0.3	0.1	0.2	0.3	0.3
55	0.1	0.8	0.1	0.5	0.8	0.8
60	0.1	1.9	0.2	0.8	1.1	1.9
65	0.2	3.8	0.4	1.2	2.2	3.8
70	0.3	6.8	0.5	1.8	3.2	6.5
75	0.5	10.6	0.9	2.5	4.6	8.8

CPS-II women, 1984-1991 (excluding prevalent disease)[2]

Risk by age	Never Smoker	Current Smoker	<40	40-49	50-59	60+
45	0.0	0.2	0.2	0.2	0.2	0.2
50	0.0	0.4	0.1	0.4	0.4	0.4
55	0.1	0.8	0.1	0.5	0.8	0.8
60	0.1	1.5	0.2	0.6	1.0	1.5
65	0.2	2.6	0.3	0.9	1.4	2.6
70	0.2	4.0	0.5	1.1	1.9	3.3
75	0.4	6.0	0.7	1.6	2.4	4.0

[1]Smoothed lung cancer death rates during years 3-6 (1984-8) of CPS-II (not excluding prevalent disease) (estimates plotted in Peto et al., 2000)

[2]Excludes first 2 years of follow-up and people who reported prevalent cancer, heart disease, or stroke at enrolment and smokers who quit within 2 years of enrollment (estimates plotted in Thun et al., 2002)

substantially lower lung cancer risk in former smokers compared to continuing smokers.

The full benefits of smoking cessation and hazards of continued smoking are underestimated, at least in absolute terms, in studies of populations where the maximum hazards of persistent lifetime smoking have not yet emerged. Individuals and policymakers who live in countries where lung cancer risk is still increasing should recognize that the maximum hazard from continuing to smoke and the maximum benefits from cessation have not yet been reached. Studies of cessation in these circumstances will seriously under-estimate the long-term benefits of cessation.

Conclusions

Many studies have shown that men and women who stop smoking have substantially lower risk of developing or dying from lung cancer than people who continue to smoke. Quitting smoking at any age avoids much of the future risk of lung cancer that would result from continued smoking. The earlier the age of cessation, the larger the long-term benefit. For individuals who have already begun to smoke, cessation is far more effective than any other measure to avoid the development of lung cancer.

Question 1: Is the risk of lung cancer lower in former smokers than in otherwise similar current smokers?

Yes. The risk of developing or dying from lung cancer is substantially lower in former smokers who quit before developing lung cancer than in those who continue to smoke. The evidence for this is sufficient.

Question 2: Does the difference in lung cancer risk between former smokers and otherwise similar current smokers become larger with time since cessation?

Yes. Within five to nine years after quitting, the lower lung cancer risk in former compared with otherwise-similar current smokers becomes apparent and diverges progressively with longer time since cessation. The evidence for this is also sufficient.

Question 3: Does the risk return to that of never smokers after a long period of abstinence?

No. There is persistent increased risk of lung cancer in former smokers compared to never smokers of the same age, even after a long duration of cessation. The evidence in support of this statement is sufficient.

Table 9. Change in relative risk of lung cancer in former smokers vs. never smokers by years since cessation and histologic type of lung cancer

Study			Adenocarcinoma			Squamous cell carcinoma		
Country	Sex	Years since cessation	Cases	RR	95% CI	Cases	RR	95% CI
Barbone et al.	Men	Current	109	8.2	(3.7, 18.0)	203	19.3	(8.4, 44.5)
(1997)		1-4	7	9.4	(3.0, 29.7)	11	18.7	(6.2, 56.3)
Italy		5-14	23	7.3	(3.0, 17.6)	31	11.9	(4.8, 29.8)
		15-24	7	4.6	(1.5, 13.8)	11	8.1	(2.8, 23.2)
		>24	4	1.8	(0.5, 6.4)	4	1.9	(0.5, 7.2)
		Never	7	1		6	1	
			157			266		
Pohlabeln et al.	Men	Current	57	*2.7*	*(1.3, 5.7)*	116	*14.3*	*(4.5, 44.9)*
(1997)		<1	40	*65.1*	*(30.5, 139.2)*	74	*285.0*	*(89.9, 904)*
Germany		1	18	*27.7*	*(12.0, 63.6)*	25	*97.7*	*(29.5, 323.6)*
		2-5	19	*4.9*	*(2.1, 11.2)*	36	*23.1*	*(7.1, 75.2)*
		6-10	13	*2.7*	*(1.1, 6.6)*	29	*14.7*	*(4.5, 48.3)*
		11-20	22	*2.3*	*(1.0, 5.2)*	18	*4.4*	*(1.3, 15.0)*
		>20	15	*1.5*	*(0.7, 3.6)*	8	*2.0*	*(0.5, 7.5)*
		Never	8	*1.0*		3	*1.0*	
			192			309		
Matos et al.	Men	Current	46	*10*	*(4.0, 25.2)*	33	*10*	*(3.1, 32.6)*
(1998)		1-5	12	*13*	*(4.6, 36.9)*	4	*7*	*(1.6, 31.3)*
Argentina		6-10	9	*10*	*(3.4, 29.8)*	5	*6*	*(1.4, 25.1)*
		≥11	12	*3*	*(1.1, 8.5)*	5	*2*	*(0.5, 8.4)*
		Never	5	*1*		3	*1*	
			84			50		
Ebbert et al.	Women	0-10	35	5.4	(3.5, 8.3)	40	21.8	(11.3, 42.4)
(2003)		11-20	9	2.3	(1.1, 4.6)	5	5.1	(1.8, 14.5)
USA		21-30	13	3.6	(1.9, 7.0)	0		
		>30	2	0.7	(0.2, 3.0)	1	1.8	(0.2, 13.4)
		All	59	3.4	(2.3, 5.0)	46	10.3	(5.4, 19.7)
		Never	27	1		8	1	
			145			100		

Estimates calculated by the Working Group are shown in italics

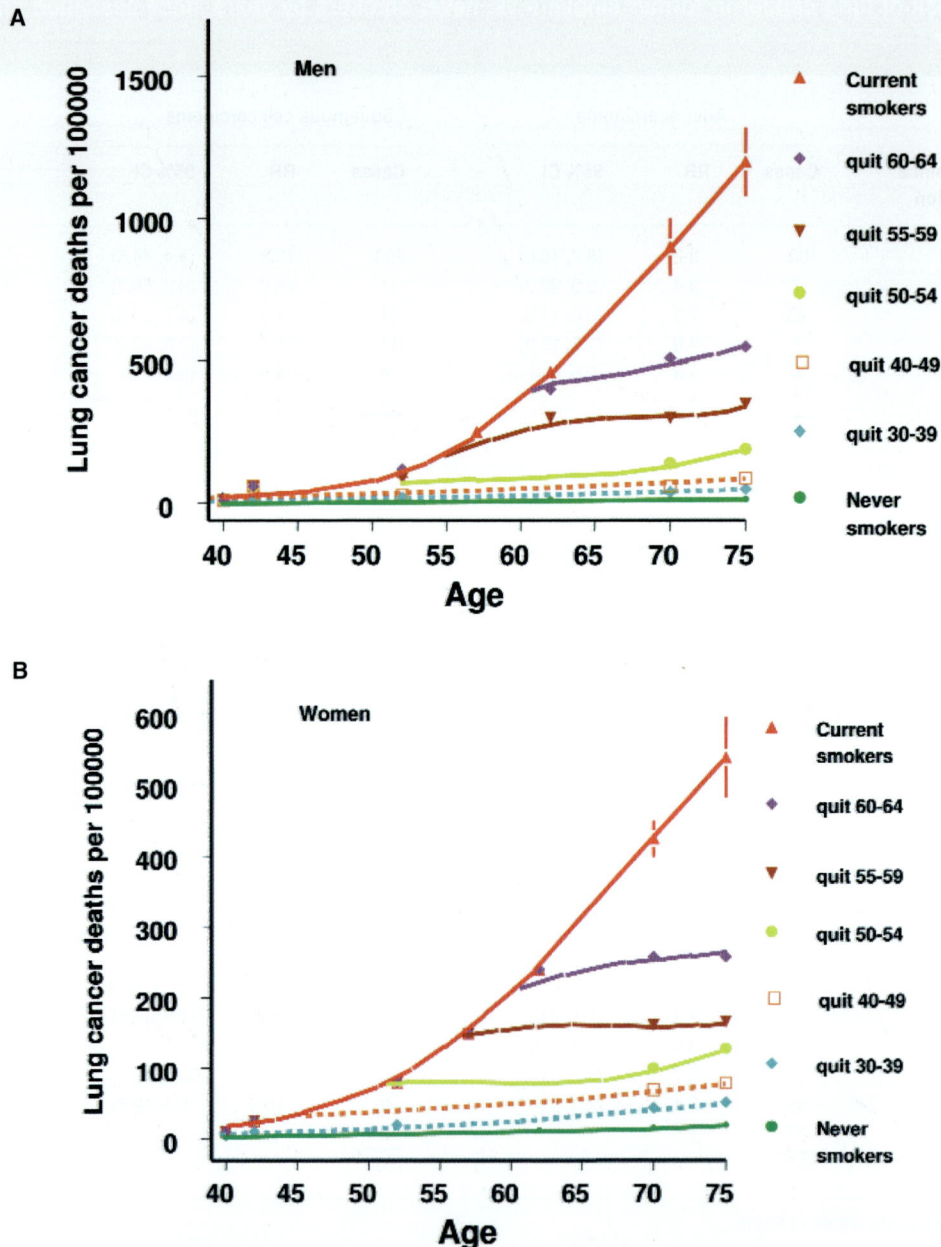

Figure 8. Model estimates of lung cancer death rates by age for men (A) and women (B) current, former, and never smokers, based on smokers who started at age 17.5 and smoked 26 cigarettes/day. Lines (from top to bottom) represent current smokers, former smokers who quit at ages 60–64, 55–59, 50–54, 40–49, 30–39 and never smokers

Adapted from Halpern *et al.* Patterns of absolute risk of lung cancer mortality in former smokers, *J. Natl Cancer Inst.*, 1993, Volume 85 (6), 457–464 by permission of Oxford University Press

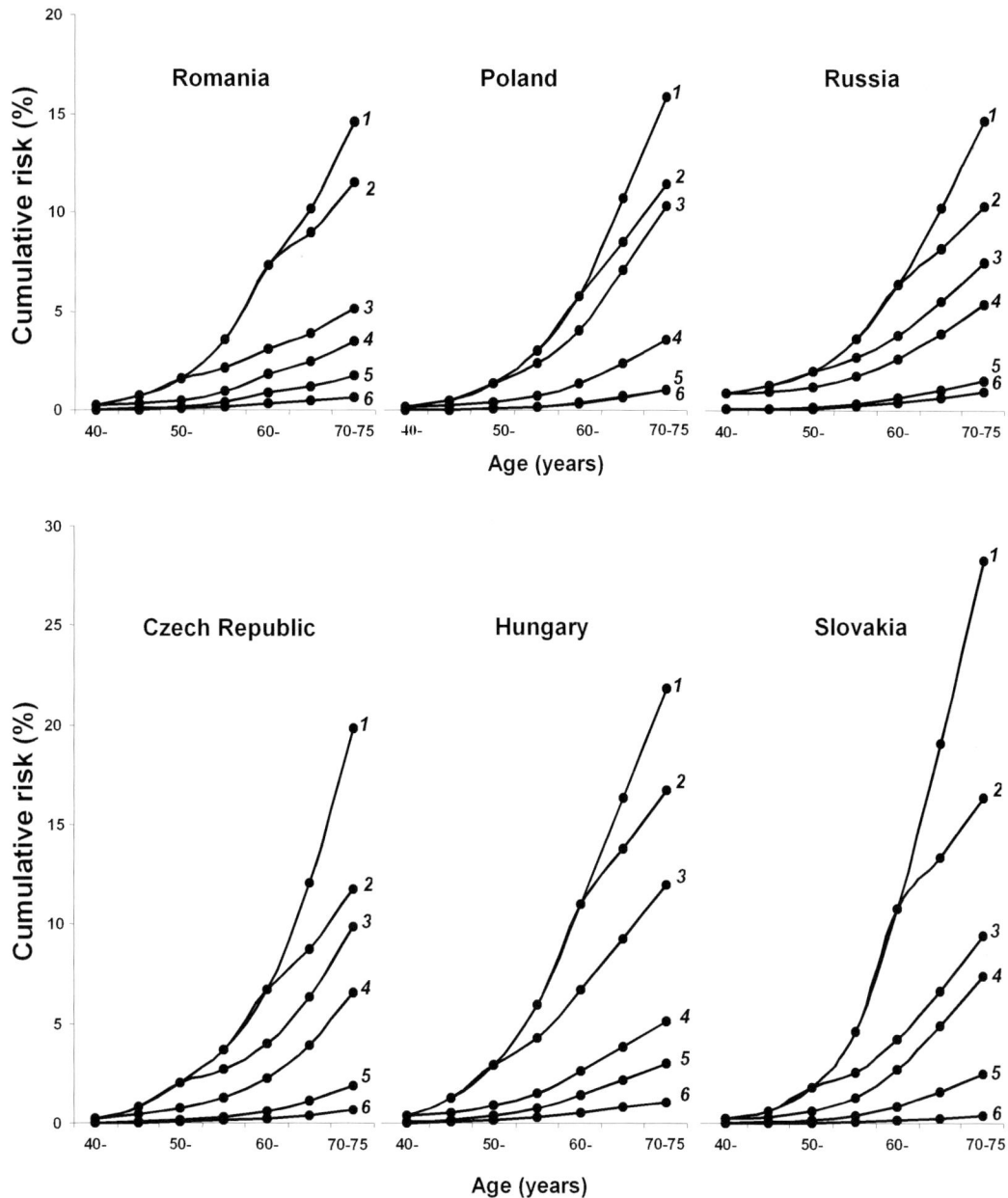

Figure 9. Cumulative risk of lung cancer death by age 75 stratified by age at quitting smoking in 6 Central European countries

1 = continuing smokers; 2 = stopped age $\geq$ 60; 3 = stopped age 50–59; 4 = stopped age 40–49; 5 = stopped age $\leq$40; 6 = lifelong non-smokers

Adapted from Brennan *et al.*, High Cumulative Risk of Lung Cancer Death among Smokers and Nonsmokers in Central and Eastern Europe, *Am. J. Epidemiol.*, Advanced access published on October 10, 2006, by permission of Oxford University Press

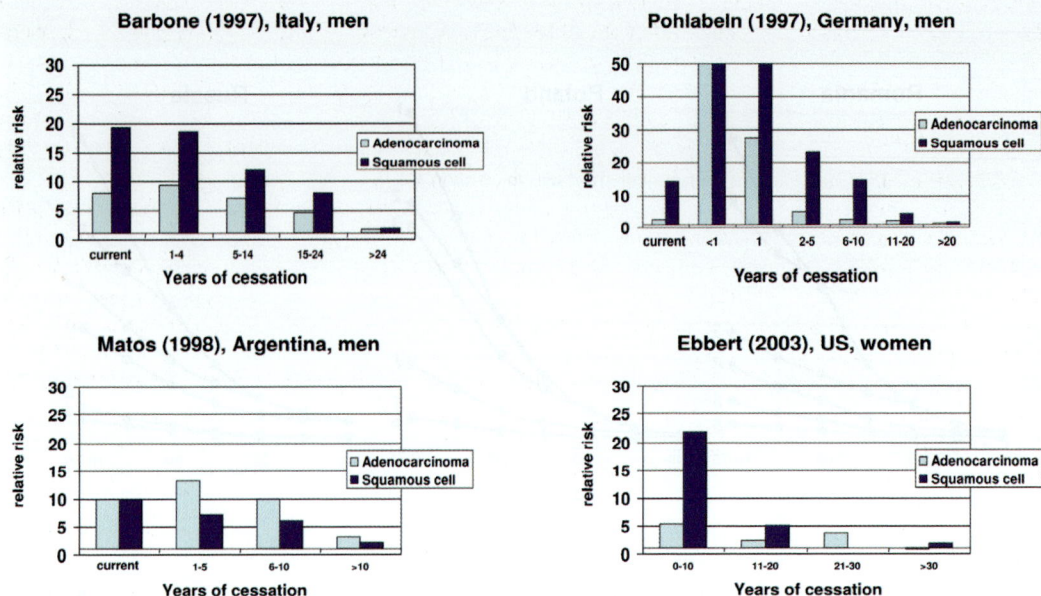

Figure 10. Decline in relative risk among former smokers with increasing time since cessation by histologic type of lung cancer

References

Agudo A, Ahrens W, Benhamou E, et al. (2000). Lung cancer and cigarette smoking in women: a multicenter case-control study in Europe. *Int J Cancer*, 88(5):820-827.

Alderson MR, Lee PN, Wang R (1985). Risks of lung cancer, chronic bronchitis, ischaemic heart disease, and stroke in relation to type of cigarette smoked. *J Epidemiol Community Health*, 39(4): 286-293.

Ando M, Wakai K, Seki N, et al. (2003). Attributable and absolute risk of lung cancer death by smoking status: findings from the Japan Collaborative Cohort Study. *Int J Cancer,* 105(2):249-254.

Anthonisen NR, Skeans MA, Wise RA, et al. (2005). The effects of a smoking cessation intervention on 14.5-year mortality: a randomized clinical trial. *Ann Intern Med*, 142(4):233-239.

Barbone F, Bovenzi M, Cavallieri F, et al. (1997). Cigarette smoking and histologic type of lung cancer in men. *Chest*, 112(6):1474-1479.

Becher H, Jockel KH, Timm J, et al. (1991). Smoking cessation and nonsmoking intervals: effect of different smoking patterns on lung cancer risk. *Cancer Causes Control,* 2(6):381-387.

Ben Shlomo Y, Smith GD, Shipley MJ, et al. (1994). What determines mortality risk in male former cigarette smokers? *Am J Public Health,* 84(8):1235-1242.

Benhamou E, Benhamou S, Auquier A, et al. (1989). Changes in patterns of cigarette smoking and lung cancer risk: results of a case-control study. *Br J Cancer,* 60(4): 601-604.

Best E (1966). *A Canadian Study of Smoking and Health.* Ottawa, Department of National Health and Welfare.

Bhurgri Y, Decullier E, et al (2002). A case control study of lung cancer in Karachi Pakistan. Int J Cancer, 98(6):952-955.

Brennan P (2006). High cumulative risk of lung cancer death among smokers and nonsmokers in Central and Eastern Europe. *Am J Epidemiol* 2006, in press. *Advanced access published on October 10, 2006.*

Carstensen JM, Pershagen G, Eklund G (1987). Mortality in relation to cigarette and pipe smoking: 16 years' observation of 25,000 Swedish men. *J Epidemiol Community Health,* 41(2):166-172.

Cederlof R, Friberg L, Hrubec Z, et al. (1975). *The Relationship of Smoking and Some Social Covariables to Mortality and Cancer Morbidity. A ten year follow-up in a probability sample of 55,000 subjects, age 18-69.* Stockholm, The Karolinska Institute, Department of Environmental Hygiene.

Chyou PH, Nomura AM, Stemmermann GN, et al. (1993). Lung cancer: a prospective study of smoking, occupation, and nutrient intake. *Arch Environ Health*, 48(2):69-72.

Correa P, Pickle LW, Fontham E, et al. (1984). The causes of lung cancer in Louisiana. In: Mizell M, Correa P, eds., *Lung Cancer: Causes and Prevention.* New York NY, Verlag Chemie International: 73-82.

Crispo A, Brennan P, Jockel KH, et al. (2004). The cumulative risk of lung cancer among current, ex- and never-smokers in European men. *Br J Cancer*, 91(7):1280-1286.

Damber LA, Larsson LG (1986). Smoking and lung cancer with special regard to type of smoking and type of cancer. A case-control study in north Sweden. *Br J Cancer,* 53(5):673-681.

Darby S, Whitley E, Silcocks P, et al. (1998). Risk of lung cancer associated with residential radon exposure in south-west England: a case-control study. *Br J Cancer,* 78(3):394-408.

De Stefani E, Fierro L, Larrinaga MT, et al. (1994). Smoking of hand-rolled cigarettes as a risk factor for small cell lung cancer in men: a case-control study from Uruguay. *Lung Cancer,* 11(3-4):191-199.

De Stefani E, Fierro L, Correa P, et al. (1996). Mate drinking and risk of lung cancer in males: a case-control study from Uruguay. *Cancer Epidemiol Biomarkers Prev,* 5(7):515-519.

Doll R, Hill AB (1950). Smoking and carcinoma of the lung; preliminary report. *Br Med J,* 2(4682):739-748.

Doll R, Hill AB (1952). A study of the aetiology of carcinoma of the lung. *Br Med J,* 2(4797):1271-1286.

Doll R, Peto R (1976). Mortality in relation to smoking: 20 years' observations on male British doctors. BMJ, 2(6051):1525-1536.

Doll R, Peto R (1978). Cigarette smoking and bronchial carcinoma: dose and time relationships among regular smokers and lifelong non-smokers. *J Epidemiol Community Health,* 32(4):303-313.

Doll R, Gray R, Hafner B, et al. (1980). Mortality in relation to smoking: 22 years' observations on female British doctors. *BMJ,* 280(6219):967-971.

Doll R, Peto R, Boreham J, et al. (2004). Mortality in relation to smoking: 50 years' observations on male British doctors. *BMJ,* 328(7455):1519.

Ebbert JO, Yang P, Vachon CM, et al. (2003). Lung cancer risk reduction after smoking cessation: observations from a prospective cohort of women. *J Clin Oncol,* 21(5):921-926.

Ebbert JO, Williams BA, Sun Z, et al. (2005). Duration of smoking abstinence as a predictor for non-small-cell lung cancer survival in women. *Lung Cancer,* 47(2):165-172.

Eberly LE, Ockene J, Sherwin R, et al. (2003). Pulmonary function as a predictor of lung cancer mortality in continuing cigarette smokers and in quitters. *Int J Epidemiol,* 32(4):592-599.

Flanders WD, Lally CA, Zhu BP, et al. (2003). Lung cancer mortality in relation to age, duration of smoking, and daily cigarette consumption: results from Cancer Prevention Study II. *Cancer Res,* 63(19):6556-6562.

Friedman GD, Tekawa I, Sadler M, et al. (1997). Smoking and mortality: The Kaiser Permanente experience. In: Burns D, Garfinkel L, Samet J, eds., *Changes in Cigarette-related Disease Risks and their Implications for Prevention and Control.* Bethesda MD, National Cancer Institute: 477-497.

Gajalakshmi V, Hung RJ, Mathew A, et al. (2003). Tobacco smoking and chewing, alcohol drinking and lung cancer risk among men in southern India. *Int J Cancer,* 107(3):441-447.

Gao CM, Tajima K, Kuroishi T, et al. (1993). Protective effects of raw vegetables and fruit against lung cancer among smokers and ex-smokers: a case-control study in the Tokai area of Japan. *Jpn J Cancer Res,* 84(6):594-600.

Gao YT, Blot WJ, Zheng W, et al. (1988). Lung cancer and smoking in Shanghai. *Int J Epidemiol,* 17(2):277-280.

Garfinkel L, Stellman SD (1988). Smoking and lung cancer in women: findings in a prospective study. *Cancer Res,* 48(23): 6951-6955.

Godtfredsen NS, Holst C, Prescott E, et al. (2002). Smoking reduction, smoking cessation, and mortality: a 16-year follow-up of 19,732 men and women from The Copenhagen Centre for Prospective Population Studies. *Am J Epidemiol,* 156(11):994-1001.

Godtfredsen NS, Prescott E, Osler M (2005). Effect of smoking reduction on lung cancer risk. *JAMA,* 294(12):1505-1510.

Graham S, Levin ML (1971). Smoking withdrawal in the reduction of risk of lung cancer. *Cancer,* 27(4):865-871.

Greenland S (1998). Meta-analysis. In:

Greenland KJRS, ed., *Modern Epidemiology.* Philadelphia PA, Lippincott-Raven: 643-673.

Halpern MT, Gillespie BW, Warner KE (1993). Patterns of absolute risk of lung cancer mortality in former smokers. *J Natl Cancer Inst,* 85(6):457-464.

Hammond EC (1966). Smoking in relation to the death rates of one million men and women. In: Haenszel W, ed., *Epidemiological Study of Cancer and Other Chronic Diseases.* (National Cancer Institute Monograph No. 19). 127-204.

Higgins IT, Wynder EL (1988). Reduction in risk of lung cancer among ex-smokers with particular reference to histologic type. *Cancer,* 62(11):2397-2401.

Hrubec Z, McLaughlin JK (1997). Former cigarette smoking and mortality among U.S. Veterans: A 26-year followup, 1954 to 1980. In: Burns D, Garfinkel L, and Samet J, eds., *Changes in Cigarette-related Disease Risks and Their Implication for Prevention and Control.* Bethesda MD, National Cancer Institute: 501-530.

IARC (1986). *IARC Monographs on the Evaluation of the Carcinogenic Risk of Chemicals to Humans, Vol. 38, Tobacco smoking.* Lyon, IARCPress.

IARC (2004). *IARC Monographs on the Evaluation of Carcinogenic Risks to Humans, Vol. 83, Tobacco Smoke and Involuntary Smoking.* Lyon, IARCPress.

Jacobs DR, Jr., Adachi H, Mulder I, et al. (1999). Cigarette smoking and mortality risk: twenty-five-year follow-up of the Seven Countries Study. *Arch Intern Med,* 159(7):733-740.

Jedrychowski W, Becher H, Wahrendorf J, et al. (1990). A case-control study of lung cancer with special reference to the effect of air pollution in Poland. *J Epidemiol Community Health,* 44(2):114-120.

Jee SH, Samet JM, Ohrr H, et al. (2004). Smoking and cancer risk in Korean men and women. *Cancer Causes Control,* 15(4):341-348.

Joly OG, Lubin JH, Caraballoso M (1983). Dark tobacco and lung cancer in Cuba. *J Natl Cancer Inst,* 70(6):1033-1039.

Jöckel KH, Ahrens W, Wichmann HE, et al.

(1992). Occupational and environmental hazards associated with lung cancer. *Int J Epidemiol,* 21(2):202-213.

Kahn HA (1966). The Dorn study of smoking and mortality among U.S. veterans: report on eight and one-half years of observation. In: Haenszel W, ed., *Epidemiolo-gical Study of Cancer and Other Chronic Diseases.* (National Cancer Institute Monograph No. 19). 1-126.

Khuder SA, Dayal HH, Mutgi AB, et al. (1998). Effect of cigarette smoking on major histo-logical types of lung cancer in men. *Lung Cancer,* 22(1):15-21.

Kreuzer M, Boffetta P, Whitley E, et al. (2000). Gender differences in lung cancer risk by smoking: a multicentre case-control study in Germany and Italy. *Br J Cancer,* 82(1):227-233.

Lam TH, He Y, Shi QL, et al. (2002). Smoking, quitting, and mortality in a Chinese cohort of retired men. *Ann Epidemiol,* 12(5):316-320.

Lubin JH, Blot WJ, Berrino F, et al. (1984). Modifying risk of developing lung cancer by changing habits of cigarette smoking. *Br Med J,* 288(6435):1953-1956.

Mao Y, Hu J, Ugnat AM, et al. (2001). Socioeconomic status and lung cancer risk in Canada. *Int J Epidemiol,* 30(4):809-817.

Matos E, Vilensky M, Boffetta P, et al. (1998). Lung cancer and smoking: a case-control study in Buenos Aires, Argentina. *Lung Cancer,* 21(3):155-163.

Miller AB, Altenburg HP, Bueno-De-Mesquita B, et al. (2004). Fruits and vegetables and lung cancer: Findings from the European Prospective Investigation into Cancer and Nutrition. *Int J Cancer,* 108(2):269-276.

Morabia A, Wynder EL (1992). Relation of bronchioloalveolar carcinoma to tobacco. *BMJ,* 304(6826):541-543.

Muscat JE, Stellman SD, Zhang ZF, et al. (1997). Cigarette smoking and large cell carcinoma of the lung. *Cancer Epidemiol Biomarkers Prev,* 6(7):477-480.

Osann KE, Lowery JT, Schell MJ (2000). Small cell lung cancer in women: risk asso-ciated with smoking, prior respiratory

disease, and occupation. *Lung Cancer,* 28(1):1-10.

Pathak DR, Samet JM, Humble CG, et al. (1986). Determinants of lung cancer risk in cigarette smokers in New Mexico. *J Natl Cancer Inst,* 76(4):597-604.

Peto R, Darby S, Deo H, et al. (2000). Smoking, smoking cessation, and lung cancer in the UK since 1950: combination of national statistics with two case-control studies. *BMJ,* 321(7257):323-329.

Petrauskaite R, Pershagen G, Gurevicius R (2002). Lung cancer near an industrial site in lithuania with major emission of airway irritant. *Int J Cancer,* 99(1):106-111.

Pohlabeln H, Jockel KH, Muller KM (1997). The relation between various histological types of lung cancer and the number of years since cessation of smoking. Lung Cancer, 18(3):223-229.

Rogot E, Murray JL (1980). Smoking and causes of death among U.S. veterans: 16 years of observation. *Public Health Rep,* 95(3):213-222.

Simonato L, Agudo A, Ahrens W, et al. (2001). Lung cancer and cigarette smoking in Europe: an update of risk estimates and an assessment of inter-country heterogeneity. *Int J Cancer,* 91(6):876-887.

Sobue T, Yamaguchi N, Suzuki T, et al. (1993). Lung cancer incidence rate for male ex-smokers according to age at cessation of smoking. *Jpn J Cancer Res,* 84(6):601-607.

Sobue T, Yamamoto S, Hara M, et al. (2002). Cigarette smoking and subsequent risk of lung cancer by histologic type in middle-aged Japanese men and women: the JPHC study. *Int J Cancer,* 99(2):245-251.

Speizer FE, Colditz GA, Hunter DJ, et al. (1999). Prospective study of smoking, antioxidant intake, and lung cancer in mid-dle-aged women (USA). *Cancer Causes Control,* 10(5):475-482.

Stellman SD, Takezaki T, Wang L, et al. (2001). Smoking and lung cancer risk in American and Japanese men: an international case-control study. *Cancer Epidemiol Biomarkers Prev,* 10(11):1193-1199.

Stellman SD, Chen Y, Muscat JE, et al. (2003).

Lung cancer risk in white and black Americans. *Ann Epidemiol,* 13(4):294-302.

Suzuki I, Hamada GS, Zamboni MM, et al. (1994). Risk factors for lung cancer in Rio de Janeiro, Brazil: a case-control study. *Lung Cancer,* 11(3-4):179-190.

Thun MJ, Henley SJ, Calle EE (2002). Tobacco use and cancer: an epidemiologic perspective for geneticists. *Oncogene,* 21(48):7307-7325.

Tverdal A, Thelle D, Stensvold I, et al. (1993). Mortality in relation to smoking history: 13 years' follow-up of 68,000 Norwegian men and women 35-49 years. *J Clin Epidemiol,* 46(5):475-487.

United States Department of Health and Human Service (USDHHS) (1990). *The Health Benefits of Smoking Cessation. A Report of the Surgeon General.* Rockville, MD, Centers for Disease Control, Office on Smoking and Health.

United States Department of Health and Human Service (USDHHS) (2004). *The Health Consequences of Smoking. A Report of the Surgeon General.* Atlanta, GA, U. S. Department of Health and Human Services, Centers for Disease Control and Prevention, Office on Smoking and Health.

Wakai K, Seki N, Tamakoshi A, et al. (2001). Decrease in risk of lung cancer death in males after smoking cessation by age at quitting: findings from the JACC study. *Jpn J Cancer Res,* 92(8):821-828.

Wen CP, Cheng TY, Lin CL, et al. (2005). The health benefits of smoking cessation for adult smokers and for pregnant women in Taiwan. *Tob Control,* 14 Suppl. 1:i56-i61.

Wigle DT, Mao Y, Grace M (1980). Relative importance of smoking as a risk factor for selected cancers. *Can J Public Health,* 71(4):269-275.

Wu AH, Henderson BE, Pike MC, et al. (1985). Smoking and other risk factors for lung cancer in women. *J Natl Cancer Inst,* 74(4):747-751.

Zhang B, Ferrence R, Cohen J, et al. (2005). Smoking cessation and lung cancer mor-tality in a cohort of middle-aged Canadian women. *Ann Epidemiol,* 15(4):302-309.

Risk of Other Cancers After Smoking Cessation

Laryngeal Cancer

Laryngeal cancer is strongly associated with tobacco smoking (IARC, 1986). In the most recent tobacco smoke *Monograph* (IARC, 2004), the risk of cancer of the larynx was reported to diminish after smoking cessation. Alcohol consumption is an important risk factor for laryngeal cancer. Here we review cohort and case–control studies on laryngeal cancer and smoking cessation published before December 2005 identified through Medline and by searching the references of the retrieved studies.

Cohort Studies

At least four cohort studies have reported data on laryngeal cancer in relation to smoking cessation (Table 1). These studies only collected information on smoking status at the enrolment of the study subjects, and not on lifetime smoking habits.

In the Life Span Study, which included over 60 000 atomic bomb survivors (Akiba *et al.,* 1994), the relative risk (RR) of laryngeal cancer was 32.1 in current smokers and 13.6 in former smokers, on the basis of information collected in the first survey conducted in 1963–1964. No reliable comparison with the data of subsequent surveys was possible.

In the 26-year follow-up of 248 046 US veterans (McLaughlin *et al.,* 1995a), the RR of laryngeal cancer was 13.7 (95% confidence interval (95% CI) = 7.0–27.1) in current smokers at the time of completion of the baseline questionnaire and 5.0 (95% CI=2.4–10.5) in former smokers compared with never smokers.

A study of data from a cohort of 1 212 906 Koreans aged 30–95 years from the National Health Insurance Corporation (Jee *et al.,* 2004), reported laryngeal cancer mortality rates of 0.8/100 000 in never smokers, 2.7 in former smokers and 4.9 in current smokers. The corresponding figures for incidence were 1.9, 6.7 and 10.3, respectively. Laryngeal cancer incidence in relation to smoking status was also covered in a smaller sub-group of the cohort insured with the National Health Insurance Corporation (Yun *et al.,* 2005). During a 4-year follow-up period (1996–2000) 11, 14 and 78 laryngeal cancer cases were identified in never, former and current smokers, respectively. Corresponding RR in former and current smokers compared with never smokers were 1.1 (95% CI=0.5–2.5) and 3.0 (95% CI=1.6–5.7) respectively.

In the 50-year follow-up of the male British Doctors Study (Doll *et al.,* 2005) including 40 deaths from cancer at this site, the laryngeal cancer mortality rates were 0.0/100 000 in never smokers, 2.6

in former smokers (defined as former smokers at the time of the original questionnaire, or smokers who quit on subsequent questionnaires) and 10.3 in current smokers. Corresponding figures for former and current smokers of other tobacco products were 2.9 and 4.7, respectively.

Case–Control Studies

At least 16 case–control studies reported information on laryngeal cancer risk after smoking cessation, and analyzed the time course of the change in risk after stopping smoking (Table 2).

In an investigation from the USA including 314 cases of laryngeal cancer (Wynder *et al.,* 1976), the risk of laryngeal cancer significantly decreased after 6 years since smoking cessation, but the odds ratio (OR) was still four times that of never smokers 16 years after cessation. In this study there was also indication that the average age at which former smokers developed laryngeal cancer was about 10 years older (68.7 years) than that of the current smokers.

In a multi-center case–control study from four European countries, including 727 men with cancer of the endolarynx

Table 1. Cohort studies: relative risk of laryngeal cancer by smoking status and/or years since quitting smoking

Author, Publication year Country	Study population	Smoking cessation/status categories	Relative risk versus never smokers	95% confidence interval	Comments
Akiba, *et al.,* (1994) Japan	Life Span Study 61 505 survivors 41 cases in men 5 cases in women	Current smokers Former smokers Never smokers	32.1 13.6 1	Could not be obtained.	Cases in men & women combined. RR reported correspond to data obtained in the first survey of smoking habits (1963-64).
McLaughlin *et al.,* (1995a) USA	US Veterans' Study 248 046 men 167 cases	Current smokers Former smokers Never smokers	13.7 5.0 1	7.0, 27.1 2.4, 10.5	RR corresponding to beginning of follow-up.
Jee *et al.,* (2004) Republic of Korea	National Health Insurance Corporation 1 212 906 adults 526 cases 223 deaths	*Mortality* Current smokers Former smokers Never smokers *Incidence* Current smokers Former smokers Never smokers	6.5 3.6 1 5.4 3.3 1	3.3, 12.8 1.8, 7.3 3.5, 8.1 2.1, 5.1	
Yun *et al.,* (2005) Republic of Korea	National Health Insurance Corporation 733 134 men 103 cases	*Incidence* Current smokers Former smokers Never smokers	3.0 1.1 1	1.6, 5.7 0.5, 2.5	Estimates adjusted for age, residence, alcohol use, body-mass index, physical activity and diet
Doll *et al.,* (2005) UK	Male British doctors 34 439 men 40 cases	*Mortality Rate* Current smokers Former smokers Never smokers	10.3 2.6 0.0		Mortality rates per 100 000

and 420 with cancer of the hypopharynx/epilarynx (Tuyns *et al.,* 1988), the OR of endolaryngeal cancer was 1.5 (95% CI=1.2–2.0) one to four years after smoking cessation as compared to current smokers, the excess risk being likely due to an effect of smokers quitting following diagnosis or early onset of symptoms of cancer. However, a 50% decreased risk was observed in subjects who had stopped smoking for 5 to 9 years (OR=0.52, 95% CI=0.3–0.8), and of about 70% in those who had stopped

10 or more years previously (OR=0.28, 95% CI=0.2–0.4). The benefit of cessation appeared earlier and stronger for cancers of the hypopharynx/epilarynx than for those of the endolarynx (OR=0.3, 95% CI=0.1–0.5 for subjects who had stopped smoking for 5 to 9 years and OR=0.3, 95% CI=0.2–0.5 for subjects with 10 or more years of abstinence).

In a case–control study conducted in Texas, USA on 151 men with laryngeal cancer (Falk *et al.* 1989), the OR for

former smokers was 3.2 (95% CI=1.3–7.8) and for current smokers 9.0 (95% CI=3.9–20.6). After allowance for the amount smoked, the OR tended to decline with passing time since cessation. However, there was still a threefold increased risk compared with never smokers among those who had smoked more than 40 cigarettes daily after 10 years of smoking cessation. The risk reduction pattern by years of smoking cessation and number of cigarettes smoked daily was examined only in this

Table 2. Case–control studies: relative risk of laryngeal cancer by years since quitting

Author Publication year Country	Study population	Smoking categories	Number of cases	Relative risk	95% confidence interval	Comments
Wynder et al., (1976) USA	314 cases (258 men/56 women) 684 controls (516 men/168 women)	*Men* Current smokers Former smokers Years since quitting	197	14.5		Former smokers included those who had stopped smoking ≥ 1 years prior to admission
		1–5		14.5		
		6–10		7.0		
		10–15		6.5		
		≥ 16		4.0		
		Never smokers	5	1[a]		
Tuyns et al., (1988) Europe (France, Italy, Spain, Switzerland)	Men 727 endolarynx 420 hypopharynx & epilarynx 3 057 controls	*Endolarynx* Current smokers Former smokers Years since quitting	470	1[a]		
		1–4	155	1.5	1.2, 2.0	
		5–9	35	0.5	0.3, 0.8	
		≥ 10	45	0.3	0.2, 0.4	
		Hypopharynx/ epilarynx Current smokers Former smokers Years since cessation	270	1[a]		
		1–4	81	1.1	0.8, 1.5	
		5–9	14	0.3	0.1, 0.5	
		≥ 10	35	0.3	0.2, 0.5	
Falk et al.,(1989) USA	Men 151 cases 235 controls	Current smokers Former smokers *3-9 years since quitting* Cigarettes/day	109	9.0	3.9, 20.6	Estimates adjusted for age, residence, alcohol use, ever employed in high-risk occupation and vegetable consumption
		1–10	1	3.0	0.2, 40.2	
		11–20	6	3.6	0.8, 15.8	
		21–30	2	4.0	0.6, 29.5	
		31–40	3	7.2	1.0, 54.3	
		> 40	4	10.9	1.8, 68.5	
		≥ 10 years since quitting Cigarettes/day				
		1–10	5	2.8	0.7, 10.7	
		11–20	6	1.2	0.4, 4.0	
		21–30	2	1.0	0.2, 6.4	
		31–40	2	3.1	0.4, 22.4	
		>40	3	3.5	0.6, 19.1	
		Never smokers	8	1[a]		

Table 2. Case-control studies laryngeal cancer (contd)

Author Publication year Country	Study population	Smoking categories	Number of cases	Relative risk	95% confidence interval	Comments
Franceschi *et al.* (1990); La Vecchia *et al.* (1990a) Italy	Men 162 cases 1 272 controls	Current smokers Former smokers Years since quitting	113	4.6	3.0, 3.2	Estimates adjusted for age, residence, education, number of alcoholic drinks/week
		1–10	32	4.6	2.0, 10.4	
		≥ 10	9	1.2	0.4, 3.3	
		Never smokers	8	1[a]		
Ahrens *et al.*, (1991) Germany	Men 85 cases 100 controls	Current smoker Former smokers Years since quitting	63	3.8	1.0, 14.7	Estimates are adjusted for age
		1–5	7	2.4	0.5, 12.9	
		6–15	6	1.4	0.3, 7.4	
		≥ 16	6	0.9	0.2, 4.3	
		Never smokers	3	1[a]		
Choi & Kahyo, (1991a) Republic of Korea	Men 94 cases 282 controls	Current smokers Former smokers Years since quitting	84	1[a]		
		1–4	4	0.7	0.2, 2.2	
		5-9	1	0.4	0.1, 3.0	
		≥ 10	1	0.2	0.03, 1.0	
Zatonski *et al.*, (1991) Poland	Men 249 cases 965 controls	Current smokers[b] Former smokers Years since quitting	227	1[a]		
		5–10	9	0.8	0.3, 1.8	
		>10	11	0.3	0.1, 0.6	
López-Abente *et al.*, (1992) Spain	Men 50 cases 103 controls	Current smokers Former smokers Years since quitting	34	1[a]		
		1	5	1.2	0.3, 5.5	
		2–5	4	0.7	0.2, 2.9	
		6–15	5	0.8	0.2, 3.0	
		>15	2	0.5	0.1, 3.2	
Muscat & Wynder, (1992) USA	Men 194 cases 184 controls	Current smokers Former smokers Years since quitting	119	13.8	2.3, 27.1	
		1–10	27	8.5	2.8, 25.4	
		>10	27	3.8	1.3, 10.8	
		Never smokers	5	1[a]		

Table 2. Case-control studies laryngeal cancer (contd)

Author Publication year Country	Study population	Smoking categories	Number of cases	Relative risk	95% confidence interval	Comments
Zheng et al., (1992a) China	Men 177 cases 269 controls	Current smokers[c] Former smokers Years since quitting	135	1[a]		Estimates adjusted for age and education
		2–4	13	1.8	0.6, 4.9	
		5–9	8	0.6	0.2, 1.5	
		≥ 10	14	0.6	0.3, 1.2	
		Never smokers	7	0.1	0.0, 0.2	
De Stefani et al., (1992) Uruguay	96 cases 273 controls	Current smokers Former smokers Years since quitting	72	1[a]		Includes smokers of manufactured or hand-rolled cigarettes
		1–4	11	0.8	0.3, 1.9	
		5–9	4	0.9	0.2, 3.6	
		≥ 10	8	0.2	0.1, 0.5	
Schlecht et al., (1999) Brazil	Brazil 194 cases 1 578 controls	Current smokers Former smokers Years since quitting	137	11.7	4.4, 31.5	Estimates based on smokers or former smokers of all tobacco products (cigarettes, black tobacco cigars, pipes). Estimates adjusted for alcohol use and tobacco consumption
		≤1	13	10.5	3.0, 36.6	
		2–5	15	7.7	2.4, 25.2	
		6–10	7	2.7	0.8, 9.6	
		11–15	6	5.9	1.4, 24.2	
		16–20	2	1.5	0.3, 8.6	
		>20	12	3.1	1.0, 9.4	
		Never smokers	5	1[a]		
Altieri et al. (2002) Talamini et al. (2002) Italy and Switzerland	527 cases 478 Men 49 Women 1 297 controls	Current smokers Former smokers Years since quitting	349	1[a]		Estimates adjusted per age, sex, alcohol use and tobacco consumption, study center, education
		1–2	29	1.3	0.7, 2.4	
		3–5	22	0.7	0.4, 1.2	
		6–9	33	0.6	0.4, 1.0	
		10–14	25	0.3	0.2, 0.5	
		14–19	18	0.2	0.1, 0.4	
		≥ 20	32	0.2	0.1, 0.3	
		Never smokers	19	0.05	0.03, 0.08	
Menvielle et al., (2004) France	Men 504 cases 242 controls	Current smokers Former smokers Years since quitting	386	1[a]		Estimates adjusted for age, alcohol use, duration of smoking and amount of tobacco smoked
		<10	68	0.4	0.2, 0.6	
		11–20	29	0.2	0.1, 0.5	
		≥ 21	6	0.1	0.03, 0.4	

[a]Reference category.
[b]Including ex-smoker for less than 4 years.
[c]Including ex-smoker for less than 2 years.

study (Falk *et al.* 1989), which indicated that there was no consistent pattern of greater reduction in risk among former smokers who had smoked fewer cigarettes per day prior to smoking cessation, particularly in those who had stopped for 10 years or more. However, the increasing magnitude of the ORs shown with increasing amount smoked among former smokers with 3–9 years of abstinence, reaching 10.9 (95% CI=1.8–68.5) for those with a past of >40 cigarettes per day, was not seen in former smokers with longer abstinence, and for those with similarly heavy smoking past (>40 cigarettes/day) the OR was 3.5 (95% CI=0.6–19.1). However, these results were based on very small number of cases (see Table 2).

A case–control study from northern Italy including 162 male cases of laryngeal cancer (Franceschi *et al.,* 1990; La Vecchia *et al.,* 1990a) reported an OR of 4.6 (95% CI=2.2–9.6) in current smokers, of 4.6 (95% CI=2.0–10.4) in former smokers with less than 10 years of abstinence and of 1.2 (95% CI=0.4–3.3) in former smokers with 10 or more years of abstinence.

In a German case–control study of 85 male laryngeal cancer cases (Ahrens *et al.,* 1991), compared to never smokers the OR was 3.8 (95% CI=1.0–14.7) in current smokers, 2.4 (95% CI=0.5, 12.9) in former smokers of 1 to 5 years, 1.4 (95% CI=0.3–7.4) in those of 6 to 15 years, and 0.9 (95% CI=0.2–4.3) for 16 or more years of abstinence. These results were based on very small number of cases, which is reflected in wide confidence intervals around the risk estimates reported.

The OR for laryngeal cancer was 5.4 (95% CI=2.1–14.3) in current smokers and 2.2 (95% CI=0.6–8.4) in former smokers in a case–control study from Korea that included 94 male laryngeal cancer cases (Choi and Kahyo, 1991a). Compared with current smokers, the OR was 0.7 (95% CI=0.2–2.2) for 1–4 years

since smoking cessation, 0.4 (95% CI=0.1–3.0) for 5–9 years and 0.2 (95% CI=0.03–1.0) for 10 or more years. After 10 or more years the RR of laryngeal cancer dropped to that of never smokers. These results are based on a small number of cases.

A Polish case–control study including 249 male laryngeal cancer cases (Zatonski *et al.,* 1991) reported an approximate 20% reduction in risk 5 to 10 years after quitting smoking as compared to current smokers (OR=0.8; 95% CI=0.3–1.8), and a 70% reduction after 10 years (OR=0.3; 95% CI=0.1–0.6).

No statistically significant decrease in the risk of laryngeal cancer with duration of abstinence was reported in a Spanish case–control study based on 50 male cases (OR=0.5; 95% CI=0.1–3.2) for quitters of ≥ 15 years (Lopez-Abente *et al.,* 1992).

A US case–control study based on 194 male cases of laryngeal cancer (Muscat and Wynder, 1992) reported a lower RR in subjects who had stopped smoking (OR=4.8) than in those who continued (OR=13.8), but the risk remained significantly elevated even after 10 or more years of having quit smoking (OR=3.8; 95% CI=1.3–10.8). A similar pattern of risk was observed for cancers of the glottis and the supraglottis in relation to time since smoking cessation.

In a case–control study from China including 177 male cases (Zheng *et al.,* 1992a), the OR of laryngeal cancer was 1.8 (95% CI=0.6–4.9) two to four years after smoking cessation as compared to current smokers. For longer abstinence the relative risk was 0.6, or a 40% reduction in relation to current smokers, but it remained six-fold higher than that in never smokers (0.6 versus 0.1) 10 or more years after quitting (Table 2).

A case–control study from Uruguay including 96 laryngeal cancer cases (De Stefani *et al.,* 1992) showed a 60%

reduction in risk in former smokers of hand-rolled cigarettes compared with current smokers, with an OR of 0.2 (95% CI=0.1–0.5) 10 years after cessation.

In a large case–control study from Brazil (194 laryngeal cancer cases, Schlecht *et al.,* 1999), in which cessation of smoking was studied also in relation to type of tobacco smoked (cigarettes, black tobacco cigars or pipe smoking), the risk of laryngeal cancer decreased, although not linearly, with time since cessation of the habit. For 20 or more years after cessation, the OR was a third of that of current smokers (11.7; 95% CI=4.4–31.5), but still threefold higher than that of never smokers (OR=3.1; 95% CI=1.0–9.4).

A case–control study from Italy including 527 cases (Altieri *et al.,* 2002) reported a reduced risk of laryngeal cancer 3–5 years after smoking cessation (OR=0.7; 95% CI=0.4–1.2) compared with current smokers, with a reduction of approximately 70% 10–19 years after smoking cessation, and of over 80% 20 or more years after. Former smokers for 20 or more years, however, still had risk increased threefold over that of never smokers (Altieri *et al.,* 2002; Talamini *et al.,* 2002).

Finally, a case–control study from France on 504 male cases of laryngeal cancer reported that the risk in former smokers was one-third that of current smokers (Menvielle *et al.,* 2004). The reduction was evident within 10 years of cessation (OR=0.4; 95% CI=0.2–0.6) and became larger with time since cessation, the OR being 0.1 (95% CI=0.03–0.4) after 20 years. The study reported that among former smokers the risk of laryngeal cancer increased linearly with amount of tobacco smoked. For each level of consumption and duration of smoking, the RR in former smokers was about three- to four-fold lower than that of current smokers. Thus, the RR for >40 g of tobacco smoked daily was 4.2 (95% CI=1.7–10.2) in former smokers who had smoked for 1–30 years, 12.1 (95% CI=5.2–28) for those who had smoked for 31–40 years and 11.1 (95% CI=4.2–29.3) for those who had smoked 40 years or longer.

Corresponding figures in current smokers were 15.2 (95% CI=5.7–40.8), 43.8 (95% CI=17.9–107) and 40.2 (95% CI=17.5–92.3), respectively.

Discussion

A large number of epidemiological studies indicate that the risk of laryngeal cancer is substantially reduced in former smokers as compared to subjects who continue to smoke. The favorable effect of stopping smoking is already evident within few years after cessation. A few studies (Wynder *et al.*, 1976; Tuyns *et al.*, 1988; Lòpez-Abente *et al.*, 1992; Altieri *et al.*, 2002; Talamini *et al.*, 2002) reported a similar or even greater relative risk in recent quitters compared with current smokers; this result is likely due to the reverse causality, when some cases could have stopped smoking because of diagnosis and early symptoms of the disease, adding cancer cases to the pool of former smokers and hence underestimating the effects of quitting.

The RR compared to current smokers steeply decreases with time since stopping smoking; reductions by about 60% were observed after 10–15 years since cessation of smoking, and even greater reductions were observed after 20 years. However, many studies, including the largest ones, showed that even after many years since stopping smoking, former smokers still had elevated risks of laryngeal cancer as compared with never smokers. There is, however, still limited evidence on the time-risk relation with reference to various levels of intensity and duration of smoking, as well as of the absolute risk function for laryngeal cancer after stopping smoking.

Some of the apparent differences across studies are likely due to the play of chance and to the variable distribution of duration of cessation and of smoking among the populations.

Oral and Pharyngeal Cancer

Tobacco smoke is causally related to oral cancer (IARC, 1986). Main confounders for the association between oro-pharyngeal cancer and tobacco smoke are use of smokeless tobacco and alcohol intake, often taken into account in those studies examining the role of smoking in the etiology of oral cancer. The effect of cessation of smoking was addressed in the most recent tobacco Monograph (IARC, 2004), which reported a rapid lowering of the risk for oral cancer after cessation.

Studies identified

Four cohort studies (Table 3) and at least 26 case–control analyses (Tables 4 and 5) reported the risk of oral or pharyngeal cancers (separately or a combination of both) in former smokers. Almost all of the studies adjusted for age and alcohol consumption. Five studies contained separate analyses for oral and pharyngeal cancers.

Former smokers versus current or never smokers

Cohort Studies

In the 26-year follow-up of 177 903 veterans aged 30 years or more during 1954–1980 (McLaughlin *et al.*, 1995a), with over 3 million accumulated person-years and 116 606 deaths, the relative risk (RR) of dying from oral cancer in current cigarette smokers was 3.4 (significant), and that in former smokers was 1.5 (95% confidence interval (CI) includes 1.0; 0.9–2.4), with former smokers having significantly less than half (44%) of the risk of current smokers and 50% more risk than never smokers. The RR for dying from pharyngeal cancer was 14.1 (95% CI=6.9–28.9) in current smokers and 2.6 (95% CI=1.1–6.2) in former smokers.

A cohort of about 120 000 persons was followed in Japan through baseline and repeated surveys. Taking information from all surveys, the RR for pharyngeal cancer among current smokers was 1.1 (95% CI=0.6–not available) and former smokers 0.4 (95% CI=0.1–1.2) (Akiba, 1994).

In a cohort of 733 134 men (aged ≥ 30 years) from South Korea, the RR for oral and pharyngeal cancer among

Table 3. Cohort studies: relative risk of oral cancer by smoking status and/or years since quitting

Author Publication year Country	Study population, Subsite and Follow-up period	Smoking categories	Cases or Deaths	Relative risk	95% confidence interval	Comments
Akiba, (1994) Japan	Life Span Study Pharynx 61 505 survivors 1966–1981	*First survey* Current smoker Former smoker *All surveys* Current smoker Former smoker	42 cases in men 27 cases in women	1.2 0.4 1.1 0.4	0.6, * 0.1, 1.4 0.6, * 0.1, 1.2	Cases in men and women combined. * 95% confidence bound could not be obtained.
McLaughlin *et al.* (1995a) USA	US Veteran's study Oral cavity Men 177 903 1954–1980 (26 years follow-up)	Current smoker Ever smoker Former smoker Never smoker	189 deaths	3.4 2.6 1.5 1.0	2.3, 5.0 1.8, 3.9 0.9, 2.4	Relative risk of oral and pharyn-geal cancer mortality at start of follow-up. Estimates refer to cigarette smoker.
	Pharynx	Current smoker Ever smoker Former smoker Never smoker	143 deaths	14.1 9.5 2.6 1.0	6.9, 28.9 4.6, 19.4 1.1, 6.2	
Doll *et al.,* (2005) U.K	British Doctors study Oral & pharynx 34 439 male doctors 1951–2001	**Oral** *Cigarette smoker* Current smoker Former smoker Never smoker	43 deaths	7.1 1.3 1.9		Mortality rate per 100 000 persons/years.
		Oro-and hypo-pharynx *Cigarette smoker* Current smoker Former smoker Never smoker	34 deaths	6.7 1.7 0.0		
Yun *et al.,* (2005) Republic of Korea	National Health Insurance Corporation Study Oral & pharynx 733 134 insured men 1996–2000	Current smoker Former smoker Never smoker	172 Cases 106 41 25	1.8 1.5 1.0	1.1, 2.7 0.9, 2.5	Estimates adjusted for age, residence, body mass index, alcohol use and physical activity.

Table 4. Case-control studies: relative risk of oral cancer and smoking cessation without specification on years since quitting

Author Publication year Country	Study population Subsite	Smoking categories	Cases	Odds ratio	95% confidence interval	Comments
Talamini et al., (1990a) Italy	Oral and pharyngeal cancer cases combined Men 291 cases Women 45 cases	Current smoker < 15 per day ≥ 15 per day Former smoker Never smoker	2 12 3 2	3.8 12.9 4.1 1.0	0.2, 58.2 2.3, 106 0.5, 93.6	Hospital based. Estimates obtained in non-drinkers. Cases in men and women combined and adjusted for age and sex.
Zheng et al., (1990) China	Incident cases ICD–9: 141; 143–145 Men 248 cases Women 156 cases	Current smoker* Former smoker Never smoker	168 22 58	2.4 1.1 1.0	1.5, 4.0 0.6, 2.1	Hospital based. Estimates adjusted for alcohol use, education, sex and age. *Cigarette and pipe smokers included. Estimates for former smokers obtained in men only; none of the women were former smokers.
Ko et al.,(1995) Taiwan	Incident cases ICD–9: 140–141; 143–145 Men 104 cases Women 3 cases	Current smoker* Former smoker Never smoker	85 11 11	4.6 3.6 1.0	1.5, 14.0 0.9, 14.6	Hospital based. Estimates adjusted for education, occupation, alcohol use and betel quid. *Cigarette smokers only
Zheng et al., (1997) China	Cancer of the tongue Men 65 cases Women 46 cases	Current smoker Former smoker Never smoker	60 3 48	2.7 0.5 1.0	1.3, 5.2 0.1, 2.2	Hospital based. Estimates adjusted for alcohol use and education.

Table 4. Case-control studies oral cancer (contd)

Author Publication year Country	Study population Subsite	Smoking categories	Cases	Odds ratio	95% confidence interval	Comments
Schildt et al., (1998) Sweden	Oral cancer ICD–9: 140; 141; 143–145 *Men* 100 cases alive 137 cases deceased *Women* 43 cases alive 74 cases deceased	Current smoker Former smoker Never smoker	122 80 152	1.8 1.0 1.0	1.1, 2.7 0.6, 1.6	Population based. Quitters within year prior to diagnosis considered current smokers. Estimates adjusted but not specified for which variables.
Bosetti et al., (2000a) Italy and Switzerland	Oral and pharyn-geal cancer Women 195 cases	Current smoker 1–14 (cigarettes/day) ≥ 15 (cigarettes/day) Former smoker Never smoker	57 47 19 72	3.6 4.6 4.6 1.6 1.0	2.3, 5.6 2.7, 7.6 0.9, 2.9	Hospital based; combines data from two studies. Estimates adjusted for education, body mass index and alcohol use.
Zavras et al., (2001) Greece	Oral and pharyn-geal cancer ICD–9: 141; 143–145; 148–149 *Men* 68 cases *Women* 42 cases	Current smoker Former smoker Never smoker	61 16 41	3.0 0.9 1.0	1.4, 6.6 0.4, 2.1	Hospital based. Cases in men and women combined. Estimates adjusted for age, sex, refering hospital and alcohol use.
Llewellyn et al., (2004) England	Lip, oral cavity, oropharynx, tonsil ICD–10: C001–06; C001–06; C09–10 *Men* 28 cases *Women* 25 cases	Current smoker Former smoker Never smoker	28 8 17	1.2 0.2 1.0	0.4, 3.8 0.5, 0.8	Population based. Cases in men and women combined. Estimates adjusted for alcohol use.

Table 5. Case-control studies: relative risk of oral cancer by years since quitting

Author Publication year Country	Study population Subsite	Smoking categories	Cases	Odds ratio	95% confidence interval	Comments
Blot et al., (1988) USA	Oral and pharyngeal	*Men*				Population based. Estimates adjusted for alcohol use, age, race, area and respondent status.
		Current smoker	485	3.4	2.3, 5.1	
	Incident cases	Ever smoker	659	1.9	1.3, 2.9	
		Former smoker				
		Years since quitting				
	ICD9:141;143–146;	1–9	64	1.1	0.7, 1.9	
	148–149	10-19	56	1.1	0.7, 1.9	
		20+	43	0.7	0.4, 1.2	
	Men 762 cases	Never smoker	50	1.0		
	Women 352 cases	*Women*				
		Current smoker	258	4.7	3.0, 7.3	
		Ever smoker	298	3.0	2.0, 4.5	
		Former smoker				
		Years since quitting				
		1–9	24	1.8	0.9, 3.6	
		10–19	10	0.8	0.4, 1.9	
		20+	4	0.4	0.1, 1.4	
		Never smoker	54	1.0		
Merletti et al., (1989) Italy	Oral and pharyngeal	*Men*	68	3.9	1.6, 9.4	Population based. Estimates adjusted for age.
		Current cigarettes	7	3.8	1.1, 12.6	
		Current pipe	11	14.6	4.7, 45.6	
	Incident cases	Current cigar				
		Former smoker				
	ICD–9: 141–146	Years since quitting	68	5.4	2.3, 16.8	
	excluding 142	0–1	11	4.4	1.6, 12.4	
		2–5	2	0.4	0.1, 2.7	
	Men 86 cases	>5	5	1.0		
		Never smoker				
	Women 36 cases	*Women*				
		Current cigarettes	23	5.4	2.4, 12.5	
		Former smoker				
		Years since quitting				
		0–1	18	7.4	3.0, 18.3	
		>2	5	3.7	1.3, 10.8	
		Never smoker	13	1.0		

Table 5. Years since quitting oral cancer (contd)

Author Publication year Country	Study population Subsite	Smoking categories	Cases	Odds ratio	95% confidence interval	Comments
Franceschi *et al.*, (1990) Italy	Oral	Current smoker Former smoker	147	11.1	3.4, 34.8	Hospital based. Estimates adjusted for age, area of residence, educa- tion, occupation, and alcohol use. Cigarette smokers
	Oral cavity	Years since quitting				
	ICD–9: 140;141;143–145	<10	20	5.7	1.6, 20.8	
		10+	5	1.1	0.3, 5.1	
		Never smoker	4	1.0		
	Men					
	157 cases	Current smoker Former smoker	132	12.9	3.1, 52.9	
	Pharyngeal	Years since quitting				
		<10	26	11.3	0.8, 18.0	
	ICD–9: 146;148;161;1	10+	10	3.7	2.6, 49.4	
		Never smoker	2	1.0		
	Men 134 cases					
Choi & Kahyo, (1991a) Korea	Oral and pharyn- geal	*Men oral*				Hospital based. Estimates adjusted for alcohol use. Linear trend for years since quitting was signifi- cant. No former smokers among women.
		Current smoker	91	2.5	1.3, 4.5	
	ICD–9: 140; 141;143–145; 146–149	Former smoker	7	0.9	0.4, 2.2	
		Years since quitting				
		1–4	2	0.7	0.1, 3.9	
		5–9	3	0.6	0.2, 2.2	
	Men 246 cases	10+	2	0.2	0.05, 0.7	
		Never smoker	15	1.0		
	Women 43 cases	*Men pharynx*				
		Current smoker	109	1.6	0.9, 3.1	
		Former smoker	10	0.9	0.3, 2.1	
		Never smoker	14	1		
		Years since quitting				
		Current smoker	109	1		
		1–4	1	0.1	0.03, 0.7	
		5–9	6	1.1	0.4, 2.8	
		10+	3	0.5	0.1, 1.6	
Oreggia *et al.*, (1991) Uruguay	Tongue	Current smoker	45	29.4	3.7, 234	Hospital based. Estimates adjusted for age, county, alcohol use, color of tobacco, age start, cigarettes per day and duration.
		Former smoker	11	11.8	1.4, 100	
	Incident cases	Never smoker	1	1.0		
	Men 57 cases	Current smoker	45	1.0		
		Years since quitting				
		1–4	5	0.4	0.1, 1.2	
		5–9	2	0.3	0.1, 1.4	
		10 +	4	0.2	0.0, 0.6	

Table 5. Years since quitting oral cancer (contd)

Author Publication year Country	Study population Subsite	Smoking categories	Cases	Odds ratio	95% confidence interval	Comments
DeStefani *et al.*, (1992) Uruguay	Oral, oropharyn- geal, hypo- pharyngeal ICD–9:141;143–145; 146;148	Current smoker Former smoker Years since quitting	84	1.0		Hospital based. Estimates adjusted for age, residence, urban status, education, time of cessation and total alcohol use.
		1–4	10	0.6	0.2, 1.4	
		5–9	7	1.1	0.4, 3.3	
	Men 109 cases	10+	5	0.1	0.0, 0.3	
Franceschi *et al.*, (1992) Italy	Tongue and mouth	*Tongue cancer* Current smoker Former smoker Years since quitting	83 15	10.5 2.1	3.2, 34.1 0.6, 7.7	Hospital based. Estimates adjusted for age, area of residence, occupation and alcohol use.
	ICD–9: 141;143–5;149	< 10	12	3.8	1.0, 14.5	
	Men 102 cases (tongue)	≥ 10 Never smoker	3 3	0.7 1.0	0.1, 3.8	
	Men and Women 104 cases (mouth)	*Mouth Cancer* Current smoker Former smoker	78 18	11.8 3.6	3.6, 38.4 1.0, 12.6	
		Years since quitting < 10	13	3.8	1.0, 14.4	
		≥ 10	3	0.7	0.1, 3.9	
		Never smoker	3	1.0		
Day *et al.*, (1993) USA	Tongue, mouth and pharynx Incident cases	*European American* Current smoker Former smoker Years since quitting	568	3.6	2.6, 4.8	Population based. Estimates adjusted for sex, age, study location and respondent status.
	Men 729 cases	1–9 10–19	70 63	1.1 1.1	0.7, 1.6 0.7, 1.6	
	Women 336 cases	≥ 20 Never smoker	41 77	0.6 1.0	0.3, 0.9	
		African American Current smoker Former smoker Years since quitting	147	2.3	1.1, 4.7	
		1–9	13	1.1	0.4, 3.1	
		10–19	1	0.1	0.0, 1.3	
		≥ 20	3	0.3	0.1, 1.7	
		Never smoker	17	1.0		

Table 5. Years since quitting oral cancer (contd)

Author Publication year Country	Study population Subsite	Smoking categories	Cases	Odds ratio	95% confidence interval	Comments
Mashberg et al., (1993) USA	Oral-oropharynx *Men* 359 cases	Minimal smoking*	9	1.0		Hospital based. Estimates adjusted by logistic regression for age, race, alcohol use, average cigarette consumption. *5 or less per day
		6–15 cig/day	41	4.0	1.9, 8.5	
		16–25 cig/day	109	4.4	2.2, 8.9	
		26–35 cig/day	61	5.6	2.7, 11.7	
		36+ cig/day	94	4.0	1.9, 8.2	
		Former smoker	9	0.8	0.3, 2.2	
		Years since quitting				
		3–10	6	1.3	0.3, 6.5	
		11+	3	0.5	0.1, 2.6	
Day et al., (1994) USA	Second cancers following oral and pharyngeal cancers ICD–9: 141;143–146; 148–149	Continuing smoker	25	1.0		Population based. Estimates adjusted for age, stage of disease and alcohol use.
		Quit at or after diagnosis	20	0.9	0.4, 2.2	
		Quit before diagnosis	7	0.5	0.2, 1.4	
		Never smoker	3	0.3	0.1, 1.5	
		Years since quitting				
	Follow-up period 1984-1989	0 (never)	25	1.0		
		1 to <3	13	0.5	0.2, 1.9	
		3 to <5	8	1.9	0.5, 6.4	
		>5	6	0.3	0.1, 1.0	
	Men 54 cases *Women* 24 cases Nested case-control in a cohort study					
Kabat et al., (1994) USA	Oral and pharyngeal *Men* 1097 cases *Women* 463 cases	*Men*				Hospital based. Estimates adjusted for age, education, alcohol use, race, time period and type of hospital.
		Current smoker	676	3.3	2.4, 4.3	
		Former smoker	246	1.1	0.8, 1.5	
		Never smoker	82			
		Current smoker				
		Years since quitting				
		0	676	1.0	0.4, 0.8	
		1–9	113	0.6	0.2, 0.5	
		10–19	59	0.3	0.3, 0.9	
		20+	70	0.5		
		Women				
		Current smoker	271	4.3	3.2, 5.9	
		Former smoker	79	1.4	1.0, 2.0	
		Never smoker	113	1		
		Current smoker	271	1.0		
		Years since quitting				
		1–9	40	0.5	0.3, 0.8	
		5–9	24	0.3	0.2, 0.5	
		10+	15	0.3	0.1, 0.8	

Table 5. Years since quitting oral cancer (contd)

Author Publication year Country	Study population Subsite	Smoking categories	Cases	Odds ratio	95% confidence interval	Comments
Macfarlane *et al.*, (1995) China Italy USA	Oral cavity ICD–9: 141;143–5 *Men* 374 *Women* 216 cases	Current smoker Years since quitting < 1 1–9 10+	Not reported	1.0 1.2 0.7 0.5	0.7, 1.8 0.5, 1.1 0.3, 0.7	Hospital based. Estimates adjusted for age, sex, centre, education, alcohol use, previous level of smoking and inter-action terms for center education and center alcohol intake
De Stefani *et al.*, (1998a) Uruguay	Oral and pharyn-geal cancer *Men* 425 cases	*Oral* Current smoker Former smoker Years since quitting 1–4 5–9 10+ Never smoker *Pharynx* Current smoker Former smoker Years since quitting 1–4 5–9 10+ Never smoker	146 36 20 12 4 24 161 44 21 15 8 14	5.7 2.2 3.2 2.7 0.7 1.0 10.2 4.3 5.9 5.1 2.1 1.0	3.4, 9.5 1.2, 3.9 1.6,3.9 1.2, 3.9 0.2, 2.1 5.5, 18.8 2.2, 8.3 2.7, 12.8 2.2, 12.0 0.8, 5.5	Hospital based. Estimates adjusted for age, residence urban/ rural status, birthplace, education and alcohol use.
Hayes *et al.*, (1999) Puerto Rico	Oral & pharyngeal ICD–9: 141; 143–6; 148, 149 *Men* 298 cases *Women* 69 cases	*Men* Years since quitting Recent use 2–9 years 10–19 years 20+ years Never smoker *Women* Years since quitting Recent use 2–9 years 10–19 years 20+ years Never smoker	183 37 20 18 16 23 8 2 2 14	7.5 4.1 2.0 1.2 1.0 14.1 8.7 2.1 0.8 1.0	3.9, 14.4 1.8, 8.9 0.9, 4.5 0.5, 2.7 4.2, 47.2 2.2, 35.2 0.3, 13.9 0.1, 4.2	Recent use is up to 2 years prior to interview. Estimates adjusted for age and alcohol use.

Table 5. Years since quitting oral cancer (contd)

Author Publication year Country	Study population Subsite	Smoking categories	Cases	Odds ratio	95% confidence interval	Comments
La Vecchia et al., (1999) Italy Switzerland	Oral and pharyngeal 638 oral cases 642 pharyngeal cases 4179 controls	*Oral cancer* Current smoker Former smoker Time since quitting	441	6.2	4.6, 8.3	Estimates adjusted for age, sex, study centre, education, and alcohol use.
		1–2 years	28	4.6	2.8, 7.8	
		3–5	38	3.9	2.5, 6.2	
		6–9	31	2.9	1.8, 4.7	
		10–14	12	0.8	0.4, 1.6	
		≥ 15	18	0.7	0.4, 1.2	
		Never smoker	70	1.0		
		Pharyngeal cancer Current smoker Former smoker Time since quitting	459	13.5	9.1, 19.8	
		1–2 years	31	9.9	5.6, 17.5	
		3–5	28	6.3	3.6, 11.0	
		6–9	27	4.8	2.7, 8.4	
		10–14	26	3.2	1.8, 5.7	
		≥ 15	39	2.9	1.7, 4.8	
		Never smoker	32	1.0		
Schlecht et al., (1999) Brazil	Oral and pharyngeal cancers ICD–9: 140; 141; 143–145; 146–149 373 oral cases 217 pharyngeal cases 1 578 controls	*Oral cancer* Commercial cigarettes: Current smoker Former smoker	214	8.0	4.3, 14.9	Multi-centre, hospital based. Estimates adjusted for alcohol use.
		≤ 5 years	19	3.1	1.3, 7.0	
		6–10 years	8	2.1	0.8, 5.7	
		11–15 years	2	0.7	0.1, 3.7	
		15 years	6	1.0	0.3, 2.9	
		Never smoker	21	1.0		
		Pharyngeal cancer Commercial cigarettes: Current smoker Former smoker	138	5.9	2.2, 15.3	
		≤ 5 years	12	2.6		
		6–10 years	2	1.2	0.8, 8.5	
		11–15 years	2	1.4	0.2, 7.0	
		15 years	2	0.9	0.2, 9.8	
		Never smoker	5	1.0	0.1, 5.5	

Table 5. Years since quitting oral cancer (contd)

Author Publication year Country	Study population Subsite	Smoking categories	Cases	Odds ratio	95% confidence interval	Comments
Lissowska et al., (2003) Poland	Oral and pharyn-geal cancer	Current smoker	78	3.4	1.5, 8.0	Hospital based; 31% cases and 56% controls lived in Warsaw (urban area). Estimates adjusted for gender age, residence and alcohol use.
		Former smoker	22	1.4	0.6, 3.3	
		Never smoker	22	1.0		
	ICD–9: 141; 143–145; 146; 149	Currently smoker Years since quitting	72	1.0		
	Men					
	78 cases	≤ 10 years	14	0.5	0.2, 1.3	
	Women	>10 years	12	0.3	0.1, 0.8	
	44 cases					
	122 controls					
Znaor et al., (2003) India	Oral and pharyn-geal cancers	Oral cancer				Hospital based – two centers. Estimates adjusted for age, center, education level, alcohol, and chewing.
		Current smoker	954	1.9	1.6, 2.3	
		Former smoker	185	0.8	0.6, 1.1	
	ICD9: 140;141;143-146;148; 149	Never smoker	424	1.0		
		Current smoker Years since quitting	954	1.0		
	Men	2–4 years	65	0.5	0.3, 0.7	
	1563 oral cases	5–9 years	46	0.5	0.3, 0.7	
	636 pharyngeal	10–14 years	25	0.3	0.2, 0.4	
	cases	≥ 15 years	49	0.5	0.3, 0.8	
	1711 cancer	Pharyngeal cancer				
	controls	Current smoker	492	4.0	3.1, 5.2	
	1927 healthy	Former smoker	57	1.2	0.8, 1.8	
	controls	Never smoker	87	1.0		
		Current smoker Years since quitting	492	1.0		
		2–4 years	24	0.4	0.2, 0.7	
		5–9 years	13	0.3	0.2, 0.6	
		10–14 years	9	0.2	0.01, 0.4	
		≥ 15 years	10	0.2	0.1, 0.5	

current smokers was 1.8 (95% CI=1.1–2.7) and former smokers 1.5 (95% CI=0.9–2.5) after adjustment for several potential confounders (Yun et al., 2005).

The follow-up of 34 439 male British doctors over a 50-year period provided a mortality rate for oral cancer among never smokers as 1.9 per 100 000, former cigarette smokers 1.3 and current cigarette smokers 7.1 (Doll et al., 2005).

For smokers of other tobacco products the mortality rate for current smokers was 6.8 versus 4.4 for former smokers. For pharyngeal cancers the mortality rates were 0.0 among never smokers and 6.7 among current cigarette smokers versus 1.7 among former cigarette smokers. Among smokers of other products the mortality rate was 7.1 for current versus 1.7 for former smokers. All four cohort studies showed reduced

relative risks for former smokers compared with current smokers.

Case–Control Studies

The odds ratio (OR) of oral cancer for former smokers as a proportion of that for current smokers varied from 16.6% in the study on men aged ≤ 45 years in the United Kingdom (Llewellyn et al., 2004) and 18.5% in the study from China on patients aged 20–80 years (Zheng *et al.*, 1997) to 78% in the study from Taiwan (Ko *et al.*, 1995). The ratio of the risks indicates proportionally, the amount of risk in current smokers present after cessation. The smaller the percentage, the greater the reduction in risk experienced by former smokers. The ratio is obtained by dividing the OR in former smokers by the OR in current smokers times 100. In four studies the proportion varied between 36% and 46% (Zheng *et al.*, 1990; Choi and Kahyo, 1991a; Oreggia *et al.*, 1991; De Stefani *et al.* 1998a). In all these studies there was an overlap between the CIs of the ORs for current and former smokers.

In these studies the excess risk of former smokers compared to never smokers was variable. The minimum residual risk was given by an OR of 0.5 for former smokers compared to never smokers in the study by Zheng *et al.* (1997) and the maximum by an OR of 11.8 (Oreggia *et al.*, 1991). In four studies, the OR for former smokers compared to never smokers was around 2 (Zheng *et al.*, 1990; Franceschi *et al.*, 1992; De Stefani *et al.*, 1998; Znaor *et al.*, 2003).

Duration of cessation

Eighteen case–control studies reported odds ratios by time since quitting smoking (Table 5). Odds ratios for any time period after quitting smoking were lower than those for current smokers, confirming the results just described on studies without specification of duration of cessation. There was generally an overlap in the 95% confidence intervals of the odds ratios for the different cessation time periods. Generally, after 10 years since quitting the OR was significantly lower than that of current smokers (no overlap of CIs). In many of the studies comparing risks of former smokers of 10 or more years duration to risks of never smokers, former smokers

could reach the level of risk of never smokers only after this duration (Franceschi *et al,* 1990; Choi and Kahyo, 1991a; Franceschi *et al,* 1992; De Stefani *et al.,* 1998a; LaVecchia, *et al.,* 1999; Schlecht *et al.,* 1999). There was no specific trend for years since quitting in one study (Znaor *et al.,* 2003).

Studies in former smokers

A study conducted in seven hospitals in Beijing, China, on 309 controls and 248 men with incident oral cancers diagnosed between 1988 and 1989, reported an OR of 1.1 for former smokers, representing a 54.2% decrease in the risk experienced by current smokers (about 85% cigarette smokers and 15% pipe or both cigarettes and pipe smokers) and a 10% increase in the risk experienced by never smokers. The study adjusted for alcohol use, education, sex and age (Zheng *et al.*, 1990; Table 4). A subsequent analysis of the subset of 111 tongue cancer patients and 111 controls showed that former smokers experienced an 81.5% reduction in the risk of cancer compared to continuing smokers (about 38% were pipe smokers among the 63 who specified type of smoke). A former smoker was defined as one who had quit smoking more than one year prior to diagnosis (Zheng *et al.*, 1997).

In Taiwan, among 104 men and 3 women oral cancer patients and 200 controls identified during 1992–93 at a hospital in Kaohsiung, the OR for former cigarette smokers was 3.6 (95% CI=0.9–14.6) compared with 4.6 (95% CI=1.5–14.0) for current cigarette smokers. Still, former smokers experienced more than 3 times the risk of never smokers, the referent group. ORs were adjusted for education, occupation, alcohol and betel quid consumption (Ko *et al.* 1995).

In a population-based study conducted in the four northern-most counties of Sweden, with 354 cancer registry cases during 1980–89 and 354 controls, former smokers had a risk equal to that of never smokers, whereas the OR for current smokers was 1.8 (95% CI=1.1–2.7). Thus former smokers had a 55% reduction in risk (Schildt *et al.,* 1998).

In an analysis of data collected on 86 male and 36 female oral cancer patients along with 385 male and 221 female controls during 1980–84 in a population-based study in Torino, Italy, men who had quit smoking for two to five years had risk reduced by 18.5% compared with smokers who had quit within one year of diagnosis, while those who had quit more than five years before had a risk reduced by 92.6%. After more than five years men had an odds ratio close to that of never smokers. Women who had quit more than two years before diagnosis experienced a 50% reduction in risk compared with those who had quit within one year (Merletti *et al.,* 1989); Table 5).

In the first-ever study from Korea on the role of tobacco and alcohol (Choi and Kahyo, 1991a), 113 men with oral cancer and 339 hospital controls were interviewed. Former smokers had a 64% lower risk than did smokers and an excess risk similar to that of never smokers after adjustment for alcohol use.

In a hospital-based study from Uruguay, with 57 male tongue cancer patients diagnosed between 1987 and 1989 and 353 controls, former smokers experienced 40% of the risk of the current smokers, but approximately 12 times greater risk than never smokers. Quitters of 1–4 years, 5–9 years and 10 years or more had their risk reduced by 60%, 70% and 80% respectively compared with continuing smokers (p for trend <0.001). Former smokers of ten years or more had a significantly reduced risk compared with those who had quit for fewer years (Oreggia *et al.,* 1991).

Among men younger than 75 years (157 oral cancer cases and 1272 controls) in a study from Italy (from 1986 until 1989), former smokers with a quitting interval of under 10 years duration had about half (51%) the risk of current smokers while those with abstinence of 10 years or more had only 10% of the risk (p for trend <0.01); their risk (OR=1.1; 95% CI=0.3–5.1) was almost the same as never smokers (Franceschi *et al.*, 1990).

In another study from Italy (1986–1990), analysing risks to men (<75 years) for tongue (101 cases) and mouth cancer (99 cases) separately with 726 controls, former smokers had an 80% reduction in risk for tongue cancer and nearly a 70% reduction in risk for mouth cancer with respect to current cigarette smokers. After 10 years or more of having stopped smoking, men had an excess risk close to never smokers, but there was a small overlap between the CIs for less than 10 years of quitting (Franceschi *et al.*, 1992).

Analysis of data on 359 men with oral cavity or oropharyngeal cancer and 2280 controls aged 37–80 years attending a Veterans hospital in New Jersey, USA (Mashberg *et al.*, 1993) collected from 1972 to 1983 showed that former smokers experience 20% less risk of oral or oropharyngeal cancer than smokers of 5 or fewer cigarettes per day (minimal smokers used as reference group). However, when stratifying by duration of cessation, those who had quit between for 3–10 years had an increased risk compared with minimal smokers (130% increase), while those who had quit for 11 or more years had only half the risk of minimal smokers (OR=0.5; 95% CI=0.1–2.6) (Mashberg *et al.*, 1993).

In a study that collected data on 425 men with oral cancer and 427 controls in Uruguay (DeStefani *et al.*, 1998a) during 1992–1996, former smokers had 2.2 times the risk of never smokers and 62% less risk than current smokers, while those who quit ten or more years previously had 88% less risk of smokers (significantly reduced) and reached the risk level of never smokers.

In an investigation that combined data collected from 1984–1997 from two case–control studies from Italy and Switzerland, on 638 men and women under 75 years with oral cancer and 4179 controls (La Vecchia *et al.*, 1999), former smokers who had quit within 1–2 years of the interview had 26% less risk than current smokers had. Those who had quit for 10–14 years had a risk significantly reduced by 87% of that of current smokers and an OR around the level of never smokers.

A study from Brazil on men and women (mean age 58 years) diagnosed during 1986–1989 with various head and neck cancers presented results by cancer site. Analysis of 270 cases of oral cancer, with 1578 never smokers as the reference group, found that the risk dropped substantially after five years of quitting to nearly one-fourth the risk of current smokers. Former smokers of over 15 years reached an odds ratio of 1.0. This paper provided graphic representation of relative risk as a function of time since quitting smoking, for mouth, pharynx and larynx cancers (Schlecht *et al.*, 1999).

In a study on 1563 male oral cancer patients and 3638 controls from India interviewed during 1993–99 (Znaor *et al.*, 2003), former smokers, defined as those who quit two or more years prior to interview, experienced a 52% reduction in risk compared with current smokers, but an 80% higher risk than never smokers. Those who quit two to four years before had half the risk of current smokers, and the risk did not appear to decrease further with time, calculated up to ≥15 years.

In summary, eighteen out of 26 case–control studies reported separate odds ratios for different time periods since quitting smoking. Odds ratios for any time period after quitting smoking were lower than those for current smokers,

confirming the results just described in studies without distinction of time periods of quitting. There was generally an overlap in the 95% confidence intervals of the odds ratios for the different time periods.

Although most participants in these studies responded that they had smoked cigarettes, the studies report on a diverse array of smoking products. Hand-rolled cigarettes containing tobaccos different from those in commercial cigarettes were used by many of the respondents (e.g., in Brazil and Uruguay). Analyses showed different odds ratios for smokers of commercial versus hand-rolled cigarettes. The fact that different proportions of smokers used filtered and non-filtered cigarettes was mentioned in two studies and differing ORs for current use were found for these types of cigarettes (Merletti *et al*, 1989; De Stefani *et al.*, 1998a). Several studies included small numbers of pipe and cigar smokers in their analyses. Smoking in India included bidis and other products along with cigarettes. Some studies analysed women separately, but as there were too few former smokers among the relatively few women smokers for analysis, results on women were rarely reported in this review.

Generally after nine or ten years since quitting, the OR for oral or pharyngeal cancer (or both) was significantly lower than that of current smokers (no overlap of 95% CIs) (Oreggia *et al.*, 1991; De Stefani *et al.*, 1992; MacFarlane *et al.*, 1995; De Stefani *et al.*, 1998a; La Vecchia *et al.*, 1999; Schlecht *et al.*, 1999; Lissowska *et al.*, 2003), or nearly so in some studies (e.g., Franceschi *et al.*, 1990; Hayes *et al.*, 1999; Schlecht *et al.*, 1999). In several other studies the ORs for former smokers after 10 years of quitting were still somewhat higher than for never smokers. Trends for time since quitting, measured in several studies, were significant (Franceschi *et al.*, 1990; Choi & Kahyo, 1991a; Oreggia *et al.*, 1991; Lissowska *et al.*, 2003).

Oesophageal Cancer

The risk of oesophageal cancer is strongly related to tobacco and alcohol consumption, with relative risks over 100 in heavy smokers and heavy drinkers (Tuyns *et al.,* 1977; Franceschi *et al.,* 1990). For both tobacco and alcohol there are strong dose-risk relations, and for tobacco there is also a strong duration of exposure-risk pattern. The risk of both squamous and adenocarcinoma of the oesophagus is associated with tobacco smoking. The proportion of each histologic type varies in different countries; the occurrence of adenocarcinoma of the oesophagus has increased over the past years (Gammon *et al.,* 1997). Several studies have been unable to distinguish between the two histologies in the cases reported.

Cohort and case–control studies published before December 2005 on oesophageal cancer and smoking cessation identified through Medline and by searching the references of the retrieved studies are reviewed here.

Cohort Studies

About 10 cohort studies (including a nested case–control study) reported data on oesophageal cancer in relation to smoking cessation (Table 6). All studies—with the exception of the nested case–control study (Guo *et al.,* 1994)—gave the RR for former smokers overall, since they collected smoking information only at the enrolment of the study subjects. No adequate information on histological type was available for these cohorts.

A cohort of 25 000 Swedish men (Carstensen *et al.,* 1987) reported a RR of 1.3 in former smokers, as compared to never smokers (death rate 4.3/100 000 person years). In current smokers the

RR was 1.1 in those smoking 1–7 g/day of tobacco, 2.5 in those smoking 8–15 g/day and 5.4 for individuals smoking >15 g/day.

In the Japanese Life Span Study, including over 60 000 atomic bomb survivors (Akiba, 1994), the RR of oesophageal cancer in current smokers as compared to never smokers was 3.1 (95% CI=1.7, upper limit not available) and 2.1 (95% CI=0.8–5.0) in former smokers on the basis of information from the first survey, and 3.3 (95% CI=1.7, upper limit not available) and 2.8 (95% CI=1.3–6.3) respectively on the basis of information from subsequent surveys.

In a nested case–control study of the Linxian Nutrition Intervention Trial including 640 oesophageal cancer cases from China (Guo *et al.,* 1994), the RR of oesophageal cancer in current smokers was similar to that of subjects who had quit smoking for less than 3 years, but was reduced by 50% in those who had quit longer (≥ 3 years).

In the 26-year follow-up of the 248 046-subject US Veterans cohort (McLaughlin *et al.,* 1995a), the RR of oesophageal cancer was 4.1 (95% CI=3.0–5.6) in current smokers and 1.5 (95% CI=1.0–2.2) in former smokers compared with never smokers.

A Swedish study on a cohort of over 26 000 women found a higher RR in former (RR=3.6; 95% CI=0.8–16) than in current smokers (RR=1.7; 95% CI=0.5–5.3) compared with never smokers (Nordlund *et al.,* 1997). These results were, however, based on a limited number of oesophageal cancer cases (n=25).

In the Reykjavik study including 22 946 subjects participating in an Icelandic cardiovascular risk factor study, the RR was 2.0 (95% CI=0.6–6.6) in former smokers, compared with never

smokers. Corresponding figures were 3.6, 4.1 and 1.5 for current smokers of 1–14 cigarettes/day, 15–24 cigarettes/day and ≥ 15 cigarettes/day, respectively, but again based on a small number of cases (n=49; Tulinius *et al.,* 1997).

In a Japanese cohort including over 220 000 adults, the adjusted RR of oesophageal cancer for former smokers was 1.9 (95% CI=0.9–3.6) in men as compared to never smokers; none of the women in the study were former smokers (Kinjo *et al.,* 1998). The RR for current smokers were 2.3 (95% CI=1.5–3.3) and 2.7 (95% CI=1.8–3.8) for male light and heavy smokers, respectively, and 1.8 (95% CI=1.1–3.0) for female light smokers.

A cohort of 1 212 906 Koreans aged 30–95 years from the Korean Medical Insurance Corporation (Jee *et al.,* 2004), gave oesophageal cancer mortality rates of 4.0/100 000 in never smokers, of 7.0 in former smokers, and of 12.4 in current smokers. Corresponding figures for incidence were 5.3, 8.4, and 16.2, respectively.

In the 50-year follow-up of the male British Doctors Study (Doll *et al.,* 2005), the mortality rates were 5.7/100 000 in never smokers, 20.1 in former cigarette smokers and 34.4 in current smokers. Corresponding figures for former and current smokers of other tobacco products were 18.9/100 000 and 25.1/100 000 respectively.

Case–Control Studies

Squamous-cell oesophageal carcinoma or without histology specified

At least 10 case–control studies reported information on squamous-cell carcinoma (or did not specify histology type) and analyzed the time pattern of

Table 6. Cohort studies: Relative risk of oesophageal cancer by smoking status and/or years since quitting

Author Publication year Country	Study population	Smoking categories	Relative risk	95% confidence interval	Comments
Carstensen et al., (1987) Sweden	Men 25 129 37 deaths	Current smoker Former smoker Never smoker	5.4 1.3 1[a]		Death rates standardized for age and residence.
Akiba, (1994) Japan	Life Span Study 61 505 survivors 103 cases	Current smoker Former smoker Never smoker	3.3 2.8 1[a]	1.7, n.a 1.3, 6.3	Estimates adjusted for city, sex, population group, atomic bomb exposure status, year of birth, age and amount smoked.
Guo et al., (1994)[b] China	Linxian Intervention Trial Study 29 584 subjects 640 cases 319 men	Current smoker Years since quitting < 3 ≥ 3	1[a] 1.1 0.5	0.6, 2.2 0.2, 1.2	Estimates adjusted for cancer history in first degree relative. Estimates reported correspond to men only.
McLaughlin et al., (1995a) USA	US Veterans' Study 248 046 men 318 deaths	Current smoker Former smoker Never smoker	4.1 1.5 1[a]	3.0, 5.6 1.0, 2.2	Estimates adjusted for attained age and calendar year period.
Nordlund et al., (1997) Sweden	Swedish Census Study 26 032 women 25 cases	Current smoker Former smoker Never smoker	1.7 3.6 1[a]	0.5, 5.3 0.8,16.0	Estimates adjusted for age and residence.
Tulinius et al., (1997) Iceland	Reykjavik Study 22 946 subjects 49 cases	Current smoker 1–14 cig/day 15–24 cig/day 25+ cig/day Former smoker Never smoker	3.6 4.1 1.5 2.0 1[a]	1.0, 12.8 1.2, 3.1 0.2, 13.2 0.6, 6.6	Values reported for male cases are age adjusted.
Kinjo et al., (1998) Japan	Six-prefecture Study 220 272 adults (100 840 men and 119 432 women) 440 deaths	Men Current smoker 1–14 cig/day 15+ cig/day Former smoker Never smoker	2.3 2.7 1.9 1[a]	1.5, 3.3 1.8, 3.8 0.9, 3.6	RR adjusted for attained age, prefecture and occupation.
		Women Current smoker 1–14 cig/day 15+ cig/day Former smoker Never smoker	1.8 1[a]	1.1, 3.0	

Table 6. Cohort studies in oesophageal cancer (contd)

Author Publication year Country	Study population	Smoking categories	Relative risk		95% confidence interval	Comments
Jee et al., (2004) Korea	Korean Medical Insurance Corporation Cohort 1 212 906 subjects 818 cases 611 deaths	*Mortality (men)*	*Mortality*			Age adjusted mortality rates per 100 000 person/year
			Rate	RR		
		Current smoker	12.4[c]	3.6	2.6, 4.9	
		Former smoker	7.0[c]	1.9	1.4, 2.7	
		Never smoker	4.0[c]	1[a]		
		Incidence (men)	*Incidence*			Age adjusted incidence rates per 100 000
			Rate	RR		
		Current smoker	16.2[c]	3.1	2.4, 4.0	
		Former smoker	8.4[c]	1.6	1.2, 2.1	
		Never smoker	5.3[c]	1		
Doll et al., (2005) United Kingdom	Male British Doctors 34 439 men 207 deaths	Current smoker Former smoker Never smoker	*Mortality* 34.4[c] 20.1[c] 5.7[c]			Age and study year standardized mortality rates

[a] Reference category.
[b] Nested case-control study.
[c] Rate per 100 000.
n.a = not available

the change in risk after stopping smoking (Table 7). In addition, five case–control studies included information on tobacco cessation and oesophageal adenocarcinoma (Table 7).

In a case–control study from coastal South Carolina, USA (Morris Brown et al., 1988), including 207 men with oesophageal cancer, those who had stopped smoking for less than 10 years had an odds ratio similar to that of current smokers (around 2), while the OR in those who had quit for 10 years or more dropped to that of never smokers.

In another case–control study from the USA on 275 oesophageal cancer cases (Yu et al., 1988), former smokers showed a reduced oesophageal cancer risk compared with current smokers, the reduction in risk increasing with increasing time since cessation of smoking. The RR was however still twofold increased in former smokers for 20 years or more, compared with never smokers.

Similarly, an Italian case–control study including 288 cancer cases (Franceschi et al., 1990; La Vecchia et al., 1990a) reported a lower oesophageal cancer risk in former smokers (OR=2.5; 95% CI=1.3–4.8 as compared to never smokers) than in current smokers (OR=5.0; 95% CI=3.0–8.5), but those who had quit smoking for 10 years or more still had a twofold increased risk compared with never smokers (95% CI=1.1–4.3).

A case–control study from the USA including 214 squamous-cell oesophageal cancers (Kabat et al., 1993) reported a significant reduction in risk in male former smokers (OR=1.3; 95% CI=0.7–2.4) in relation to current smokers (OR=4.5; 95% CI=2.5–8.1). When using current smokers as a reference group, the reduction in risk was evident within a few years after smoking cessation (OR=0.5 for those quitting 1–5 years earlier), and got larger with increasing number of years since

quitting smoking (OR=0.2 for over 20 years; Table 7). Among women, the OR was 2.2 (95% CI=1.1–4.3) in former smokers and 6.8 (95% CI=3.7–12.1) in current smokers. Using current smokers as the reference group, the OR was reduced by 70% (OR=0.3) after 10 years since quitting.

In a study from Paraguay on 131 cases (Rolón et al., 1995), the OR of oesophageal cancer was still elevated up to 7 years after smoking cessation (OR=5.2 as compared to never smokers), and dropped thereafter, although a two-fold increased risk persisted after 20 years since stopping smoking.

A similar pattern of risk reduction after stopping smoking was found in a US case–control study based on 221 cases with squamous-cell oesophageal cancer (Gammon et al., 1997), which reported an OR of 5.1 (95% CI=2.8–9.2) in current smokers and 5.6 (95% CI=2.9–10.8) in former smokers up to 10

Table 7. Case-control studies: relative risk of oesophageal cancer by years since quitting

Author Publication year Country	Study population	Smoking categories	Number of cases	Relative risk	95% confidence interval	Comments
Squamous-Cell or not specified						
Morris-Brown *et al.*, (1988) USA	Men 207 cases 422 controls	Current smoker Former smoker Years since cessation	128	1.8	1.0, 3.0	Estimates adjusted for study series (incidence or mortality) and alcohol use. Data presented correspond to cases directly interviewed (47%), all other case interviews were conducted by proxy family members.
		1–9 years	34	2.0	1.0, 3.7	
		≥ 10 years	8	1.0	0.5, 2.1	
		Never smoker	25	1[a]		
Yu *et al.*, (1988) USA	Subjects 275 cases 275 controls	Current smoker				
		1 pack/day	39	6.6	2.3, 19.3	
		2 packs/day	32	9.1	2.9, 29.0	
		3 + packs/day Former smoker Years since cessation	14	5.1	1.5, 16.9	
		<5	3	4.1	0.6, 28.6	
		5–9	9	3.3	0.8, 12.8	
		10–19	9	2.0	0.6, 7.2	
		≥ 20	7	1.9	0.5, 6.6	
		Never smoker	11	1[a]		
Franceschi *et al.*, (1990) La Vecchia *et al.*, (1990a) Italy	Men 288 cases 1 272 controls	Current smoker Former smoker Years since cessation	200	5.0	3.0, 8.5	Estimates adjusted for age, area of residence, education, occupation and alcohol use.
		<10	41	2.5	1.3, 4.8	
		≥ 10	29	2.2	1.1, 4.3	
		Never smoker	17	1[a]		
Kabat *et al.*, (1993) USA	Men 136 cases 4540 controls* Women 78 cases 2228 controls*	*Men* Current smoker Former smoker Years since cessation	68 43	1[a]		Estimates adjusted for age, education, alcohol use, hospital and time period.
		1–5		0.5	0.3, 1.0	* Controls for SCC, ADO and ADS.
		6–10		0.4	0.2, 0.8	
		11–20		0.3	0.2, 0.6	
		≥ 21		0.2	0.1, 0.3	
		Never smoker	15			
		Women Current smoker	41	1[a]		
		Former smoker Years since cessation	21			
		1–10		0.4	0.2, 0.9	
		≥ 11		0.3	0.1, 0.5	
		Never smoker	16			

Table 7. Case-control studies: oesophageal cancer (contd)

Author Publication year Country	Study population	Smoking categories	Number of cases	Relative risk	95% confidence interval	Comments
Rolón et al., (1995) Paraguay	Men 110 cases 318 controls Women 21 cases 63 controls	Current smoker Former smoker Years since cessation 1–7 8–19 ≥ 20 Never smoker	78 25 6 4 18	4.5 5.2 2.0 2.0 1[a]	2.2, 9.1 2.2, 2.4 0.6, 6.7 0.5, 7.9	Cases in men and women combined. Estimates adjusted for age, sex, hospital and alcohol use.
Gammon et al., (1997) USA	Subjects 221 cases 695 controls*	Current smoker Former smoker Years since cessation <11 11–20 21–30 >30 Never smoker	108 47 24 8 12 22	5.1 5.6 2.3 1.0 1.8 1[a]	2.8, 9.2 2.9, 10.8 1.1, 4.8 0.4, 2.7 0.8, 4.2	* Controls to SCC, ADO, GAD.
Launoy et al., (1997) France	Men 208 cases 399 controls	Current smoker Former smoker Years since cessation 1–5 6–10 ≥ 11	106 35 17 40	1[a] 1.4 0.7 0.5	0.8, 2.6 0.3, 1.5 0.3, 1.0	Estimates adjusted for interviewer, age, residence, occupation, education and marital status.
Castellsagué et al., (1999) Castellsagué et al., (2000) Argentina, Brazil, Paraguay & Uruguay	Men 655 cases 1407 controls Women 175 cases 372 controls	Men Current smoker Former smoker Years since cessation 1–4 5–9 ≥ 10 Never smoker Women Current smoker Former smoker Years since cessation 1–9 ≥ 10	415 68 39 101 32 43 11 9	1[a] 0.7 0.5 0.5 0.2 1[a] 1.0 0.4	0.5, 1.0 0.3, 0.8 0.4, 0.7 0.1, 0.4 0.3, 3.1 0.1, 1.2	Estimates adjusted for age, hospital, education and alcohol use.
Lagergren et al., (2000) Sweden	Subjects 167 cases 820 controls	Current smoker Former smoker Years since cessation <2 3–10 11–25 >25 Never smoker	101 93 18 15 13 22	9.3 10.3 5.2 2.1 1.9 1[a]	5.1, 17.0 5.6, 19.1 2.4, 11.3 1.0, 4.7 0.8, 4.0	Cases in men and women combined. Adjustment for age, sex, alcohol use, education, body mass index, physical activity, energy intake, fruit and vegetable consumption.

Table 7. Case-control studies: oesophageal cancer (contd)

Author Publication year Country	Study population	Smoking categories	Number of cases	Relative risk	95% confidence interval	Comments
Zambon et al., (2000) Bosetti et al., (2000b) Italy	Men 275 cases 593 controls	Former smoker Years since cessation				Estimates adjusted for age, area of residence, education and alcohol use.
		<5	27	7.7	3.2, 18.5	
		5–9	27	4.1	1.8, 9.1	
		≥ 10	51	1.5	0.8, 3.0	
		Never smoker	19	1[a]		
Znaor et al., (2003) India	Men 566 cases 1711 controls	Current smokers (cigarettes, bidi & other)	373	1[a]		Estimates adjusted for age, center, education, alcohol use and chewing.
		Former smoker Years since cessation				
		2–4	28	0.6	0.4, 0.9	
		5–9	23	0.6	0.4, 1.1	
		10–14	15	0.5	0.2, 0.8	
		> 15	19	0.5	0.3, 0.9	

Adenocarcinoma

Author Publication year Country	Study population	Smoking categories	Number of cases	Relative risk	95% confidence interval	Comments
Kabat et al, (1993) USA	Men 173 cases 4540 controls* Women 21 cases 2228 controls*	Men Current smoker Former smoker Years since cessation		2.3	1.4, 3.9	* Controls for SSC, ADO, ADS.
		1–5 years		0.5	0.2, 1.1	
		6–10 years		1.1	0.6, 1.9	
		11-20 years		1.2	0.8, 1.9	
		≥ 21 years		0.5	0.3, 0.9	
		Never smoker		1[a]		
		Women Current smoker Former smoker Years since cessation		4.8	1.7, 14.0	
		1–10 years		0.3	0.1, 1.7	
		≥ 11 years		0.3	0.1, 1.7	
		Never smoker		1[a]		
Morris Brown et al., (1994) USA	Men 174 cases 750 controls	Current smoker Former smoker Years since cessation	47	1.7	0.9, 3.2	Estimates adjusted or age, area, alcohol use and income.
		1–9	26	2.0	1.0, 4.1	
		10–19	28	2.4	1.2, 4.9	
		20–29	21	2.2	1.0, 4.7	
		≥ 30	23	3.1	1.5, 6.6	
		Never smoker	16	1[a]		

Table 7. Case-control studies: oesophageal cancer (contd)

Author Publication year Country	Study population	Smoking categories	Number of cases	Relative risk	95% confidence interval	Comments
Gammon et al., (1997) USA	293 cases 695 controls*	Current smoker Former smoker Years since cessation	86	2.2	1.4, 3.3	Estimates adjusted for age, sex, center, race, body mass index, income and alcohol use
		<11	44	2.7	1.6, 4.4	
		11–20	43	2.3	1.4, 3.8	* Controls to SCC, ADO, GAD.
		21–30	31	1.9	1.1, 3.2	
		>30	26	1.2	0.7, 2.2	
		Never smoker	63	1[a]		
Lagergren et al., (2000) Sweden	189 cases 820 controls*	Current smoker Former smoker Years since cessation	43	1.6	0.9, 2.7	* Controls to SCC, ADO, GAD.
		0–2	40	1.7	1.0, 3.0	
		3–10	20	2.4	1.2, 4.8	
		11–25	29	1.6	0.9, 2.5	
		>25	30	1.6	0.9, 2.8	
		Never smoker	57	1[a]		
Wu et al., (2001) USA	Subjects 222 cases 1356 controls	Current smoker Former smoker Years since cessation	68 106	2.8	1.8, 4.3	Adjusted for age, sex, race, birth place and education
		1–5		2.2	1.2, 3.9	
		6–10		1.1	0.5, 2.3	
		11–19		1.7	1.1, 2.9	
		≥ 20		1.3	0.8, 2.1	
		Never smoker	48	1[a]		

[a] Reference category.
SCC Squamous cell carcinoma
ADO Adenocarcinoma of the oesophagus
ADS Adenocarcinoma of the stomach
GAD Gastric cardia adenocarcinoma

years after cessation. The magnitude of the odds ratio decreased to 1.8 (95% CI=0.8–4.2) more than 30 years after cessation.

In a French case–control study including 208 squamous-cell oesophageal cancer cases (Launoy et al., 1997), the OR in former smokers compared with current smokers was 0.7 (95% CI=0.3–1.5) for subjects who had stopped for 6–10 years and 0.5 (95% CI=0.3–1.0) for those with longer abstinence.

A large case–control study of more than 800 squamous-cell oesophageal cancer cases from South America (Castellsagué et al., 1999, 2000) reported a OR of 5.1 (95% CI=3.4–7.6) for male current smokers and of 2.8 (95% CI=1.8–4.3) for former smokers. A reduction of risk with increasing time since cessation was evidenced in men when comparing former with current smokers (OR=0.7, 95% CI=0.5–1.0, one to four years after smoking cessation and 0.5, 95% CI=0.4–0.7, after 10 years

of cessation). A combined analysis of time since quitting smoking and past number of cigarettes smoked in men showed that the reduction in risk with time since cessation was higher in those with a greater average amount smoked per day (OR=5.1 1–4 years after quitting versus OR=2.8 ≥ 10 years after quitting in men who had smoked 15–24 cigarettes per day, while the corresponding figures in men who used to smoke 1–7 cigarettes per day were OR=1.5 and 2.0 respectively). In women, the ORs were

3.1 in current and 1.6 in former smokers as compared to never smokers, and a similar reduction of risk was observed with years since cessation, although the risk estimates were based on a limited number of cases (9 cases, OR=0.4, 95% CI=0.1–1.2, ten years or more after quitting smoking).

In a Swedish case–control study on 167 oesophageal squamous-cell carcinomas (Lagergren *et al.*, 2000), the risk of former smokers was about a third of that of current smokers as compared with never smokers (OR= 2.5 and 9.3, respectively). The risk reduction was evident after 3 years of cessation, tending to further decline with longer cessation (OR=1.9 for >25 years since smoking cessation).

An Italian case–control study including 275 men with squamous-cell oesophageal cancer (Bosetti *et al.*, 2000b; Zambon *et al.*, 2000) reported a reduction in risk following smoking cessation, dropping from 7.7 (95% CI=3.2–18.5) within 2 years after quitting to 1.5 (95% CI=0.8–3.0) 10 or more years after quitting.

A hospital-based case–control study conducted in Chennai and Trivandrium, India between 1993 and 1999 and including 566 male oesophageal cancer patients and 1927 controls found an overall OR of 2.8 (95% CI=2.2–3.7) in current and of 1.6 (95% CI=1.1–2.2) in former smokers of cigarettes, bidi and other types of tobacco products compared with never smokers (Znaor *et al.*, 2003). Using current smokers as a comparison group, the relative risk declined with increasing time since quitting from 0.6 2–9 years after quitting to 0.5 for longer periods of abstinence. The OR was 2.1 (95% CI=1.6–2.6) for current tobacco chewers and 1.6 (95% CI=1.05–2.5) for former chewers. In this group of tobacco users, the risk also declined with time since stopping, with an OR of 0.7 2–9 years after

quitting and 0.5 10 or more years since stopping chewing as compared with non-quitters.

Adenocarcinoma of the oesophagus

With reference to adenocarcinoma of the oesophagus, in a case–control study from the USA including 194 cases (Kabat *et al.*, 1993), the OR in current smokers was 2.3 (95% CI=1.4–3.9) and 1.9 (95% CI=1.2–3.0) in former smokers as compared to never smokers among men, and 4.8 (95% CI=1.7–14) and 1.4 (95% CI=0.4–4.4) in women. No trend in risk reduction over time was observed either in men or in women.

Another study from the USA including 174 cases in men (Morris-Brown *et al.*, 1994) showed no reduction in risk following smoking cessation on adeno-carcinoma of the oesophagus. Similarly, in a US case–control study on 293 adenocarcinoma cases (Gammon *et al.*, 1997) former and current smokers had similar OR (around 2), and the OR levelled to that of never smokers only 30 years after smoking cessation.

A Swedish case–control study on 189 oesophageal adenocarcinomas (Lagergren *et al.*, 2000) showed similar increased risks in both current (OR=1.6; 95% CI=0.9–2.7) and former smokers (OR=1.9; 95% CI=1.2–2.9) compared with never smokers, with no trend with time since smoking cessation.

Conversely, in a case–control study from the USA including 222 cases (Wu *et al.*, 2001), former smokers had a lower RR risk of oesophageal adeno-carcinoma than current smokers (OR=1.5; 95% CI=1.0–2.2 and 2.8; 95% CI=1.8–4.3, respectively). The pattern of decreased risk with increasing time since cessation was not monotonic, however, and the relative risk levelled to that of never smokers only after 20 years of abstinence.

Discussion

Epidemiological studies on smoking cessation and squamous-cell oeso-phageal cancer indicate that former smokers have a lower risk of oesophageal cancer than do current smokers. The risk of oesophageal can-cer remains elevated several years after cessation of smoking. After 10 years of smoking abstinence, former smokers still have a cancer risk twice that of never smokers.

Alcohol is the other major risk factor for oesophageal cancer (IARC, 1988). The fall in risk is larger after stopping both tobacco and alcohol consumption, and—compared with current smokers and drinkers—reaching an OR of 0.11 ten or more years after cessation of both habits in an Italian study (Bosetti *et al.*, 2000b).

The few studies which investigated the effect of smoking in adenocarcinoma of the oesophagus (Kabat *et al.*, 1993; Morris-Brown *et al.*, 1994; Gammon *et al.*, 1997; Lagergren *et al.*, 2000; Wu *et al.*, 2001) did not report a clear reduction in risk following smoking cessation. Some decline of risk, if any, was suggested only after 20–30 years of cessation. These results would indicate therefore that smoking may affect an early stage in the process of carcino-genesis for adenocarcinoma of the oesophagus (Day and Brown, 1980). The less clear decline in the risk of oesophageal adenocarcinoma after smoking cessation may help explain the fact that mortality trends for adeno-carcinoma do not parallel trends in smoking prevalence, and that they differ from those for squamous-cell oesophageal cancer (Blot and McLaughlin, 1999). The data on adeno-carcinoma are however too limited to provide adequate inference on any time-risk relation with time since smoking cessation.

Likewise, there is inadequate evidence on the time-risk relation with reference to various levels of intensity and duration of smoking, as well as on the absolute risk function for oesophageal cancer after stopping smoking. A combined analysis of time since cessation of smoking and number of cigarettes smoked in men enrolled in a South American case–control study (Castellsagué et al., 1999, 2000) showed that the reduction in the risk of squamous-cell oesophageal cancer following smoking cessation was greater for higher quantities smoked per day. Likewise, an Italian case–control study (Zambon et al., 2000) showed that among former smokers—as in current smokers—squamous-cell oesophageal cancer linearly increased with increasing number of cigarettes smoked per day and with years of duration of the habit, but no relation was found according to age at starting smoking.

Stomach Cancer

A causal association between tobacco smoking and stomach cancer was established recently (IARC, 2004). The relative risk for current smokers compared with never smokers is in the order of 2. A large body of evidence also supports a causative role for Helicobacter pylori in stomach cancer. However, assessment of the role of H. pylori in studies considering the effect of smoking cessation on the risk of stomach cancer was not available. Alcohol consumption is also a known risk factor for this neoplasm.

Relative risks in former smokers have been examined in 18 cohort studies; 10 found a lower relative risk in former smokers than in current smokers (Table 8). Two studies have assessed a number of factors that may influence the reduction in risk (Guo et al., 1994; Chao et al., 2002). Increasing number of years since cessation and younger age at cessation were associated with a significant trend in decreasing risk (Chao et al., 2002).

Twenty-four reports of case–control studies detailed in Table 9 have described results regarding the influence of smoking cessation on stomach cancer risk. Fourteen studies were hospital-based and 10 studies were population-based. In most studies, odds ratios were adjusted for variables such as sex, age, residence, socioeconomic status, income, diet and consumption of fresh fruits and vegetables. Odds ratios were adjusted for alcohol consumption in 11 studies (Correa et al., 1985; Ferraroni et al., 1989; De Stefani et al., 1990; Kabat et al., 1993; Ji et al., 1996; Gammon et al., 1997; De Stefani et al., 1998b; Inoue et al., 1999; Ye et al., 1999; Lagergren et al., 2000; Zaridze et al., 2000). In 19 of the 24 studies examined, quitting smoking was found to decrease the risk for stomach cancer.

Eleven studies also examined the effect of the duration of smoking cessation on stomach cancer risk (De Stefani et al., 1990; Kabat et al., 1993; Hansson et al., 1994; Inoue et al., 1994; Ji et al., 1996; Gammon et al., 1997; De Stefani et al., 1998b; Chow et al., 1999; Ye et al., 1999; Lagergren et al., 2000; Wu et al., 2001). A significant negative trend for increasing number of years since cessation was reported in seven studies (De Stefani et al., 1990; Hansson et al., 1994; Inoue et al., 1994; Gammon et al., 1997; De Stefani et al., 1998b; Lagergren et al., 2000), whereas two studies found no linear trend (Kabat et al., 1993; Ji et al., 1996). However, in examining temporal trends in risk with time since cessation, some studies did not exclude persons who had quit recently, among whom increased risk may reflect cessation due to smoking-attributable disease.

Several case–control studies presented studies for various subsites (cardia, antrum) (De Stefani et al., 1990; Wu-Williams et al., 1990; Saha, 1991; Palli et al., 1992; Kabat et al., 1993; Inoue et al., 1994; Gammon et al., 1997; De Stefani et al., 1998b; Ye et al., 1999; Zaridze et al., 2000; Wu et al., 2001). Dose–response relationships were observed between time since quitting and cancer of both cardia and distal stomach.

In synthesis, epidemiological studies show that former smokers have a lower risk for stomach cancer compared with current smokers. Increasing number of years since cessation was associated with decreasing risk in most studies.

Table 8. Cohort studies on tobacco smoking and stomach cancer

Reference Country and years of study	No. of subjects	No. of cases	Exposure estimates	Relative risk (95% CI)	Comments
Kahn (1966) USA 1954ñ62	US Veteransí Study 293 658 men 2 265 674 personñ years	420 deaths		Mortality ratio	Crude mortality ratio *Current and former cigarette smokerírefer to combined use of cigarettes and other forms of tobacco
			Current cigarette smoker* Former cigarette smoker*	1.5 (p < 0.01) 1.0	
			Cigarettes/day 1ñ9 10ñ20 21ñ39 ≥ 40	1.0 0.8 1.1 2.0	
			Former cigarette only-smoker	0.9	
			Past cigarettes/day 1ñ9 10ñ20 21ñ39 ≥ 40 Non- or occasional smoker	1.0 0.7 0.8 2.1 1.0	
McLaughlin et al. (1990a) USA 1954ñ80	US Veteransí Study 293 916 men 4 531 000 personñ years	1520 deaths	Current smoker Former smoker Never smoker	1.4 (1.2, 1.6) 1.0 (0.9, 1.2) 1	
Nomura et al. (1990a,b) USA 1965ñ84	American Men of Japanese Ancestry Study 7990 men 140 190 personñ years	150 cases	Current smoker Former smoker all quitters quitting ≤ 5 years	2.7 (1.8, 4.1) 1.0 (0.6, 1.7) 0.9 (0.4, 2.0)	Relative risks adjusted for age.
Kneller et al. (1991) USA 1966ñ86	Lutheran Brotherhood Insurance Study 17 633 men 287 000 personñ years	75 deaths	Ever smoker Current smoker Occasional smoker Former smoker Never smoker	2.1 (0.98, 4.4) 2.4 (1.1, 5.8) 0.7 (0.2, 2.8) 2.2 (1.0, 4.9) 1	Response rate, 68%; 23% of cohort lost to follow-up. Diagnosis not confirmed histologically.
Kato et al. (1992a) Japan 1985ñ91	9753 men and women 55 284 personñyears	57 deaths (35 men, 22 women)	Current smoker Former smoker	Men 2.3 (1.2, 4.6) 2.6 (1.0, 7.0)	Information on smoking habits taken from another survey unrelated to study. Small number of observations. Relative risks adjusted for age and sex. Multivariate analysis adjusted for alcohol intake, diet, cooking methods and family history of stomach cancer
			Current smoker Former smoker	Women 1.7 (0.4, 7.3) 4.9 (0.6, 36.8)	
			Current smoker Former smoker Never smoker	Multivariate analysis 2.2 (1.1, 4.4) 2.6 (1.0, 7.1) 1	

Table 8. Cohort studies stomach cancer (contd)

Reference Country and years of study	No. of subjects	No. of cases	Exposure estimates	Relative risk (95% CI)	Comments
Kato et al. (1992b) Japan 1985–89	3194 patients (1851 men, 2063 women) 17 289 person-years	45 cases (35 men, 10 women)	Former smoker ≤ 19 cigarettes/day ≥ 20 cigarettes/day Never smoker	1.2 (0.5, 2.9) 1.1 (0.4, 3.3) 2.2 (0.9, 5.4) 1	Relative risk adjusted for age, sex and residence
Tverdal et al. (1993) Norway 1972–88	Norwegian Screening Study 44 290 men, 24 535 women	98 deaths (78 men, 20 women)	Current smoker Former smoker Never smoker	Mortality rate *Men* *Women* 18.8 4.1 7.5 10.5 6.9 7.3	Mortality rate/100 000 person-years adjusted for age and area. No statistical analysis performed.
Guo et al. (1994) China 1985–91	Linxian Intervention Trial Study 29 584 men and women	539 cases in men	Ever smoker Current smoker *Years since quitting* ≥ 3 < 3	1.0 (0.7, 1.3) 1 0.8 (0.4, 1.7) 1.0 (0.4, 2.3)	Nested case-control study. Analysis for men only. Odds ratios adjusted for participation in intervention group and cancer history in first-degree relatives
McLaughlin et al. (1995) USA 1954–80	US Veterans Study 177 903 men 3 252 983 person years	1058 deaths	Ever smoker Current smoker Former smoker Never smoker	1.3 (1.1, 1.4) 1.4 (1.2, 1.6) 1.0 (0.9, 1.2) 1	Relative risks adjusted for attained age and calendar-year time-period.
Nomura et al. (1995) USA 1965–94	American Men of Japanese Ancestry Study 7972 men 177 080 person years	250 cases	Current smoker Former smoker Never smoker	2.3 (1.7, 3.2) 1.1 (0.7, 1.6) 1	Adjusted for age and alcohol intake.
Engeland et al. (1996) Norway 1966–93	Norwegian Cohort Study 11 863 men, 14 269 women About 540 000 Person-years	417 cases (258 men, 159 women)	Current smoker Former smoker Never smoker	*Men* *Women* 1.3 (0.9, 1.9) 1.0 (0.6, 1.4) 1.3 (0.9, 2.0) 0.8 (0.4, 1.6) 1	Response rate, 76%. Relative risks adjusted for age.
Nordlund et al. (1997) Sweden 1963–89	Swedish Census Study 26 032 women Almost 600 000 person-years	226 cases	Current smoker Former smoker Never smoker	1.3 (0.8, 1.9) 0.2 (0.0, 1.3) 1	Relative risks adjusted for age and place of residence.

Table 8. Cohort studies stomach cancer (contd)

Reference Country and years of study	No. of subjects	No. of cases	Exposure estimates	Relative risk (95% CI)	Comments
Tulinius et al. (1997) Iceland 1968–95	Reykjavik Study 11 366 men, 11 580 women	246 cases (171 men, 75 women)	Current smoker 1–14 cig./day 15–24 cig./day 25+ cig./day Former smoker Never smoker	1.5 (0.8, 2.5) 1.9 (1.1, 3.1) 1.0 (0.4, 203) 1.2 (0.8, 1.8) 1	Analysis for men only because of small no. of deaths in women. Relative risks adjusted for age.
Mizoue et al. (2000) Japan	Fuknoma Study 4054 men 35 785 person years		Current smoker Former smoker	SMR 2.2 (0.8, 5.7) 2.2 (0.8, 6.0)	SMR adjusted for study area, age and alcohol consumption.
Chao et al. (2002) USA 1982–96	Cancer Prevention Study II 467 788 men, 588 053 women	1505 deaths (996 men, 509 women)	Current smoker Former smoker Years since cessation ≥ 20 1–19 ≤10 p for trend Age at quitting smoking (years) ≤ 30 31–40 41–50 ≥ 51 p for trend	Men 2.2 (1.8, 2.7) 1.6 (1.3, 1.9) 1.2 (0.95, 1.6) 1.6 (1.3, 2.1) 1.9 (1.5, 2.5) 0.0015 1.2 (0.8, 1.7) 1.3 (0.9, 1.7) 1.6 (1.2, 2.1) 1.9 (1.5, 2.4) 0.0015 — Women 1.5 (1.2, 1.9) 1.4 (1.1, 1.7) 1.3 (0.95, 1.6) 1.5 (1.00, 2.1) 1.3 (0.9, 1.9) 0.683 1.1 (0.7, 1.9) 1.8 (1.2, 2.7) 1.3 (0.8, 2.0) 1.3 (0.9, 1.8) 0.68	Multivariate models include age, race, education, family history of stomach cancer, consumption of high-fibre cereal products, vegetables, citrus fruits and juices, and use of vitamin C, multivitamins and aspirin. Estimates of p for trend excluded non-users of tobacco.
Doll et al., 2005 UK 1951–2001	British Doctors' Study 34 439 men		Current smoker Former smoker Never smoker	Mortality rate 41.9 25.4 28.1	Mortality rate per 100 000/year
Koizumi et al. 2004 Japan 1984–1992 1990–1997	Pooled analysis of 2 cohorts studies 129 392 men	451 cases	Current smoker Former smoker Years since quitting < 5 5–14 ≥15 Never smoker	1.8 (1.4, 2.4) 1.8 (1.3, 2.4) 1.7 (1.1, 2.6) 2.1 (1.4, 3.1) 1.3 (0.8, 2.2) 1.0	
Fujino et al. 2005 Japan 1988–1999	JACC Study 43 482 men 54 580 women 970 251 person-years	757 deaths	Current smoker Former smoker Never smoker	Men 1.3 (1.0, 1.7) 1.2 (1.0, 1.6) 1.0 — Women 0.8 (0.4, 1.5) 1.2 (0.5, 2.7) 1.0	Estimates presented are adjusted hazard ratios.

CI, confidence interval
SMR, standardized mortality ratio

Table 9. Case-control studies on tobacco smoking and stomach cancer

Reference Country Years of study	Subjects	Exposure estimates	Relative risk (95% CI) versus never smokers		Comments
Correa et al. (1985) USA 1979–83	Hospital based study *Men* 264 cases 264 controls *Women* 127 cases 127 controls	*Cigarette smoker* Ever smoker Current smoker Former smoker	*Whites* 1.3 (0.8, 2.2) 1.4 (0.8, 2.4) 1.0 (0.5, 2.0)	*Blacks* 2.6 (1.4, 5.0) 2.7 (1.3, 5.3) 1.9 (0.8, 4.2)	No response rate for cases or controls. No definition of smoking habit. High proportion of interviews with proxies. Odds ratios adjusted for age, sex, current alcohol consumption, respondent type, education and income. About 30% of controls had cardiac or respiratory diseases.
Jedrychowski et al. (1986) Poland 1980–81	Hospital and population based study *Men* 70 cases 140 controls *Women* 40 cases 80 controls	Current smoker Former smoker	0.7 (0.4, 1.2) 0.8 (0.3, 2.1)		No definition of smoking habit. Analysis performed with hospital controls only. Odds ratio adjusted for residence only. Risk estimate could be underestimated because hospital controls included patients with smoking-related diseases
Ferraroni et al. (1989) Italy 1983–88	Hospital based study *Men* 243 cases 1334 controls *Women* 154 cases 610 controls	Former smoker *Cigarettes/day* <15 15–20 > 25	*Univariate* 0.9 0.9 1.0 1.1	*Multivariate* 0.9 1.0 1.0 1.1	No participation rate for cases or controls. Univariate analysis adjusted for age and sex. Multivariate analysis adjusted for age, sex, social class, education, marital status, alcohol and coffee consumption.
De Stefani et al. (1990) Uruguay 1985–88	Hospital based study *Men* 138 cases 414 controls *Women* 72 cases 216 controls	Current smoker Former smoker *p* for trend Years since quitting ≥ 10 5–9 1–4 *p* for trend	*All subsites* 2.7 (1.3, 5.5) 1.9 (0.9, 3.8) 0.004 0.6 (0.3, 1.0) 0.5 (0.2, 1.1) 1.2 (0.6, 2.3) 0.028	*Cardia and corpus* (*n* = 46) 5.3 (1.2, 24.1) 1.8 (0.4, 8.8) 0.002	Analysis for men only because there were few women who smoked. No participation rate for controls. Odds ratios adjusted for age, area of residence, wine intake and vegetable consumption.

Table 9. Case–control studies stomach cancer (contd)

Reference Country Years of study	Subjects	Exposure estimates	Relative risk (95% CI) versus never smokers		Comments
			Men	Women	
Kato et al. (1990) Japan 1985–89	Hospital based study Men 289 cases 2013 controls Women 138 cases 2415 controls	All types Using healthy controls Cigarettes/day 1–19 ≥ 20 Former smoker	1.9 (1.1, 3.3) 2.8 (1.8, 4.3) 1.8 (1.2, 2.8)	0.6 (0.2, 1.8) 1.5 (0.6, 3.7) 1.3 (0.5, 3.1)	Many more cases than controls were aged ≥ 55 years. Odds ratios adjusted for age and residence.
		Atrophic gastritis controls Cigarettes/day 1–19 ≥ 20 Former smoker	2.5 (1.5, 4.4) 3.5 (2.3, 5.5) 2.1 (1.4, 3.3)	0.6 (0.2, 1.8) 2.5 (0.9, 6.9) 1.1 (0.4, 2.9)	
		Diffuse type Using healthy controls Cigarettes/day 1–19 ≥ 20 Former smoker	(n = 117) 1.8 (0.7, 4.2) 3.3 (1.7, 6.4) 2.7 (1.4, 5.5)	(n = 86) 0.5 (0.1, 2.1) 1.1 (0.3, 3.6) 1.0 (0.3, 3.4)	
		Intestinal type Using healthy controls Cigarettes/day 1–19 ≥ 20 Former smoker	(n = 166) 2.3 (1.2, 4.3) 3.0 (1.7, 5.1) 1.6 (0.9, 2.8)	(n = 49) 0.8 (0.2, 3.6) 2.7 (0.8, 9.9) 1.2 (0.3, 5.3)	
		Atrophic gastritis controls Cigarettes/day 1–19 ≥ 20 Former smoker	3.1 (1.6, 6.0) 3.8 (2.2, 6.6) 2.0 (1.2, 3.4)	0.7 (0.2, 3.2) 6.4 (1.5, 27.4) 0.9 (0.2, 4.3)	

Table 9. Case–control studies stomach cancer (contd)

Reference Country Years of study	Subjects	Exposure estimates	Relative risk (95% CI) versus never smokers		Comments
WuñWilliams et al. (1990) USA 1975ñ82	Population based study *Men* 137 cases 137 controls		*All pairs*	*Excl. proxies*	Very small study. Very low response rate for cases. High proportion of interviews with proxies (42% of cases, 12% of controls). Numbers in analyses by subsites too small for meaningful conclusion. Matched analysis made without adjustment.
		Current smoker (packs/day) 1 2 ≥ 3 Former smoker Never smoker	2.2 (1.1ñ4.7) 2.1 (1.0ñ4.5) 5.2 (1.4ñ8.6) 1.3 (0.6ñ2.5) 1	5.4 4.0 17.7 1.8 1	
			Cardia	*Fundus/body*	
		Current smoker (packs/day) 1 2 ≥ 3 Former smoker Never smoker	2.3 2.2 7.0 1.0 1	2.0 4.4 9.3 3.4 1	
			Antrum/pylorus	*All others*	
		Current smoker (packs/day) 1 2 ≥ 3 Former smoker Never smoker	4.0 4.1 7.2 0.8 1	1.7 1.8 1.8 1.4 1	
Boeing et al. (1991) Germany 1985ñ87	Hospital based study 143 cases 579 controls	Current smoker Former smoker Never smoker	0.5 (0.3, 0.9) 0.6 (0.3, 1.2) 1		Higher proportion of nonsmokers in cases from two study centres; higher proportion of smokers in hospital controls than in visitor controls; 47% of hospital controls had tobacco-related diseases. Odds ratios adjusted for age, sex and hospital.
Saha (1991) UK 8 years	Hospital based study *Men* 81 cases 162 controls *Women* 36 cases 72 controls	Current smoker Former smoker Never smoker	2.6 (1.2, 5.5) 1.4 (1.7, 3.6) 1		Small size study. Odds ratios not adjusted.

Table 9. Case–control studies stomach cancer (contd)

Reference Country Years of study	Subjects	Exposure estimates	Relative risk (95% CI) versus never smokers	Comments
Agudo et al. (1992) Spain 1987ñ89	Hospital based study *Men* 235 cases 235 controls *Women* 119 cases 119 controls	Current smoker Former smoker Never smoker	0.9 (0.6, 1.5) 0.9 (0.5, 1.7) 1	Analysis for men only because few women smoked. No participation rate for cases or controls. Odds ratios adjusted for total caloric intake (including alcohol) and consumption of fruit, vegetables, cold cuts and preserved fish.
Hoshiyama & Sasaba (1992) Japan 1984ñ90	Population based study *Men* 251 cases 483 controls	Current smoker Former smoker Never smoker	*Single* 1.5 (0.9, 2.6) 1.1 (0.6, 1.8) 1	No definition of smoking status. Very low response rate for controls. Odds ratios adjusted for sex, age and administrative division.
Palli et al. (1992) Italy 1985ñ87	Population based study *Men* 597 cases 705 controls *Women* 326 cases 454 controls	Current smoker Former smoker Never smoker	*Gastric cardia* 1.1 (0.6, 2.3) 1.1 (0.5, 2.2) 1	*Other subsites* 0.9 (0.7, 1.1) 1.1 (0.8, 1.4) 1	Study population from Buatti et al. (1989, 1991). Odds ratios adjusted for age, sex, area and place of residence, migration from the south, socioeconomic status, family history of stomach cancer and Quetelet index.
Kabat et al. (1993) USA 1981ñ90	Hospital based study *Men* 295 cases 4544 controls *Women* 52 cases 2228 controls	*Men* Current smoker Former smoker Never smoker *Years since quitting* ≥ 21 11ñ20 6ñ10 1ñ5 *Women* Current smoker Former smoker Never smoker *Years since quitting* 1ñ10 ≥ 11	*Distal stomach* 1.7 (1.0, 3.0) 1.4 (0.9, 2.4) 1 (reference) 0.6 (0.3, 1.2) 1.1 (0.6, 1.9) 1.1 (0.6, 2.4) 1.0 (0.5, 2.0) 3.2 (1.3, 7.7) 2.0 (0.8, 4.9) 1 0.7 (0.2, 2.2) 0.7 (0.2, 2.1)	Analysis limited to Caucasians. No participation rate for controls. Odds ratios adjusted for age, education, alcohol consumption, hospital and time of interview.

Table 9. Case–control studies stomach cancer (contd)

Reference Country Years of study	Subjects	Exposure estimates	Relative risk (95% CI) versus never smokers	Comments
Hansson et al. (1994) Sweden 1989–92		Current smoker Former smoker	1.7 (1.2, 2.5) 1.1 (0.8, 1.6)	Odds ratios adjusted for age, sex, socioeconomic status and use of other tobacco
		Years since quitting > 31 > 21-31 > 11-20 ≤ 10 Current smoker p for trend	0.9 (0.5-1.7) 0.9 (0.5-1.7) 1.2 (0.7-2.1) 1.3 (0.7-2.2) 1.7 (1.2-2.5) 0.02	
Inoue et al. (1994) Japan 1988–91	Hospital based study Men 420 cases 420 controls Women 248 cases 248 controls	Men Ever smoker Current smoker Former smoker Years since quitting ≥ 10 1–9 < 1	Cardia (n = 79) All 2.6 (1.7, 3.8) 4.4 (1.8, 11.3) 2.7 (1.8, 4.1) 4.7 (1.8, 12.3) 2.4 (1.6, 3.6) 4.1 (1.6, 11.0) 2.3 (1.4, 3.7) 2.8 (0.9, 8.6) 2.5 (1.5, 4.1) 4.7 (1.6, 13.7) 2.6 (1.2, 5.2) 6.9 (1.9, 25.0)	No definition of smoking habit. Odds ratios adjusted for age (continuous) and intake of fresh vegetables. According to the authors, prevalence of smoking in general population in Japan is slightly higher than in hospital controls used (81.6% vs 77% in men)
		Current smoker Former smoker Never smoker Years since quitting ≥ 10 1–9 < 1	Middle (n = 133) Antrum (n = 170) 1.9 (1.1, 3.4) 3.0 (1.7, 5.4) 1.6 (0.9, 2.9) 2.7 (1.5, 5.0) 1 1 1.7 (0.9, 3.4) 2.7 (1.4, 5.4) 1.4 (0.7, 3.0) 3.0 (1.5, 6.1) 3.6 (0.8, 5.8) 2.1 (0.7, 6.1)	
Gajalakshmi & Shanta (1996) India 1988–90	Hospital based study Men 287 cases 287 controls Women 101 cases 101 controls	Any tobacco Ever smoker Current smoker Former smoker Current cigarette smoker Never smoker	Model 1 Model 2 2.5 (1.7, 3.6) 2.2 (1.3, 3.8) 2.7 (1.8, 4.1) 2.5 (1.4, 4.4) 1.8 (1.1, 3.1) 1.5 (0.7, 3.5) 2.0 (1.1, 3.6) 1 1	Any tobacco included bidi, cigarette and/or chutta. Conditional logistic regression models: Model 1, adjusted for income, education and area of residence; Model 2, additionally adjusted for betel-quid chewing habit and significant dietary factors.

Table 9. Case–control studies stomach cancer (contd)

Reference Country Years of study	Subjects	Exposure estimates	Relative risk (95% CI) versus never smokers		Comments
Ji et al. (1996) China 1988–89	Population based study *Men* 770 cases 819 controls *Women* 354 cases 432 controls		*Men*	*Women*	Odds ratios adjusted for age, education and income (and alcohol drinking for men only)
		Current smoker	1.4 (1.1, 1.7)	0.9 (0.5, 1.4)	
		Former smoker	1.3 (0.9, 1.8)	2.0 (0.7, 5.6)	
		Years since quitting			
		≥ 20	0.7 (0.3, 1.6)	≥ 10 3.7 (0.9, 14.7)	
		10–19	1.5 (0.8, 2.7)	< 10 0.7 (0.1, 4.1)	
		5–9	0.9 (0.5, 1.9)		
		< 5	2.7 (1.4, 5.4)		
		p for trend	0.10	0.48	
			Cardia (n = 145)	*Distal (n = 530)*	
		Men			
		Current smoker	1.2 (0.8, 1.9)	1.4 (1.1, 1.9)	
		Former smoker	1.8 (0.97, 3.4)	1.1 (0.7, 1.7)	
		Years since quitting			
		≥ 20	1.5 (0.5, 5.2)	0.5 (0.2, 1.5)	
		10–19	1.3 (0.5, 4.0)	1.4 (0.7, 2.8)	
		5–9	1.3 (0.4, 4.3)	0.7 (0.3, 1.8)	
		< 5	5.5 (1.9, 15.9)	2.5 (1.1, 5.4)	
		p for trend	0.01	0.10	
Gammon et al. (1997) USA 1993–95	Population based study *Men* 477 cases 555 controls *Women* 152 cases 140 controls		*Cardia*	*Other*	Odds ratios adjusted for age, sex, geographical area, race, body-mass index, income and alcohol intake
		Current smoker	2.6 (1.7, 4.0)	1.8 (1.2, 2.7)	
		Former smoker	1.9 (1.3, 2.9)	1.5 (1.1, 2.1)	
		Years since quitting			
		> 30	1.1 (0.6, 2.0)	1.0 (0.6, 1.8)	
		21–30	2.2 (1.3, 3.7)	1.5 (0.9, 2.4)	
		11–20	1.6 (0.9, 2.8)	1.7 (1.0, 2.7)	
		< 10	2.9 (1.8, 4.8)	1.8 (1.2, 2.9)	
		p for trend	< 0.05	< 0.05	
De Stefani et al. (1998b) Uruguay 1992–96	Hospital based *Men* 311 cases 622 controls	Ever smoker	1.8 (1.2, 2.8)		Odds ratios adjusted for age, residence, urban/rural status, total alcohol consumption and vegetable intake
		Current smoker	2.6 (1.6, 3.1)		
		Former smoker	1.3 (0.8, 2.2)		
		Never smoker	1		
		Years since quitting			
		≥ 15	1.1 (0.7, 1.9)		
		10–14	1.0 (0.5, 2.1)		
		5–9	1.5 (0.8, 2.9)		
		1–4	2.4 (1.3, 4.3)		
		Current smoker	2.6 (1.6, 4.1)		
		p for trend	< 0.001		

Table 9. Case–control studies stomach cancer (contd)

Reference Country Years of study	Subjects	Exposure estimates	Relative risk (95% CI) versus never smokers	Comments
Chow et al. (1999) Poland 1994–97	Population based study *Men* 302 cases 314 controls *Women* 162 cases 166 controls	Ever smoker Current smoker Former smoker *Years since quitting* ≥ 30 20–29 10–19 < 10	*Men* 1.2 (0.8, 1.8) 1.7 (1.1, 2.7) 0.9 (0.6, 1.4) 0.7 (0.4, 1.5) 0.8 (0.4, 1.6) 0.9 (0.5, 1.7) 1.0 (0.5, 1.8) / *Women* 1.8 (1.1, 3.0) 1.8 (1.0, 3.3) 1.8 (0.9, 3.7) 3.0 (1.0, 9.2) 1.5 (0.5, 4.3) 1.3 (0.4, 4.0)	Odds ratios adjusted for age, education, years lived on a farm, family history of cancer
Inoue et al. (1999) Japan 1988–95	Hospital based study *Men* 651 cases 12 041 controls *Women* 344 cases 31 805 controls	Current smoker Former smoker < 60 years old (n = 314) Current smoker Former smoker ≥ 60 years old (n = 337) Current smoker Former smoker	*Men* 2.5 (1.9, 3.3) 1.7 (1.3, 2.3) 3.3 (2.2, 4.9) 2.2 (1.4, 3.4) 1.9 (1.3, 2.7) 1.4 (0.9, 2.0) / *Women* 1.7 (1.3, 2.4) 1.4 (0.8, 2.3) (n = 182) 1.7 (1.1, 2.5) 2.1 (1.1, 4.1) (n = 162) 2.0 (1.2, 3.2) 0.8 (0.3, 2.0)	Odds ratios adjusted for age, year and season at first hospital visit, family history of gastric cancer, alcohol drinking, preference for salty food and fruit intake
Ye et al. (1999) Sweden 1989–95	Population based study *Men* 348 cases 779 controls *Women* 166 cases 385 controls	Current former *Cigarettes/day* 1–10 11–15 ≥ 16 Former smoker *Years since quitting* ≥ 21 11–20 ≤ 10	*Cardia*: 1.7 (0.7, 3.8), 1.2 (0.4, 3.8), 2.2 (1.0, 4.8), 0.8 (0.4, 1.5), 0.7 (0.3, 1.6), 0.6 (0.2, 1.5), 0.9 (0.4, 2.2); *Distal (intestinal)*: 1.6 (0.9, 2.8), 1.8 (0.9, 3.7), 2.0 (1.1, 3.9), 1.4 (0.9, 2.0), 1.4 (0.9, 2.2), 1.4 (0.8, 2.3), 1.4 (0.8, 2.3); *Distal (diffuse)*: 1.9 (1.0, 3.4), 2.5 (1.2, 5.5), 2.7 (1.4, 5.1), 1.2 (0.8, 2.0), 0.9 (0.5, 1.9), 1.8 (1.0, 3.3), 1.1 (0.5, 2.2)	Odds ratios adjusted for age, sex, residence area, body-mass index 20 years before interview, socioeconomic status, use of smokeless tobacco and use of beer, wine and spirits. About 30% of eligible cases died or became too ill to be interviewed. Data on cessation from ex-smokers of cigarettes, pipe and cigar
Lagergren et al. (2000) Sweden 1995–97	Population based study *Men* 223 cases 681 controls *Women* 39 cases 139 controls	Current smoker Former smoker Never smoker *Years since quitting* > 25 11–25 3–10 0–2 *p* for trend	*Univariate*: 3.9 (2.6, 5.8), 3.1 (2.1, 4.5), 1, 1.9 (1.1, 3.1), 3.7 (2.3, 5.8), 4.1 (2.4, 7.0), 4.2 (2.8, 6.4); *Multivariate*: 4.5 (2.9, 7.1), 3.4 (2.2, 5.2), 1, 2.1 (1.2, 3.6), 4.2 (2.6, 7.0), 4.9 (2.8, 8.7), 5.0 (3.2, 8.0), < 0.0001	Smokers include cigarette, cigar and pipe smokers. Univariate analysis adjusted for age and sex; multivariate analysis further adjusted for alcohol use, educational level, body-mass index, reflux symptoms, intake of fruit and vegetables, energy intake and physical activity.

Table 9. Case–control studies stomach cancer (contd)

Reference Country Years of study	Subjects	Exposure estimates	Relative risk (95% CI) versus never smokers		Comments
Zaridze et al. (2000) Russia 1996-97	Hospital based study Men 248 cases 292 controls Women 200 cases 318 controls	Current smoker Former smoker Never smoker	*All types* 1.4 (0.9, 2.2) 1.1 (0.6, 1.9) 1	*Cardia* 2.0 (0.9, 4.5) 1.2 (0.5, 3.1) 1	Controls significantly younger and better educated than cases (p < 0.01). Odds ratios adjusted for age, education and vodka consumption. Relative risk may be underestimated because of substantial proportion of controls had smoking-associated diseases (> 20%).
Wu et al. (2001) USA 1992-97	Population based study Men 402 cases 999 controls Women 228 cases 357 controls	Current smoker *Cigarettes/day* 1-19 ≥ 20 Former smoker Never smoker	*Cardia* 2.1 (1.5, 3.1) 1.1 (0.7, 1.6) 1.3 (0.9, 1.8) 1.2 (0.9, 1.6) 1	*Distal stomach* 1.5 (1.1, 2.1) 1.1 (0.8, 1.6) 1.0 (0.7, 1.5) 1.1 (0.8, 1.5) 1	Very low participation rate for cases. Odds ratios adjusted for age, sex, race, birthplace and education
		Years since quitting ≥ 20 11-19 6-10 1-5 *p* for trend	1.1 (0.7, 1.7) 1.2 (0.8, 1.9) 1.6 (0.9, 2.7) 1.4 (0.8, 2.4) 0.08	1.1 (0.8, 1.6) 0.9 (0.6, 1.4) 1.4 (0.9, 2.2) 1.2 (0.7, 2.0) 0.31	

CI, confidence interval

Liver Cancer

The major risk factors for liver cancer include chronic infection with hepatitis B and C virus (HBV and HCV) (IARC, 1994) and heavy alcohol consumption (IARC, 1988). An association between smoking and increased risk of liver cancer was identified in numerous cohort and case–control studies, particularly the largest ones from Asia, Greece and the USA (IARC, 2004). Two cohort studies from the Republic of Korea, one case–control study from Italy and an update of the British Doctors' cohort, subsequently published, have reported on the association between smoking and liver cancer including data in former smokers (Jee et al., 2004; Doll et al., 2005; Yun et al., 2005; Franceschi et al., 2006).

Cohort studies and case–control studies providing information on the relative risk for liver cancer in former smokers are shown in Tables 10 and 11 respectively. Several of the studies originally appearing in the IARC Monograph on tobacco smoke (IARC, 2004) showed a lower risk for liver cancer among former smokers than in current smokers but did not look at time since cessation. In the 50-year follow-up of the British Doctors Study, liver cancer mortality rates were 4.4/100 000 in never smokers, 5.7/100 000 in former smokers and 13.6/100 000 in current smokers (Doll et al., 2005).

Jee et al. (2004) and Yun et al. (2005) reported elevated risk of liver cancer in current and former smokers as compared with never smokers, but no reduction in risk in former over current smokers. In the study by Franceschi et al. (2006), current and former smokers did not show increased liver cancer risk as compared with never smokers.

The only study that examined the relative risks by number of years since quitting showed some decrease in risk with time since cessation in women but not in men (Goodman et al., 1995) (Table 10).

Covariates that may potentially confound or modify the relationship between smoking and liver cancer include alcohol consumption and chronic infection with HBV/HCV. Exposure to aflatoxin as a confounder in the association between smoking and liver cancer has not been assessed.

In synthesis, the risk of cancer of the liver appears to be lower in former than in current smokers, but the data are inconsistent across studies in different geographic areas. There is no adequate information to assess the effect of time since stopping.

Pancreas Cancer

Smokers have about twice as high a risk for pancreas cancer as never smokers, and the risk increases with duration of smoking and number of cigarettes smoked daily (IARC, 2004).

In 19 out of 23 cohort studies (Table 12) and in 17 out of 21 case–control studies (Table13) the relative risk of developing or dying from pancreatic cancer was lower for former smokers than for current smokers. The risk reduction for former smokers was confirmed in the 50-year follow-up of the British Doctors Study when it reported 39.4, 30.5 and 20.6 age-standardized pancreas cancer mortality rates per 100 000 in current, former and never smokers respectively (Doll et al., 2005). A recent cohort study of 446 407 Korean men who had a medical evaluation in 1992 and were followed up for ten years (Yun et al., 2006) included 863 incident cases of pancreatic cancer. Compared with never smokers, the relative risk of pancreas cancer in current smokers was 1.7 (95% CI: 1.6–1.9), and the RR of dying from pancreas cancer was 1.6 (95% CI: 1.4–1.7). Corresponding figures for former smokers were 1.3 (95% CI=1.2–1.5) and 1.2 (95% CI=1.0–1.3) respectively. Former smokers had significantly lower risks than current smokers but higher risks than never smokers. This study provided detailed information on the risk of pancreatic cancer incidence and mortality in relation to smoking intensity and duration but did not offer data according to duration of abstinence.

Five of eight early studies reporting on the risk of pancreatic cancer according to the number of years since quitting smoking found a decreasing monotonic trend in risk associated with the number of years for which the subjects had stopped smoking (Mack et al. 1986; Howe et al. 1991; Silverman et al. 1994; Ji et al. 1995; Partanen et al. 1997) (Table 14). An additional study (Fuchs et al. 1996) reported that the excess risk in former smokers disappeared after less

Table 10. Cohort studies on cigarette smoking including former smokers and liver cancer

Reference Country and years of study	Cohort No. of subjects	No. deaths/ incident cancers	Smoking categories and other variables	Relative risk	(95% CI)	Adjustment factors/ comments
Carstensen et al. (1987) Sweden 1963ñ79	Swedish Census Study 25 129 men	54 deaths	Current smoker	3.0		Relative death rates Categories in grams of any tobacco/day combined: 1 cigarette = 1 g; 1 small cigar = 3 g; 1 large cigar = 5 g
			Cigarettes/day			
			1ñ7	1.6		
			8ñ15	3.3		
			> 15	4.1		
			Former smoker	1.7		
			Never smoker	1		
Hsing et al. (1990) USA 1954ñ80	US Veterans Study 293 916 men	289 deaths	Current smoker	2.4	1.6, 3.5	Adjusted for age and calendar period
			Cigarettes/day			
			< 10	2.2	1.2, 3.8	
			10ñ20	2.0	1.3, 3.0	
			21ñ39	2.9	1.8, 4.5	
			> 39	3.8	1.9, 8.0	
			Former smoker	1.9	1.2, 2.9	
			Never smoker	1		
Shibata et al. (1990) Japan 1960ñ86 (II)	Cohort II 677 men 17 172 personñ years	22 deaths	Current smoker	3.6	0.6, 22.3	Adjusted for age and alcohol use
			Cigarettes/day			
			1ñ9	11.9	1.5, 96.8	
			10ñ19	1.1	0.1, 10.6	
			20ñ29	2.7	0.4, 19.2	
			$\geq$ 30	3.2	0.4, 23.7	
			1ñ19	2.1	0.4, 10.0	
			$\geq$ 20	1.9	0.4, 9.4	
			Former smokers	2.9	0.3, 29	
			Never smoker	1		

Table 10. Cohort studies in liver cancer (contd)

Reference Country and years of study	Cohort No. of subjects	No. deaths/ incident cancers	Smoking categories and other variables	Relative risk	(95% CI)	Adjustment factors/ comments
Kato et al. (1992) Japan 1987ñ90	1441 patients with decompensated liver cirrhosis, 343 with post-transfusion hepatitis 4386 personñ years	122 cases	Current smoker	1.0	0.5, 1.8	Adjusted for sex and age. Record linkage study. Patients at high risk for development of hepatocellular carcinoma
			Pack–years			
			< 30	0.8	0.4, 1.7	
			≥ 30	0.9	0.5, 1.9	
			Former smoker	0.9	0.4, 2.0	Adjusted for HBV, alcohol consumption, aflatoxin exposure and education
			Never smoker	1		
Goodman et al. (1995) Japan 1980ñ89	Life Span Study 36 133 men and women 311 086 personñ years	252 cases (156 men, 86 women)	**Men**			Adjusted for city, age at time of bombing and radiation dose to liver. Relative risk among non-drinkers of alcohol for ever smoking, 1.9 (95% CI, 1.2ñ2.9); among men, 7.2 (95% CI, 1.0ñ 53.3); among women, 1.3 (95% CI, 1.0ñ1.7). [CIs calculated by the Working Group Volume 83]
			Current smoker	4.3	1.9, 9.7	
			Former smoker	4.2	2.0, 10.7	
			Never smoker	1		
			Years since quitting			
			≥ 24	4.0	1.5, 10.6	
			14ñ23	4.1	1.6, 10.7	
			< 14	5.6	2.2, 14.6	
			Women			
			Current smokers	1.6	0.9, 2.9	
			Former smokers	1.7	0.8, 3.6	
			Never smoker	1		
			Years since quitting			
			≥ 25	2.3	0.7, 7.4	
			10ñ24	1.0	0.3, 4.2	
			< 10	10.4	2.5, 43.5	

Table 10. Cohort studies in liver cancer (contd)

Reference Country and years of study	Cohort No. of subjects	No. deaths/ incident cancers	Smoking categories and other variables	Relative risk	(95% CI)	Adjustment factors/ comments
McLaughlin et al. (1995) USA 1954–80	US Veterans' Study 248 046 men 3 252 983 person–years	363 deaths	Current smokers *Cigarettes/day* 1–9 10–20 21–30 ≥ 40	1.8 1.8 1.4 2.3 2.6	1.4, 2.3 1.1, 2.8 1.1, 2.0 1.6, 3.1 1.4, 4.6	Adjusted for age and calendar-year time-period
			Former smokers Never smoker	1.5 1	1.4, 2.3	
Mizoue et al. (2000) Japan 1986–96	Fukuoka Study 4050 men 35 785 person– years	59 deaths	Current smoker *Cigarettes/day* 1–24 ≥ 25 Former smoker Never smoker	3.3 3.5 2.8 2.9 1	1.2, 9.5 1.2, 10.2 0.8, 9.6 1.0, 8.4	Adjusted for age, alcohol use and area of residence
Mori et al. (2000) Japan 1992–97	974 men, 2078 women 13 984 person– years	22 (14 men, 8 women)	Current smoker *Pack–years* < 10 ≥ 10 Former smoker Never smoker	3.3 2.0 2.1 1	0.4, 28.2 0.6, 6.9 0.6, 7.2	Adjusted for age and sex

Table 10. Cohort studies in liver cancer (contd)

Reference Country and years of study	Cohort No. of subjects	No. deaths/ incident cancers	Smoking categories and other variables	Relative risk	(95% CI)	Adjustment factors/ comments
				Men	*Women*	
Jee et al. (2004) Republic of Korea 1992-1995	Korean Cancer Prevention Study Cohort, participants of a national insurance program; 1 212 906 men and women	4 149 deaths in men 528 deaths in women	*Mortality*			Death rate in never smokers: 48.4 per 100 000 in men and 14.3 per 100 000 in women
			Current smoker	1.2 (1.1, 1.3)	1.0 (0.7, 1.3)	
			Former smoker	1.3 (1.2, 1.5)	1.3 (0.9, 1.8)	
			Never smoker	1	1	
			Incidence			
			Current smoker	1.1 (1.0, 1.2)		
			Former smoker	1.3 (1.2, 1.4)		
			Never smoker	1		
Doll et al. (2005) 1951-2001	British Doctors' study 34 439 men	74 deaths	Current smoker	13.6		Mortality per 100 000
			Former smoker	5.7		
			Never smoker	4.4		
Yun et al. (2005) Republic of Korea 1996-2000	National Health Insurance Corporation Study 733 134 men, 30 years or older in 1996 3 590 872 person-years	1434 incident cases	Current smoker	1.5	1.3, 1.7	Estimates adjusted for age, residence, alcohol use, body mass index, physical activity and dietary factors.
			Cigarettes / day			
			1-9	2.2	1.8, 2.7	
			10-19	1.5	1.3, 1.7	
			≥ 20	1.0	0.8, 1.2	
			Former smokers	1.5	1.3, 1.8	
			Never smokers	1		

HBV, hepatitis B virus; HCV, hepatitis C virus

Table 11. Case–control studies: relative risk of liver cancer in former smokers

Reference Country and years of study	No. of cases and controls	Smoking categories	Relative risk (95% CI)		Adjustment/comments
Yu et al. (1983) USA 1975–79		Current smoker			Population-based study among black and white non-Asians; Incident cases histologically confirmed (70.6%); aged ≥70 years. Adjusted for alcohol. Never smokers and former smokers combined.
		≤ 20 cigarettes/day	1.2	0.6, 2.5	
		> 20 cigarettes/day	2.6	1.0, 6.7	
		Former smoker	1.1	0.3, 4.0	
		Never smoker	1		
Austin et al. (1986) USA	86/172	Current smoker	1.5	0.7, 3.7	Adjusted for HBsAg status and alcohol consumption
		Former smokers	0.9		
		Never smokers	1		
La Vecchia et al. (1988) Italy 1984–87	151/1051	Current smoker	0.9	0.6, 1.5	Hospital-based study; cases aged 24-74 years. Adjusted for age, sex, geographical area, hepatitis, cirrhosis and alcohol consumption
		Former smoker	0.7	0.4, 1.0	
		Never smoker	1		
Tsukuma et al. (1990) Japan 1983–87	229/266	*Men and women*			Hospital-based study. Adjusted for age and sex
		Current smoker	2.5	1.4, 4.5	
		Former smoker	0.7		
		Never smoker	1		
		Men			
		Current smoker	2.3	1.1, 4.8	Adjusted for age
		Former smoker	0.8		
		Never smoker	1		
		Women			
		Current smoker	2.9	1.1, 7.9	Crude risk estimates
		Never smoker	1		

Table 11. Case–control studies in liver cancer (contd)

Reference Country and years of study	No. of cases and controls	Smoking categories	Relative risk (95% CI)	Adjustment/comments
Choi & Kahyo (1991b) Republic of Korea 1986ñ90	216/648	Current smoker Former smoker Never	1.0 0.7, 1.6 0.7 0.4, 1.2 1	Hospital-based study. Cases had average age 79 years. Adjusted for HBV status, age, alcohol consumption, education and marital status
Yu et al. (1991) USA 1984ñ90	74/162	Current smoker Former smoker Never smoker	*All* 2.1 (1.1, 4.3) 1.1 (0.4, 2.6) 1	*Men* 2.2 (0.8, 6.0) 1.1 (0.4, 3.3) 1	*Women* 2.4 (0.9, 6.7) 0.8 (0.1, 8.9) 1	Population-based study. Cases histologically confirmed (100%); aged 18-74 years. Adjusted for alcohol consumption
Tanaka et al. (1992) Japan 1985ñ89	204/410	Current smoker Former smoker Never smoker	*All* 1.5 (0.5, 2.5) 1.6 (0.9, 2.8) 1	*Men* 1.7 (0.9, 3.2) 1.8 (0.9, 3.5) 1	*Women* 1.0 (0.3, 3.2) 1.7 (0.4, 7.1) 1	Hospital-based study: Cases histologically confirmed (40%); aged 40-69 years. Adjusted for age and sex. Subjects with chronic hepatitis and cirrhosis excluded from control group. Histologically confirmed cases (82) did not differ from the remaining cases of liver cancer in their smoking habits.

Table 11. Case–control studies in liver cancer (contd)

Reference Country and years of study	No. of cases and controls	Smoking categories	Relative risk (95% CI)	Adjustment/comments
Tanaka et al. (1995) Japan 1983ñ89	120/257	Current smokers Male ever-smokers Former smokes Never smoker	2.8 (1.1, 6.9) 1.9 (1.2, 2.8) 2.2 (1.2, 4.1) 1	Hospital-based study. Cases aged 35-74 years. Adjusted for age, study category (except for ever-smokers), HBV, history of transfusion, family history of liver cancer and alcohol consumption. Combined analysis of 3 studies; partial overlap with Tanaka et al. (1992)
Kuper et al. (2000) Greece 1995ñ98	333/360	Current smoker Former smoker Never smoker	< 40 cigarettes/day / ≥ 40 cigarettes/day 1.2 (0.8, 1.9) / 1.6 (0.9, 2.9) 1.2 (0.7, 1.9) / 1.5 (0.7, 3.0) 1 / 1	Hospital-based study. Cases histologically confirmed (47%) Adjusted for age and sex Adjusted for age, sex and HBV and HCV status
		Current smoker HBV- and HCV-negative HBV- and/or HCV-positive All, adjusted for HBV/HCV	1.8 (0.9, 3.6) 1.3 (0.3, 5.6) 1.6 (0.8, 2.9)	2.8 (1.1, 6.9) 2.1 (0.3, 17.1) 2.5 (1.1, 5.5)	Adjusted for age, sex, education and HBV and HCV status
Franceschi et al. (2006) Italy 1999ñ2000	229/431	Current smoker Former smoker Never smoker	1.1 0.8 1	0.6, 2.2 0.5, 1.5	Hospital-based study. Cases histologically confirmed (72.8%). Cases under 85 years. Adjusted for age, sex, hospital, education and HbsAg or anti-HCV positivity

CI, confidence interval; NS, not significant; HBsAg, hepatitis B surface antigen; HBV, hepatitis B virus; HCC, hepatocellular carcinoma; HCV, hepatitis C virus

Table 12. Cohort studies: relative risk of pancreas cancer by smoking status without specification of years since quitting

Reference Country Years of follow-up	Subjects	Number of cases or deaths	Smoking status	Relative risks and 95% confidence interval (CI)						Comments
				Men	CI	Women	CI	Men and Women	CI	
Kahn (1966) USA 1954–62	US Veteransi Study 293 958 men	415 deaths	Current smoker Cigarettes/day 1–9 10–20 21–39 ≥ 40 Former smoker Never smoker	1.4 1.8 2.2 2.7 1.3 1						
Cederlof et al. (1975) Sweden 1963–72	Swedish Census Study 25 444 men 26 467 women	Men 46 deaths Women 37 deaths	Current smoker Cigarettes/day 1–7 8–15 ≥ 16 Former smoker Never smoker	1.6 3.4 5.9 4.8 1	$p < 0.05$	2.4 2.5 3.0 5.5 1				
Doll & Peto (1976) UK 1951–71 Doll et al. (1980) UK 1951–73	British Doctorsi Study 34 440 men 6194 women	Men 78 deaths Women 14 deaths	Current smoker Tobacco (g)/day 0 1–14 15–24 ≥ 25 Former smoker	Mortality rate 14 14 18 27 12		Mortality rate 9 4 24 16 11				
Hirayama (1981) Japan 1965–79	Six-prefecture Study 122 261 men 142 857 women	Men 251 deaths	Current smoker Cigarettes/day 1–9 10–19 ≥ 20 Former smoker Never smoker					Mortality rate 14.7 19.8 20.3 15.4 13.3		Annual death rates per 100 000 standardized for age
Hiatt et al. (1988) USA 1978–85	Kaiser Permanente Medical Care Program Study II 122 894 persons	49 cases	Current smoker < .5 pack/day .5 –1 pack/day 1–2 packs/day > 2 packs/day Former smoker Never smoker					1.8 1.9 2.1 6.6 0.8 1	0.4, 8.1 0.6, 6.2 0.6, 8.2 1.4, 31.8 0.4, 2.0	Annual death rates per 100 000 adjusted for age

Table 12. Cohort studies in pancreas cancer (contd)

Reference Country Years of follow-up	Subjects	Number of cases or deaths	Smoking status	Relative risks and 95% confidence interval						Comments
				Men	CI	Women	CI	Men and Women	CI	
Mills et al. (1988) USA 1976-82	Adventistsi Health Study 34 198 persons	40 cases	Current smoker Former smoker Never smoker					5.4 1.5 1	1.8, 16.5 0.7, 3.4	
Friedman & van den Eeden (1993) USA 1964-88	Kaiser Permanente Medical Care Program Study I 175 000 persons	450 cases 2687 controls	Current smoker > 20 years < 1 pack/day 1ñ2 packs/day > 2 packs/day Former smoker Never smoker					1.6 1.8 1.6 3.0 1.3 1	1.1, 2.2 $p < 0.01$ $p < 0.01$ $p < 0.01$	
Tverdal et al. (1993) Norway 1972-88	Norwegian Screening Study 44 290 men 24 535 women	57 deaths	Current smoker Former smoker Never smoker					Mortality rate 13.5 6.3 4.4	personñyears 248 159 144 776 127 325	
Zheng et al. (1993a) USA 1966-86	Lutheran Brotherhood Insurance Study 17 633 men 286 731 personñyears	57 deaths	Current smoker < 25 cigarettes/day ≥ 25 Former smoker Never smoker	1.4 3.9 1.0 1	0.6, 3.2 1.5, 10.3 0.4, 2.2					
Doll et al. (1994) UK 1951-91	British Doctorsi Study 34 439 men	205 deaths	Current smoker Former smoker Never smoker	Mortality rate 35 23 16						
Shibata et al. (1994) USA 1981-90	Leisure World Study 13 979 persons 100 921 personñyears	65 cases 28 men 37 women	Current smoker & Recent quitter (quit < 20 years) Former smoker (quit ≥ 20 years) Never smoker					1.2 1.4 1	0.7, 2.2 0.7, 2.6	
McLaughlin et al. (1995a) USA 1954-80	US Veteransi Study 248 046 men 3 252 983 personñ years	1264 deaths	Current smoker Former smoker Never smoker	1.7 1.1 1	1.5, 1.9 0.9, 1.3					

Table 12. Cohort studies in pancreas cancer (contd)

Reference Country Years of follow-up	Subjects	Number of cases or deaths	Smoking status	Relative risks and 95% confidence interval						Comments
				Men	CI	Women	CI	Men and Women	CI	
Engeland et al. (1996) Norway 1966–93	Norwegian Cohort Study 11 857 men and 14 269 women	224 cases 109 men 115 women	Current smoker			0.9	0.4, 1.8			55% histologically verified
			1–4 cigarettes/day	0.9	0.5, 1.8	1.8	1.1, 3.0			
			5–9	1.0	0.5, 1.8					
			10–14	1.3	0.7, 2.4					
			≥ 15	1.6	0.8, 3.2					
	Personñyears: about 230 000 men and 310 000 women		Former smoker	0.9	0.6, 1.5	0.6	0.2, 1.5			
			Never smoker	1		1				
			Unknown consumption	7.9	1.1, 5.8					
Fuchs et al. (1996) USA 1980–92	Nurses' Health Study (1976–92) and Health Professionals Follow Up Study (1986–94) 49 428 men 118 339 women 2 116 229 personñ years	186 cases	Current smoker	3.0	1.6, 6.3	2.4	1.6, 3.6			
			Former smoker	1.3	0.7, 2.3	1.1	0.7, 1.7			
			Never smoker	1		1				
Harnack et al. (1997) USA 1986–94	Iowa Women's Health Study 33 976 women 291 598 personñ years	66 cases	Current smoker			2.3	1.3, 4.2			
			Former smoker			1.1	0.6, 2.1			
			Never smoker			1				
Nordlund et al. (1997) Sweden 1963–89	Swedish Census Study 26 032 women 600 000 personñ years	144 cases	Current smoker			1.8	1.1, 2.9			
			Former smoker			2.5	1.1, 5.3			
Tulinius et al. (1997) Iceland 1968–95	Reykjavik Study 11 366 men, 11 580 women	101 cases 65 men 36 women	Current smoker							
			1–14 cigarettes/day	7.2	2.3, 22.3	1.5	0.7, 3.5			
			15–24	10.2	3.4, 30.6	1.7	0.6, 4.4			
			≥ 25	12.5	3.7, 41.7	4.5	1.0, 0.1			
			Former smoker	2.4	0.7, 7.6	0.9	0.3, 2.8			
			Never smoker	1		1				

Table 12. Cohort studies in pancreas cancer (contd)

Reference Country Years of follow-up	Subjects	Number of cases or deaths	Smoking status	Relative risks and 95% confidence interval (CI)						Comments
				Men	CI	Women	CI	Men and Women	CI	
Coughlin et al. (2000) USA 1982–96	American Cancer Society's Cancer Prevention 483 109 men 619 199 women	3751 deaths	Current smoker Former smoker Never smoker	2.1 1.1 1	1.9, 2.4 1.0, 1.3	2.0 1.2 1	1.8, 2.3 1.0, 1.3			
Nilsen et al. (2000) Norway 1984–96	National Health Screening Service Survey in North-Trondelag 31 000 men 32 374 women	166 cases	Current smoker Former smoker Never smoker	2.1 1.3 1	1.2, 3.6 0.8, 2.4	2.1 1.8 1	1.1, 4.2 0.8, 4.2			
Isaksson et al. (2002) Sweden 1958-1997	Swedish twin registry 9 680 men 12 204 women	176 cases	Current smoker Former smoker Never smoker	1.4 0.8 1	1.0, 2.0 0.4, 1.4					
Lin et al. (2002) Japan 1988–97	JACC study 110 792 subjects	225 deaths	Current smoker Former smoker Never smoker	1.6 1.1 1	1.0, 2.6 0.6, 1.9	1.7 1.8 1	0.9, 3.4 0.7, 5.0			
Doll et al. (2005) UK 1951–2001	British Doctors' Study 34 439 men	272 deaths	Current smoker Former smoker Never smoker	Mortality rate 39.4 30.5 20.6						Annual death rate per 100 000 standardized for age
Larsson et al. (2005) Sweden 1987–2004	Swedish Mammo-graphy Cohort (SMC) and the Cohort of Swedish Men COSM) 45 906 men 37 147 women	136 cases	Current smoker Former smoker Never smoker	2.5 1.0 1	1.3, 4.6 0.6, 1.7	3.8 1.4 1	2.1, 7.0 0.7, 2.8			
Gallicchio et al. (2006) USA 1963–78 and 1975–94	Two cohorts established in Washington County 45 749 subjects 48 172 subjects	133 cases	Cohorts: Current smoker Former smoker Never smoker	1963 2.0 1.9 1	1.0, 4.1 0.8, 4.2	1975 1.8 1.6 1	1.0, 3.1 0.9, 2.8			
Yun et al. (2006) Republic of Korea 1992–2003	446 407 men	863 cases	Current smoker Former smoker Never smoker	1.7 1.3 1	1.6, 1.9 1.2, 1.5					

Table 13. Case–control studies: relative risk of pancreas cancer by smoking status without specification of years since quitting

Reference Country Years of study	Study population	Smoking status	Relative risks and 95% confidence intervals (CI)					
			Men	CI	Women	CI	Men and Women	CI
MacMahon et al. (1981) USA 1974–79	369 cases 644 controls	Current smoker Cigarettes/day						
		1–19	1.1	0.5, 2.2	1.5	0.8, 2.8		
		≥ 20	1.4	0.9, 2.4	1.6	0.9, 2.9		
		Former smoker	1.4	0.9, 2.3	1.3	0.8, 2.2		
		Never smoker	1		1			
Wynder et al. (1983) USA 1977-1981	275 cases 7994 controls	Current smoker Cigarettes/day						
		1–10	0.9		1.8			
		11–20	2.1	$p < 0.05$	1.5			
		21–30	2.3	$p < 0.05$	2.0	$p < 0.05$		
		> 31	3.0	$p < 0.05$				
		Former smoker	1.7	$p < 0.05$	1.4			
		Never smoker	1		1			
Hsieh et al. (1986) USA 1981–84	176 cases 273 controls	Current smoker						
		<1 pack/day					1.8	0.8, 3.9
		≥ 1 pack/day					1.9	1.1, 3.3
		Former smoker					1.0	0.6, 1.7
		Never smoker					1	
Wynder et al. (1986) USA 1981–84	Men 127 cases 371 controls Women 111 cases 325 controls	Current smoker Cigarettes/day						
		1–20	3.5	1.8, 6.5	1.5	0.8, 2.7		
		≥ 21	2.9	1.5, 5.7	4.8	2.4, 9.5		
		Former smoker	1.3	0.7, 2.4	1.2	0.7, 2.1		
		Never smoker	1		1			
Clavel et al. (1989a) France 1982–85	161 cases 268 controls	Current smoker Cigarettes/day						
		1–20	1.7	0.8, 3.7	1.0	0.3, 3.3		
		≥ 21	1.4	0.6, 3.5	0.8	0.3, 2.5		
		Former smoker	1.0	0.5, 2.14	2.7	0.5, 14.1		
		Never smoker	1		1			

Table 13. Case–control studies in pancreas cancer (contd)

Reference Country Years of study	Study population	Smoking status	Relative risks and 95% confidence intervals (CI)					
			Men	CI	Women	CI	Men & Women	CI
Ferraroni et al. (1989) Italy 1983-88	214 cases 1944 controls	Current smoker						
		Cigarettes/day						
		< 15					0.8	
		15ñ24					1.2	
		≥ 25					1.4	
		Former smoker					1.2	
		Never smoker					1	
Baghurst et al. (1991) Australia 1984-87	104 cases 253 controls	Current smoker					1.8	0.9, 3.3
		Former smoker					1.1	0.6, 2.2
		Never smoker					1	
Bueno de Mesquita et al. (1991) The Netherlands 1984-88	176 cases 487 controls	Cigarettes lifetime						
		Current smoker						
		Low ≤ 111 200					1.6	0.7, 3.8
		High > 111 200					2.0	1.0, 4.0
		Former Smoker						
		Low ≤ 111 200					1.4	0.7, 2.6
		High > 111 200					1.1	0.4, 2.7
		Never smoker					1	
Howe et al. (1991) Canada 1983-86	249 cases 505 controls	Current smoker						
		Packs/year						
		0ñ17.9	0.9	0.4, 1.9	1.4	0.7, 2.8	2.1	1.0, 4.5
		17.9ñ37.5	1.6	0.8, 3.1	3.4	1.5, 7.5	2.9	1.6, 5.4
		> 37.5	1.6	0.8, 3.2	4.7	2.0, 11.4	3.4	1.9, 6.1
		Former smoker						
		Packs/year						
		0ñ17.9					0.7	0.4, 1.3
		17.9ñ37.5					1.6	0.8, 3.2
		> 37.5					1.2	0.6, 2.6
		Never smoker	1		1		1	
Vioque & Walker (1991) Multinational 1960ñ1980s	108 cases 374 controls	Current smoker					2.3	0.7, 7.3
		Former smoker					0.9	0.4, 1.7
		Never smoker					1	

Table 13. Case–control studies in pancreas cancer (contd)

Reference Country Years of study	Study population	Smoking status	Relative risks and 95% confidence intervals (CI)					
			Men	CI	Women	CI	Men and Women	CI
Mizuno et al. (1992) Japan 1989–90	68 cases 68 controls	Current smoker	4.5	1.5, 13.2				
		Cigarettes/day						
		1–12	2.6	1.0, 6.5				
		13–22	2.7	0.9, 7.0				
		≥ 23	1.2	0.4, 3.4				
		Former smoker						
		Never smoker	1					
Silverman et al. (1994) USA 1986–89	526 cases 2153 controls	Ever smoker	1.7	1.3, 2.2				
		Current smoker	2.0	1.5, 2.6				
		Former smoker	1.4	1.1, 1.9				
		Never smoker	1					
Gullo et al. (1995) Italy 1987–89	570 cases 570 controls	Current smoker						
		Cigarettes/day						
		≤ 20	0.9	0.6, 1.5	2.2	1.3, 3.7		
		> 20	1.6	0.9, 2.8	0.6	0.1, 2.7		
		Former smoker	0.6	0.4, 0.9	1.0	0.5, 1.9		
		Never smoker	1		1			
Ji et al. (1995) China 1990–93	451 cases 1552 controls	Current smoker	1.6	1.1, 2.2	1.4	0.9, 2.4		
		Former smoker	1.2	0.8, 2.0	1.6	0.6, 4.0		
		Never smoker	1		1			
Fernandez et al. (1996) Italy 1983–92	362 cases 1408 controls	Current smoker	1.3	0.9, 1.9	1.3	0.8, 2.2		
		Former smoker	1.4	0.9, 1.2	0.9	0.4, 2.0		
		Never smoker	1		1			
Ohba et al. (1996) Japan 1987–92	141 cases 282 controls	Current smoker	1.3	0.8, 2.0				
		Former smoker	1.3	0.7, 2.1				
		Never smoker	1					
Fryzek et al. (1997) USA 1994–95	66 cases 131 controls	Current smoker	2.5	1.1, 5.4				
		Former smoker	1.8	0.9, 3.6				
		Never smoker	1					
Muscat et al. (1997) USA 1985–93	484 cases 954 controls	Current smoker	1.6	1.1, 2.4	2.3	1.4, 3.5		
		Former smoker	1.0	0.7, 1.5	1.9	1.3, 2.9		
		Never smoker	1		1			

Table 13. Case–control studies in pancreas cancer (contd)

Country Years of study			Men	CI	Women	CI	Men and Women	CI
Chiu et al. (2001) USA 1986-89	376 cases 2434 controls	Current smoker Former smoker Never smoker	2.5 1.5 1	1.2, 4.1 1.0, 2.4	2.4 1.7 1	1.5, 3.9 1.0, 2.9		
Bonelli et al. (2003) Italy 1992-96	202 cases 406 controls	Current smoker Former smoker Never smoker					2.4 1.0 1	1.2, 4.6 0.6, 1.7
Inoue et al. (2003) Japan 1988-99	200 cases 2000 controls	Current smoker Former smoker Never smoker	1.0 0.6 1	0.6, 1.6 0.3, 1.0	1.8 0.3 1	0.8, 3.8 0.04, 2.4		

than 10 years since quitting, but did not provide quantitative estimates. More recently, results from four large prospective cohort studies conducted in three different continents added important detailed information on the relation between smoking cessation and pancreatic cancer risk:

The American Cancer Society's (ACS) Cancer Prevention Study II (CPS II), which followed 483 109 men and 619 199 women from 1982, was used to assess the predictors of pancreatic cancer mortality (Coughlin et al., 2000). During 14 years of follow-up 3 751 persons died of pancreatic cancer, making of this study one of the largest ever conducted. The risk of pancreatic cancer was doubled for current smokers but was just marginally elevated in former smokers (men RR=1.1; 1.0, 1.3; women RR=1.2; 1.0, 1.3), although the association was statistically significant due to the important power of the study. Among smokers, the risk of dying from pancreatic cancer decreased with increasing number of years since quitting smoking. The risk was still increased by 30% in men and 70% in women 10 years after quitting smoking, but returned to the risk of never smokers 20 years after quitting.

A large health-survey in the county of Nord-Trøndelag was conducted by the National Health Screening Service in Norway, following-up 31 000 men and 32 374 women for almost 12 years and contributing to 622 721 person-years of observation (Nilsen et al., 2000). The risk of pancreatic cancer was doubled for men and women who were current smokers at entry compared with never smokers. In contrast, former smokers did not have significantly elevated risk. Compared to current smokers, men and women who quit smoking less than 5 years before inclusion experienced no significant reduction in risk. However, cessation of smoking more than 5 years before study entry reduced the risk of pancreatic cancer to nearly half the risk of current smokers, thus approaching the risk for never smokers.

The Japan Collaborative Cohort Study for Evaluation of Cancer Risk (the JACC study; Lin et al., 2002) began in 1988, and enrolled 110 792 inhabitants aged 40–79 years (46 465 men and 64 327 women) from 45 areas throughout Japan. Subjects were followed-up for mortality to the end of 1997. Because of the small number of smokers among women, detailed results were provided only for men. Compared with never smokers, male former smokers did not experience a significant elevation in mortality from pancreatic cancer (RR=1.1). A significant decreasing trend in risk with increasing years after cessation was observed, though it took more than ten years for the risk among former smokers to approach the level of never smokers.

A pooled analysis of the Swedish Mammography Cohort (SMC) and the Cohort of Swedish Men (COSM; Larsson et al., 2005) was conducted in order to assess the relation between obesity, diabetes and cigarette smoking and the risk of pancreatic cancer. In these two cohorts assembling 37 147 women and 45 906 men residing in central Sweden, smoking was associated with a three-fold excess risk of developing pancreatic cancer. The risk in former smokers was not significantly elevated (RR=1.16; 95% CI=0.75–1.80). Compared with current smokers, the RR among former smokers diminished steeply and approached the RR for never smokers within 5–10 years following smoking cessation.

Only a few studies have assessed the effect of smoking cessation in relation to other aspects of the smoking history. In a study conducted in China, Ji et al. (1995) found that the decreasing risk associated with increasing number of years of cessation was not affected substantially by the number of past cigarettes smoked per day

Table 14. Studies on pancreas cancer and cessation by years since quitting

Reference Country Year of study	Study Type Population	Smoking category Number of years since quitting	Relative Risk or Odds Ratio (95% CI)		
Mack et al. (1986) USA 1976–81	Case-Control study Los Angeles County 490 cases 490 controls		Men and Women		
		Current smoker			
		≤1 pack/day	2.4 (1.7, 3.6)		
		>1 pack/day	2.1 (1.4, 3.2)		
		Former smoker			
		Years since quitting			
		0–4	3.3 (1.6,6.9)		
		5–9	2.3 (1.2, 4.3)		
		≥ 10 (smoked ≤ 1 pack/day)	1.1 (0.7, 1.8)		
		(smoked > 1 pack/day)	0.9 (0.5, 1.7)		
		Never smoker	1		
Cuzick & Babiker (1989) UK 1983–86	Case-Control study Leeds, London, Oxford 216 cases 279 controls		Men	Women	Men and women
		Current smoker			
		< 10 cigs/day	1.3	0.8	1.1
		10–20 cigs/day	1.7	1.1	1.3
		> 20 cigs/day	4.1 ($p < 0.01$)	5.5 ($p<0.1$)	4.4 ($p<0.01$)
		Former smoker			
		Years since quitting			
		< 10 years	3.6 ($p < 0.01$)	0.8	1.7
		10–20	3.6 ($p < 0.05$)	1.0	1.8
		> 20	1.3	1.1	1.0
		Never smoker	1	1	1
		χ^2 for trend	8.64 ($p < 0.01$)	0.23	3.14 ($p < 0.1$)
Bueno de Mesquita et al. (1991) Netherlands 1984–88	Population based Case-Control study 176 cases 487 controls		Low consumption (≤ 111 200 cigarettes in lifetime)	High consumption (> 111 200 cigarettes in lifetime)	
		Current smoker	1.6 (0.7, 3.8)	2.0 (1.0, 4.0)	
		Former smoker			
		Years since quitting			
		2–14	2.0 (0.8, 5.0)	1.7 (0.6, 4.6)	
		≥ 15	1.0 (0.5, 2.2)	–	
		Never smoker	1	1	

Table 14. Years since quitting: pancreas cancer (contd)

Reference Country Year of study	Study Type Population	Smoking category Number of years since quitting	Relative Risk or Odds Ratio (95% CI)
Howe et al. (1991) Canada 1983ñ86	Population based Case-Control study Toronto 249 cases 505 controls		Men and Women
		Current smoker	2.5
		Former smoker	
		Years since quitting	
		2ñ9	1.8
		10ñ19	1.4
		≥ 20	0.7
		Never smoker	1.0
Silverman et al. (1994) USA 1986ñ89	Population based Case-Control study Atlanta, Detroit, 10 counties-New Jersey 526 cases 2153 controls		Men and Women
		Current smoker	2.0 (1.5, 2.6)
		Former smoker	
		Years since quitting	
		1ñ2	3.1 (2.0, 5.0)
		3ñ5	2.0 (1.1, 3.5)
		6ñ10	1.8 (1.1, 2.9)
		11ñ20	1.2 (0.8, 1.9)
		> 20	1.3 (0.8, 1.9)
		Never smoker	1
Ji et al. (1995) China 1990ñ93	Case-Control study Shanghai Men only 451 cases 1552 controls		Men
		Current smoker	1.6 (1.1-2.2)
		Former smoker	
		Years since quitting	
		≤ 1	3.8 (1.4, 10.2)
		2ñ9	1.6 (0.8, 3.0)
		≥ 10	0.7 (0.3, 1.5)
		Never smoker	1
		p for trend	0.02

Table 14. Years since quitting: pancreas cancer (contd)

Reference Country Year of study	Study Type Population	Smoking category Number of years since quitting	Relative Risk or Odds Ratio (95% CI)	
Muscat et al. (1997) USA 1985–93	Hospital-based Case-Control study 484 cases 954 controls		*Men*	*Women*
		Current smoker	1.6 (1.1, 2.4)	2.3 (1.4, 3.5)
		Former smoker		
		Years since quitting		
		1–2	1.7 (0.8, 3.7)	10.6 (2.9, 39.2)
		3–5	0.5 (0.2, 1.1)	1.5 (0.6, 3.7)
		6–10	1.2 (0.6, 2.3)	2.1 (0.9, 4.5)
		> 10	1.1 (0.7, 1.6)	1.6 (1.0, 2.7)
		Never smoker	1	1
		p for trend	>0.05	< 0.05
Partanen et al. (1997) Finland 1984–87	Population-based Case-Control study 662 decedent cases 1770 cancer controls		*Any tobacco*	*Cigarette*
		Current smoker	2.5 (1.9, 3.2)	2.5 (1.9, 3.3)
		Early quitters (before 1975)	1.2 (0.9, 1.6)	1.2 (0.9, 1.5)
		Late quitters (quit 1975–83)	1.8 (1.3, 2.6)	1.8 (1.3, 2.5)
		Never smoker	1	1
Coughlin et al. (2000) USA 1982–1996	CPS II Cohort 483 109 men 619 199 women 3751 pancreas cancer deaths		*Men*	*Women*
		Current smoker	2.1 (1.9, 2.4)	2.0 (1.8, 2.3)
		Former smoker		
		Years since quitting		
		<10	1.6 (1.2, 2.0)	1.3 (1.0, 1.8)
		10-19	1.3 (1.0, 1.5)	1.7 (1.4, 2.0)
		≥ 20	1.0 (0.9, 1.2)	0.9 (0.8, 1.1)
		Never smoker	1	1
Nielsen et al. (2000) Norway 1984-1996	Cohort study 31 000 men 32 374 women 166 incident cases		*Men*	*Women*
		Current smoker	1	1
		Former smoker		
		Years since quitting		
		1-5	1.0 (0.5, 2.2)	1.3 (0.4, 4.6)
		>5	0.6 (0.3, 1.0)	0.5 (0.2, 1.9)
		Never smoker	0.5 (0.3, 0.8)	0.5 (0.2, 1.0)
		p for trend	0.004	0.03

Table 14. Years since quitting: pancreas cancer (contd)

Reference Country Year of study	Study Type Population	Smoking category Number of years since quitting	Relative Risk or Odds Ratio (95% CI)	
Lin et al. (2002) Japan 1988ñ1997	Cohort study 46 465 men 64 327 women 225 pancreas cancer deaths		*Men*	*Women*
		Current smoker	1.6 (1.0, 2.7)	1.7 (0.9, 3.4)
		Former smoker	1.1 (0.6, 1.9)	1.8 (0.7, 5.0)
		Years since quitting		Only 4 deaths in former smokers
		<10	1.4 (0.7, 2.6)	
		10-19	0.9 (0.4, 2.0)	
		≥ 20	0.9 (0.4, 2.0)	
		Never smoker	1	
		p for trend	0.04	
Bonelli et al. (2003) Italy 1992ñ1996	Hospital-based Case-Control study 202 cases 406 controls			*Men and Women*
		Current smoker >20 cigs/day		2.4 (1.5, 3.6)
		Former smoker		1.0 (0.6, 1.7)
		Years since quitting		
		<5		2.7 (0.8, 9.4)
		5-14		2.7 (0.9, 8.2)
		≥ 15		0.6 (0.2, 1.6)
		Never smoker		1
Larsson et al. (2005) Sweden 1987ñ2004	Cohort of Swedish Men Swedish Mammography Cohort 45 906 men 37 147 women 136 incident pancreas cases			*Men and Women*
		Current smoker		1
		Former smoker		
		Years since quitting		
		<5		0.5 (0.2, 1.3)
		5-9		0.3 (0.1, 0.9)
		≥ 10		0.4 (0.2, 0.6)
		Never smoker		0.3 (0.2, 0.5)

(Table 15). In a multi-center case–control study of the SEARCH (Surveillance of Environmental Aspects Related to Cancer in Humans) programme of the IARC, the authors assessed the association between lifetime cigarette consumption and pancreatic cancer risk in former smokers, according to the duration of cessation (Boyle *et al.,* 1996). Significant elevated risks were still observed for moderate and heavy smokers who ceased smoking for less than 5 years and for heavy smokers who ceased smoking for 5–15 years, providing some evidence that the duration of abstinence necessary to reduce the risk of pancreatic cancer is inversely proportional to the lifetime cigarette consumption (Table 15). In this and in another case–control study from Italy (Bonelli *et al.,* 2003), the magnitude of the risk reduction was larger among individuals with the highest lifetime cigarette consumption, but these results are based on limited data.

In synthesis, the risk of pancreatic cancer is lower in former than in current smokers and declines with time since stopping, but remains higher than that in never smokers for at least 15 years after cessation.

Table 15. Effect of smoking cessation on the risk of pancreas cancer in relation to lifetime or daily cigarette consumption

Reference	Odds ratio	Lifetime cigarette consumption		
Ji *et al.* (1995)	Years since quitting	**< 20 cigarettes/day**	**20+ cigarettes/day**	
	<10	2.2 (1.0, 4.9)	1.8 (0.9, 3.6)	
	≥ 10	0.8 (0.2, 2.3)	0.7 (0.3, 1.7)	
	Never smoker	1	1	
		1st tertile	**2nd tertile**	**3rd tertile**
Boyle *et al.* (1996)	Former smoker	1.2	1.3	2.0
	Years since quitting			
	≤ 4	2.3	2.7	3.8
	5–14	1.2	1.4	2.1
	≥ 15	1.1	0.8	0.6
	Never smoker	1	1	1
Bonelli *et al.* (2003)	Years since quitting			
	≤ 4	1.6 (0.5, 5.6)	1.7 (0.4, 7.5)	9.4 (0.9, 103)
	5–14	2.5 (1.0, 6.2)	2.4 (0.8, 6.9)	1.1 (0.3, 3.7)
	≥ 15	0.5 (0.2, 1.2)	1.6 (0.1, 19)	0.3 (0.1, 1.4)
	Never smoker	1	1	1

Bladder Cancer

The lower urinary tract comprises the renal pelvis, ureter, bladder and urethra. Cancers originating in the urothelium at these sites are mostly transitional-cell carcinomas or squamous-cell carcinomas. Bladder cancer represents the large majority of cancer of the lower urinary tract. In both IARC monographs on tobacco smoking (IARC, 1986, 2004), cancer of the lower urinary tract was identified as being causally associated with cigarette smoking. Most studies found clear evidence demonstrating that the risk for cancer of the lower urinary tract increases with daily cigarette consumption (with a levelling-off of the dose response attributable either to an underestimation of consumption by heavy smokers or to the saturation of metabolic enzymes). Also, both duration of cigarette smoking and age at starting smoking have been found to be positively associated with risk. It has been estimated that bladder cancer was responsible for approximately 175 000 deaths worldwide in 2001, and that 48 000 of these (28%) were attributable to tobacco smoking (Danaei *et al.*, 2005).

At least 13 cohort studies and 11 case–control studies reported data on bladder cancer risk in relation to smoking cessation, providing separate risk estimates for current and former smokers (Table 16). In all but one cohort study (Nordlund *et al.* 1997) and an early case–control study (Anthony & Thomas, 1970), the risk of bladder cancer was lower in former smokers than in current smokers. Combined analyses of the original data from selected case–control studies (Fortuny *et al.*, 1999; Puente *et al.*, 2006) provided more precise quantification of the decline of the relative risk in former smokers: compared with never smokers, the pooled relative risks for current smokers were between 3.6 and 3.9, both for men and women, and between 1.4 and 2.2, both for men and women, in former smokers (Table 17). A comprehensive meta-analysis of 35 case–control and 8 cohort studies (Zeegers *et al.*, 2000) reported summary odds ratios of 2.6 (95% CI=2.2–3.0) and 1.7 (95% CI=1.5–1.9) in current and former smokers respectively. To better characterize the association between smoking and bladder cancer, a pooled analysis of 11 case–control studies from six European countries reported results in men (Brennan *et al.*, 2000) and in women (Brennan *et al.*, 2001) (Table 17). In both men and women, bladder cancer risk declined sharply after cessation, by approximately 30% after 1-4 years; however, even after 25 years the odds ratio did not reach the level of non-smokers. Duration of cessation was also addressed in the meta-analysis by Zeegers and collaborators (2000), in which men who stopped smoking for less than 10 years had higher risks of urinary tract cancer than did men who stopped smoking for longer than 10 years (summary odds ratio, 1.23; 95% CI, 0.80–1.87). Similarly, 16 of 20 studies reporting on the risk of bladder cancer according to the number of years of cessation found a decreasing trend in risk associated with the number of years for which the subjects had stopped smoking (Table 18).

Only a few studies on the relation between smoking and cancer of the bladder have been published more recently:

The Iowa Women's Health Study included 37 459 postmenopausal women who were followed 13 years for bladder cancer incidence (Tripathi *et al.*, 2002). A higher than three-fold risk was observed in women who were current smokers compared with those who had never smoked (Table 18). The relative risk declined as years since quitting increased (RR=2.89, 95% CI=1.25–6.66 for women who quit smoking for less than 5 years, RR=1.69, 95% CI=0.67–4.25 for women who quit smoking for 5–15 years and RR=1.06, 95% CI=0.44–2.54, for women who quit smoking for more than 15 years).

The association between smoking different tobacco products and bladder cancer was studied in a population-based prospective cohort study of 120 852 adults in the Netherlands using a case–cohort approach (Zeegers *et al.*, 2002). Compared to never smokers, the adjusted incidence relative risks for former and current cigarette smokers were 2.1 (95% CI=1.5–3.0) and 3.3 (95% CI=2.4–4.0) respectively. The risk decreased with increasing duration of cessation and became not significantly different from never smokers only after 30 years of cessation (RR $_{>30\ years\ of\ cessation\ versus\ never\ smokers}$ = 0.8; 95% CI=0.4–1.6).

The National Health Insurance Corporation Study (Yun *et al.*, 2005) included 733 134 Korean men who had a medical evaluation in 1996 and were followed up through 2000 for cancer incidence. Current cigarette smokers had a 2.2-fold risk of developing bladder cancer (95% CI=1.5–3.4) in relation to never smokers, while the risk was reduced in former smokers (OR=1.3; 95% CI=0.8–2.1) (Table 16). Among former smokers, significant elevated risk of bladder cancer was observed in individuals who had previously smoked for more than 20 years (RR=2.3; 95% CI=1.2–4.6).

A hospital case–control study conducted in the USA from 1994 to 1997 with patients having pathologically confirmed bladder carcinoma (Cao *et al.*, 2005) examined cigarette smoking and metabolic genes. The adjusted OR revealed an elevated risk within 10 years of quitting (3.0; 95% CI=1.3–7.1) and decreasing after longer periods of abstinence (Table 18).

In the few studies that looked at the effect of smoking cessation in relation to the amount of tobacco smoked, the magnitude of the risk reduction was somewhat greater among men with the highest lifetime consumption, but these results are based on limited data (Table 19). The reduction in risk seen with increasing cessation time was preserved when stratifying by duration of past smoking (Table 19).

In synthesis, the risk of cancer of the lower urinary tract is lower in former than in current smokers. The relative risk declines with time since stopping, but remains higher than that in never smokers for at least 25 years after cessation.

Table 16. Studies on the relative risk of bladder cancer in former smokers

Reference Country Years of study	Subjects	Smoking Status	Relative risk (95% CI) Versus Never Smokers	
			Men	Women
Cohort Studies			*Mortality ratio (Deaths)*	
Kahn (1966) USA 1954–62	US Veterans' Study 293 958 men	Current Former	2.2 (82) 1.6 (51)	
Doll & Peto (1976) UK 1957–71	British Doctors' Study 34 440 men	Current Former	*Mortality ratio* [2.1] (80) [1.2]	
Rogot & Murray (1980) USA 1954–69	US Veterans Study 293 958 men	Current Former	*SMR* 2.2 (326) 1.4 (126)	
Steineck et al. (1988) Sweden 1967–82	Swedish Twin Registry 16 477 persons	Ever-smoker Former	*Men and Women* 3.3 (1.7, 6.7) 1.9 (0.8, 4.7)	
Mills et al. (1991) USA 1976–82	Adventist Health Study 34 198 men and women	Current Former	*Men and Women* 5.7 (1.7, 18.6) 2.4 (1.3, 4.7)	
Chyou et al. (1993) USA 1965–95	American Men of Japanese Ancestry Study 8006 men	Current Former	2.9 (1.7, 4.9) 1.4 (0.7, 2.6)	
Doll et al. (1994) UK 1951–91	British Doctors' Study 34 439 men	Current Former	*Mortality rate per 100 000/yrs* 21 13	
Mc Laughlin et al. (1995a) USA 1954–80	US Veterans' Study 293 958 men	Current Former	2.2 (1.9, 2.6) 1.3 (1.1, 1.6)	
Engeland et al. (1996) Norway 1966–93	Norwegian Cohort Study 11 857 men, 14 269 women	>15cigs/day Former	5.1 (3.1, 8.4) 2.1 (1.3, 3.2)	7.9 (3.3, 19.0) 1.5 (0.6, 3.5)
Nordlund et al. (1997) Sweden 1963–89	Swedish Census Study 25 829 women	Current Former		2.3 (1.4, 3.8) 2.5 (1.1, 5.9)
Tulinius et al. (1997) Iceland 1968–95	Reykjavík Study 11 580 men	15–24 cigs/day Former	2.6 (1.4, 4.7) 2.3 (1.4, 3.9)	
Doll et al. (2005) UK 1951–2001	British Doctors' Study 34 439 men	Current Former	*Mortality rate per 100 000/yrs* 38.8 22.6	
Yun et al. (2005) Republic of Korea 1996-2000	National Health Insurance Corporation Study 733 134 men	Current Former	2.2 (1.5, 3.4) 1.3 (0.8, 2.1)	

Table 16. Risk of bladder cancer in former smokers (contd)

Reference Country Years of study	Subjects	Smoking Status	Relative risk (95% CI) Versus Never Smokers	
			Men	Women
Case-Control Studies				
Anthony & Thomas (1970) UK 1958-67	Hospital-based study Men: 381 cases and 275 controls	Current Former	0.9 1.2	
Morrison et al. (1984) Japan and UK, 1976–78 USA, 1976–77	Population-based study Boston area	Current Former	1 0.5 (0.4, 0.8)	1 0.7
Harris et al. (1990) USA 1969 onwards	Men, 1114 cases, White 3252 controls Women, 420 cases, 1289 controls	Current Former	3.2 (2.6, 3.9) 2.1 (1.7, 2.6)	3.2 (2.4, 4.1) 1.3 (1.0, 1.8)
	Men, 84 cases, 271 Blacks controls W, 84 cases, 271 controls	Current Former	2.0 (1.0, 3.9) 1.6 (0.8, 3.4)	
Mc Carthy et al. (1995) USA 1975–92	Population-based study 301 cases and 1196 controls	Current Former	*Men and Women* 1.7 (1.2, 2.3) 1.3 (1.0, 1.7)	
Donato et al. (1997) Italy 1991–92	Hospital-based study 172 cases and 578 controls	Current Former	8.4 (3.7,19) 4.8 (2.2, 10.7)	
Pommer et al. (1999) Germany 1990–94	Population-based study Men, 415 cases and 415 controls Women, 232 cases and 232 controls	Current Former	*Men and Women* 3.2 (2.3, 4.5) 1.6 (1.1, 2.2)	
Pohlabeln et al. (1999) Germany 1989-92	Hospital-based study 300 cases, 300 controls	Current Former (1–9) Former (>10)	5.2 (2.7, 9.7) 3.4 (1.6, 6.9) 1.7 (0.9, 3.0)	5.6 (1.1, 27.3) 5.2 (1.3, 20.2)
Castelao et al. (2001) USA 1987–96	Population-based study Men: 415 cases and 415 controls Women: 232 cases and 232 controls	Current Former	3.6 (2.8, 4.6) 1.7 (1.4, 2.1)	4.6 (3.0, 7.0) 1.5 (1.0, 2.4)
Pelucchi et al. (2002) Italy 1985–92	Hospital-based study Women: 110 cases and 298 controls	Current Former		2.9 (1.6, 5.1) 1.1 (0.4, 3.6)
Zeegers et al. (2002) Netherlands 1986–92	Nested case–control study Men: 532 cases Women: 87 cases	Current Former	*Men and Women* 3.3 (2.4, 4.0) 2.1 (1.5, 3.0)	
Kellen et al. (2006) Belgium 1999–2004	Population-based study 200 cases and 385 controls	Current Former	*Men and Women* 6.00 (3.3, 11.0) 2.22 (1.4, 3.6)	

SMR = standardized mortality ratio
Values in brackets calculated by the Working Group of Volume 83 (IARC, 2004)

Table 17. Pooled analyses and meta-analyses of studies on the association of smoking and risk of bladder cancer

Reference Country Years of study	Type of analysis	Smoking status	Summary Relative Risk (95% CI)	
Fortuny et al. (1999) Europe 1983–85	Pooled analyses of case–control studies		*Non-cancer controls*	*Cancer controls*
		Current	3.6 (2.1, 6.3)	0.8 (0.4, 1.4)
		Former	1.4 (0.8, 2.5)	0.6 (0.3. 1.3)
Zeegers et al. (2000) Multinational 1968-1998	Meta-analysis of cohort and case-control studies		*Men*	*Women*
		Current	2.8 (2.3, 3.4)	2.3 (1.8, 3.)
		Former	2.0 (1.6, 2.6)	1.7 (1.1, 2.4)
			Men and women	
		Current	2.6 (2.2, 3.0)	
		Former	1.7 (1.5, 1.9)	
Brennan et al. (2000, 2001) Europe 1976–96	Pooled analyses of 11 case-control studies and 1 unpublished study	Current smoker Years quitting	*Men* 1	*Women* 1
		1–4	0.7 (0.5, 0.8)	0.6 (0.3, 1.1)
		5–9	0.7 (0.6, 0.8)	0.6 (0.3, 1.1)
		10–14	0.6 (0.5, 0.8)	0.5 (0.3, 1.0)
		15–19	0.5 (0.4, 0.6)	1.1 (0.5, 2.2)
		20–24	0.5 (0.4, 0.6)	0.5 (0.2, 1.2)
		> 24	0.4 (0.3, 0.5)	0.8 (0.5, 1.5)
		Never smoker	0.2 (0.17, 0.24)	0.7 (0.5, 0.9)
Puente et al. (2006) Multinational 1976–96	Pooled analyses of case–control studies	Current Former	*Men* 3.9 (3.5, 4.3) 2.2 (2.0, 2.4)	*Women* 3.6 (3.1, 4.1) 2.2 (1.9, 2.6)

Table 18. Studies on the risk of bladder cancer by years since quitting

Reference Country Years of study	Study Population	No. of years since quitting	Odds ratio (relative to Never Smokers) (95% CI)	
Tyrell *et al.* (1971) Ireland 1967–68	Hospital-based case-control study Men: 200 cases, 200 controls	0 0.1–3.9 4.0–6.9 7.0–12.9 13.0–21.9 ≥ 22.0	*Men* 3.9 (129) 1.5 (3) 2.9 (5) 4.1 (6) 6.2 (9) 2.7 (11)	Crude relative risks calculated by the IARC Monograph Working Group (Volume 83, 2004)
Wynder & Goldsmith (1977) 1969–74	Hospital-based case-control study Men: 574 cases, 574 controls	1–3 4–6 7–9 10–12 13–15 ≥ 16	*Men* 2.6 (1.6, 4.5) 2.9 (1.7, 5.2) 1.5 (0.8, 3.0) 1.6 (0.8, 3.1) 1.2 (0.6, 2.5) 1.1 (0.7, 1.8)	
Howe *et al.* (1980) Canada 1974–76	Population-based case-control study Men: 480 cases, 480 controls Women: 152 cases, 152 controls	Current smoker Former smoker 2–15 > 15	*Men* 1.0 0.6 (0.4, 0.9) 0.5 (0.4, 0.8)	*Women* 1.0 0.2 (0.1, 0.5)
Cartwright *et al.* (1983) UK 1978–81	Hospital and Population-based case-control study Men: 932 cases, 1402 controls	≤ 5 6–15 16–25 26–35 > 35 and never-smoker	*Men* 1.7 1.0 1.1 0.9 1.0 (reference)	
Vineis *et al.* (1984) Italy 1978–83	Hospital-based case-control study Men: 512 cases, 596 controls	0–2 3–9 10–14 ≥ 15	*Men aged < 60* 10.2 (5.0, 21.2) 3.3 (1.2, 9.2) 1.6 (0.3, 8.2) 1.9 (0.5, 7.9)	*Men aged > 60* 3.8 (2.0, 7.2) 2.8 (1.2, 6.6) 2.4 (0.9, 6.3) 2.5 (1.0, 5.8)
Clavel *et al.* (1989) France 1984–87	Hospital-based case-control study Men: 477 cases, 477 controls	0–2 (reference) 3–9 10–14 ≥ 15	1.0 1.0 (0.6, 1.3) 0.7 (0.4, 1.2) 0.4 (0.3, 0.6)	
Burch *et al.* (1989b) Canada 1979–82	Population-based case-control study Men: 627 cases Women: 199 cases Controls: 792 controls	1–5 >5–10 >10 Current	*Men* 1.1 (0.6, 1.9) 0.8 (0.4, 1.7) 1.4 (0.7, 2.8) 1.6 (0.8, 3.0)	*Women* 0.4 (0.2, 1.2) 0.7 (0.1, 4.1) 0.8 (0.2, 3.7) 1.0 (0.3, 3.4)
D'Avanzo *et al.* (1990) Italy 1985–89	Hospital-based case-control study 337 cases, 392 controls	>15 5–14 2–14	*Men and women* 1.2 (0.6, 2.5) 1.8 (1.0, 3.2) 3.1 (1.6, 6.2)	
De Stefani *et al.* (1991) Uruguay 1987–89	Hospital-based case-control study Men: 91 cases, 182 controls	1–4 5–9 ≥ 10	*Men* 0.5 (0.2, 1.3) 0.5 (0.2, 1.3) 0.4 (0.2, 0.8)	
López–Abente *et al.* (1991) Spain 1983–86	Hospital and population-based case-control study 430 cases, 405 hospital controls, 386 population controls	0–5 6–15 ≥ 16	*Men* 4.4 (2.8, 7.0) 3.0 (1.7, 5.2) 2.4 (1.3, 4.3)	

Table 18. Years since quitting bladder cancer (contd)

Reference Country Years of study	Study Population	No. of years since quitting	Odds ratio (relative to Never Smokers) (95% CI)	
Kunze et al. (1992) Germany 1977–85	Hospital-based case-control study Men: 531 cases, 531 controls Women:144 cases, 144 control	1–9 10–19 ≥ 20	*Men* 1.3 (0.9,1.8) 0.7 (0.5, 1.0) 0.6 (0.4, 0.9)	*Women* 0.8 (0.3, 2.7) 1.7 (0.4, 7.0) 2.2 (0.8, 6.3)
Momas et al. (1994) France 1987–89	Population-based case-control study 219 cases, 794 controls	≤ 2 3–15 > 15	*Men* 5.0 (2.6, 9.7) 7.1 (3.6, 13.9) 4.6 (2.3, 9.1)	
Sorahan et al. (1994) UK 1985–87	Case-control study 989 cases 1059 population controls 1599 patients from practitioners as controls	Current smoker 1–9 10–19 ≥ 20	*Men* 3.1 (2.4, 4.1) 1.9 (1.4, 2.6) 1.5 (1.1, 2.1) 1.2 (0.9, 1.7)	
Bedwani et al. (1998), Egypt, 1994–96	Hospital-based case-control study Men: 151 cases, 157 controls	< 10 ≥ 10	*Men* 5.8 (1.6, 21.0) 3.4 (1.0, 10.7)	
Pohlabeln et al. (1999) Germany 1989–1992	Hospital-based case-control study Men: 239 cases, 239 controls Women: 61 cases, 61 controls	Current smoker Former (1–9 years) (>10 years)	*Men* 5.2 (2.7, 9.7) 3.4 (1.6, 6.9) 1.7 (0.9, 3.0)	*Women* 5.6 (1.1, 27.3) 5.2 (1.3, 20)
Castelao et al. (2001), USA, 1987–96	Population-based case-control study 1514 cases, 1514 controls	Current smoker < 10 10–19 ≥ 20	*Men* 3.6 (2.8, 4.6) 2.3 (1.8, 2.9) 1.9 (1.5, 2.5) 1.1 (0.9, 1.5)	*Women* 4.6 (3.0, 7.0) 2.7 (1.5, 4.8) 1.1 (0.6, 2.1) 1.1 (0.6, 2.0)
Zeegers et al. (2002), Netherlands, 1986–92	Cohort study 120 852 subjects 619 cases	Current smoker Former smoker <1 1–9 10–19 20–29 30+	*Men and women* 3.3 (2.4, 4.0) 2.1 (1.5, 3.0) 3.4 (2.5, 4.7) 2.9 (2.0, 4.3) 1.7 (1.1, 2.5) 1.9 (1.2, 2.9) 0.8 (0.4, 1.6) p<0.01	
Tripathi et al. (2002) USA, 1987-97	Cohort study 37459 women 112 cases	The Iowa Women's Health Study Current Former Quit >5 years Quit 5–15 years Quit >15 years		*Women* 5.5 (3.6–8.4) 2.1 (1.3–3.5) 3.8 (1.9-7.5) 2.4 (1.1-5.3) 1.2 (0.5-2.8)
Cao et al. (2005) USA, 1994–97	Hospital case-control study 233 cases, 204 controls	Ever smoker Former Quit >10 years Quit 10–20 years Quit >20 years	*Men and women* 3.1 (1.7, 5.9) 3.0 (1.3, 7.1) 1.1 (0.5, 24) 0.6 (0.3, 1.4)	

Table 19. Effect of smoking cessation on bladder cancer risk in relation to lifetime cigarette consumption and smoking duration

Reference Country Years of Study	Smoking category	Odds Ratio (95% CI) Lifetime cigarette consumption		
		<21.5 pack-yrs*	**21.5-40.5 pack-yrs**	**>40.5 pack-yrs**
Fortuny *et al.* (1999) Europe, 1983–85	*Men and women*			
	Non cancer controls			
	Current smoker	2.2 (1.0, 4.8)	2.7 (1.3, 5.6)	7.0 (3.6, 13.7)
	Former smoker	1.6 (0.8, 3.0)	1.4 (0.6, 3.3)	1.6 (0.7, 3.9)
	Never smoker	1	1	1
	Cancer controls			
	Current smoker	0.9 (0.4, 1.9)	0.5 (0.2, 1.0)	1.1 (0.5, 1.9)
	Former smoker	0.9 (0.4-1.7)	0.4 (0.2, 1.0)	0.4 (0.2 -1.0)
	Never smoker	1	1	1
		<20 tob-yrs**	**20-40 tob-yrs**	**>40 tob-yrs**
Gaertner *et al.* (2004) Canada	*Men*			
	Current smoker	1.3 (0.7, 2.2)	2.9 (1.9, 4.5)	4.2 (2.8, 6.0)
	Former smoker	1.2 (0.9, 1.8)	2.2 (1.5, 3.3)	2.8 (1.8, 4.2)
	Never smoker	1	1	1
	Women			
	Current smoker	3.0 (1.9, 4.8)	4.6 (3.1, 6.9)	5.4 (3.4, 8.8)
	Former smoker	1.2 (0.9, 1.8)	2.1 (1.3, 3.5)	3.4 (1.4, 8.2)
	Never smoker	1	1	1
			Duration of smoking	
	Men	**1–19 years**	**20–39 years**	**>39 years**
Brennan *et al.* (2000) Europe, 1976–96	Current smoker	1	1	1
	Years since quitting			
	< 5	1.01 (0.36, 2.82)	0.62 (0.43, 0.89)	0.67 (0.52, 0.86)
	5–9	0.21 (0.05, 0.95)	0.63 (0.47, 0.85)	0.87 (0.66, 1.16)
	10–14	0.57 (0.25, 1.28)	0.65 (0.49, 0.86)	0.76 (0.54, 1.08)
	15–19	0.61 (0.29, 1.27)	0.57 (0.41, 0.79)	0.33 (0.17, 0.65)
	20–24	0.50 (0.25, 1.01)	0.58 (0.39, 0.78)	0.82 (0.27, 2.47)
	>24	0.57 (0.34, 0.97)	0.49 (0.34, 0.70)	0.65 (0.24, 1.78)
	Never smoker	0.34 (0.21, 0.55)	0.21 (0.17, 0.26)	0.20 (0.16, 0.23)

* pack-yrs=cumulative pack-years of cigarettes categorized in tertiles
** tob-yrs= tobacco years, calculated as number of packs of 20 cigarettes smoked per day times the number of years smoked

Renal Cell Carcinoma (Kidney Cancer)

Tobacco smoking has been shown to be associated with renal cell carcinoma (RCC) in both men and women (McLaughlin *et al.,* 1990b; 1995a; Doll, 1996; Yuan *et al,* 1998; IARC, 2004). More recently, a combined analysis of the Nurses' Health Study and of the Health Professionals Follow-up Study (Flaherty *et al.,* 2005) showed only a modest increase in risk in men, limited to current smokers with ≥ 40 pack-years of exposure. A precise assessment of the relationship between various aspects of smoking history and RCC is difficult to obtain because the risk of RCC associated with smoking is only modest and could easily be obscured by the use of inappropriate controls in case–control studies. The incidence of RCC is also rather low, conferring limited statistical power to cohort studies.

Hunt and colleagues (2005) performed a meta-analysis on the risk of RCC and cigarette smoking that included 19 case–control and 5 cohort studies. The relative risk for ever-smokers compared with never smokers was 1.4 (95% CI 1.3–1.5) with a strong dose-dependent increase risk observed both in men and in women. The advantages of smoking cessation were confirmed by a reduction in relative risk for those who had quit smoking for >10 years (1.2; 0.9–1.7) as compared to those who had quit smoking for 1–10 years (1.8; 1.4–2.2). In the 3 studies published subsequently to this meta-analysis (Flaherty *et al.,* 2005; Hu *et al.,* 2005; Yun *et al.,* 2005), the risk of kidney cancer in former smokers was of similar magnitude to that of current smokers (Table 20).

Results from a recent large case–control study conducted in eight Canadian provinces (Hu *et al.,* 2005) support the association between cigarette smoking and the risk of RCC. In this, as in most previous studies (McLaughlin *et al.,* 1995b; Yuan *et al.,* 1998), the risk decreases with increasing years since quitting, with a 25–30% reduction in risk after 10–15 years of cessation (Table 21). A study specially designed to characterize the association of smoking cessation and RCC development (Parker *et al.,* 2003) suggested an inverse linear trend between years of cessation and risk of RCC, but indicated that the benefit may not be sizeable until more than 20 years following cessation (Table 21). The 50-year follow-up of the British Doctors Study of kidney cancer death showed a lower risk among former smokers compared to current smokers (Doll *et al.,* 2005).

The risk of RCC according to lifetime cigarette consumption in former smokers is shown in Table 22.

In synthesis, the risk of renal cell cancer is lower in former smokers than in current smokers, and the relative risk appears to decline with time since stopping but remains higher than that in never smokers for at least 20 years after cessation.

Table 20. Studies on the risk of renal-cell carcinoma in former smokers

Reference Country, years of study	Study	Status (current / former)	Relative risk (95% CI) versus Never Smokers	
			Men	Women
McLaughlin et al. (1990) USA 1954ñ80	US Veteransí Study	Current	1.5 (1.2, 1.8)	
		Former	1.1 (0.9, 1.4)	
Doll et al. (1994) UK 1951ñ91	British Doctorsí Study	Current	1.4	Mortality Rate
		Former	1.2	
McLaughlin et al. (1995) USA 1954ñ80	US Veteransí Study	Current	1.5 (1.2, 1.9)	
		Former	1.1 (0.9, 1.4)	
Engeland et al. (1996) Norway 1966ñ93	Norwegian Cohort Study	Current	1.4 (0.8, 2.5)	1.1(0.6, 2.0)
		Former	1.3 (0.8, 2.4)	0.2 (0.0, 1.7)
Heath et al. (1997) USA 1982ñ89	Cancer Prevention Study II	Current	1.7 (1.2, 2.6)	1.4 (0.9, 2.3)
		Former	1.7 (1.1, 2.4)	1.2 (0.7, 1.9)
Nordlund et al. (1997) Sweden 1963ñ89	Swedish Census Study	Current	1.1 (0.6, 2.0)	
		Former	1.9 (0.8, 4.7)	
Chow et al. (2000) Sweden 1971ñ92	Swedish Construction Worker Cohort	Current	1.6 (1.3,1.9)	
		Former	1.3 (1.0, 1.6)	
Doll et al. (2005) UK 1951-2001	British Doctorsí Study	Current Former Never	16.2 / 100 000 13.2 / 100 000 9.3 / 100 000	Mortality Rate
Flaherty et al. (2005) USA 1976-2000, NHS 1986-1998 HPFS	Nurses' Health Study and the Health Professionals Follow-up Study	Current Former	Men 1.3 (0.6, 2.9) 1.4 (0.9, 2.2)	Women 0.9 (0.6,1.5) 1.3 (0.9,1.8)
Yun et al. (2005) Korea 1996-2000	National Health Insurance Corporation	Current	0.94 (0.66, 1.32)	
		Former	0.96 (0.65, 1.42)	
La Vecchia et al. (1990) Italy 1985ñ89	Case-control study	15-24 cig/day	1.9 (1.0, 3.6)	
		Former	1.7 (1.0, 3.1)	

Table 20. Studies on the risk of renal-cell carcinoma in former smokers (contd)

Reference Country, years of study	Study	Status (current/ former)	Relative risk (95% CI) versus Never Smokers	
			Men	Women
Talamini *et al.* (1990) Italy 1986–89	Case-control study	15-24 cig/day	1.3 (0.8, 2.1)	
		Former	1.4 (0.8, 2.2)	
McCredie & Stewart (1992) Australia 1989-90	Case-control study	Current	*Renal-cell* 2.9 (1.8, 4.8)	1.6 (1.0, -2.6)
		Former	1.5 (1.0, 2.4)	1.3 (0.8, 2.2)
		Current	*Renal-pelvis* 5.9 (2.5, 13.5)	3.3 (1.7, 6.6)
		Former	1.2 (0.5, 2.7)	1.7 (0.7, 3.8)
McLaughlin *et al.* (1995b) Multinational 1989-92	Case-control study	Current Former	*Men and Women* 1.4 (1.2, 1.7) 1.2 (1.0, 1.4)	
Schlehofer *et al.* (1995) Germany 1989-91	Case-control study	Current	1.4 (0.8, 2.5)	0.8 (0.4, 1.8)
		Former	1.1 (0.6, 1.9)	1.0 (0.4, 1.4)
Yuan *et al.* (1998) USA 1986–94	Case-control study	Current	1.6 (1.2, 2.1)	1.5 (1.0, 2.1)
		Former	1.3 (1.1, 1.7)	1.1 (0.8, 1.5)
Hu *et al.* (2005) Canada 1994-1997	Case-control study	Current	0.9 (0.7, 1.2)	0.9 (0.7, 1.2)
		Former	1.2 (1.0, 1.5)	1.3 (1.0, 1.6)
Hunt *et al.* (2005)	Meta-Analysis	Current	1.6 (1.4, 1.8)	1.3 (1.0, 1.6)
		Former	1.4 (1.2, 1.6)	1.1 (0.9, 1.3)

Table 21. Studies on the risk of renal cell carcinoma by time since quitting smoking

Reference Country and years of study	Years since quitting	Odds ratio (relative to Never Smokers) (95% CI)	
McLaughlin *et al.* (1984) USA 1974–79		Men	Women
	Current smokers	1.8	2.0
	≤ 10	1.1	1.6
	> 10	1.7	1.7
La Vecchia *et al.* (1990) Italy 1985–89		*Univariate*	*Multivariate*
	<10	2.6 (1.1, 5.7)	2.2 (1.1, 4.4)
	≥ 10	*1.3 (0.6, 3.0)*	1.3 (0.6, 2.7)
McCredie & Stewart (1992) Australia 1989–90	Current smokers	*Model 1** reference	*Model 2**
	1–12	0.9 (0.5, 1.4)	0.9 (0.5, 1.4)
	13–24	0.9 (0.5, 1.5)	0.8 (0.5, 1.4)
	≥ 25	0.5 (0.2, 1.0)	0.4 (0.2, 0.7)
	p for trend	0.13	0.003
Kreiger *et al.* (1993) Canada 1986–87		*Men*	Women
	1–4	2.1 (1.2, 3.8)	1.4 (0.6, 2.9)
	5–9	1.8 (1.0, 3.3)	1.6 (0.7, 3.7)
	10–19	2.1 (1.3, 3.4)	1.9 (0.8, 4.2)
	≥ 20	1.3 (0.8, 2.1)	1.5 (0.7, 3.1)
McLaughlin *et al.* (1995) Australia, Denmark, Germany, Sweden, USA 1989–92	*Relative to current smokers*	*Men and women*	
	≤ 5	0.90 (0.7, 1.2)	
	6–15	0.84 (0.7, 1.1)	
	16–25	0.75 (0.6, 1.0)	
	> 25	0.85 (0.6, 1.1)	
	p for trend	0.09	
Yuan *et al.* (1998) USA 1986–94		*Men*	*Women*
	1–9	1.6 (1.2, 2.3)	0.9 (0.6, 1.4)
	10–19	1.3 (0.9, 1.8)	1.2 (0.7, 2.0)
	≥ 20	1.2 (0.9, 1.6)	1.2 (0.7, 2.0)
	Current smokers 1–9	*Men and Women* reference	
	10–19	0.8 (0.6, 1.1)	
	≥ 20	0.7 (0.5, 1.0)	
		0.7 (0.5, 1.0)	
Parker *et al.* (2003) USA 1986–89 Case-control	Relative to current smokers	*Men and women*	
	<10	0.7 (0.4, 1.1)	
	10–19	0.8 (0.5, 1.2)	
	20–29	0.7 (0.4, 1.1)	
	≥ 30	0.5 (0.3, 1.0)	
	never smokers	0.6 (0.4, 0.9)	
	p for trend	0.005	
Hu *et al.* (2005) Canada 1994–97		*Men*	*Women*
	Current smokers	0.9 (0.7, 1.2)	Current 0.9 (0.7, 1.2)
	≤ 10	1.5 (1.0, 2.3)	≤ 10 1.5 (0.8, 2.6)
	11–20	1.1 (0.8, 1.5)	11–20 0.6 (0.4, 1.1)
	21–30	1.2 (0.8, 1.6)	≥ 20 1.1 (0.7, 1.6)
	≥ 31	1.0 (0.7, 1.4)	

* Model 1 included duration of smoking prior to quitting, amount smoked (cigarettes per day), and length of cessation in ever smokers.
Model 2 included age at smoking initiation, amount smoked (cigarettes per day) and length of cessation in ever smokers.

Table 22. Effect of smoking cessation on the risk of renal-cell cancer in relation to lifetime cigarette consumption

Renal-cell cancer	Stratum	Cigarette consumption		
		Odds Ratio (relative to Never Smokers)		
Schlehofer et al. (1995) Germany 1989–91	Men	<20 pack-years	20–40 pack-years	>40 pack-years
	Current smoker	1.4 (0.7, 3.0)	1.1 (0.5, 2.1)	2.2 (0.99, 4.7)
	Former smoker	0.9 (0.5, 1.8)	1.0 (0.4, 2.2)	2.3 (0.9, 6.2)
	Women	<10 pack-years	10–20 pack-years	>20 pack-years
	Current smoker	0.5 (0.1, 1.9)	0.3 (0.1, 1.2)	2.2 (0.7, 6.8)
	Former smoker	0.9 (0.3, 2.3)	0.7 (0.1, 4.7)	3.0 (0.3, 30.2)

Cervical Cancer

Chronic infection with selected high-risk types of human papilloma virus (HPV), which are sexually transmitted viruses, is the main cause of cervical cancer, both cervical intraepithelial neoplasia (CIN) and invasive cancer (IARC, 1995). There are however, additional recognized risk factors, including high parity, oral contraceptive use, and tobacco smoking.

At least 7 cohort studies and 29 case–control studies have provided some information on the risk of cervical cancer on former smokers (IARC, 2004). Although most estimates have been influenced by large random variation, the relative risk among former smokers appears to be intermediate between that of never and of current smokers. For individual studies, data for the analysis of elapsed time since quitting smoking and cervical cancer risk are scarce.

The quantitative information on stopping smoking in cervical neoplasia comes from a collaborative re-analysis of individual data on 13 541 women with carcinoma of the cervix and 23 017 women without carcinoma of the cervix from 23 epidemiological studies (International Collaboration of Epidemi-

ological Studies of Cervical Cancer, 2006). That collaborative re-analysis included data on 8 cohort studies (Gram et al., 1992; Schiffman et al., 1993; Kjaer et al., 1996a; Ylitalo et al., 1999; Deacon et al., 2000; Hildesheim et al., 2001; Beral et al., 2003; Vessey et al., 2003), 9 population-based (Brinton et al., 1986; Peters et al., 1986; Cuzick et al., 1990; Bosch et al., 1992; Cuzick et al., 1996; Daling et al., 1996; Kjaer et al., 1996b; Ursin et al., 1996; Lacey et al., 2001; Madeleine et al., 2001; Green et al., 2003); and 6 hospital-based case–control studies (La Vecchia et al., 1986; Herrero et al., 1989; Parazzini et al., 1992; Muñoz et al., 1993; WHO, 1993; Eluf-Neto et al., 1994; Chaouki et al., 1998; Chichareon et al., 1998; Ngelangel et al., 1998 ; Rolon et al., 2000; Sitas et al., 2000; Santos et al., 2001; Thomas et al., 2001; Bayo et al., 2002; Rajkumar et al., 2003; Hammouda et al., 2005). It found a pooled relative risk of invasive squamous cell carcinoma, adjusted for age, parity, oral contraceptive use, number of sexual partners and age at sexual debut, of 1.46 (95% CI = 1.35–1.58) in current smokers compared with never smokers

and of 1.05 (95% C=0.92–1.19) in former smokers (Figure 1). The RR of invasive squamous cell carcinoma seemed to drop rapidly 1–4 years after smoking cessation (1.05; 95% CI=0.87–1.28) (Figure 2).

The multivariate pooled RR of carcinoma in situ CIN 3 for current (1.83: 95% CI=1.68–1.99) and former smokers (1.32; 95% CI=1.12–1.56) were somewhat greater than for invasive carcinoma of the cervix (Figure 1). When combining invasive and in situ cases, the pooled RR of squamous cell carcinomas of the cervix was 1.60 (95% CI=1.48–1.73) in current smokers and 1.12 (95%, CI 1.01–1.25) in former smokers (Figure 3). Estimates of the relative risk of combined invasive squamous cell and in situ/CIN3 carcinomas of the cervix in former smokers compared with never smokers by study design were 1.49 (95% CI=1.10–2.01) in 4 cohort studies, 1.21 (95% CI=1.04–1.41) in 9 population-based case–control studies and 1.07 (95% CI=0.90–1.29) in 6 hospital-based case–control studies (Figure 3).

The collaborative re-analysis showed lack of association of current smoking (pooled multivariate RR versus never

INVASIVE CANCER   **CARCINOMA IN SITU/CIN3**

a: SQUAMOUS CELL CARCINOMA♦

Smoking status	Cases/Controls	RR[1]	RR[2] (95% FCI)*	RR[2] (95% FCI)*	Cases/Controls	RR[1]	RR[2] (95% FCI)*	RR[2] (95% FCI)*
never	5151/11929	1.00	1.00 (0.94-1.06)		1501/9972	1.00	1.00 (0.91-1.10)	
past	759/1552	1.17	1.05 (0.94-1.17)		315/1286	1.50	1.32 (1.12-1.56)	
current	1653/2764	1.69	1.46 (1.35-1.58)		1444/2892	2.18	1.83 (1.68-1.99)	

0.5 1.0 1.5 2.0   0.5 1.0 1.5 2.0

b: ADENOCARCINOMA

Smoking status	Cases/Controls	RR[1]	RR[2] (95% FCI)*	RR[2] (95% FCI)*	Cases/Controls	RR[1]	RR[2] (95% FCI)*	RR[2] (95% FCI)*
never	779/11929	1.00	1.00 (0.89-1.13)		141/9972	1.00	1.00 (0.81-1.24)	
past	152/1552	0.97	0.84 (0.68-1.03)		63/1286	1.08	1.04 (0.77-1.41)	
current	260/2764	1.12	0.92 (0.78-1.07)		68/2892	1.05	0.81 (0.61-1.08)	

0.5 1.0 1.5 2.0   0.5 1.0 1.5 2.0

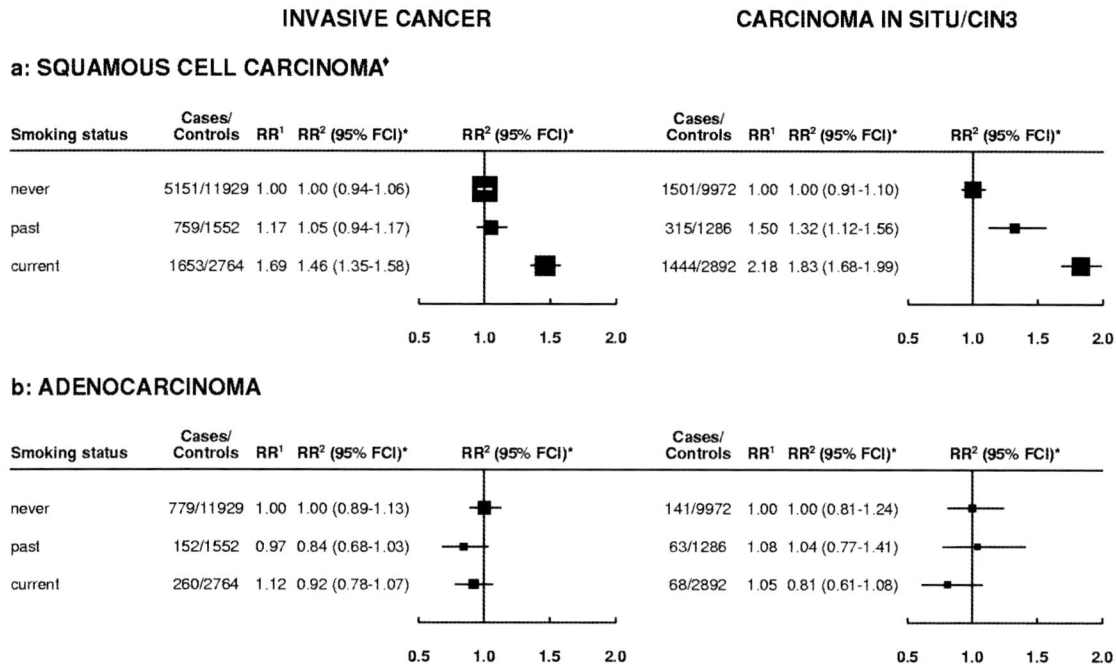

* RR[1] stratified by study and age at diagnosis only. RR[2] stratified by study, age at diagnosis, number of sexual partners, duration of oral contraceptive use, age at first intercourse and number of births, 95% floated confidence intervals (FCIs) for RR[2]. Women with no information of sexual partners are excluded from these analyses.

♦ includes all non-adenocarcinomas

From International Collaboration of Epidemiological Studies of Cervical Cancer (2006)

Figure 1. Relative risk (RR)* of carcinoma of the cervix by histological type in relation to smoking status

smokers: 0.92; 95% CI=0.78–1.07) or past smoking (pooled multivariate RR=0.84; 95% CI=0.68–1.03) and adenocarcinoma of the cervix (Figure 1 lower panel).

The Working Group noted that HPV prevalence among cancer-free control women was not associated with tobacco smoking. Thus, the adverse effect of smoking on cervical cancer is likely due to the effects of smoking on the progres-

sion of HPV infection into preneoplastic and neoplastic cervical lesions. Rapid reduction of the relative risk of squamous cell carcinoma among former smokers suggests, therefore, that such effects are probably reversible.

In synthesis, the pooled relative risk for squamous-cell carcinoma of the cervix, adjusted for age, parity, oral contraceptive (OC) use and sexual habits, among former smokers

compared with never smokers (1.12, 95% CI=1.01–1.25) is lower than the RR for current smokers (1.60, 95% CI=1.48–1.73). The risk in former smokers decreases rapidly following cessation to that of the never smokers. There is no association between smoking (any type) and adenocarcinoma of the cervix.

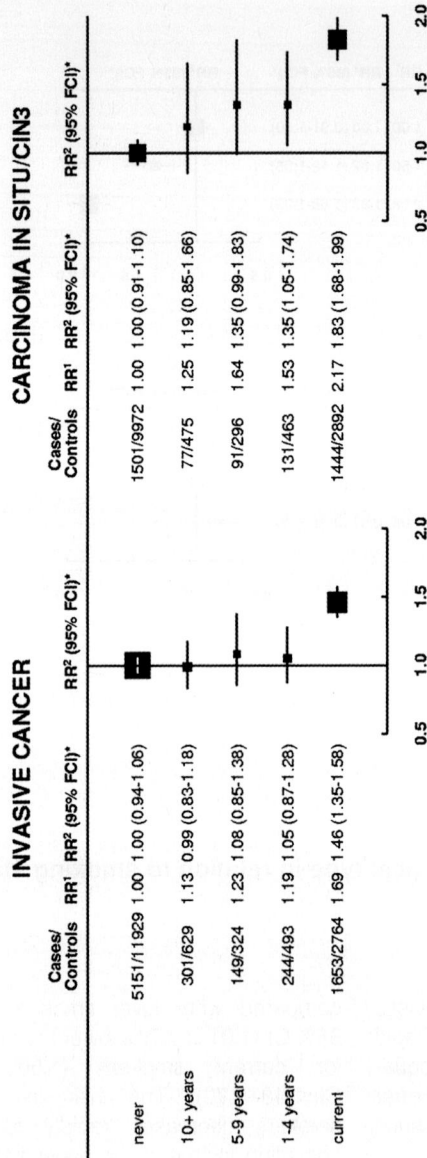

INVASIVE CANCER

	Cases/Controls	RR[1]	RR[2] (95% FCI)*
never	5151/11929	1.00	1.00 (0.94-1.06)
10+ years	301/629	1.13	0.99 (0.83-1.18)
5-9 years	149/324	1.23	1.08 (0.85-1.38)
1-4 years	244/493	1.19	1.05 (0.87-1.28)
current	1653/2764	1.69	1.46 (1.35-1.58)

CARCINOMA IN SITU/CIN3

	Cases/Controls	RR[1]	RR[2] (95% FCI)*
never	1501/9972	1.00	1.00 (0.91-1.10)
10+ years	77/475	1.25	1.19 (0.85-1.66)
5-9 years	91/296	1.64	1.35 (0.99-1.83)
1-4 years	131/463	1.53	1.35 (1.05-1.74)
current	1444/2892	2.17	1.83 (1.68-1.99)

* RR[1] stratified by study and age at diagnosis only. RR[2] stratified by study, age at diagnosis, number of sexual partners, duration of oral contraceptive use, age at first intercourse and number of full-term pregnancies; 95% floated confidence intervals (FCIs) for RR[2]. Women with no information of sexual partners are excluded from these analyses.

Trends in past smokers = 0.6 (invasive cancer) and 0.5 (carcinoma in situ/CIN3).

◆ includes all non-adenocarcinomas

From International Collaboration of Epidemiological Studies of Cervical Cancer (2006)

Figure 2. Relative risk (RR)* of squamous cell carcinoma of the cervix◆ in relation to time since stopping smoking

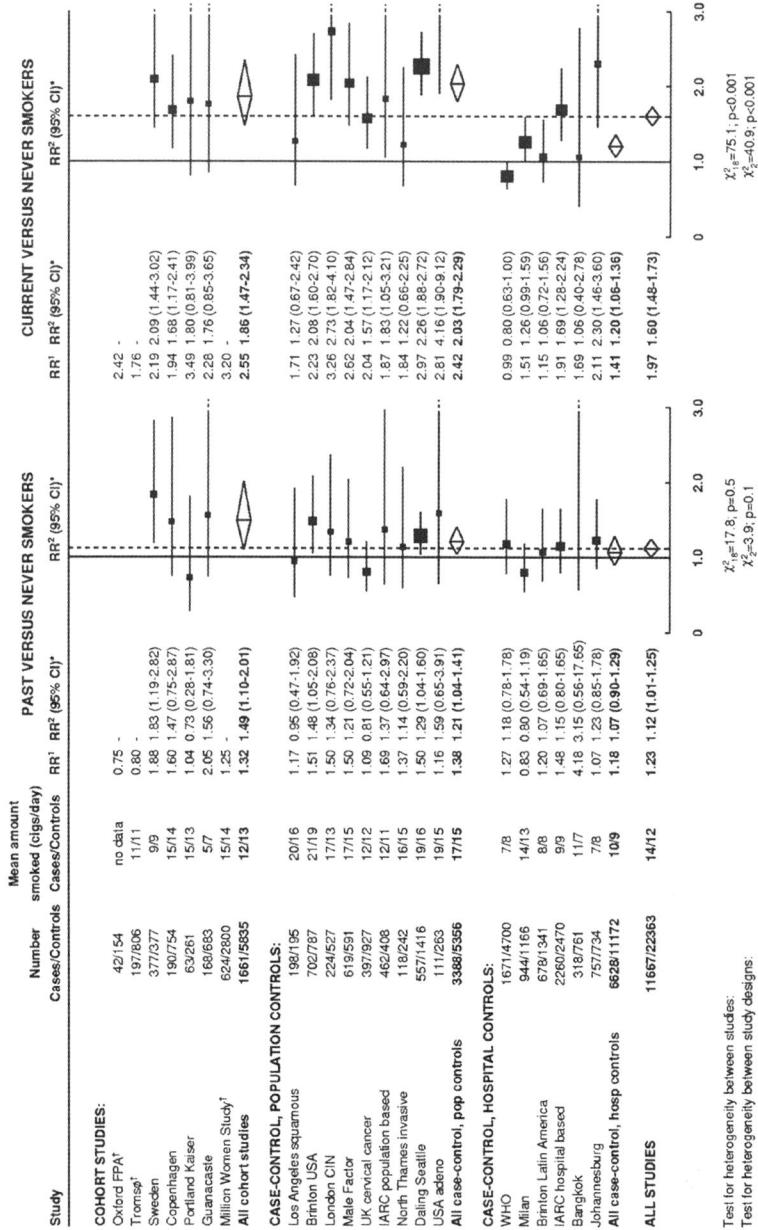

Figure 3. Relative risk (RR)* of squamous cell carcinoma of the cervix♦ in relation to smoking status by study

* RR[1] stratified by study and age at diagnosis only (includes studies with no data on number of sexual partners and so risks may differ from those in Figure 1). RR[2] stratified by study, age at diagnosis, number of sexual partners, duration of oral contraceptive use, age at first intercourse and number of full-term pregnancies. CI – confidence interval.

◇ no adjustment for number of sexual partners (data not available)

♦ invasive and carcinoma in situ/CIN3 (includes all non-adenocarcinomas)

From International Collaboration of Epidemiological Studies of Cervical Cancer (2006)

Myeloid Leukaemia

There is sufficient evidence in adults that tobacco smoking is causally related to myeloid leukaemia (IARC, 2004). No clear evidence of an increased risk in relation to smoking was seen for lymphoid leukaemia/lymphoma. A reduced number of studies on myeloid leukaemia and smoking include data on former smokers and are summarized in Tables 23 (cohort studies) and 24 (case–control studies).

Three incidence cohort studies report results on the risk of acute myeloid leukaemia (AML) and past smoking (Mills *et al.*, 1990; Friedman & van den Eeden, 1993; Adami et al., 1998). Two of these studies report elevated, but not statistically significant, risk in former smokers when compared with never smokers (Mills *et al.*, 1990; Friedman &

van den Eeden, 1993). Male former smokers in the study by Friedman (1993) show a decreased risk of AML when compared with current smokers although not significant. Three of the four cohort studies on mortality report a somewhat lower risk in former than in current smokers but higher than in never smokers (McLaughlin *et al.*, 1989; Garfinkel & Boffetta, 1990 (CPS-I and CPS-II estimates)). In Doll's study (2005), the mortality rate in heavy smokers ($\geq$ 25 cigarettes per day), but not in overall current smokers, was higher than that reported in former smokers (18.3 per 100 000 versus 12.6 per 100 000 respectively; current smokers 11.3 per 100 000). Three case–control studies (Mele *et al.*, 1994; Stagnaro *et al.*, 2001; Kasim *et al.*, 2005)

report a non-significant increased risk of AML among former smokers compared with never smokers. In these studies (Mele *et al.*, 1994; Stagnaro *et al.*, 2001; Kasim *et al.*, 2005) the confidence intervals of former and current smokers overlap considerably. The only study including data on time since quitting (Kane *et al.*, 1999) does not report a significant trend but shows a lower risk in former smokers with prolonged abstinence (over 20 years, OR=0.7; 95% CI=0.5–1.0) than in current smokers (OR=1.4; 95% CI=1.1–1.8).

The data presented here offer conflicting results of a decreased risk among former smokers compared to current smokers.

Sinonasal and Nasopharyngeal Cancers

One study (Zheng *et al.*, 1993b) examined the residual risk after cessation of smoking and found a significant decrease in risk for sinonasal cancer associated with increasing number of years since cessation (Table 25). In a previous study, the same authors had

found a negative, non-significant association (Zheng *et al.*, 1992b).

Two studies investigated the effect of quitting smoking (Nam *et al.*, 1992; Vaughan *et al.*, 1996) and found that the risk of nasopharyngeal carcinoma decreased with increasing time since

quitting (Table 26). The reduction was statistically significant within 5 years of smoking (OR=0.1; 95% CI=0.0–0.6) in the study by Vaughan and colleagues (1996).

Table 23. Cohort studies on tobacco smoking and myeloid leukemia

Reference, Country	Study type population	Sex	Status/Quantity		Relative risk	95 % CI
Cohort Incidence studies						
Mills *et al.*, 1990 USA	Adventists' Health Study	Men Women	Current smokers 1–14 cig/day 15–24 ≥ 25 Former smokers Never smokers	N=12 N=10 N=1	2.0 1.9 1.5 3.6 2.2 1.0	0.3, 16.7 0.6, 6.3 0.3, 7.0 1.1, 11 0.9, 5.5
Friedman, 1993 USA	Kaiser Permanente Medical Care Program Cohort I	Men	Current smokers Former smokers Never smokers	N=26 N=13 N=7	2.8 2.3 1.0	1.2, 6.4 0.9, 5.7
		Women	Current smokers Former smokers Never smokers	N=14 N=8 N=27	0.9 1.3 1	0.4, 1.7 0.6, 2.8
Adami *et al.,* 1998 Sweden	Swedish Construction workers	Men	Current smokers Former smokers Never smokers	N=83 N=30 N=58	1.0 0.7 1.0	0.7, 1.4 0.5, 1.2
Cohort Mortality studies						
McLaughlin *et al.*, 1989 USA	Veterans' Study	Men	Current smokers Cigarettes/day <10 10-20 >20 Former smokers Never smokers	N=142 N=62 N=71	1.6* 1.5 1.5 2.0 1.3 1.0	
Garfinkel & Boffetta 1990 USA	Cancer Prevention Study I	Men	Current smokers Cigarettes/day 1–29 ≥ 20 Formers smokers Never smokers		2.5* 2.3 2.9 2.2* 1	
		Women	Current smokers Cigarettes/day 1–29 ≥ 20 Former smokers Never smokers		0.7 0.6 0.7 0.4 1	

Table 23. Cohort studies on tobacco smoking and myeloid leukemia (contd)

Reference, Country	Study type population	Sex	Status/Quantity	Relative risk	95 % CI
Cohort Mortality studies					
Garfinkel & Boffetta, 1990 USA	Cancer Prevention Study II	Men	Current smokers	1.7*	
			Cigarettes/day		
			1–19	1.7	
			≥ 20	1.8	
			Former smokers	1.2	
			Never smokers	1	
		Women	Current smokers	1.2	
			Cigarettes/day		
			1–19	1.5	
			≥ 20	1.0	
			Former smokers	1.3	
			Never smokers	1	
Doll *et al.* 2005 UK	British Doctors' Study	Men (100 deaths)	Current smokers	11.3	Mortality rates per 100 000 / year
			Cigarettes/day		
			1–14	2.8	
			15–24	14.0	
			≥ 25	18.3	
			Former smokers	12.6	
			Never smokers	6.3	

* p < 0.05

Table 24. Case-control studies on tobacco smoking cessation and myeloid leukemia

Reference Country Years of study	Study characteristics	Smoking Categories	AML Relative Risk	95% CI	Adjustment variable
Mele *et al.*1994 Italy	118 cases 467 controls	Current smokers	1.4	0.8, 2.5	Age, sex, education level, residence outside study town
		Former smokers	1.6	0.9, 2.8	
		Never smokers	1.0		
Kane *et al.* 1999 UK	695 cases 1374 controls	Current smokers	1.4	1.1, 18	Deprivation
		Former smokers	0.9	0.7, 1.2	
		Years since quitting			
		21+	0.7	0.5, 1.0	
		11–20	1.0	0.7, 1.5	
		1–10	1.0	0.7, 1.4	
		Never smokers	1.0		
Stagnaro *et al.* 2001 Italy	220 cases 1765 controls	Current smokers	0.9	0.6, 1.4	Sex, age, area of residence, education level, type of interview
		Former smokers	1.2	0.8, 1.9	
		Never smokers	1.0		
Kasim *et al.* 2005 Canada	307 cases 5039 controls	Current smokers	1.4	1.1, 1.8	ORs also adjusted for sex, body mass index, pack-years of smoking
		Former smokers	1.2	0.9, 1.6	
		Never smokers	1.0		

Table 25. Case-control studies: relative risk of sinonasal cancer and smoking cessation

Reference Country Years of study	Number of cases	Cancer subsite ICD code	Exposure categories	Relative Risk	95% CI	Comments
Zheng et al. (1993b) USA	147 deaths 449 controls	Nasal cavity, paranasal sinuses, middle ear ICD–9: 160	Current smoker Years since quitting <5 5-9 >10	1.0 1.3 1.2 0.4	 0.7–2.2 0.5–2.8 0.2–0.7	 P for trend <0.01

Table 26. Case-control studies: relative risk of nasopharyngeal carcinoma and smoking cessation

Reference Country Years of study	Number of cases	Smoking categories	Relative Risk	95% CI	Comments
Nam et al. (1992) USA	204 cases 408 controls	*Men* Current smoker Never smoker	 1.5 1	 0.9, 2.6	
		Current smoker *Years since quitting* <5 ≥ 5	1.0 (reference) 1.2 0.6	 0.7, 2.2 0.3, 1.1	
		Women Current smoker Never smoker	 2.0 1	 1.0, 4.0	
		Current smoker *Years since quitting* <5 ≥ 5	1.0 (reference) 1.3 0.3	 0.5, 3.4 0.1, 1.3	 p for trend <0.001
Vaughan et al. (1996) USA	231 cases 246 controls	Current smoker *Packs/year* 1–4 35–59 60+ Former smoker Never smoker	 1.9 3.0 4.3 1.3 1	 0.9, 4.0 1.3, 6.8 1.5, 12.4 0.7, 2.3	
		Current smoker *Years since quitting* < 5 5–14 ≥ 15	1.0 (reference) 0.1 0.2 0.2	 0.0, 0.6 0.1, 0.7 0.0, 0.8	 p for trend = 0.003

References

Adami J, Nyren O, Bergstrom R, et al. (1998). Smoking and the risk of leukemia, lymphoma, and multiple myeloma (Sweden). *Cancer Causes Control*, 9(1):49-56.

Agudo A, Gonzalez CA, Marcos G, et al. (1992). Consumption of alcohol, coffee, and tobacco, and gastric cancer in Spain. *Cancer Causes Control*, 3(2):137-143.

Ahrens W, Jockel KH, Patzak W, et al. (1991). Alcohol, smoking, and occupational factors in cancer of the larynx: a case-control study. *Am J Ind Med*, 20(4):477-493.

Akiba S (1994). Analysis of cancer risk related to longitudinal information on smoking habits. *Environ Health Perspect*, 102(Suppl 8):15-19.

Altieri A, Bosetti C, Talamini R, et al. (2002). Cessation of smoking and drinking and the risk of laryngeal cancer. *Br J Cancer*, 87(11):1227-1229.

Anthony HM, Thomas GM (1970). Bladder tumours and smoking. *Int J Cancer*, 5(2):266-272.

Austin H, Delzell E, Grufferman S, et al. (1986). A case-control study of hepatocellular carcinoma and the hepatitis B virus, cigarette smoking, and alcohol consumption. *Cancer Res*, 46(2):962-966.

Baghurst PA, McMichael AJ, Slavotinek AH, et al. (1991). A case-control study of diet and cancer of the pancreas. *Am J Epidemiol*, 134(2):167-179.

Bayo S, Bosch FX, de Sanjose S, et al. (2002). Risk factors of invasive cervical cancer in Mali. *Int J Epidemiol*, 31(1):202-209.

Bedwani R, Renganathan E, El Kwhsky F, et al. (1998). Schistosomiasis and the risk of bladder cancer in Alexandria, Egypt. *Br J Cancer*, 77(7):1186-1189.

Beral V (2003). Breast cancer and hormone-replacement therapy in the Million Women Study. *Lancet*, 362(9382):419-427.

Blot WJ, McLaughlin JK, Winn DM, et al. (1988). Smoking and drinking in relation to oral and pharyngeal cancer. *Cancer Res*, 48(11):3282-3287.

Blot WJ, McLaughlin JK (1999). The changing epidemiology of esophageal cancer. *Semin Oncol*, 26(5 Suppl 15):2-8.

Boeing H, Frentzel-Beyme R, Berger M, et al. (1991). Case-control study on stomach cancer in Germany. *Int J Cancer*, 47(6):858-864.

Bonelli L, Aste H, Bovo P, et al. (2003). Exocrine pancreatic cancer, cigarette smoking, and diabetes mellitus: a case-control study in northern Italy. *Pancreas*, 27(2):143-149.

Bosch FX, Munoz N, de Sanjose S, et al. (1992). Risk factors for cervical cancer in Colombia and Spain. *Int J Cancer*, 52(5):750-758.

Bosetti C, Negri E, Franceschi S, et al. (2000a). Risk factors for oral and pharyngeal cancer in women: a study from Italy and Switzerland. *Br J Cancer*, 82(1):204-207.

Bosetti C, Franceschi S, Levi F, et al. (2000b). Smoking and drinking cessation and the risk of oesophageal cancer. *Br J Cancer*, 83(5):689-691.

Boyle P, Maisonneuve P, Bueno de Mesquita, et al. (1996). Cigarette smoking and pancreas cancer: a case control study of the search programme of the IARC. *Int J Cancer*, 67(1):63-71.

Brennan P, Bogillot O, Cordier S, et al. (2000). Cigarette smoking and bladder cancer in men: a pooled analysis of 11 case-control studies. *Int J Cancer*, 86(2):289-294.

Brennan P, Bogillot O, Greiser E, et al. (2001). The contribution of cigarette smoking to bladder cancer in women (pooled European data). *Cancer Causes Control*, 12(5):411-417.

Brinton LA, Schairer C, Haenszel W, et al. (1986). Cigarette smoking and invasive cervical cancer. *JAMA*, 255(23):3265-3269.

Bueno de Mesquita HB, Maisonneuve P, Moerman CJ, et al. (1991). Life-time history of smoking and exocrine carcinoma of the pancreas: a population-based case-control study in The Netherlands. *Int J Cancer*, 49(6):816-822.

Burch JD, Rohan TE, Howe GR, et al. (1989). Risk of bladder cancer by source and type of tobacco exposure: a case-control study. *Int J Cancer*, 44(4):622-628.

Cao W, Cai L, Rao JY, et al. (2005). Tobacco smoking, GSTP1 polymorphism, and bladder carcinoma. *Cancer*, 104(11):2400-2408.

Carstensen JM, Pershagen G, Eklund G (1987). Mortality in relation to cigarette and pipe smoking: 16 yearsí observation of 25,000 Swedish men. *J Epidemiol Community Health*, 41(2):166-172.

Cartwright RA, Adib R, Alppleyard I, et al. (1983). Cigarette smoking and bladder cancer: an epidemiological inquiry in West Yorkshire. *J Epidemiol Community Health*, 37:256-263.

Castelao JE, Yuan JM, Skipper PL, et al. (2001). Gender- and smoking-related bladder cancer risk. *J Natl Cancer Inst*, 93(7):538-545.

Castellsague X, Munoz N, De Stefani E, et al. (1999). Independent and joint effects of tobacco smoking and alcohol drinking on the risk of esophageal cancer in men and women. *Int J Cancer*, 82(5):657-664.

Castellsague X, Munoz N, De Stefani E, et al. (2000). Smoking and drinking cessation and risk of esophageal cancer (Spain). *Cancer Causes Control*, 11(9):813-818.

Cederlof R, Friberg L, Hrubec Z, et al. (1975). *The Relationship of Smoking and Some Social Covariables to Mortality and Cancer Morbidity. A ten year follow-up in a probability sample of 55,000 subjects, age 18-69*. Stockholm, The Karolinska Institute, Department of Environmental Hygiene.

Chao A, Thun MJ, Henley SJ, et al. (2002). Cigarette smoking, use of other tobacco products and stomach cancer mortality in US adults: The Cancer Prevention Study II. *Int J Cancer*, 101(4):380-389.

Chaouki N, Bosch FX, Munoz N, et al. (1998). The viral origin of cervical cancer in Rabat, Morocco. *Int J Cancer*, 75(4):546-554.

Chichareon S, Herrero R, Munoz N, et al. (1998). Risk factors for cervical cancer in Thailand: a case-control study. *J Natl Cancer Inst*, 90(1):50-57.

Chiu BC, Lynch CF, Cerhan JR, et al. (2001). Cigarette smoking and risk of bladder, pancreas, kidney, and colorectal cancers in Iowa. *Ann Epidemiol*, 11(1):28-37.

Choi SY, Kahyo H (1991a). Effect of cigarette smoking and alcohol consumption in the aetiology of cancer of the oral cavity, pharynx and larynx. *Int J Epidemiol*, 20(4):878-885.

Choi SY, Kahyo H (1991b). Effect of cigarette smoking and alcohol consumption in the etiology of cancers of the digestive tract. *Int J Cancer*, 49(3):381-386.

Chow WH, Swanson CA, Lissowska J, et al. (1999). Risk of stomach cancer in relation to consumption of cigarettes, alcohol, tea and coffee in Warsaw, Poland. *Int J Cancer*, 81(6):871-876.

Chow WH, Gridley G, Fraumeni JF, Jr., et al. (2000). Obesity, hypertension, and the risk of kidney cancer in men. *N Engl J Med*, 343(18):1305-1311.

Chyou PH, Nomura AM, Stemmermann GN (1993). A prospective study of diet, smoking, and lower urinary tract cancer. *Ann Epidemiol*, 3(3):211-216.

Clavel F, Benhamou E, Auquier A, et al. (1989a). Coffee, alcohol, smoking and cancer of the pancreas: a case-control study. *Int J Cancer*, 43(1):17-21.

Clavel J, Cordier S, Boccon-Gibod L, et al. (1989b). Tobacco and bladder cancer in males: increased risk for inhalers and smokers of black tobacco. *Int J Cancer*, 44(4):605-610.

Correa P, Fontham E, Pickle LW, et al. (1985). Dietary determinants of gastric cancer in south Louisiana inhabitants. *J Natl Cancer Inst*, 75(4):645-654.

Coughlin SS, Calle EE, Patel AV, et al. (2000). Predictors of pancreatic cancer mortality among a large cohort of United States adults. *Cancer Causes Control*, 11(10):915-923.

Cuzick J, Babiker AG (1989). Pancreatic cancer, alcohol, diabetes mellitus and gall-bladder disease. *Int J Cancer*, 43(3):415-421.

Cuzick J, Singer A, De Stavola BL, et al. (1990). Case-control study of risk factors for cervical intraepithelial neoplasia in young women. *Eur J Cancer*, 26(6):684-690.

Cuzick J, Sasieni P, Singer A (1996). Risk factors for invasive cervix cancer in young women. *Eur J Cancer*, 32A(5):836-841.

Daling JR, Madeleine MM, McKnight B, et al. (1996). The relationship of human papillomavirus-related cervical tumors to cigarette smoking, oral contraceptive use, and prior herpes simplex virus type 2 infection. *Cancer Epidemiol Biomarkers Prev*, 5(7):541-548.

Danaei G, Vander HS, Lopez AD, et al. (2005). Causes of cancer in the world: comparative risk assessment of nine behavioural and environmental risk factors. *Lancet*, 366(9499):1784-1793.

DiAvanzo B, Negri E, La Vecchia C, et al. (1990). Cigarette smoking and bladder cancer. *Eur J Cancer*, 26(6):714-718.

Day GL, Blot WJ, Austin DF, et al. (1993). Racial differences in risk of oral and pharyngeal cancer: alcohol, tobacco, and other determinants. *J Natl Cancer Inst*, 85:465-473.

Day GL, Blot WJ, Shore RE, et al. (1994). Second cancers following oral and pharyngeal cancers: role of tobacco and alcohol. *J Natl Cancer Inst*, 86(2):131-137.

Day NE, Brown CC (1980). Multistage models and primary prevention of cancer. *J Natl Cancer Inst*, 64(4):977-989.

De Stefani E, Correa P, Fierro L, et al. (1990). Alcohol drinking and tobacco smoking in gastric cancer. A case-control study. *Rev Epidemiol Sante Publique*, 38(4):297-307.

De Stefani E, Correa P, Fierro L, et al. (1991). Black tobacco, mate, and bladder cancer. A case-control study from Uruguay. *Cancer*, 67(2):536-540.

De Stefani E, Oreggia F, Rivero S, et al. (1992). Hand-rolled cigarette smoking and risk of cancer of the mouth, pharynx, and larynx. *Cancer*, 70:679-682.

De Stefani E, Boffetta P, Oreggia F, et al. (1998a). Smoking patterns and cancer of the oral cavity and pharynx: a case-control study in Uruguay. *Oral Oncol*, 34(5):340-346.

De Stefani E, Boffetta P, Carzoglio J, et al. (1998b). Tobacco smoking and alcohol drinking as risk factors for stomach cancer: a case-control study in Uruguay. *Cancer Causes Control*, 9(3):321-329.

Deacon JM, Evans CD, Yule R, et al. (2000). Sexual behaviour and smoking as determinants of cervical HPV infection and of CIN3 among those infected: a case-control study nested within the Manchester cohort. *Br J Cancer*, 83(11):1565-1572.

Doll R, Peto R (1976). Mortality in relation to smoking: 20 yearsí observations on male British doctors. *BMJ*, 2(6051):1525-1536.

Doll R, Peto R, Wheatley K, et al. (1994). Mortality in relation to smoking: 40 yearsí observations on male British doctors. *BMJ*, 309(6959):901-911.

Doll R (1996). Cancers weakly related to smoking. *Br Med Bull*, 52(1):35-49.

Doll R, Peto R, Boreham J, et al. (2005). Mortality from cancer in relation to smoking: 50 years observations on British

Donato F, Boffetta P, Fazioli R, et al. (1997). Bladder cancer, tobacco smoking, coffee and alcohol drinking in Brescia, northern Italy. *Eur J Epidemiol*, 13(7):795-800.

Eluf-Neto J, Booth M, Munoz N, et al. (1994). Human papillomavirus and invasive cervical cancer in Brazil. *Br J Cancer*, 69(1):114-119.

Engeland A, Andersen A, Haldorsen T, et al. (1996). Smoking habits and risk of cancers other than lung cancer: 28 yearsí follow-up of 26,000 Norwegian men and women. *Cancer Causes Control*, 7(5):497-506.

Falk RT, Pickle LW, Brown LM, et al. (1989). Effect of smoking and alcohol consumption on laryngeal cancer risk in coastal Texas. *Cancer Res*, 49(14):4024-4029.

Fernandez E, La Vecchia C, Decarli A (1996). Attributable risks for pancreatic cancer in northern Italy. *Cancer Epidemiol Biomarkers Prev*, 5(1):23-27.

Ferraroni M, Negri E, La Vecchia C, et al. (1989). Socioeconomic indicators, tobacco and alcohol in the aetiology of digestive tract neoplasms. *Int J Epidemiol*, 18(3):556-562.

Flaherty KT, Fuchs CS, Colditz GA, et al. (2005). A Prospective Study of Body

Mass Index, Hypertension, and Smoking and the Risk of Renal Cell Carcinoma (United States). *Cancer Causes Control*, 16(9):1099-1106.

Fortuny J, Kogevinas M, Chang-Claude J, et al. (1999). Tobacco, occupation and non-transitional-cell carcinoma of the bladder: an international case-control study. *Int J Cancer*, 80(1):44-46.

Franceschi S, Talamini R, Barra S, et al. (1990). Smoking and drinking in relation to cancers of the oral cavity, pharynx, larynx, and esophagus in northern Italy. *Cancer Res*, 50(20):6502-6507.

Franceschi S, Barra S, La Vecchia C, et al. (1992). Risk factors for cancer of the tongue and the mouth. A case-control study from northern Italy. *Cancer*, 70(9):2227-2233.

Franceschi S, Montella M, Polesel J, et al. (2006). Hepatitis viruses, alcohol, and tobacco in the etiology of hepatocellular carcinoma in Italy. *Cancer Epidemiol Biomarkers Prev*, 15(4):683-689.

Friedman GD (1993). Cigarette smoking, leukemia, and multiple myeloma. *Ann Epidemiol*, 3(4):425-428.

Friedman GD, van den Eeden SK (1993). Risk factors for pancreatic cancer: an exploratory study. *Int J Epidemiol*, 22(1):30-37.

Fryzek JP, Garabrant DH, Harlow SD, et al. (1997). A case-control study of self-reported exposures to pesticides and pancreas cancer in southeastern Michigan. *Int J Cancer*, 72(1):62-67.

Fuchs CS, Colditz GA, Stampfer MJ, et al. (1996). A prospective study of cigarette smoking and the risk of pancreatic cancer. *Arch Intern Med*, 156(19):2255-2260.

Fujino Y, Mizoue T, Tokui N, et al. (2005). Cigarette smoking and mortality due to stomach cancer: findings from the JACC Study. *J Epidemiol*, 15 Suppl 2:S113-S119.

Gaertner RR, Trpeski L, Johnson KC (2004). A case-control study of occupational risk factors for bladder cancer in Canada. *Cancer Causes Control*, 15(10):1007-1019.

Gajalakshmi CK, Shanta V (1996). Lifestyle and risk of stomach cancer: a hospital-based case-control study. *Int J Epidemiol*, 25(6):1146-1153.

Gallicchio L, Kouzis A, Genkinger JM, et al. (2006). Active cigarette smoking, household passive smoke exposure, and the risk of developing pancreatic cancer. *Prev Med*, 42(3):200-205.

Gammon MD, Schoenberg JB, Ahsan H, et al. (1997). Tobacco, alcohol, and socioeconomic status and adenocarcinomas of the esophagus and gastric cardia. *J Natl Cancer Inst*, 89(17): 1277-1284.

Garfinkel L, Boffetta P (1990). Association between smoking and leukemia in two American Cancer Society prospective studies. *Cancer*, 65(10):2356-2360.

Goodman MT, Moriwaki H, Vaeth M, et al. (1995). Prospective cohort study of risk factors for primary liver cancer in Hiroshima and Nagasaki, Japan. *Epidemiology*, 6(1):36-41.

Gram IT, Austin H, Stalsberg H (1992). Cigarette smoking and the incidence of cervical intraepithelial neoplasia, grade III, and cancer of the cervix uteri. *Am J Epidemiol*, 135(4):341-346.

Green J, Berrington dG, Sweetland S, et al. (2003). Risk factors for adenocarcinoma and squamous cell carcinoma of the cervix in women aged 20-44 years: the UK National Case-Control Study of Cervical Cancer. *Br J Cancer*, 89(11):2078-2086.

Gullo L, Pezzilli R, Morselli-Labate AM (1995). Coffee and cancer of the pancreas: an Italian multicenter study. The Italian Pancreatic Cancer Study Group. *Pancreas*, 11(3):223-229.

Guo W, Blot WJ, Li JY, et al. (1994). A nested case-control study of oesophageal and stomach cancers in the Linxian nutrition intervention trial. *Int J Epidemiol*, 23(3):444-450.

Hammouda D, MuÒoz N, Herrero R, et al. (2005). Cervical carcinoma in Algiers, Algeria: human papillomavirus and lifestyle risk factors. *Int J Cancer*, 113(3):483-489.

Hansson LE, Baron J, Nyren O, et al. (1994). Tobacco, alcohol and the risk of gastric cancer. A population-based case-control study in Sweden. *Int J Cancer*, 57(1):26-31.

Harnack LJ, Anderson KE, Zheng W, et al. (1997). Smoking, alcohol, coffee, and tea intake and incidence of cancer of the exocrine pancreas: the Iowa Womenís Health Study. *Cancer Epidemiol Biomarkers Prev*, 6(12):1081-1086.

Harris RE, Chen-Backlund JY, Wynder EL (1990). Cancer of the urinary bladder in blacks and whites. A case-control study. *Cancer*, 66(12):2673-2680.

Hayes RB, Bravo-Otero E, Kleinman DV, et al. (1999). Tobacco and alcohol use and oral cancer in Puerto Rico. *Cancer Causes Control*, 10(1):27-33.

Heath CWJ (1997). Hypertension diuretics and antihypertensive medications as possible risk factor for renal cancer. *Am J Epidemiol*, 145:607-613.

Herrero R, Brinton LA, Reeves WC, et al. (1989). Invasive cervical cancer and smoking in Latin America. *J Natl Cancer Inst*, 81(3):205-211.

Hiatt RA, Klatsky AL, Armstrong MA (1988). Pancreatic cancer, blood glucose and beverage consumption. *Int J Cancer*, 41(6):794-797.

Hildesheim A, Herrero R, Castle PE, et al. (2001). HPV co-factors related to the development of cervical cancer: results from a population-based study in Costa Rica. *Br J Cancer*, 84(9):1219-1226.

Hirayama T (1981). A large-scale cohort study on the relationship between diet and selected cancers of digestive organs. In: Bruce WR, Correa P, Lipkin M, et al., eds., *Gastrointestinal Cancer: Endogenous Factors (Banbury Report 7)*. 409-426.

Hoshiyama Y, Sasaba T (1992). A case-control study of single and multiple stomach cancers in Saitama Prefecture, Japan. *Jpn J Cancer Res*, 83(9):937-943.

Howe GR, Burch JD, Miller AB, et al. (1980). Tobacco use, occupation, coffee, various nutrients, and bladder cancer. *J Natl Cancer Inst*, 64(4):701-713.

Howe GR, Jain M, Burch JD, et al. (1991). Cigarette smoking and cancer of the pancreas: evidence from a population-based case-control study in Toronto, Canada. *Int J Cancer*, 47(3):323-328.

Hsieh CC, MacMahon B, Yen S, et al. (1986). Coffee and pancreatic cancer (Chapter 2). *N Engl J Med*, 315(9):587-589.

Hsing AW, McLaughlin JK, Hrubec Z, et al. (1990). Cigarette smoking and liver cancer among US veterans. *Cancer Causes Control*, 1(3):217-221.

Hu J, Ugnat AM (2005). Active and passive smoking and risk of renal cell carcinoma in Canada. *Eur J Cancer*, 41(5):770-778.

Hunt JD, van der Hel OL, McMillan GP, et al. (2005). Renal cell carcinoma in relation to cigarette smoking: meta-analysis of 24 studies. *Int J Cancer*, 114(1):101-108.

IARC (1986). *IARC Monographs on the Evaluation of the Carcinogenic Risk of Chemicals to Humans, Vol. 38, Tobacco smoking*. Lyon, IARCPress.

IARC (1988). *IARC Monographs on the Evaluation of Carcinogenic Risks to Humans, Vol. 44, Alcohol Drinking*. Lyon, IARCPress.

IARC (1994). *IARC Monographs on the Evaluation of Carcinogenic Risks to Humans, Vol. 59, Hepatitis Viruses*. Lyon, IARCPress.

IARC (1995). *IARC Monographs on the Evaluation of Carcinogenic Risks to Humans, Vol. 64, Human papillomaviruses*. Lyon, IARCPress.

IARC (2004). *IARC Monographs on the Evaluation of Carcinogenic Risks to Humans, Vol. 83, Tobacco Smoke and Involuntary Smoking*. Lyon, IARCPress.

Inoue M, Tajima K, Hirose K, et al. (1994). Life-style and subsite of gastric cancerójoint ef fect of smoking and drinking habits. *Int J Cancer*, 56(4): 494-499.

Inoue M, Tajima K, Yamamura Y, et al. (1999). Influence of habitual smoking on gastric cancer by histologic subtype. *Int J Cancer*, 81(1):39-43.

Inoue M, Tajima K, Takezaki T, et al. (2003). Epidemiology of pancreatic cancer in Japan: a nested case-control study from the Hospital-based Epidemiologic Research Program at Aichi Cancer Center (HERPACC). *Int J Epidemiol*, 32(2):257-262.

International Collaboration of Epidemiological Studies of Cervical Cancer (2006). Carcinoma of the cervix and tobacco smoking: Collaborative reanalysis of individual data on 13,541 women with carcinoma of the cervix and 23,017 women without carcinoma of the cervix from 23 epidemiological studies. *Int J Cancer*, 118(6):1481-1495.

Isaksson B, Jonsson F, Pedersen NL, et al. (2002). Lifestyle factors and pancreatic cancer risk: a cohort study from the Swedish Twin Registry. *Int J Cancer*, 98(3):480-482.

Jedrychowski W, Wahrendorf J, Popiela T, et al. (1986). A case-control study of dietary factors and stomach cancer risk in Poland. *Int J Cancer*, 37(6):837-842.

Jee SH, Samet JM, Ohrr H, et al. (2004). Smoking and cancer risk in Korean men and women. *Cancer Causes Control*, 15(4):341-348.

Ji BT, Chow WH, Dai Q, et al. (1995). Cigarette smoking and alcohol consumption and the risk of pancreatic cancer: a case-control study in Shanghai, China. *Cancer Causes Control*, 6(4):369-376.

Ji BT, Chow WH, Yang G, et al. (1996). The influence of cigarette smoking, alcohol, and green tea consumption on the risk of carcinoma of the cardia and distal stomach in Shanghai, China. *Cancer*, 77(12):2449-2457.

Kabat GC, Ng SK, Wynder EL (1993). Tobacco, alcohol intake, and diet in relation to adenocarcinoma of the esophagus and gastric cardia. *Cancer Causes Control*, 4(2):123-132.

Kabat GC, Chang CJ, Wynder EL (1994). The role of tobacco, alcohol use, and body mass index in oral and pharyngeal cancer. *Int J Epidemiol*, 23(6):1137-1144.

Kahn HA (1966). The Dorn study of smoking and mortality among U.S. veterans: report on eight and one-half years of observation. In: Haenszel W, ed., *Epidemiological Study of Cancer and Other Chronic Diseases*. 1-126.

Kane EV, Roman E, Cartwright R, et al. (1999). Tobacco and the risk of acute leukaemia in adults. *Br J Cancer*, 81(7):1228-1233.

Kasim K, Levallois P, Abdous B, et al. (2005). Lifestyle factors and the risk of adult leukemia in Canada. *Cancer Causes Control*, 16(5):489-500.

Kato I, Tominaga S, Ito Y, et al. (1990). A comparative case-control analysis of stomach cancer and atrophic gastritis. *Cancer Res*, 50(20):6559-6564.

Kato I, Tominaga S, Ito Y, et al. (1992a). A prospective study of atrophic gastritis and stomach cancer risk. *Jpn J Cancer Res*, 83(11):1137-1142.

Kato I, Tominaga S, Matsumoto K (1992b). A prospective study of stomach cancer among a rural Japanese population: a 6-year survey. *Jpn J Cancer Res*, 83(6):568-575.

Kato I, Tominaga S, Ikari A (1992c). The risk and predictive factors for developing liver cancer among patients with decompensated liver cirrhosis. *Jpn J Clin Oncol*, 22(4):278-285.

Kellen E, Zeegers M, Paulussen A, et al. (2006). Fruit consumption reduces the effect of smoking on bladder cancer risk. The Belgian case control study on bladder cancer. *Int J Cancer*, 118(10):2572-2578.

Kinjo Y, Cui Y, Akiba S, et al. (1998). Mortality risks of oesophageal cancer associated with hot tea, alcohol, tobacco and diet in Japan. *J Epidemiol*, 8(4):235-243.

Kjaer SK, van den Brule AJ, Bock JE, et al. (1996a). Human papillomavirusóthe most significant risk determinant of cervical intraepithelial neoplasia. *Int J Cancer*, 65(5):601-606.

Kjaer SK, Engholm G, Dahl C, et al. (1996b). Case-control study of risk factors for cervical squamous cell neoplasia in Denmark. IV: role of smoking habits. *Eur J Cancer Prev*, 5(5):359-365.

Kneller RW, McLaughlin JK, Bjelke E, et al. (1991). A cohort study of stomach cancer in a high-risk American population. *Cancer*, 68(3):672-678.

Ko YC, Huang YL, Lee CH, et al. (1995). Betel quid chewing, cigarette smoking and alcohol consumption related to oral cancer in Taiwan. *J Oral Pathol Med*, 24(10):450-453.

Koizumi Y, Tsubono Y, Nakaya N, et al. (2004). Cigarette smoking and the risk of gastric cancer: a pooled analysis of two prospective studies in Japan. *Int J Cancer*, 112(6):1049-1055.

Kreiger N, Marrett LD, Dodds L, et al. (1993). Risk factors for renal cell carcinoma: results of a population-based case-control study. *Cancer Causes Control*, 4(2):101-110.

Kunze E, Chang-Claude J, Frentzel-Beyme R (1992). Life style and occupational risk factors for bladder cancer in Germany. A case-control study. *Cancer*, 69(7):1776-1790.

Kuper H, Tzonou A, Kaklamani E, et al. (2000). Tobacco smoking, alcohol consumption and their interaction in the causation of hepatocellular carcinoma. *Int J Cancer*, 85(4):498-502.

La Vecchia C, Franceschi S, Decarli A, et al. (1986). Cigarette smoking and the risk of cervical neoplasia. *Am J Epidemiol*, 123(1):22-29.

La Vecchia C, Negri E, Decarli A, et al. (1988). Risk factors for hepatocellular carcinoma in northern Italy. *Int J Cancer*, 42(6):872-876.

La Vecchia C, Bidoli E, Barra S, et al. (1990a). Type of cigarettes and cancers of the upper digestive and respiratory tract. *Cancer Causes Control*, 1(1):69-74.

La Vecchia C, Negri E, DíAvanzo B, et al. (1990b). Smoking and renal cell carcinoma. *Cancer Res*, 50(17):5231-5233.

La Vecchia C, Franceschi S, Bosetti C, et al. (1999). Time since stopping smoking and the risk of oral and pharyngeal cancers. *J Natl Cancer Inst*, 91(8):726-728.

Lacey JV, Jr., Frisch M, Brinton LA, et al. (2001). Associations between smoking and adenocarcinomas and squamous cell carcinomas of the uterine cervix (United States). *Cancer Causes Control*, 12(2):153-161.

Lagergren J, Bergstrom R, Lindgren A, et al. (2000). The role of tobacco, snuff and alcohol use in the aetiology of cancer of the oesophagus and gastric cardia. *Int J Cancer*, 85(3):340-346.

Larsson SC, Permert J, Hakansson N, et al. (2005). Overall obesity, abdominal adiposity, diabetes and cigarette smoking in relation to the risk of pancreatic cancer in two Swedish population-based cohorts. *Br J Cancer*, 93(11):1310-1315.

Launoy G, Milan CH, Faivre J, et al. (1997). Alcohol, tobacco and oesophageal cancer: effects of the duration of consumption, mean intake and current and former consumption. *Br J Cancer*, 75(9):1389-1396.

Lin Y, Tamakoshi A, Kawamura T, et al. (2002). A prospective cohort study of cigarette smoking and pancreatic cancer in Japan. *Cancer Causes Control*, 13(3):249-254.

Lissowska J, Pilarska A, Pilarski P, et al. (2003). Smoking, alcohol, diet, dentition and sexual practices in the epidemiology of oral cancer in Poland. *Eur J Cancer Prev*, 12(1):25-33.

Llewellyn CD, Johnson NW, Warnakulasuriya KA (2004). Risk factors for oral cancer in newly diagnosed patients aged 45 years and younger: a case-control study in Southern England. *J Oral Pathol Med*, 33(9):525-532.

Lopez-Abente G, Gonzalez CA, Errezola M, et al. (1991). Tobacco smoke inhalation pattern, tobacco type, and bladder cancer in Spain. *Am J Epidemiol*, 134(8):830-839.

Lopez-Abente G, Pollan M, Monge V, et al. (1992). Tobacco smoking, alcohol consumption, and laryngeal cancer in Madrid. *Cancer Detect Prev*, 16(5-6):265-271.

Macfarlane GJ, Zheng T, Marshall JR, et al. (1995). Alcohol, tobacco, diet and the risk of oral cancer: a pooled analysis of three case-control studies. *Eur J Cancer B Oral Oncol*, 31B(3):181-187.

Mack TM, Yu MC, Hanisch R, et al. (1986). Pancreas cancer and smoking, beverage consumption, and past medical history. *J Natl Cancer Inst*, 76(1):49-60.

MacMahon B, Yen S, Trichopoulos D, et al. (1981). Coffee and cancer of the pancreas. *N Engl J Med*, 304(11):630-633.

Madeleine MM, Daling JR, Schwartz SM, et al. (2001). Human papillomavirus and long-term oral contraceptive use increase the risk of adenocarcinoma in situ of the cervix. *Cancer Epidemiol Biomarkers Prev*, 10(3):171-177.

Mashberg A, Boffetta P, Winkelman R, et al. (1993). Tobacco smoking, alcohol drinking, and cancer of the oral cavity and oropharynx among U.S. veterans. *Cancer*, 72(4):1369-1375.

McCarthy PV, Bhatia AJ, Saw SM, et al. (1995). Cigarette smoking and bladder cancer in Washington County, Maryland: ammunition for health educators. *Md Med J*, 44(12):1039-1042.

McCredie M, Stewart JH (1992). Risk factors for kidney cancer in New South Walesól. Cigarette smoking . *Eur J Cancer*, 28A(12):2050-2054.

McLaughlin JK, Mandel JS, Blot WJ, et al. (1984). A populationñbased case control study of renal cell carcinoma. *J Natl Cancer Inst*, 72(2):275-284.

McLaughlin JK, Hrubec Z, Linet MS, et al. (1989). Cigarette smoking and leukemia. *J Natl Cancer Inst*, 81(16):1262-1263.

McLaughlin JK, Hrubec Z, Blot WJ, et al. (1990a). Stomach cancer and cigarette smoking among U.S. veterans, 1954-1980. *Cancer Res*, 50(12):3804.

McLaughlin JK, Hrubec Z, Heineman EF, et al. (1990b). Renal cancer and cigarette smoking in a 26-year followup of U.S. veterans. *Public Health Rep*, 105(5):535-537.

McLaughlin JK, Hrubec Z, Blot WJ, et al. (1995a). Smoking and cancer mortality among U.S. veterans: a 26-year follow-up. *Int J Cancer*, 60(2):190-193.

McLaughlin JK, Lindblad P, Mellemgaard A, et al. (1995b). International renal-cell cancer study. I. Tobacco use. *Int J Cancer*, 60(2):194-198.

Mele A, Szklo M, Visani G, et al. (1994). Hair dye use and other risk factors for leukemia and pre-leukemia: a case-control study. Italian Leukemia Study Group. *Am J Epidemiol*, 139(6):609-619.

Menvielle G, Luce D, Goldberg P, et al. (2004). Smoking, alcohol drinking and cancer risk for various sites of the larynx and hypopharynx. A case-control study in France. *Eur J Cancer Prev*, 13(3):165-172.

Merletti F, Boffetta P, Ciccone G, et al. (1989). Role of tobacco and alcoholic beverages in the etiology of cancer of the oral cavity/oropharynx in Torino, Italy. *Cancer Res*, 49(17):4919-4924.

Mills PK, Beeson WL, Abbey DE, et al. (1988). Dietary habits and past medical history as related to fatal pancreas cancer risk among Adventists. *Cancer*, 61(12):2578-2585.

Mills PK, Newell GR, Beeson WL, et al. (1990). History of cigarette smoking and risk of leukemia and myeloma: results from the Adventist health study. *J Natl Cancer Inst*, 82(23):1832-1836.

Mills PK, Beeson WL, Phillips RL, et al. (1991). Bladder cancer in a low risk population: results from the Adventist Health Study. *Am J Epidemiol*, 133(3):230-239.

Mizuno S, Watanabe S, Nakamura K, et al. (1992). A multi-institute case-control study on the risk factors of developing pancreatic cancer. *Jpn J Clin Oncol*, 22(4):286-291.

Mizoue T, Tokui N, Nishisaka K, et al. (2000). Prospective study on the relation of cigarette smoking with cancer of the liver and stomach in an endemic region. *Int J Epidemiol*, 29(2):232-237.

Momas I, Daures JP, Festy B, et al. (1994). Relative importance of risk factors in bladder carcinogenesis: some new results about Mediterranean habits. *Cancer Causes Control*, 5(4):326-332.

Mori M, Hara M, Wada I, et al. (2000). Prospective study of hepatitis B and C viral infections, cigarette smoking, alcohol consumption, and other factors associated with hepatocellular carcinoma risk in Japan. *Am J Epidemiol*, 151(2):131-139.

Morris-Brown LM, Blot WJ, Schuman SH, et al. (1988). Environmental factors and high risk of esophageal cancer among men in coastal South Carolina. *J Natl Cancer Inst*, 80(20):1620-1625.

Morris-Brown LM, Silverman DT, Pottern LM, et al. (1994). Adenocarcinoma of the esophagus and esophagogastric junction in white men in the United States: alcohol, tobacco, and socioeconomic factors. *Cancer Causes Control*, 5(4):333-340.

Morrison AS, Buring JE, Verhoek WG, et al. (1984). An international study of smoking and bladder cancer. *J Urol*, 131(4):650-654.

Muñoz N, Bosch FX, de Sanjose S, et al. (1993). Risk factors for cervical intraepithelial neoplasia grade III/carcinoma in situ in Spain and Colombia. *Cancer Epidemiol Biomarkers Prev*, 2(5):423-431.

Muscat JE, Wynder EL (1992). Tobacco, alcohol, asbestos, and occupational risk factors for laryngeal cancer. *Cancer*, 69(9):2244-2251.

Muscat JE, Stellman SD, Hoffmann D, et al. (1997). Smoking and pancreatic cancer in men and women. *Cancer Epidemiol Biomarkers Prev*, 6(1):15-19.

Nam JM, McLaughlin JK, Blot WJ (1992). Cigarette smoking, alcohol, and nasopharyngeal carcinoma: a case-control study among U.S. whites. *J Natl Cancer Inst*, 84(8):619-622.

Ngelangel C, Muñoz N, Bosch FX, et al. (1998). Causes of cervical cancer in the Philippines: a case-control study. *J Natl Cancer Inst*, 90(1):43-49.

Nilsen TI, Vatten LJ (2000). A prospective study of lifestyle factors and the risk of pancreatic cancer in Nord-Trondelag, Norway. *Cancer Causes Control*, 11(7):645-652.

Nomura A, Grove JS, Stemmermann GN, et al. (1990a). A prospective study of stomach cancer and its relation to diet, cigarettes, and alcohol consumption. *Cancer Res*, 50(3):627-631.

Nomura A, Grove JS, Stemmermann GN, et al. (1990b). Cigarette smoking and stomach cancer. *Cancer Res*, 50(21):7084.

Nomura AM, Stemmermann GN, Chyou PH (1995). Gastric cancer among the Japanese in Hawaii. *Jpn J Cancer Res*, 86(10):916-923.

Nordlund LA, Carstensen JM, Pershagen G (1997). Cancer incidence in female smokers: a 26-year follow-up. *Int J Cancer*, 73(5):625-628.

Ohba S, Nishi M, Miyake H (1996). Eating habits and pancreas cancer. *Int J Pancreatol*, 20(1):37-42.

Oreggia F, De Stefani E, Correa P, et al. (1991). Risk factors for cancer of the tongue in Uruguay. *Cancer*, 67(1):180-183.

Palli D, Bianchi S, Decarli A, et al. (1992). A case-control study of cancers of the gastric cardia in Italy. *Br J Cancer*, 65(2):263-266.

Parazzini F, La Vecchia C, Negri E, et al. (1992). Risk factors for cervical intraepithelial neoplasia. *Cancer*, 69(9):2276-2282.

Parker AS, Cerhan JR, Janney CA, et al. (2003). Smoking cessation and renal cell carcinoma. *Ann Epidemiol*, 13(4):245-251.

Partanen TJ, Vainio HU, Ojajarvi IA, et al. (1997). Pancreas cancer, tobacco smoking and consumption of alcoholic beverages: a case-control study. *Cancer Lett*, 116(1):27-32.

Pelucchi C, La Vecchia C, Negri E, et al. (2002). Smoking and other risk factors for bladder cancer in women. *Prev Med*, 35(2):114-120.

Peters RK, Thomas D, Hagan DG, et al. (1986). Risk factors for invasive cervical cancer among Latinas and non-Latinas in Los Angeles County. *J Natl Cancer Inst*, 77(5):1063-1077.

Pohlabeln H, Jockel KH, Bolm-Audorff U (1999). Non-occupational risk factors for cancer of the lower urinary tract in Germany. *Eur J Epidemiol*, 15(5):411-419.

Pommer W, Bronder E, Klimpel A, et al. (1999). Urothelial cancer at different tumour sites: role of smoking and habitual intake of analgesics and laxatives. Results of the Berlin Urothelial Cancer Study. *Nephrol Dial Transplant*, 14(12):2892-2897.

Puente D, Hartge P, Greiser E, et al. (2006). A pooled analysis of bladder cancer case-control studies evaluating smoking in men and women. *Cancer Causes Control*, 17(1):71-79.

Rajkumar T, Franceschi S, Vaccarella S, et al. (2003). Role of paan chewing and dietary habits in cervical carcinoma in Chennai, India. *Br J Cancer*, 88(9):1388-1393.

Rogot E, Murray JL (1980). Smoking and causes of death among U.S. veterans: 16 years of observation. *Public Health Rep*, 95(3):213-222.

Rolon PA, Castellsague X, Benz M, et al. (1995). Hot and cold mate drinking and esophageal cancer in Paraguay. *Cancer Epidemiol Biomarkers Prev*, 4(6):595-605.

Rolon PA, Smith JS, Munoz N, et al. (2000). Human papillomavirus infection and invasive cervical cancer in Paraguay. *Int J Cancer*, 85(4):486-491.

Saha SK (1991). Smoking habits and carcinoma of the stomach: a case-control study. *Jpn J Cancer Res*, 82(5):497-502.

Santos C, Munoz N, Klug S, et al. (2001). HPV types and cofactors causing cervical cancer in Peru. *Br J Cancer*, 85(7):966-971.

Schiffman MH, Bauer HM, Hoover RN, et al. (1993). Epidemiologic evidence showing that human papillomavirus infection causes most cervical intraepithelial neoplasia. *J Natl Cancer Inst*, 85(12):958-964.

Schildt EB, Eriksson M, Hardell L, et al. (1998). Oral snuff, smoking habits and alcohol consumption in relation to oral cancer in a Swedish case-control study. *Int J Cancer*, 77(3):341-346.

Schlecht NF, Franco EL, Pintos J, et al. (1999). Effect of smoking cessation and tobacco type on the risk of cancers of the upper aero-digestive tract in Brazil. *Epidemiology*, 10(4):412-418.

Schlehofer B, Heuer C, Blettner M, et al. (1995). Occupation, smoking and demographic factors, and renal cell carcinoma in Germany. *Int J Epidemiol*, 24(1):51-57.

Shibata A, Fukuda K, Toshima H, et al. (1990). The role of cigarette smoking and drinking in the development of liver cancer: 28 years of observations on male cohort members in a farming and fishing area. *Cancer Detect Prev*, 14(6):617-623.

Shibata A, Mack TM, Paganini-Hill A, et al. (1994). A prospective study of pancreatic cancer in the elderly. *Int J Cancer*, 58(1):46-49.

Silverman DT, Dunn JA, Hoover RN, et al. (1994). Cigarette smoking and pancreas cancer: a case-control study based on direct interviews. *J Natl Cancer Inst*, 86(20):1510-1516.

Sitas F, Pacella-Norman R, Carrara H, et al. (2000). The spectrum of HIV-1 related cancers in South Africa. *Int J Cancer*, 88(3):489-492.

Sorahan T, Lancashire RJ, Sole G (1994). Urothelial cancer and cigarette smoking: findings from a regional case-controlled study. *Br J Urol*, 74(6):753-756.

Stagnaro E, Ramazzotti V, Crosignani P, et al. (2001). Smoking and hematolymphopoietic malignancies. *Cancer Causes Control*, 12(4):325-334.

Steineck G, Norell SE, Feychting M (1988). Diet, tobacco and urothelial cancer. A 14-year follow-up of 16,477 subjects. *Acta Oncol*, 27(4):323-327.

Talamini R, Franceschi S, Barra S, et al. (1990a). The role of alcohol in oral and pharyngeal cancer in non-smokers, and of tobacco in non-drinkers. *Int J. Cancer*, 46(3):391-393.

Talamini R, Baron AE, Barra S, et al. (1990b). A case-control study of risk factor for renal cell cancer in northern Italy. *Cancer Causes Control*, 1(2):125-131.

Talamini R, Bosetti C, La Vecchia C, et al. (2002). Combined effect of tobacco and alcohol on laryngeal cancer risk: a case-control study. *Cancer Causes Control*, 13(10):957-964.

Tanaka K, Hirohata T, Takeshita S, et al. (1992). Hepatitis B virus, cigarette smoking and alcohol consumption in the development of hepatocellular carcinoma: a case-control study in Fukuoka, Japan. *Int J Cancer*, 51(4):509-514.

Thomas DB, Qin Q, Kuypers J, et al. (2001). Human papillomaviruses and cervical cancer in Bangkok. II. Risk factors for in situ and invasive squamous cell cervical carcinomas. *Am J Epidemiol*, 153(8):732-739.

Tripathi A, Folsom AR, Anderson KE (2002). Risk factors for urinary bladder carcinoma in postmenopausal women. The Iowa Womenís Health Study. *Cancer*, 95(11):2316-2323.

Tsukuma H, Hiyama T, Oshima A, et al. (1990). A case-control study of hepatocellular carcinoma in Osaka, Japan. *Int J Cancer*, 45(2):231-236.

Tulinius H, Sigfusson N, Sigvaldason H, et al. (1997). Risk factors for malignant diseases: a cohort study on a population of 22,946 Icelanders. *Cancer Epidemiol Biomarkers Prev*, 6(11):863-873.

Tuyns AJ, Pequignot G, Jensen OM (1977). [Esophageal cancer in Ille-et-Vilaine in relation to levels of alcohol and tobacco consumption. Risks are multiplying]. *Bull Cancer*, 64(1):45-60.

Tuyns AJ, Esteve J, Raymond L, et al. (1988). Cancer of the larynx/hypopharynx, tobacco and alcohol: IARC international case-control study in Turin and Varese (Italy), Zaragoza and Navarra (Spain), Geneva (Switzerland) and Calvados (France). *Int J Cancer*, 41(4):483-491.

Tverdal A, Thelle D, Stensvold I, et al. (1993). Mortality in relation to smoking history: 13 yearsí follow-up of 68,000 Norwegian men and women 35-49 years. *J Clin Epidemiol*, 46(5):475-487.

Tyrrell BA, MacAirt JG, McCaughey WT (1971). Occupational and non-occupational factors associated with vesical neoplasm in Ireland. *J Irish Med Assoc*, 64:213-217.

Ursin G, Pike MC, Preston-Martin S, et al. (1996). Sexual, reproductive, and other risk factors for adenocarcinoma of the cervix: results from a population-based case-control study (California, United States). *Cancer Causes Control*, 7(3):391-401.

Vaughan TL, Shapiro JA, Burt RD, et al. (1996). Nasopharyngeal cancer in a low-risk population: defining risk factors by histological type. *Cancer Epidemiol Biomarkers Prev*, 5(8):587-593.

Vessey M, Painter R, Yeates D (2003). Mortality in relation to oral contraceptive use and cigarette smoking. *Lancet*, 362(9379):185-191.

Vineis P, Esteve J, Terracini B (1984). Bladder cancer and smoking in males: types of cigarettes, age at start, effect of stopping and interaction with occupation. *Int J Cancer*, 34:165-170.

Vioque J, Walker AM (1991). [Pancreatic cancer and ABO blood types: a study of cases and controls]. *Med Clin (Barc)*, 96(20):761-764.

WHO (1993). Invasive squamous-cell cervical carcinoma and combined oral contraceptives: results from a multinational study. WHO Collaborative Study of Neoplasia and Steroid Contraceptives. *Int J Cancer*, 55(2):228-236.

Wu AH, et al (2001). A multiethnic population based study of smoking alcohol and body sixe and risk of adenocarcinomas of the stomach and esophagus. *Cancer Causes Control*, 12:721-732.

Wu-Williams AH, Yu MC, Mack TM (1990). Life-style, workplace, and stomach cancer by subsite in young men of Los Angeles County. *Cancer Res*, 50(9):2569-2576.

Wynder EL, Covey LS, Mabuchi K, et al. (1976). Environmental factors in cancer of the larynx: a second look. *Cancer*, 38(4):1591-1601.

Wynder EL, Goldsmith JR (1977). The epidemiology of bladder cancer. *Cancer*, 40:1246-1268.

Wynder EL, Hall NE, Polansky M (1983). Epidemiology of coffee and pancreatic cancer. *Cancer Res*, 43(8):3900-3906.

Wynder EL, Dieck GS, Hall NE (1986). Case-control study of decaffeinated coffee consumption and pancreatic cancer. *Cancer Res*, 46(10):5360-5363.

Ye W, Ekstrom AM, Hansson LE, et al. (1999). Tobacco, alcohol and the risk of gastric cancer by sub-site and histologic type. *Int J Cancer*, 83(2):223-229.

Ylitalo N, Sorensen P, Josefsson A, et al. (1999). Smoking and oral contraceptives as risk factors for cervical carcinoma in situ. *Int J Cancer*, 81(3):357-365.

Yu MC, Mack T, Hanisch R, et al. (1983). Hepatitis, alcohol consumption, cigarette smoking, and hepatocellular carcinoma in Los Angeles. *Cancer Res*, 43(12 Pt 1):6077-6079.

Yu MC, Garabrant DH, Peters JM, et al. (1988). Tobacco, alcohol, diet, occupation, and carcinoma of the esophagus. *Cancer Res*, 48(13):3843-3848.

Yuan JM, Castelao JE, Gago-Dominguez M, et al. (1998). Tobacco use in relation to renal cell carcinoma. *Cancer Epidemiol Biomarkers Prev*, 7(5):429-433.

Yun JE, Jo I, Park J, et al. (2006). Cigarette smoking, elevated fasting serum glucose, and risk of pancreatic cancer in Korean men. *Int J Cancer*, 119(1):208-212.

Yun YH, Jung KW, Bae JM, et al. (2005). Cigarette smoking and cancer incidence risk in adult men: National Health Insurance Corporation Study. *Cancer Detect Prev*, 29(1):15-24.

Zambon P, Talamini R, La Vecchia C, et al. (2000). Smoking, type of alcoholic beverage and squamous-cell oesophageal cancer in northern Italy. *Int J Cancer*, 86(1):144-149.

Zaridze D, Borisova E, Maximovitch D, et al. (2000). Alcohol consumption, smoking and risk of gastric cancer: case-control study from Moscow, Russia. *Cancer Causes Control*, 11(4):363-371.

Zatonski W, Becher H, Lissowska J, et al. (1991). Tobacco, alcohol, and diet in the etiology of laryngeal cancer: a population-based case-control study. *Cancer Causes Control*, 2(1):3-10.

Zeegers MP, Tan FE, Dorant E, et al. (2000). The impact of characteristics of cigarette smoking on urinary tract cancer risk: a meta-analysis of epidemiologic studies. *Cancer*, 89(3):630-639.

Zeegers MP, Goldbohm RA, van Den Brandt PA (2002). A prospective study on active and environmental tobacco smoking and bladder cancer risk (The Netherlands). *Cancer Causes Control*, 13(1):83-90.

Zheng TZ, Boyle P, Hu HF, et al. (1990). Tobacco smoking, alcohol consumption, and risk of oral cancer: a case-control study in Beijing, Peopleís Republic of China. *Cancer Causes Control*, 1(2):173-179.

Zheng T, Holford T, Chen Y, et al. (1997). Risk of tongue cancer associated with tobacco smoking and alcohol consumption: a case-control study. *Oral Oncol*, 33(2):82-85.

Zheng W, Blot WJ, Shu XO, et al. (1992a). Diet and other risk factors for laryngeal cancer in Shanghai, China. *Am J Epidemiol*, 136(2):178-191.

Zheng W, Blot WJ, Shu XO, et al. (1992b). Risk factors for oral and pharyngeal cancer in Shanghai, with emphasis on diet. *Cancer Epidemiol Biomarkers Prev*, 1(6):441-448.

Zheng W, McLaughlin JK, Gridley G, et al. (1993a). A cohort study of smoking, alcohol consumption, and dietary factors for pancreatic cancer (United States). *Cancer Causes Control*, 4(5):477-482.

Zheng W, McLaughlin JK, Chow WH, et al. (1993b). Risk factors for cancers of the nasal cavity and paranasal sinuses among white men in the United States. *Am J Epidemiol*, 138(11):965-972.

Znaor A, Brennan P, Gajalakshmi V, et al. (2003). Independent and combined effects of tobacco smoking, chewing and alcohol drinking on the risk of oral, pharyngeal and esophageal cancers in Indian men. *Int J Cancer*, 105(5):681-686.

Risk of Cardiovascular Diseases After Smoking Cessation

Coronary Heart Disease (CHD)

Introduction

Coronary heart disease (CHD), also called Ischaemic Heart Disease (IHD), is the largest disease entity within the group of cardiovascular diseases (CVD) and is estimated to be the leading cause of mortality in the world (World Health Organization, 1999). WHO has estimated that CHD is responsible for 13% of all male deaths and 12% of all female deaths, 56% of which occur before age 75. There are a number of well-established risk factors for development of CVD, most of them related to lifestyle. These include smoking, dyslipidemia, hypertension, diabetes, obesity, physical inactivity, psychosocial factors and genetic factors. Risk of CHD increases with increasing age, with women developing disease approximately 10 years later than men.

The relationship between smoking and CHD is well established, with cigarette smokers having 1.5–4 times higher risk than never smokers, depending on quantity smoked, age and gender (USDHHS, 1990; Doll *et al.*, 1994; Prescott *et al.*, 1998a; Asia Pacific Cohort Studies Collaboration, 2005). This has been shown in numerous studies comprising study populations of all races. In recent years experimental studies on both animals and humans have focused on the mechanisms through which cigarette smoking causes CHD, and findings have supported results from observational studies. Smoking has been estimated to cause as much as 22% of cardiovascular disease mortality in European and North American societies, with lower fractions in societies with lower smoking prevalence (WHO, 2002).

Is the risk of disease lower in former smokers than in current smokers?

The risk of CHD has consistently been shown to be lower in former smokers than in continued smokers. In 1990, after an extensive review of the literature, the US Surgeon General concluded that smoking cessation reduces the risk of CHD substantially in men and women of all ages. The excess risk was estimated to be reduced by half after 1 year of abstinence, followed by a gradual decline. Risk reduction was seen both in disease-free subjects and subjects with established disease (USDHHS, 1990).

To evaluate the relationship between smoking cessation and CHD we describe findings from previous reviews (the US Surgeon General's Report from 1990) and meta-analysis (Cochrane Report from 2003), prospective cohort studies of low-risk populations (Table 1), randomized controlled trials (Table 2), cohort studies including time-course of risk reduction (Table 3) and case-control studies reporting on risk by duration of smoking abstinence (Table 4). Since effect of smoking cessation may differ according to pre-existing disease, findings are reported separately for high-risk (pre-existing CHD) and low-risk subjects (without established disease). Findings on effect of smoking cessation in epidemiological studies have been supplemented by laboratory studies of cardiovascular disease mechanisms, as described earlier in this Handbook.

Because of the abundance of studies addressing risk of CHD in relation to smoking habits, we rely on data included in already-published reviews and meta-analyses, and update these when possible. Studies were limited to those with CHD morbidity and CHD mortality as outcomes. These endpoints were chosen because they are the most commonly used study outcomes in CHD, thus allowing for comparison between different studies. In addition they are less subject to bias and misclassification. Studies were included based mainly on quality of data, sample size and representation of different populations around the world. The associations of smoking

Table 1. Cohort studies: risk of coronary heart disease (CHD) and smoking cessation in low-risk populations							
Reference Country	Study population	Proportion former smokers at baseline (%)	Number of deaths or event of CHD	Duration follow-up (years)	CHD-mortality RR* (95% CI)		Comments
					Current vs never	Former vs never	
Rogot & Murray (1980) USA	US Veterans Study (Dorn Study) 293 958 veterans	[16]	107 563 deaths	16	1.6	1.2	Smoking status assessed at baseline
Cook et al. (1986) UK	British Regional Heart Study (Random sample) 7 735 men Age 40–59	35	333 events	6.2	Men [3.2]	Men [2.3]	Smoking status assessed at baseline
Willet et al. (1987) USA	Nurses' Health Study 119 404 female nurses Age 30–55	36	307 events 65 fatal 242 non-fatal	6	Women Cig/day 1–4 2.4 (1.1, 5.0) 15–14 4.2 (3.1, 5.6) 25–34 5.4 (3.8, 7.7)	Women 1.5 (1.0, 2.1)	Smoking status updated regularly
Lacroix et al. (1991) USA	Three communities Study (Random sample) 7 178 subjects 62% women Age ≥ 65	[20]	729 deaths	5	Men 1.9 (1.2, 3.0) Women 1.5 (0.9, 2.5)	Men 1.2 (0.8, 2.0) Women 0.5 (0.3, 1.1)	Subjects with history of CVD or cancer excluded. Smoking status assessed at baseline. Adjustment for CVD risk factors
Ben Shlomo et al. (1994) UK	Whitehall Study 18 370 male civil cadre Age 40–69	26	1 695 deaths	18	1.90 (1.6, 2.2)	[1.09]	Smoking status assessed at baseline
Doll et al. (1994) UK	British Doctors Study 34 439 male doctors Age>20	13	6 438 deaths	40	Men 1.6	Men 1.2	Smoking status updated regularly
Friedman et al. (1997) USA	Kaiser-Permanente 25 000 Age 20–79	11	31 deaths in former smokers	4	1.6	0.9	Smoking status assessed at baseline

Table 1. Cohort studies in CHD (contd)

Reference Country	Study population	Proportion former smokers at baseline (%)	Number of deaths or event of CHD	Duration follow-up (years)	CHD-mortality RR* (95% CI)		Comments
					Current vs never	Former vs never	
Prescott et al. (1998) Denmark	Copenhagen Prospective Population Studies (Random sample) 30 917 subjects 44% Women Age ≥ 20	18	1 943 events	15 (mean)	*Men* 1.8 *Women* 1.8	*Men* 1.4 *Women* 1.3	Adjusted risk of MI in former smokers: Men 1.11 (0.86, 1.42) Women 1.05 (0.74, 1.50). Smoking data updated regularly
Jee et al. (1999) Republic of Korea	Korea Medical Insurance Corporation Study 106 745 men Age 35–59	21	1006 events	6	2.2 (1.8, 2.8)	2.1 (1.6, 2.7)	Smoking status assessed at baseline
Glynn et al. (2005) USA	Male Physicians Health Study 18 662 male physicians	Not given	1 348 events	20	1.8 (1.6, 2.1)	1.1 (1.0, 1.2)	No history of CVD or cancer, RR multivariate adjusted
Iso et al. (2005) Japan	Japan Collaborative Cohort Study for Evaluation of Cancer Risk (JACC) 94 683 subjects 44% women Age 40–79	25	547 deaths	9.9	*Men* 2.5 (1.8, 3.5) *Women* 1.7 (1.2, 2.3)	*Men* 1.7 (1.2, 2.4) *Women* 0.9 (0.3, 2.5)	Subjects with history of CVD or cancer excluded. Smoking assessed at baseline. Based on 4 deaths among female former smokers.
Wen et al. (2005) Taiwan	Taiwan civil servants 30 244 men Age>35	14	57 deaths in former smokers	11	2.3 (1.4, 3.5)	1.0 (0.5, 1.8)	Smoking status assessed at baseline
Woodward et al. (2005) Asian countries Australia New Zealand	Asia Pacific Cohort Studies Collaboration 463 674 Asians 33% female 98 664 Australasians 45% female Mean age 42–79	[0–62]	8 490 deaths	3–25	1.6 (1.5, 1.7)	[1.24]	Pooling of 40 cohort studies. No significant difference between Asian and Australian populations. Smoking assessed at baseline

In brackets [ ]: values calculated by the Working Group
*Age-adjusted relative risk estimates are provided

Table 2. Randomised controlled trials of smoking cessation and coronary heart disease by level of risk

Reference Country	Study Population	Cessation rate Intervention (I)/ Usual care (UC) %	Number of deaths from CHD	Duration Follow-up (Years)	Intervention	CHD-mortality OR (95% CI)		Comments
						I vs UC	Quitters vs continued smokers	
High-risk subjects								
Rose et al. (1982, 1992) UK	Whitehall Study 1445 male smokers Age 40–59	At 9 years: 55 / 41	231	20	Anti-smoke advice	0.87 (0.67, 1.13)	Not applicable	Smokers with high CHD-risk selected from the Whitehall Study
Hjermann et al. (1986) Norway	Oslo Study Diet and anti smoking trial 1 232 men Age 40-49 80% smokers	At 5 years: 25 / 17	24	8–9	Diet and anti-smoke advice	0.53	Not applicable	
Ockene et al. (1990) MRFIT (1990) USA	MRFIT (Multiple Risk Factor Intervention Trial) 12 866 men Age 35–57 64% smokers	At 6 years: 49 / 29	428 787	10.5 16	Diet and anti-smoke advice, hypertension and weight control	0.89 (0.76, 1.05) 0.80 (0.66, 0.97)	0.35 (0.20, 0.63) Not applicable	From 36-month visit
Low-risk subjects								
Anthonisen et al. (2005) USA	5 887 smokers, 63% men Age 35–60	At 5 years: 21.7 / 5.4	161	14.5	2 groups: anti-smoking advice and nicotine gum +/- ipratropium and UC	[0.77]	[0.3] p=0.02	Asymptomatic smokers with mild to moderate COPD

OR = odds ratio
95% CI = 95% confidence interval
I = Intervention group
UC = Usual care group
In brackets [ ]: values calculated by the Working Group

cessation with other CHD manifestations such as angina, revascularization procedures, severity of disease assessed from angiography, single photon emission computed tomography (SPECT) scan, etc., were not included.

In subjects without established disease
Prospective cohort studies
There is no doubt that risk of CHD decreases after smoking cessation (USDHHS, 1990). However, the risk reduction following smoking cessation may differ according to pre-existing cardiovascular disease, with different importance of the atherogenic and the more reversible thrombogenic effects of smoking. There are numerous prospective observational studies of healthy and low-risk subjects documenting this, as summarized in the US Surgeon General's Report from 1990 (USDHHS, 1990). Results from the largest and the most recent cohort studies are presented in Table 1.

In 1951 all British doctors, the majority of whom were male, were invited to join the British Doctors' Study. At study onset in 1951, 13% were former smokers; this number had increased to 60% in 1990. Relative CHD-mortality risk in former smokers was 1.2 compared with 1.6 in continued smokers (Doll *et al.*, 1994). In the British Regional Heart study based on 7 735 middle-aged men, the relative risk (RR) of a CHD event was 3.2 in current smokers and approximately 2 in former smokers (Cook *et al.*, 1986). In the Copenhagen Prospective Population Studies, which followed 30 917 subjects with an equal gender distribution for a mean of 15 years, relative CHD-mortality risk was 1.4 in men and 1.3 in women (Prescott *et al.*, 1998b). RR in continued smokers was 1.8 in both sexes. However, in the same study population, the adjusted risk of myocardial infarction (MI) in former smokers did not differ from the RR in never smokers, and results were similar in women and men (Prescott *et al.*, 1998a). In the Whitehall

study, 18 379 male civil servants were followed for 18 years for CHD-mortality (Ben Shlomo *et al.*, 1994). Age-adjusted relative CHD mortality risk was 1.74 in continuous smokers and 1.09 in former smokers (values calculated by the Working Group). This mortality risk increased with amount and duration of smoking in former smokers. Former smokers who had quit 1–9, 10–29 and ≥ 30 years earlier and accruing 20 or more years of smoking had a RR of CHD death of 1.3 (95% CI=0.8–2.2), 1.2 (95% CI=0.9–1.5), and 0.9 (95% CI=0.5–1.8) if smoking 1–19 cigarettes per day and 1.6 (95% CI=1.0–2.5), 1.4 (95% CI=1.1–1.8) and 1.5 (95% CI=0.9–2.5) if smoking ≥ 20 cigarettes per day, respectively. Counterparts who had quit 10–29 and ≥ 30 years earlier and having smoked for a shorter duration (up to 19 years) had a RR of CHD death of 0.6 (95% CI=0.3–1.0) and 1.04 (95% CI=0.8–1.4) if smoking 1–19 cigarettes per day and 0.7 (95% CI=0.4–1.3) and 1.3 (95% CI=0.9–2.0) if smoking ≥ 20 cigarettes per day, respectively.

Similar results have been reported from USA-based studies. In the Kaiser-Permanente study of 25 000 subjects, relative risk of CHD death after 4 years of follow-up was 0.9 in former smokers and 1.6 in continued smokers (USDHHS, 1990). In the US veterans study of more than 200 000 subjects, the relative risks of CHD mortality were 1.58 in current smokers and 1.15 in former smokers after 16 years of follow-up (USDHHS, 1990). In the Nurses' Health Study based on 120 000 women the overall RR after 6 years of follow-up for nonfatal MI and CHD-deaths was 2.1 to 6.0 depending on the quantity smoked; RR in former smokers was 1.5 (95% CI=1.0-2.1) (Willett *et al.*, 1987). In the US physicians study, which followed 18 662 male physicians for 20 years, the adjusted RR of a CHD-event was 1.84 (95% CI=1.62–2.08) in current smokers and 1.11 (95% CI=0.01-1.22) in former

smokers. In a USA-based random sample consisting of 2 709 men and 4 469 women aged 65 years or older followed for 5 years, CVD and CHD mortality risk in former smokers at baseline did not differ significantly from that of never smokers (LaCroix *et al.*, 1991). Relative mortality risk of CHD was 1.2 (95% CI=0.8-2.0) in men and 0.5 (95% CI=0.3-1.1) in women. The RR was not affected by adjustment for other cardiovascular risk factors and was similar to the never smokers regardless of the number of years since they had last smoked.

Large studies based on non-Caucasian populations are mostly limited to studies from Asia, mainly China and Japan. Smoking rates in Asian populations are high in men, and quitting rates are low (Asia Pacific Cohort Studies Collaboration, 2005). In contrast, smoking rates in women are low, and often it is not possible to analyse women's risk associated with smoking in detail. In addition to differences in smoking behaviour, including types of cigarettes smoked, there may also be genetic differences in susceptibility to the effects of smoking. A large Japanese study based on 94 683 men and women followed from 1989 to 1999 yielded relative risks for CHD among current smokers similar to those found in Western studies: RR of 2.51 (95% CI=1.79-3.51) in men and 3.35 (95% CI=2.23-5.02) in women. Former smokers generally had a risk that was intermediate between current- and never smokers: in men the adjusted risk of CHD was 1.66 (95% CI=1.15-2.39), in women there were too few cases among former smokers to calculate valid risk estimates (Iso *et al.*, 2005).

A study from Taiwan included 71 361 government employees from 1989 and followed them for an average of 11 years. Overall, the relative CHD mortality risk in smokers compared with never smokers was 2.25 (95% CI=1.44-3.53). The risk in former smokers was much lower than in continued smokers (RR=0.46; 95% CI=0.25-0.84) and did not differ from never smokers, although the estimate was not precise (wide confidence interval): RR=1.0 (95% CI=0.54-1.84) (Wen *et al.*, 2005). In contrast, in a study from Korea of 106 745 men, risk of an IHD event during an average of 6 years of follow-up was 2.2 (95% CI=1.8-2.8) in current smokers and 2.1 (95% CI=1.6-2.7) in former smokers (Jee *et al.*, 1999). However, for CVD mortality the RR was 1.6 (95% CI=1.5, 1.8) in current smokers and 1.1 (95% CI=0.9–1.3) in former smokers. In the Asia Pacific Cohort Studies Collaboration, which pooled data from 40 cohort studies comprising 463 674 Asians and 98 664 Australasians, RR for current smokers for all CHD events, fatal and non-fatal, was 1.75 (95% CI=1.60-1.90) as compared with never smokers. The risk in former smokers was significantly lower, 0.71 (95% CI=0.64-0.78), when compared with current smokers (Asia Pacific Cohort Studies Collaboration, 2005). The majority of the Asian studies were from China and Japan but also South Korea, Taiwan and Thailand were also represented. When these Asian studies were subdivided by country, no statistical differences were noted.

Light smokers tend to quit more easily than heavy smokers (Osler *et al.*, 1999) which may lead to overestimation of the beneficial effect of cessation because the population that quits have lower intensities of smoking and shorter durations of smoking at the time of cessation than do continuing smokers (USDHHS, 1990). Thus, at any age of quitting, former smokers have had on average less accumulated exposure to cigarette smoke. However, the differences between quitters and continuing smokers persist even when differences in intensity and duration of smoking are controlled in the analyses (USDHHS, 1990; Kawaki *et al.*, 1994, 1997).

In summary, risk of CHD in former smokers differs between studies as does risk in current smokers. When no adjustment for accumulated exposure or time since quitting is done, the vast majority of studies find risk in former smokers to be intermediate between current and never smokers, which is similar to the risk reduction found in observational cohort studies of high-risk subjects.

In high-risk subjects
Randomised intervention trials
A number of clinical trials in patients with established CHD or at high risk have attempted to intervene on smoking, but most have done this in conjunction with interventions aimed at other risk factors for CHD. Thus, it is difficult to isolate the effect on CHD risk due to smoking cessation. Table 2 shows intervention trials of subjects at high risk for CHD that have succeeded in achieving differences in smoking rates between intervention and usual care groups.

One of the first studies with a smoking intervention in subjects with high risk of CHD was based on 1 441 smokers from the Whitehall Study (Rose *et al.*, 1982). The sole intervention was anti-smoking advice, with smoking habits recorded at 1, 3 and 9 years after randomization. Smoking rates did not differ much in the two groups: after 9 years 55% in the intervention group and 41% in the reference group had quit smoking, but some of the participants had changed to smoking pipes or cigars. The net reduction in the number of cigarettes smoked was 30% after 10 years. Neither CHD mortality nor all-cause mortality differed between the two groups. At the 10-year follow-up CHD mortality risk was 7.3% in the intervention group versus 8.9% in the usual care group, equivalent to a RR of 0.82 (95% CI=0.57-1.18). After 20 years the RR was 0.87 (95% CI=0.67-1.13). For all-cause mortality the 20-year RR was 0.93 (95% CI=0.80-1.09) (Rose *et al.*, 1982; Rose & Colwell, 1992).

The Multiple Risk Factor Intervention (MRFIT) study included approximately 12 000 middle-aged men (age 35–57) with high risk of CHD. The multiple intervention tested in the trial consisted of advice on changes in diet, weight control by reducing caloric intake, hypertension treatment and smoking cessation. Subjects were randomised to intervention on all of these factors or to usual care. Participants were seen annually, thus minimizing the risk of misclassification of smoking status. Overall smoking rate was 64% at study onset. Cessation rates were higher in the intervention group: After 6 years 49% had quit in the intervention group, versus 29% in the usual care group. When comparing smokers who had quit for at least 1 year with persistent smokers, the adjusted RR of CHD death was 0.58 (95% CI=0.40-0.84), and after at least 3 years of smoking cessation the RR was 0.35 (95% CI=0.20-0.63) (Ockene *et al.*, 1990). This difference was found despite the fact that cigarette smokers switching to cigar or pipe smoking were counted as former smokers (Neaton *et al.*, 1981). After 6 and 8 years of follow-up, all cause mortality and CHD mortality did not differ between the intervention and the usual care groups. However, after 10.5 years of follow-up there was a reduction of 10.6% in CHD-mortality and of 7.7% in all-cause mortality in an intention to treat analyses (MRFIT, 1990). After 16 years the RR of acute MI in the intervention group was 0.80 (95% CI=0.66-0.97) and for all-cause mortality was 0.89 (95% CI=0.77-1.02) compared with the usual care group.

In the Oslo study, 1 232 healthy men aged 40–49 at high risk of CHD based on lipid levels, blood pressure and smoking habits were randomised to receive interventions on diet and smoking or to usual care and followed during 60 months for CHD-events (fatal and non-fatal MI and sudden cardiac death). The intervention group was seen every 6 months, the usual care group annually. At study onset 80% in both groups were smokers. After five years of follow-up, 25% in the intervention group had quit, compared with 17% in the usual care group, and overall tobacco consumption was reduced by 45% in the intervention group. The study reported an inverse relationship between smoking reduction and CHD incidence but this association was not statistically significant. After five years the intervention group had a 47% decline in risk of CHD events, 25% of which could be explained by changes in smoking (Hjermann *et al.*, 1986). After eight to nine years all-cause mortality was reduced by 33%, with greater risk reductions for CHD-related events: The intervention group had significantly reduced risk of fatal CHD (RR= 0.41), total CHD-events (RR=0.56) and CVD-events (RR=0.39).

In summary, the controlled trials in high-risk populations have yielded greater risk-reduction in quitters compared to continuing smokers with risk reductions similar to those reported in observational studies. Although risk reduction estimates from the intention-to-treat analyses are based on a multi-factorial intervention and not exclusively on tobacco control, the results are consistent with those of studies focusing simply on smoking cessation. However, with the relatively small differences in smoking cessation rates achieved in the studies, the differences between intervention group and usual care groups may have been caused by other components of the intervention 'package' received, rather than by smoking cessation per se.

In populations not at high risk
Intervention trials
The Lung Health Study was performed on 5 887 middle-aged smokers with mild chronic obstructive pulmonary disease

but not clinical disease. Subjects were randomised to one of three groups: intervention groups receiving a smoking cessation programme or the cessation programme and medical treatment (ipratropium), and a usual care group. Smoking status was assessed biannually for 10 years. After 5 years, 51% in the intervention groups and 28.7% in the usual care group were either intermittent or sustained quitters. At 14.5 years of follow-up relative mortality risk in the usual care group was 1.18 (95% CI=1.02-1.37) compared with the intervention groups combined. CHD mortality rates were higher in the usual care group (1.2 versus 0.9 per 1 000 person-years) but the difference was not statistically significant. When survival was analysed according to smoking habits, CHD death rates were significantly related to smoking: the RR for sustained quitters in comparison with continuing smokers was approximately 0.3 and 0.6 for all-cause mortality. The authors concluded that the lower mortality recorded in the intervention group was caused by the difference in smoking cessation registered between this and the usual care groups (Anthonisen *et al.*, 2005).

In subjects with clinically evident disease
Observational cohort studies of patients with CHD
Most studies have shown that 30–60% of smokers give up smoking after MI (Rea *et al.*, 2002; Critchley & Capewell, 2003; Quist-Paulsen *et al.*, 2005). A meta-analysis conducted by the Cochrane Collaboration (Critchley & Capewell, 2003, 2004) on risk reduction associated with smoking cessation in patients with established coronary heart disease included all prospective observational studies with sufficient ascertainment of smoking status and follow-up. The review focused on all-cause mortality, which has been most extensively studied, but also reported findings on

CHD mortality for the studies in which this had been included. All-cause mortality as an end point has the advantage that it is a very relevant outcome and not subject to bias in disease classification. After screening 665 papers, 20 studies were included in the meta-analysis (Sparrow & Dawber, 1978; Salonen, 1980; Baughman *et al.*, 1982; Aberg *et al.*, 1983; Daly *et al.*, 1983; Bednarzewski, 1984; Johansson *et al.*, 1985; Perkins & Dick, 1985; Hallstrom *et al.*, 1986; Vlietstra *et al.*, 1986; Burr *et al.*, 1992; Sato *et al.*, 1992; Gupta *et al.*, 1993; Hedback *et al.*, 1993; Tofler *et al.*, 1993; Herlitz *et al.*, 1995; Greenwood *et al.*, 1995; Voors *et al.*, 1996; Hasdai *et al.*, 1997; van Domburg *et al.*, 2000). The most common reasons for exclusion include uncertainty about timing of smoking cessation, presentation of smoking status at baseline only, study designs other than prospective cohorts (e.g. retrospective cohorts), and presenting outcomes for former smokers and never smokers together. As the minimum follow-up required for inclusion was 2 years, this review could not examine risk reduction within the first two years of cessation. Most studies ranged in follow-up time from 3 to 7 years with a mean of 5 years (Critchley & Capewell, 2003, 2004). Eighteen studies originated from the USA and Europe (Scandinavia, United Kingdom, Ireland, Poland, the Netherlands) and ranged in size from 77 to 4 165 smokers at baseline. Two studies were from Asia, one from Japan (n=87) and one from India (n=225). The largest studies were from the USA, comprising approximately 50% of the population covered in the meta-analysis. In most studies subjects were included a few weeks after a coronary event. The study thus only includes patients surviving their first cardiac event. The combined study population consisted of 12 603 smokers at baseline (20% women) of whom 5 659 quit and 6 944 continued smoking. The all-cause mortality risk in former smokers compared to continued smokers in the included studies ranged from 0.34 to 0.81 with a pooled relative risk (RR) for all 20 studies of 0.64 (95% CI=0.58-0.71) (Figure 1). This estimate was stable after exclusion of studies based on the main cardiac event (MI, coronary artery bypass graft, angioplasty, other), quality criteria or period when conducted. No indications of differences between studies done in Western countries and non-Western studies were found, although the vast majority of studies were Western. Since women and older patients were under-represented, it was concluded that results may not be applicable to these groups.

An earlier meta-analysis including 12 studies, of which 10 were also included in the Cochrane Report, estimated a slightly larger all-cause mortality risk reduction after smoking cessation with an OR of 0.54 (95% CI=0.46-0.62) (Wilson et al., 2000). This analysis did not include the largest study in the Cochrane report, a US study of 4 165 patients in which RR in former smokers was 0.68 (95% CI=0.59-0.78) (Vlietstra et al., 1986). In this meta-analysis, subgroup analysis showed greater risk reduction in women than in men: OR=0.36 (95% CI=0.23-0.54) and 0.52 (95% CI=0.45-0.58), respectively. However, the analysis of women was based

on only 185 patients because several of the studies included did not present data for each sex separately. The Cochrane meta-analysis did not report sex-specific results. The overall risk reduction reported in this study is of similar magnitude to the ones reported in prospective cohort studies of low-risk populations.

Eight of the studies in the Cochrane report also reported RR for nonfatal re-infarctions. Crude RR's ranged from 0.10 to 3.87 with a pooled RR of 0.68 (95% CI=0.57-0.82) (Critchley & Capewell, 2003, 2004). A study not included in the Cochrane review followed 808 active smokers with an MI, and estimated their risk of a recurrent

Review : Smoking cessation for the secondary prevention of coronary heart disease

Comparison : 01 Ceased v continued smoking

Outcome: 01 total deaths

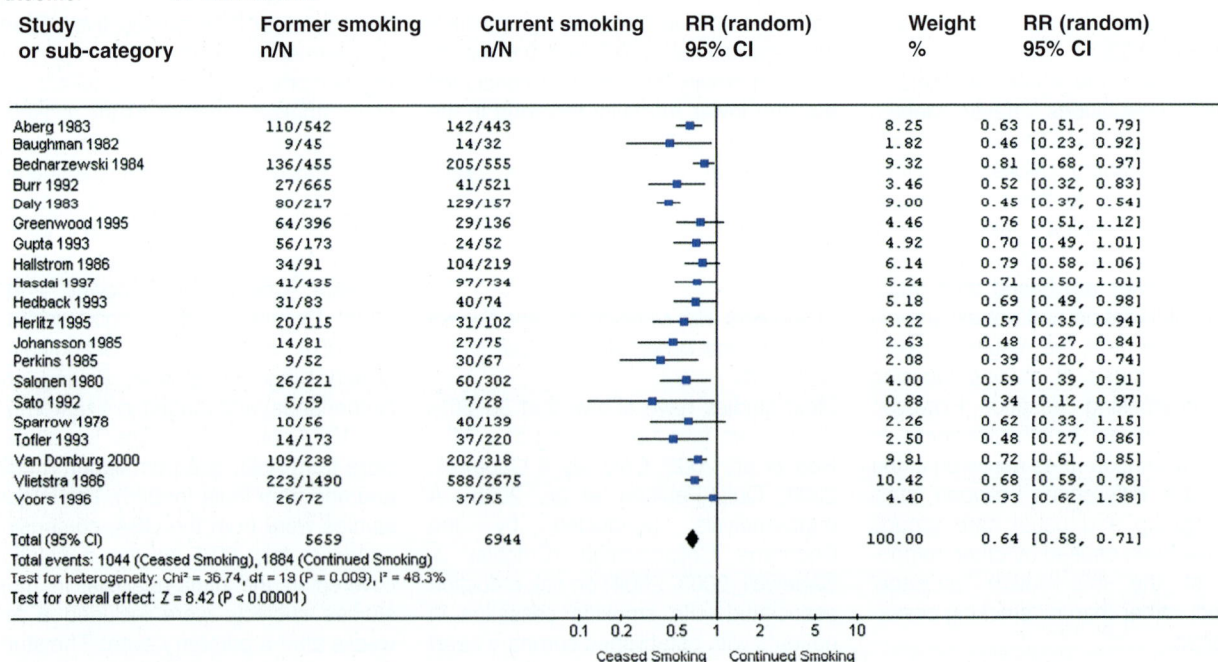

Study or sub-category	Former smoking n/N	Current smoking n/N	RR (random) 95% CI	Weight %	RR (random) 95% CI
Aberg 1983	110/542	142/443		8.25	0.63 [0.51, 0.79]
Baughman 1982	9/45	14/32		1.82	0.46 [0.23, 0.92]
Bednarzewski 1984	136/455	205/555		9.32	0.81 [0.68, 0.97]
Burr 1992	27/665	41/521		3.46	0.52 [0.32, 0.83]
Daly 1983	80/217	129/157		9.00	0.45 [0.37, 0.54]
Greenwood 1995	64/396	29/136		4.46	0.76 [0.51, 1.12]
Gupta 1993	56/173	24/52		4.92	0.70 [0.49, 1.01]
Hallstrom 1986	34/91	104/219		6.14	0.79 [0.58, 1.06]
Hasdai 1997	41/435	97/734		5.24	0.71 [0.50, 1.01]
Hedback 1993	31/83	40/74		5.18	0.69 [0.49, 0.98]
Herlitz 1995	20/115	31/102		3.22	0.57 [0.35, 0.94]
Johansson 1985	14/81	27/75		2.63	0.48 [0.27, 0.84]
Perkins 1985	9/52	30/67		2.08	0.39 [0.20, 0.74]
Salonen 1980	26/221	60/302		4.00	0.59 [0.39, 0.91]
Sato 1992	5/59	7/28		0.88	0.34 [0.12, 0.97]
Sparrow 1978	10/56	40/139		2.26	0.62 [0.33, 1.15]
Tofler 1993	14/173	37/220		2.50	0.48 [0.27, 0.86]
Van Domburg 2000	109/238	202/318		9.81	0.72 [0.61, 0.85]
Vlietstra 1986	223/1490	588/2675		10.42	0.68 [0.59, 0.78]
Voors 1996	26/72	37/95		4.40	0.93 [0.62, 1.38]
Total (95% CI)	5659	6944		100.00	0.64 [0.58, 0.71]

Total events: 1044 (Ceased Smoking), 1884 (Continued Smoking)
Test for heterogeneity: Chi² = 36.74, df = 19 (P = 0.009), I² = 48.3%
Test for overall effect: Z = 8.42 (P < 0.00001)

```
      0.1  0.2   0.5   1    2    5   10
       Ceased Smoking   Continued Smoking
```

Figure 1. Smoking cessation for the secondary prevention of coronary heart disease: Total mortality

Critchley J. & Capewell S. Smoking cessation for the secondary prevention of coronary heart disease. The Cochrane Database of Systematic Reviews 2003; Issue 4. Copyright Cochrane Library, reproduced with permission.

CHD event up to 6 months, 6–18 months, 18–36 months, and more than 36 months after cessation (Rea *et al.*, 2002). The study found that risk in former smokers was comparable to that in continued smokers up to 36 months after cessation, at which point the risk did not differ from that in never smokers (RR=1.02; 95% CI=0.54-1.86). [However, this study was small with estimates with wide confidence intervals, and the RR in continued smokers compared with never smokers differed from that in most other studies in being only 1.51 (95% CI=1.1-2.1)].

In the Heart Outcomes Prevention Evaluation trial (HOPE), with a population comprising 5 241 current, former and never smokers mainly with ischemic heart disease and who did not change their smoking status during the trial, former smokers did not have a higher risk of all-cause mortality (RR= 0.93;95% CI=0.80-1.08) or of a new MI (RR=0.90; 95% CI=0.77-1.05) than never smokers. (Dagenais *et al.*, 2005). In this study, however, continued smokers also had low RR of MI (1.26; 95% CI=1.01-1.58), suggesting that there may have been selection bias.

Among patients with CHD there seems to be an increased risk of sudden cardiac death among current smokers (RR=2.47, 95% CI=1.46-4.10) compared with never smokers, but the risk in former smokers is not increased compared with never smokers (Goldenberg *et al.*, 2003). Similarly, in a study of patients at high risk of arrhythmic death followed for 16 months (the Cardiac Arrhythmia Suppression Trial or CAST study), risk of arrhythmic death was significantly lower in former smokers compared to continued smokers (Peters *et al.*, 1995). These findings are consistent with the acute effects of nicotine or CO (carbon monoxide) in causing arrhythmias, in addition to the reduced risk of thrombosis observed following cessation.

Absolute risk reduction

Despite the low magnitude in the relative risks of developing CHD associated with smoking, due to the high baseline risk of CHD events in never smokers, smoking causes more deaths from CHD than from any other disease. As opposed to cancer (in particular lung cancer) and COPD, the etiology of CHD is multifactorial with several contributing risk factors of comparable importance to smoking. As mentioned above, these risk factors include age, gender, genetic predisposition, diet, physical activity, lipids, hypertension, diabetes, BMI and social and psychosocial factors. In the absence of interaction with other risk factors, the absolute risk associated with smoking and smoking cessation can be calculated directly from knowledge of the baseline risk. It can be inferred from the evidence presented above that the absolute risk following smoking cessation will be lower than the risk that would manifest had the smoking habit been continued. Whether the absolute risk will decrease following smoking cessation compared to the risk prior to quitting does not have a unique answer, but it will depend on the baseline risk and thus on presence of the other risk factors contributing to the development of CHD. It will also depend on duration of follow-up due to the strong association between age and risk of developing CHD. However, the relevant comparison for the individual contemplating smoking cessation is with the risk the person would have had he continued being a smoker. With similar risk reduction in relative terms, the higher the baseline risk the greater the risk reduction after smoking cessation in absolute risk. Thus subjects at high risk of CHD, e.g. because of older age, diabetes or previous myocardial infarction, have more to gain in absolute risk reduction than do subjects at low risk of CHD.

Among former smokers, is the risk of disease lower with more prolonged abstinence?

Based on a review of the available data, the US Surgeon General's Report in 1990 concluded that excess risk of CHD caused by smoking is reduced by about half after 1 year of smoking abstinence and then declines gradually (USDHHS, 1990). After 15 years of abstinence the risk of CHD is similar to that of persons who have never smoked. The report concluded that among persons with diagnosed CHD, smoking cessation also markedly reduces the risk of recurrent infarction and cardiovascular death. In many studies this reduction was 50% or more.

Well-designed cohort studies have a number of advantages over case–control studies, and they are useful for estimating the long-term benefit of quitting smoking. However, the number of adverse outcomes in cohort studies is small, and very large studies with wide time intervals are needed to register enough events to detect a significant difference in risk between former and continued smokers. In addition, in cohort studies there are the methodological issues of reverse-causality and stability of smoking cessation (smoking habit changing over time), which are of particular importance to risk estimation within the first years of cessation. For this reason many prospective cohort studies choose to exclude the first years of cessation, thus eliminating the possibility of examining the precise risk reduction immediately following cessation. Case–control studies have the advantage of involving a larger number of adverse outcomes, and are less susceptible to misclassification resulting from resumption of smoking among former smokers. However, case–control studies may be subject to recall bias, and hence evoking smoking habits in case–control studies does not eliminate the problem of reverse causality. In addition, the lack of detailed smoking data on fatal cases is a limitation of these studies. When analysing the impact of time since smoking cessation, the inverse correlation between the latter and lifetime accumulated duration of smoking is also a methodological concern.

In the NIH monograph on smoking and tobacco control from 1997, the time course of risk of CHD after smoking cessation in subjects free of disease was examined in several large US studies: Cancer Prevention Study I (CPS I)(Burns et al., 1997), US Veteran's Cohort (Hrubec et al., 1997), Kaiser-Permanente (Friedman et al., 1997) and the Nurses' Health Study (Kawachi et al.,1994, 1997). Most studies have included former smokers with a minimum smoking abstinence of 1-2 years because of the high probability of relapse in the first months following smoking cessation. This requirement has the additional benefit of limiting the effects of reverse causality in study estimates. Only in the Nurses' Health Study (NHS) and the CPS II were the risks immediately following smoking cessation estimated.

In the NHS, there was a rapid decline in adjusted risk of total CHD upon smoking cessation, removing 25% of risk (RR=0.75; 95% CI=0.49-1.15) within the first 2 years, although the risk was still more than double that of never smokers (RR=0.24). This rapid decline was followed by a slow decline, with risk reaching the level of never smokers within 10–14 years after quitting. Notably, adjustment for other cardiovascular risk factors did not markedly change this estimate. Total CVD mortality risk decrease was similar (RR=0.76; 95% CI=0.43-1.32). Risk estimates may be biased by the 'ill-quitter effect', i.e. that some smokers quit due to development of disease. To avoid this bias, the analyses were repeated with exclusion of CVD cases occurring at the beginning of each 2-year follow-up. The results of

this re-analysis indicated that risk reduction might be greater with a relative risk estimate among former smokers of 0.63 (95% CI=0.28-1.45) within the two first years of cessation. However, although the risk reduction was greater, the two estimates did not differ significantly. The initial rapid decline found in the NHS was consistent with previous reports from prospective studies (USDHHS, 1990). In CPS II the risk of CHD death within the first year after quitting was also assessed, but results were mixed, with both higher and lower risks reported in former smokers than in continued smokers (see Table 3), probably reflecting the fact that a number of smokers quit due to pre-existing or sub-clinical disease (USDHHS, 1990).

In the very large CPS-I study, which included more than 1 000 000 subjects, CHD mortality risk in former smokers could be analysed in detail. In female former smokers risk reached the level of never smokers after 10 years of cessation, in men after 20 years (Burns et al., 1997). Results were similar irrespective of quantity smoked daily. The Kaiser-Permanente study followed 60 000 subjects for 18 years and reported that CHD-mortality risk in women who used to smoke was still higher than in never smokers, even after 20 years of cessation (RR=1.1). In men the risk reached the level of never smokers after 20 years (RR= 1.0) (Friedman et al., 1997). In a 26-year follow-up of the US Veterans Study comprising 248 000 men at baseline, the CHD-mortality risk remained slightly increased after more than 30 years (RR=1.1) of smoking abstinence. Risk also increased with number of cigarettes formerly smoked, even up to 30 years after smoking cessation (Hrubec et al., 1997). In the CPS-II study, risk of CHD in men smoking ≤1 pack a day reached the level of never smokers after 10 years of cessation, whereas in men smoking >1 pack a day the time-span reported for a reduction in risk reaching

the level of never smokers was more than 15 years. In women the risk remained elevated even after >15 years for both levels of former consumption (RR=1.17 and 1.12, respectively) (USDHHS, 1990).

Other prospective studies have reported increased risk even many years after smoking cessation: in the British Doctors Study risk of CHD in men was 1.3–1.4 at 5–9 years after cessation and was still increased after 15 years of abstention (RR= 1.1 to 1.3) (Doll & Peto, 1976). In the British Regional Heart Study, the risk of CHD among men also remained elevated (RR=1.7) more than 20 years after cessation, although there were only 11 cases in this group (Cook et al., 1986). In a Danish population study, the overall risk of MI in former smokers did not differ from that of never smokers (Prescott et al., 1998a). However, when restricting analyses to recent quitters followed for approximately 14 years, the RR of MI in former smokers was 0.82 (95% CI=0.64-1.03) compared with continued heavy smokers and thus did not reach the level of never smokers within this time-span (Godtfredsen et al., 2003).

The Whitehall Study also examined the time-course of risk reduction following smoking cessation (Ben Shlomo et al., 1994). They found a fall in mortality in the first 19 years after quitting. However, after this period there appeared to be little further reduction in risk, and there was no significant trend with years since quitting. Heavy smokers showed a significant elevated risk up to 30 years after quitting.

In a Japanese study comprising approximately 95 000 persons with 10 years of follow-up, the adjusted risk declined after smoking cessation, but was still 0.91 (95% CI=0.59-1.40) in former smokers compared to continuing smokers after 2–4 years and 0.83 (95% CI=0.56-1.24) after 5–9 years. However, the risk reached the level of never

Table 3. Cohort studies: Time-course of CHD risk reduction following smoking cessation

Reference Country	Study Population	Outcome	Smoking Category	Relative Risk (95%)		Comments
Cederlof et al. (1975) Sweden	Swedish Study 51 911 men age 18–69	IHD mortality	Current smoker Years since quitting 1–9 <20 cig/day ≥ 20 cig/day ≥ 10 <20 cig/day ≥ 2 0 cig/day Never smoker	1.7 1.5 0.9 0.6 1.0 0.9 1.1 1	Not reported	Smoking assessed at baseline 10 years follow-up
Doll & Peto (1976) UK	British Doctors' Study 34 439 males age 55-64	CHD mortality	Current smoker Years since quitting <5 5–9 10–14 >15 Never smoker	1.7 1.9 1.4 1.7 1.3 1		Smoking data updated regularly 20 years follow-up
Cook et al. (1986) UK	British Regional Heart Study 7735 men age 40-59	CHD event	Current smoker Years since quitting ≤ 5 6–10 11–20 >20 Never smoker	3.2 3.1 1.9 2.3 1.7 1		Smoking assessed at baseline 6.2 years follow-up Ischaemic heart disease in men 55–64 years
USDHHS (1990) Unpublished tabulations	Cancer Prevention Study (CPS II) >1 200 000 men and women	CHD mortality		*Men* *<20 cig/day*	*Women* *<20 cig/day*	
			Current smoker Years since quitting <1 1–2 3–5 6–10 11–15 ≥ 16	1.93 1.43 1.61 1.49 1.28 0.99 0.88	1.76 2.13 0.87 1.31 0.74 1.20 1.17	
				≥ 20 cig/day	*≥ 20 cig/day*	
			Current smoker Years since quitting <1 1–2 3–5 6–10 11–15 ≥ 16 Never smoker	2.02 2.56 1.57 1.41 1.63 1.16 1.09 1	2.27 1.41 1.16 0.96 1.88 1.37 1.12 1	

Table 3. Cohort studies: Time-course of CHD risk reduction (contd)

Reference Country	Study Population	Outcome	Smoking Category	Relative Risk (95% CI)			Comments
LaCroix et al. (1991) USA	Three communities 7 178 62% women age ≥ 65	CHD mortality		Men		Women	Subjects with history of CVD, or cancer excluded
			Current smoker	1.7	1.3, 2.3	1.6	
			Years since quitting				Smoking assessed at baseline
			≤ 5	1.1	0.7, 1.8	1.0 0.5, 2.1	
			6–10	0.9	0.5, 1.5	1.0 0.5, 2.0	
			11–20	1.1	0.8, 1.6	0.5 0.2, 1.1	
			>20	1.0	0.7, 1.4	0.8 0.4, 1.4	
			Never smoker	1			
BenSchlomo et al. (1994) UK	Whitehall Study 18 370 male civil employees age 40–69	CHD mortality	Current smoker	1.7			Smoking assessed at baseline
			Years since quitting				
			1–9	1.4	1.0, 2.0		
			10–19	1.2	0.9, 1.5		18 years follow-up
			20–29	1.1	0.9, 1.4		
			≥ 30	1.1	0.9, 1.5		Mortality rate ratio
			Never smoker	1			
Burns et al. (1997) USA	Cancer Prevention Study (CPS I) >1 000 000 59% women	CHD mortality		Men		Women	Smoking assessed at baseline, 12 years follow-up
			Years since quitting				
			2–4	2.66		2.23	
			5–9	1.64		1.53	
			10–14	1.37		0.98	Estimates are mortality rate ratios from CHD
			15–19	1.13		0.84	
			20–24	0.99		0.88	
			25–29	0.96		0.96	
			30–34	0.93		0.63	
			35–39	0.55		0.63	
			Never smoker	1		1	
Friedman et al. (1997) USA	Kaiser-Permanente 60 000 59% women age ≥35	CHD mortality		Men		Women	Smoking assessed at baseline
			Current smoker	2.0		2.2	
			Years since quitting				
			2–10	1.3		1.4	18 years follow-up
			11–20	1.3		1.4	
			>20	1.0		1.1	Current smokers ≥ 20 cig/day
			Never smoker	1		1	
Hrubec & McLaughlin (1997) USA	US Veterans' Cohort 248 046 men	CHD mortality	Current smoker	1.2			Smoking assessed at baseline
			Years since quitting				
			<5	1.7			
			5–9	1.5			26 years follow-up
			10–19	1.4			
			20–29	1.2			
			30–39	1.1			
			40+	1.0			
			Never smoker	1			

Table 3. Cohort studies: Time-course of CHD risk reduction (contd)

Study Reference Country	Study Population	Outcome	Smoking Category	Relative Risk (95% CI)				Comments
Kawachi et al. (1997) USA	Nurses' Health Study 117 000 women age 30-55	CHD mortality	Current smoker	3.74	2.86, 4.89			Smoking data updated
			Former smoker	1.57	1.17, 2.12			
			Years since quitting					
			0	1	reference			12 years follow-up
			<2	0.76	0.43, 1.32			
			2–4	0.90	0.54, 1.51			Total CVD
			5–9	0.75	0.47, 1.18			
			10–14	0.29	0.13, 0.63			
			≥ 15	0.42	0.27, 0.66			
			Never smoker	0.30	0.24, 0.37			
Iso et al. (2005) Japan	Japan Collaborative Cohort Study Evaluation of Cancer Risk (JACC) 94 683 44% women age 40–79	CHD mortality		Men		Women		Smoking assessed at baseline
			Current smoker	2.4	1.7, 3.4	3.6	2.5, 5.3	
			Former smoker	1.7	1.2,2.4	1.0	0.4, 2.7	
			Never smoker	1		1		10 years follow-up
			Years since quitting	Men				
			0	1				
			<1	0.3	0.1, 0.9			
			2–4	0.9	0.6, 1.4			
			5–9	0.8	0.6, 1.2			
			10–14	0.5	0.3, 0.8			
			≥ 15	0.4	0.3, 0.6			
Wen et al. (2005) Taiwan	Taiwan civil employees 30 244 men age >35		Current smoker	2.25	1.44, 3.53			Smoking assessed at baseline
			Former smoker	1.0	0.50, 1.84			
			Never smoker	1				
								11 years follow-up
			Years since quitting					
			Current	1				
			0-5	0.62	0.24, 1.58			
			0-16	0.43	0.19, 0.96			
			≥ 17	0.54	0.17, 0.78			

IHD = Ischaemic Heart Disease

smokers after 10–14 years (0.47; 95% CI=0.27–0.83) (Iso et al., 2005). In another large study from Taiwan that included 30 244 male civil employees, the time-course of CHD mortality risk reduction after cessation in male former smokers was estimated with different duration of quitting. The RR of CHD 5 years after quitting was 0.62 (95% CI=0.24–1.58) and within the first 16 years was 0.43 (95% CI=0.19–0.96), thus reaching the level of never smokers

somewhere within that time-span (Wen et al., 2005). In a Swedish study of 51 911 men with 183 deaths among former smokers during 10 years of follow-up, relative risk of CHD compared to never smokers was 1.5 within the first 1–9 years of quitting and 1.0 after more than 9 years, thus reaching the level of never smokers (Cederlof et al., 1975)

Hurley et al. (2005) modelled the time course of MI risk after quitting in disease-free subjects based on several of

the studies above (Willett et al., 1981; Rosenberg et al., 1985, 1990; Kawachi et al., 1994; McElduff et al., 1998). In this study the risk of MI in current male smokers was 3.4 and in female smokers 4.1. The reduction in risk was modelled with the number of months since cessation, showing a rapid decrease within the first 1–2 years followed by a slow decline. In long-time abstinent former smokers (200 months [approximately 17 years]), the RR was 1.1 in men and 1.3

in women compared with never smokers. The model may have overestimated risk reduction because it is based on thousands of observations from case–control studies (Rosenberg *et al.*, 1985, 1990; McElduff *et al.*, 1998) and cohort studies (Willett *et al.*, 1981; Kawachi *et al.*, 1994). The smaller risk reduction modelled in women is probably the result of model-assumptions, as the results finds little support in the large studies that include women (showing larger reductions; see Table 3).

Most observational cohort studies use only baseline information on smoking habits and calculate risk reduction in former smokers from their baseline information on when they quit. The difficulty of tracking smoking habits in patients with CHD was demonstrated in a study of patients with angina who were followed for changes in smoking habits during 5 years. Eleven percent changed smoking habits at either the 2- or 5-year follow-up visits, and 34 of 92 smokers (37%) were abstinent at some time during follow-up (Corrigan *et al.*, 2002). Another methodological issue of particular concern in studies that rely exclusively on baseline information is the inability to detect if smokers who succeed in quitting are the persons that have greater success in changing their life-style in other ways conducive to reduction of their risk of new events, i.e. change of diet, modifications of the level of cholesterol, increase physical activity, excess weight loss and compliance with medical treatments. These additional changes, unrecorded, would tend to bias the results attributed to smoking habits in direction of overestimating the benefits of smoking cessation. However, results regarding differences in former smokers and continued smokers in studies of the prevalence of other cardiovascular risk factors do not indicate systematic trends to support this possibility (Wilson *et al.*, 2000), and the benefits of cessation persist when these other

factors are controlled for in the analyses. Most studies have found very little difference between adjusted and unadjusted estimates of risk reduction. Some studies have even found that adjusted estimates of risk reduction are greater than the crude estimates (Johansson *et al.*, 1985; Greenwood *et al.*, 1995; Wilson *et al.*, 2000; Critchley & Capewell, 2004).

Risk of CHD increases with accumulated exposure to cigarette smoking, although not to the same extent as other smoking-related diseases such as COPD and lung cancer. The fact that not only smoking exposure but also duration of smoking are predictive of CHD would indicate that risk reduction after smoking cessation would also depend on accumulated exposure. This was seen in both CPS I and II, in which CHD mortality risks diminished more rapidly in former smokers with previous consumption of less than 20 cigarettes per day ('light smokers') as compared with former smokers who had smoked a greater daily quantity but with comparable length of cessation ('heavy smokers', USD-HHS, 1990; Burns *et al.*, 1997). In light smokers risk reached the level of never smokers after 10 years of smoking abstinence, whereas the risk remained slightly elevated even after >20 years in heavy smokers. Similar results were reported from the US Veterans Study, in which light smokers reached the CHD-mortality level of never smokers 30 years after cessation whereas in heavy smokers risks continued to be higher (Hrubec *et al.*, 1997).

Another issue of concern regarding the time-course of changes in risk is that most smokers started to smoke at a similar age. Therefore, among former cigarette smokers, for any given age, duration of smoking will determine the number of years since quitting. Hence, these two variables will be highly (negatively) correlated and also correlated with age and age at initiation.

It has been difficult to establish that the risk associated with smoking also depends on age at smoking initiation. Attempts have been made to determine an independent contribution of younger age at initiation with higher risk of lung cancer, in which timing of exposure to carcinogens in relation to organ growth may be of importance, but this has not been methodologically possible. In the NHS the risk for CHD in former smokers did not depend on age at starting to smoke, with the exception of the women who began before age 15, who had very high risks (Kawachi *et al.*, 1997). Based on the largest available dataset, the CPS study, it was concluded that the major contribution of age of initiation to increased risk was through longer duration of smoking at any given age and an independent effect of age of initiation would be small (Burns *et al.*, 1997). Risk of CHD is not likely to be affected in the long term by differences in age of smoking initiation, other than the effect on duration of smoking. As a consequence, risk reduction after smoking cessation will not be affected by age at initiation.

Case–control studies have generally been more optimistic regarding how fast risk reaches the level of never smokers. In three such studies risks were similar to that of never smokers within 2–4 years (Rosenberg *et al.*, 1985, 1990; Dobson *et al.*, 1991). The largest case-control study was conducted in Australia and New Zealand and comprised approximately 12 000 subjects (McElduff *et al.*, 1998). Risk reduction following cessation was similar in men and in women in the two populations included and was also present irrespective of whether the study outcome was a fatal or a non-fatal event or whether results were adjusted for other cardiovascular risk factors. Results were consistent with a rapid decline within the first year of smoking cessation, followed by a more moderate decline with risk approaching the level of never smokers within 4–6 years (Table 4). The lack of decrease in risk or even increased risk within the first 5 months is likely to be related to the methodological issues mentioned above (in the study by Rosenberg *et al.*, 1990). In an Italian case–control study of subjects with acute myocardial infarction, the odds ratio was 2.9 in current smokers and 1.6 in former smokers within the first year after quitting, and continued to decline but remained higher than in never smokers after 10 years, although the difference was not statistically significant (Negri *et al.*, 1994). Another Italian study reported relative risk reduction of similar magnitude within the first 5 years following cessation, with continued slightly elevated risk compared with life-long never smokers with prolonged follow up (Bosetti *et al.*, 1999). Two USA-based studies of women under age 65 and men under age 55 found significant risk reduction within the first 2 years, with risks approaching the level of never smokers shortly thereafter (Rosenberg *et al.*, 1985, 1990). Similar patterns of decline were seen irrespective of former daily consumption or duration of smoking in both studies.

In subjects with clinically evident disease

In the Cochrane Report the available information from each study included was not detailed enough to determine the time-course of risk reduction (Critchley & Capewell, 2003, 2004). The authors argued that if risk in former smokers continues to decline after smoking cessation, one would expect risk in former smokers to vary with length of follow-up. This was unexpectedly not found in the Cochrane meta-analysis, and several explanations were offered: the timing of the majority of risk reduction occurs relatively quickly after stopping smoking among those with evident disease, i.e. before the minimum length of follow-up of two years required for study inclusion in the Cochrane review; the variation in length of follow-up—mostly 3–7 years—was not large enough to explore differences. The combined risk reduction in the meta-analysis study was 36% with a mean follow-up of 5 years. The meta-analysis did not include risk among never smokers, but a risk reduction of 36% compared with continued smokers is not likely to be equivalent to reaching the level of never smokers.

Summary

Cigarette smoking is a major cause of coronary heart disease. The risk is manifest both as an increased risk for thrombosis and degree of atherosclerosis in coronary vessels. The cardiovascular risk owing to cigarette smoking increases with the amount smoked and with the duration of smoking. Former smokers have considerably reduced risk of CHD compared with continued smokers.

Evidence from studies of patients with manifest CHD point towards risk reduction in the order of 35% compared with continued cigarette smokers of similar accumulated exposure within the first 2–4 years of smoking cessation. Findings from case-control studies and cohort studies of subjects without diagnosed CHD are compatible with this conclusion and point toward similar relative risk reduction following smoking cessation.

Methodological issues of particular concern when assessing risk reduction within the first 1–2 years after smoking cessation include the issue of reverse causation and constancy of smoking habits. These issues are of such importance that the risk reduction in healthy subjects immediately following cessation cannot be accurately assessed based on observational cohort studies or case–control studies.

Detection of risk reduction following prolonged abstinence is less subject to the methodological concerns delineated above, and can rely more on the very large observational cohort studies available to shed light on the time-course question. Some studies find the risk to be similar to that in never smokers after 10–15 years abstinence, whereas others find a persistent increased risk of 10–20% even after 10–20 years. The main methodological issue in this type of study is misclassification of both current and former smokers with prolonged follow-up. An additional concern is self-selection of former smokers causing the risk associated with smoking cessation to be overestimated with prolonged period of observations. With these methodological issues taken into account, the body of evidence points toward the risk of CHD asymptotically approaching the risk of never smokers.

Table 4. Case-control studies: Time-course of CHD risk reduction following smoking cessation

Reference Country	Study Population	Number of Cases/ Controls	Smoking status	RR (95%)	Comments
Rosenberg et al. (1985) USA	First MI, non-fatal, Men age<55	Cases 1873 Controls 2775	Current smoker Former smoker Years since quitting < 2 2-3 4-9 10-12 > 12 Never smoker	2.9 (2.4, 3.4) 2.0 1.1 1.4 1.0 1.0 1	Current smoker defined as men smoking up to one year prior to MI onset Estimates derived from a graph
Rosenberg et al. (1990) USA	First MI, non-fatal, Women age<65	Cases 910 Controls 2375	Current smoker Years since quitting < 6 months 6–12 months 1–3 4–6 7–9 10–12 Never smoker	3.6 (3.0, 4.4) 3.2 2.3 1.5 0.9 1.1 1.0 1	RR <2 years of abstinence=2.6 (1.8, 3.8) Estimates derived from a graph
Negri et al. (1994) Italy	Non-fatal MI	Cases 916 Controls 1106	Current smoker Years since quitting 1 > 1-5 6–9 > 10 Never smoker	2.9 (2.2, 3.9) 1.6 (0.8, 3.2) 1.4 (0.9, 2.1) 1.2 (0.7, 2.1) 1.1 (0.8, 1.8) 1	Adjusted for CVD risk factors RR former versus continued smokers: p<0.05 for all intervals
Bosetti et al. (1999) Italy	Non-fatal MI	Cases 1230 Controls 1839	Men Current smoker Years since quitting < 5 ≥ 5 Never smoker Women Current smoker Years since quitting < 5 ≥ 5 Never smoker	3.3 (2.4, 4.6) 1.5 (0.9, 2.5) 1.2 (0.8, 1.7) 1 4.1 (2.3, 5.7) 2.9 (1.3, 6.7) 1.3 (0.6, 2.7) 1	Combining data from two studies, adjusted for CVD risk factors

Table 4. Case-control studies: Time course of CHD risk reduction (contd)

Reference Country	Study Population	Number of Cases/ Controls	Smoking status	RR (95%)	Comments
Dobson et al. (1991) McElduff et al. (1998) Australia, New Zealand	Non-fatal MI Age 35-69	Cases 5572 Controls 6268	*Men* Current smoker	3.5 (3.0, 4.1)	Part of MONICA, results similar after adjustment for CVD risk factors
			Years since quitting		
			1–5 months	7.4 (4.4, 12.6)	
			6–12 months	3.1 (1.9, 5.2)	
			1–3 years	1.6 (1.2, 2.1)	
			4–6	1.1 (0.8, 1.5)	
			7–9	1.0 (0.7, 1.4)	
			10–12	1.3 (0.9, 1.8)	
			> 12	1.1 (0.9, 1.3)	
			Women Current smoker	5.6 (4.5, 7.0)	
			Years since quitting		
			1–5 months	4.7 (2.4, 9.1)	
			6–12 months	2.7 (1.2, 6.4)	
			1–3 years	2.1 (1.3, 3.3)	
			4–6	1.0 (0.6, 1.9)	
			7–9	1.6 (0.9, 3.1)	
			10–12	1.7 (0.9, 3.1)	
			> 12	1.0 (0.7, 1.4)	
			Never smoker	1	

MI = Myocardial Infarction
RR = Relative risk
95% = 95% confidence interval

Cerebrovascular Disease

Introduction

According to the World Health Organization, cardiovascular diseases are the leading cause of death and a major cause of disability in the world. Coronary heart disease is the dominant type of vascular disease in Caucasian populations, whereas cerebrovascular diseases are more important in most Asian populations (World Health Organization, 2006). Cerebrovascular diseases consist of three major disease entities: subarachnoidal haemorrhage, intracerebral haemorrhage and ischaemic stroke. Transient ischaemic attack (TIA), characterised by transient neurological symptoms, is a strong predictor of subsequent ischaemic stroke onset (Johnston et al., 2000). The pathophysiological settings of these three major sub-types of stroke are different, but they share many of the same risk factors; high blood pressure is the most important, followed by tobacco smoking (Stegmayer et al., 1997; Jacobs et al., 1999). Other risk factors that have been reported include high serum cholesterol and low high-density lipoprotein (HDL) cholesterol levels, left ventricular hypertrophy, atrial fibrillation, alcohol drinking, sedentary lifestyle, obesity, diabetes, systemic low-level inflammation measured by serum C-reactive protein (CRP) level, and haemostatic factors such as plasma fibrinogen level. The role of these factors in haemorrhagic stroke is to some extent different than in ischaemic stroke.

Numerous studies have shown an association between smoking and the risk of stroke (Abbott et al., 1986; Colditz et al., 1988; Shinton & Beevers, 1989; Donnan et al., 1989; Kuller et al., 1991; Kawachi et al., 1993; Robbins et al., 1994; Bonita et al., 1999; Anderson et al., 2004; Mannami et al., 2004; Ueshima et al., 2004; Doll et al., 2004; Asia Pacific Cohort Studies Collaboration, 2005).

Current smokers have a relative risk of stroke of 1.5 to 4 compared with never smokers, and many studies have demonstrated a clear dose-response relationship between the amount of tobacco smoking and the risk of stroke. Smoking-associated risk of stroke, however, varies markedly between different studies, populations, sexes and stroke subtypes. In Asian populations the smoking-associated relative risk of stroke may be lower than in Caucasian populations (Iso *et al.,* 2005; Asia Pacific Cohort Studies Collaboration, 2005). On the other hand, because cerebrovascular disease is more common in many Asian populations, compared to the Caucasian populations, their smoking-related absolute risk may be similar or even higher due to higher background risk.

Depending on the underlying mechanisms, the effects of tobacco smoke on stroke risk are both acute and cumulative. The effect of smoking on arteriosclerosis is most probably cumulative and only partly reversible, whereas the effects of smoking on the haemostatic system appear soon after the start of the exposure, and the effects diminish gradually after the exposure has stopped (Hamsten, 1993).

The effect of smoking cessation on the risk of cerebrovascular disease can be assessed using the following epidemiological study designs: randomised clinical (or population) trials, observational cohort studies, case–control (or cohort/referent) studies and cross-sectional analysis. Randomised trials can provide the strongest evidence on the causal relationship between exposure and outcome. However, because the harmful health effects of smoking are well known, strict individual randomisation of smoking or smoking cessation is not possible. Several intervention studies have assessed the effect of different types of smoking cessation programs on cessation. In these studies, smoking

cessation rate may be larger in the intervention group, but not all of the smokers in the intervention group quit, and many smokers in the control group do. Therefore, most of the evidence about the effect of smoking cessation on cerebrovasculalar disease risk is based on the data from observational studies. Cohort studies can assess the effect of smoking cessation based on smoking status at baseline, and also change of smoking status if the smoking data is updated during the follow-up. Case–control studies look at the smoking status and history of smoking prior to the stroke event, but the data are collected in both the diseased and the control groups, only after the event in the diseased has occurred. This study design is prone to both selection and information bias. Data on smoking cessation trials can be used, but it is questionable whether the data can be analysed based on the "intention to treat" principle. If the data are analysed based on the actual smoking status of participants, the study approach does not differ, in principle, from that of cohort studies. Cross-sectional studies can assess the relationship of smoking status or smoking history to the development of subclinical arteriosclerosis in cerebral arteries but preclude establishing a temporal relationship between smoking and biological determinations. Furthermore, the effect of smoking cessation on cerebrovascular disease risk can be expressed as a change in relative risk or absolute risk difference.

Is there a reduction in cerebrovascular disease risk following smoking cessation?

Subjects without clinically evident cerebrovascular disease
Relative risk
In a meta-analysis including 13 cohort and case–control studies with separate data on former smokers (from a total of

32 studies examined), the overall risk of stroke was 1.5 (95% CI=1.4-1.6) among current smokers and 1.17 (95% CI=1.05-1.30) among former smokers compared with never smokers (Shinton & Beevers 1989). Current and past smoking was associated with higher relative risk in a subset of studies with stroke occurring before age 75. The authors concluded that although a modest elevation in stroke risk persisted among younger former smokers, this relative risk was substantially less than that observed among current smokers. Studies published since 1989 or which include detailed data on smoking cessation (repeated assessments of smoking status during follow-up or detailed data on smoking history at base-line) are reviewed here and summarised in Tables 5 and 6.

In the Honolulu Heart Study, which included 8 006 men of Japanese ancestry, smoking status was assessed both at baseline and after 6 years of follow-up (Abbott *et al.,* 1986). In 12 years of follow-up, smokers had 2.5 times higher (95% CI=2.0–3.3) risk of stroke compared with the never smokers after adjusting for age, diastolic blood pressure, serum cholesterol, hematocrit, body mass and alcohol use. Subjects who stopped smoking before the sixth year of the follow-up reduced their risk of stroke considerably. Compared to the never smokers, they had 1.5-fold (95% CI=1.0-2.3) risk, whereas those men who continued to smoke in the course of follow-up had 3.5-fold (95% CI=2.3-5.5) risk.

The Framingham Heart Study cohort included 4 255 men and women aged 36–68 years and free of stroke or history of TIA at baseline. Smoking increased the risk of any incident stroke event, and the risk of ischemic stroke both in men and women independent of other major risk factors in 26 years of follow-up (Wolf *et al.,* 1988). Smokers had about 1.5 fold (RR=1.4 in men and 1.6 in women)

Table 5. Risk of cerebrovascular disease risk and smoking cessation

Reference	Study	Population	Outcome	Duration Follow-up (Years)	Risk Category	Relative risk (95% CI) Never smokers as reference group		Comments
						Current smoker	Former smokers	
Shinton & Beevers (1989)		Meta-analyses of data from 18 studies	Risk of total stroke & by sub-type	Varying by study		1.47 (1.15, 1.88)	1.17 (1.05, 1.30)	
Kawachi et al. (1993)	Nurses' Health Study	117 006 female nurses Age 3055	Non-fatal and fatal stroke 495 events	12	Total stroke SAH Ischaemic stroke Cerebral haemorrhage	2.73 (2.18, 3.41) 4.85 (2.90, 8.11) 2.53 (1.91, 3.35) 1.24 (0.64, 2.42)	1.35 (0.98, 1.85) 2.26 (1.16, 4.42) 1.27 (0.85, 1.89) 1.24 (0.64, 2.42)	
Robbins et al. (1994)	US Physicians Health Study	22 071 male physicians Age 40-84	Incidence of stroke 312 events	10	<20 cigarettes daily ≥20 cigarettes daily	1.86 (1.04, 3.33) 2.71 (1.84, 3.98)	1.25 (0.95, 1.63)	
Wannamethee et al. (1995)	British Regional Heart Study	7 735 men Age 4059	Any stroke (43 fatal and 124 non-fatal)	13	1-19 cig./day ≥20 cig./day	3.7 (2.0, 6.7)	1.0 (0.4, 2.5) 2.2 (1.1, 4.3) 2.3	
Hart et al. (1999)	Renfrew-Paisley Study	7 052 men and 8354 women Age 45-64	Stroke mortality 689 deaths	20	Men Women	1.36* (1.12, 1.65) 1.77* (1.42, 2.20)	0.63 (0.47, 0.84) 0.79 (0.53, 1.18)	*per 20 cigarettes per day
Doll et al. (2004)	British Doctors Study	34 439 male doctors Age over 20 years	Stroke mortality 3307 deaths	50		4.32 per 1 000 person years	3.18 per 1 000 person years	Never-smokers 2.75 per 1 000 person years
Glynn & Rosner (2005)	US Physicians Health Study	18 662 male physicians Age 4084	Incidence of stroke 902 events	20		1.83 (1.50, 1.26)	1.09 (0.94, 1.26)	Extended follow-up of the previous study by Robbins et al.
Ueshima et al. (2004)	NIPPON DATA80	9 639 men and women Age 30 years or more	Stroke mortality 203 deaths	14	Men, 1-20 cigarettes daily Men, > 20 cigarettes daily Women, 1-20 cigarettes daily Women, > 20 cigarettes daily	1.60 (0.91, 2.79) 2.17 (1.06, 4.30) 1.42 (0.72, 2.78) 3.91 (1.18, 12.9)	1.56 (0.84, 2.90) 1.31 (0.50, 3.39)	

Table 5. Risk of cerebrovascular disease (contd)

Reference	Study	Population	Outcome	Duration Follow-up (Years)	Risk Category	Relative risk (95% CI) Never smokers as reference group		Comments
						Current smoker	Former smokers	
Mannami et al. (2004)	Japan Public Health Center-based Prospective Study on Cancer Cardiovascular Diseases (JPCH Study)	19 782 men and 21500 women Age 40-59	Risk of total stroke & by sub-type (702 events)	10	Total stroke, men	1.27(1.05, 1.54)	0.82 (0.65, 1.04)	
					Total stroke, women	1.98 (1.42, 277)	1.47 (0.80, 2.70)	
					SAH, men	3.60 (1.62, 8.01)	1.12 (0.40, 3.10)	
					SAH, women	2.70 (1.45, 5.02)	Not available	
					Cerebral haemorrhage, men	0.90 (0.65, 1.25)	0.72 (0.49, 1.07)	
					Cerebral haemorrhage, women	1.53 (0.86, 4.25)	1.54 (0.56, 4.25)	
					Ischaemic stroke, men	1.56 (1.17, 2.10)	0.87 (0.60, 1.25)	
					Ischaemic stroke, women	1.57 (0.86, 2.87)	1.10 (0.35, 49)	
JACC, (2005)	Japan Collaborative Cohort Study for Evaluation of Cancer Risk	41 782 men and 52901 women Age 40-79	Stroke mortality 698 deaths	10	Total stroke, men	1.39 (1.13, 1.70)	0.95 (0.76, 1.20)	
					Total stroke, women	1.65 (1.21, 2.25)	1.20 (0.71, 2.03)	
					SAH, men	2.98 (1.34, 6.63)	1.67 (0.68, 4.14)	
					SAH, women	3.35 (1.92, 5.52)	0.90 (0.22, 3.69)	
					Cerebral haemorrhage, men	1.48 (0.97, 2.24)	1.05 (0.66, 1.68)	
					Cerebral haemorrhage, women	1.10 (0.51, 2.40)	1.20 (0.38, 3.83)	
					Ischaemic stroke, men	1.52 (1.07, 2.15)	0.84 (0.59, 1.19)	
					Ischaemic stroke, women	1.64 (0.97, 2.79)	1.24 (0.54, 2.88)	
Asia Pacific Cohort Studies Collaboration (2005)		Meta-analyses of 33 cohort studies From Asia and Australia	Incidence of CHD and stroke	3-25		1.43 (1.32, 1.54)	0.84*(0.76, 0.92)	* Former smokers compared with current smokers. Current smokers compared with never smokers

SAH = Subarachnoid hemorrhage

Table 6. Summary of studies assessing the time-course of cerebrovascular disease risk reduction following smoking cessation

Study and reference	Population	Outcome and duration of follow-up	Relative Risk Current smokers Versus Never smokers (95% CI)	Relative Risk Former smokers Time since quitting (years) (95% CI)	Comments
Honolulu Heart Study Abbott et al. (1986)	8006 men of Japanese ancestry Average age 55 No history of stroke at baseline	Incidence of stroke 12 year follow-up 289 events	*Men* 3.5 (2.3, 5.5)	< 6 → 1.5 (1.0, 2.3) Never smoker → 1	Smoking status assessed at baseline and after 5 years of follow-up. RR adjusted for age, diastolic blood pressure, serum cholesterol, alcohol consumption, hematocrit and body mass. Subjects with myocardial infarction excluded.
Nurses Health Study Kawachi et al. (1993)	117 006 women Age 30–55 Free of coronary heart disease Stroke and cancer at baseline	Non-fatal and fatal stroke combined 12 year follow-up 448 events	*Women* 2.73 (2.18, 3.41)	Current smoker → 1.0 < 2 → 0.73 (4.40, 1.33) 2–4 → 0.59 (0.28, 1.21) 5–9 → 0.39 (0.20, 0.77) 10–14 → 0.60 (0.32, 1.12) ≥ 15 → 0.39 (0.24, 0.64) Never smoker → 0.37 (0.29, 0.46)	Smoking status assessed every two years. RR adjusted for age, follow-up period, history of hypertension, diabetes, high cholesterol, body mass index, past use of oral contraceptives, postmenopausal estrogen therapy and daily number of cigarettes consumed.
British Regional Heart Study Wannamethee et al. (1995)	7 264 men Age 40–59 No recall of ischemic heart disease or stroke at baseline	Non-fatal and fatal stroke 13 year follow-up 167 events	3.7 (2.0, 6.9)	1–5 → 1.8 (0.8, 4.4) 6–10 → 1.2 (0.4, 3.3) 11–19 → 1.8 (0.8, 4.4) ≥ 20 → 2.1 (0.9, 4.8)	Smoking history at baseline. RR adjusted for age, body mass index, physical activity, alcohol intake, social class, diabetes, indication of ischemic heart disease (questionnaire and ECG), antihypertensive treatment, systolic blood pressure and cholesterol level.
Cancer Prevention Study (CPS I) Burns et al. (1997)	1 078 894 men and women, Age 30 years or more (93% white)	Stroke mortality	*Duration smoking (yr)* 　　　Men　Women 15–19　1.59　1.33 20–24　1.28　1.69 25–29　1.74　1.55 30–34　1.51　1.60 35–39　1.62　1.61 40–44　1.85　1.49	Men　Women 2–4　1.62　2.28 5–9　1.16　1.18 10–14　1.05　1.25 15–19　1.01　1.01 20–24　0.93　1.11	Smoking history at baseline. The mortality risk ratios are for the white population.
Japan Collaborative Cohort Study for Evaluation of Cancer Risk (JACC) Iso et al. (2005)	94683 men and women Age 40–79 years Free of history of stroke Coronary heart disease or cancer at baseline	Stroke mortality 10 year follow-up 1250 deaths	*Men Total stroke* 1.39 (1.13, 1.70) *Women Total stroke* 1.45 (1.21, 2.25)	Current smoker → 1 0–1 → 1.03 (0.66, 1.60) 2–4 → 0.73 (0.50, 1.06) 5–9 → 0.75 (0.54, 1.04) 10–14 → 0.48 (0.31, 0.74) ≥ 15 → 0.71 (0.55, 0.92) Never smoker → 0.53 (0.37, 0.76)	Smoking history at baseline. RR adjusted for sex, age, body mass index, alcohol intake, physical activity, hours of sleep, education, mental stress, fruit and fish intake, history of diabetes and hypertension, number of cigarettes smoked daily, age at starting smoking.

adjusted risk compared with never smokers, and a clear dose-response relationship was found between the amount of cigarettes smoked daily and the risk of stroke. The study subjects were contacted and their smoking status updated every two years. About half of the smokers quit during the 26 years of follow-up of the study (a quitter was any individual who was a cigarette smoker in 1950 and in 1956 and who stopped definitively some time after that interval). The risk of stroke decreased markedly after two years of abstinence, and after five years the risk did not differ from that of never smokers. Furthermore, the risk of stroke among past smokers returned to that of never smokers both among normotensive and hypertensive subjects.

The Nurses' Health Study consisted of 117 006 female registered nurses aged 30–55 years and free of coronary heart disease, stroke and cancer at baseline (Kawachi *et al.*, 1993). The cohort was followed 12 years and the information on smoking habits was updated every two years. Smokers had 2.7 (95% CI=2.2-3.4) and former smokers 1.3 (95% CI=1.0-1.8) multifactorially adjusted relative risks of stroke compared to never smokers. The smoking-associated risk was higher in subarachnoid haemorrhage than in ischaemic stroke or intra-cerebral haemorrhage. The risk increased with the increase number of cigarettes smoked daily. The relative risk was 2.0 (95% CI=1.3-3.1) among light smokers (1-14 cigarettes daily) and 4.5 (95% CI=2.8-7.2) among heavy smokers (≥ 35 cigarettes daily). Smoking cessation during the follow-up reduced the risk of stroke markedly. In two years of abstinence, the adjusted relative risk of stroke among the quitters was 0.82 (95% CI=0.45-1.51), compared with those who continued smoking during the follow-up, and in four years the risk was reduced to 0.39 (95% CI=0.17-0.87), which was practically the same as

in never smokers (0.37, 95% CI=0.29-0.46). The risk of subarachnoid haemorrhage also decreased after quitting, but still remained higher than in those who had never smoked. Due to relatively small number of former smokers, there was some variation in the risk ratios during the course of follow-up, particularly in the stroke type-specific analyses. Among former smokers, the age of starting smoking also affected the risk reduction after quitting, and the risk decline was smaller among those who had started smoking before 18 years of age, compared with those who had started at an older age (Kawachi *et al.,* 1993).

The British Regional Heart Study consisted of 7 264 men aged 40–59 years at baseline with no recall of previous ischemic heart disease or stroke (Wannamethee *et al.,* 1995). During a 13-year follow-up, current cigarette smokers had nearly fourfold (RR=3.7, 95% CI=2.0-6.9) adjusted risk of stroke compared with never smokers. Light smokers (1–19 cigarettes daily) had a risk ratio of 3.3 (95% CI=1.6-7.1), and heavy smokers (≥ 21 cigarettes daily) had a risk ratio of 4.2 (95% CI=2.2-8.2). Former smokers showed lower risk than current smokers, but their risk was still higher (RR 1.7, 95% CI=0.9-3.3) than that in never smokers. The benefit of giving up smoking completely was seen within five years of quitting. The risk reduction was dependant on the amount of tobacco smoked prior to cessation. Light smokers (<20 cigarettes daily) reported a risk level similar to those who had never smoked, but the heavier smokers retained a more than twofold risk compared with never smokers (RR=2.2, 95% CI=1.1–4.3). The risk of stroke in those who quit during the first 5 years of follow-up (recent quitters; RR=1.8, 95% CI=0.7–4.6) was reduced also markedly compared to those who continued smoking (RR=4.3, 95% CI=2.1–8.8). The benefit of quitting smoking was observed in both

normotensive and hypertensive men, but the absolute risk reduction was greater among the hypertensive subjects.

The American Cancer Society Cancer Prevention Study (CPS-I) is the largest prospective mortality study of diseases caused by tobacco use (Burns *et al.,* 1997). The study started in 1959 and continued until 1972, enrolling 1 078 894 men and women. Smoking status and detailed smoking history was assessed at the beginning of the study. The 12-year follow-up of the study cohort includes more than 11 million person-years. Smoking men and women had approximately 1.5-fold risk of stroke compared to never smokers. The risk varied considerably by age group and duration of smoking. Male former smokers had 1.6-fold and female former smokers 2.4-fold risk of stroke during the first 2-4 years of abstinence; thereafter the risk reduced markedly, and 10 years after quitting the risk was at the same level with never smokers.

The researchers of the Japan Collaborative Cohort Study for Evaluation of Cancer Risk (JACC Study) followed for 10 years 95 000 Japanese men and women aged 40 to 79 years at baseline (Iso *et al.,* 2005). Smoking status was assessed at baseline and included data on the number of cigarettes smoked among smokers and the time since quitting among former smokers. Smoking men had 1.4-fold (95% CI=1.1-1.7) and smoking women had 1.6-fold (95% CI=1.2-2.2) adjusted risk of stroke mortality compared with never smokers. In former smokers the relative risks were 0.9 (95% CI=0.8-1.2) in men and 1.2 (95% CI= 0.71-2.03) in women. Stroke mortality decreased markedly in the two to four years after quitting, and after 10 years of abstinence the risk did not differ from the risk of never smokers. The risk reduction was faster and returned to that of never smokers in the group aged 40–64 years, but some residual risk was left in the group aged 65–79 years.

Sub-clinical markers of cerebrovascular disease

Thickness of the carotid artery wall is a sub-clinical measure and a predictor of increased risk of ischaemic stroke. Tell and colleagues found nearly 20 years ago that the wall was thicker among smokers than among never smokers (Tell *et al.*, 1989). Former smokers had a thinner wall compared with current smokers, but they had thicker walls compared with never smokers. The differences were significant also after adjustment for age, sex, race, hypertension and diabetes. However, because the study was based on cross-sectional data, the effect of smoking cessation on the progression of atherosclerosis could not be directly evaluated, possible only with the availability of repeated measurements over time. A year later, in 1990, Whisnant and colleagues reported a strong association between the number of years of smoking and the risk of having severe carotid atherosclerosis after adjustment for other risk factors (Whisnant *et al.*, 1990). Age was the strongest factor affecting this risk, but duration of smoking was also associated with the risk of carotid atherosclerosis in all age groups. Based on mathematical modelling, quitting at the age of 40 markedly decreased the risk of severe carotid atherosclerosis in subsequent years.

In accordance with the two previous cross-sectional studies, Kiechl and colleagues reported a dose response relationship between smoking history, measured as pack-years, and incidence of severe premature arteriosclerosis in internal and common carotid arteries within five years of follow-up (Kiechl *et al.*, 2002). The risk of early atherogenesis was strongly associated with lifetime smoking exposure, and remained elevated after cessation of smoking.

Current and former smokers, however, faced an increased atherosclerosis risk only in the presence of chronic infections (chronic bronchitis, chronic obstructive pulmonary disease, urinary infection, other chronic infections) or increased C-reactive protein (CRP) (>1mg/L). Among those who did not have chronic infections and whose CRP was below 1 mg/L, the risk of carotid arteriosclerosis did not differ significantly between current and former smokers and never smokers. Smoking alone increased the risk only slightly (RR ≈ 1.2 [derived from a figure]), but if the smoker had also chronic infection and increased CRP, the risk was about six-fold that of never smokers without chronic infections or inflammation. Relative risk of early arteriosclerosis, associated with smoking and chronic infections and inflammation, was highest among those who were free of carotid arteriosclerosis at study baseline (RR ≈ 6 [derived from figure]).

Absolute risk

The etiology of cerebrovascular diseases, as with other cardiovascular and chronic diseases, is multifactorial. The causes, or risk factors, include non-modifiable factors (age, sex, race and other genetic factors), partly modifiable environmental factors (socio-economic position), a large number of modifiable behavioural factors (smoking, diet and physical activity) and biological mediating factors (body weight, blood pressure and blood lipids) that are determined by genetic, environmental and behavioural factors. These factors determine the absolute risk, and the effect of smoking cessation on the cerebrovascular disease risk must be assessed in the context of these other factors. In addition, the absolute risk in a defined population depends on the length of the follow-up.

A few studies have assessed the effect of smoking cessation on the absolute stroke risk at different levels of other risk factors, particularly hyperten-

sion. In the 26-year follow-up of the Framingham cohort, age-adjusted incidence of stroke was 80/1000 among normotensive never smoking men, 82/1 000 among normotensive former smoking men and 119/1000 among normotensive smoking men. Among hypertensive men the incidences were 190/1 000, 152/1000 and 246/1000, respectively. Among women the incidences were 61/1000, 59/1000 and 91/1000 in normotensive subjects, and 168/1000, 188/1000 and 273/1000 in hypertensive subjects, respectively (Wolf *et al.*, 1988). Thus, the relative risk of stroke among former smokers compared with current smokers was fairly similar among both normotensive and hypertensive subjects, but the absolute risk difference was larger among hypertensive subjects. In the British Regional Heart Study, in accordance with the Framingham results, the benefit of quitting smoking was observed in both normotensive and hypertensive men, but the absolute risk reduction was greater among the hypertensive subjects (Wannamethee *et al.*,1995).

The role of other risk factors

Other risk factors may also modify the association of smoking and smoking cessation on the risk of cerebrovascular disease. If the effect of other risk factors on stroke risk is similar in different smoking categories (no interaction), the effect of these factors when evaluating the association between smoking and stroke can be controlled by multifactorial adjustment. In most studies, adjustment for other risk factors did not markedly affect the smoking- and cessation-associated risk of stroke. Data on the possible effect modification of other risk factors are scarce. In the study published by Kiechl and colleagues, however, current and former smokers faced an increased atherosclerosis risk only in the presence of chronic infections, particularly if the CRP was increased (Kiechl *et al.,* 2002). This finding is interesting but needs to be confirmed in other populations.

The effect of smoking cessation among cerebrovascular disease patients

Data on the effect of smoking cessation on the prognosis of patients with existing cerebrovascular disease are scarce. Mast and colleagues assessed the effect of smoking on the risk of high-grade carotid artery stenosis among TIA and stroke patients (Mast *et al.,* 1998). Smoking was an independent determinant of severe stenosis in patients. The association differed by ethnicity, and the greatest effect was observed among whites. However, the authors did not assess the effect of smoking cessation on the risk of severe carotid artery stenosis.

In a recent British study, current smoking was a strong predictor (RR = 2.3, 95% CI=1.1-4.6 compared with never smokers) of total mortality among 308 stroke patients who were followed on average 7.5 years (Myint *et al.,* 2006). Also, former smokers had an increased but non-significant risk (RR=1.5, 95% CI= 0.9-2.4), but the study did not assess the effect of duration of smoking cessation on mortality.

The Heart Outcomes Prevention Evaluation (HOPE) clinical trial assessed the impact of cigarette smoking in high-risk patients (stable cardio-vascular disease or diabetes with at least one additional risk factor) (Dagenais *et al.,* 2005). Current smokers had a 1.4 fold risk of stroke in 4.5 years of follow-up compared with never smokers. The risk of stroke among former smokers did not differ from the risk among never smokers.

In their review of the scientific evidence for stroke prevention, Straus and colleagues estimated that smoking cessation among secondary prevention patients would reduce the risk of a new stroke event by 33% (95% CI = 29–38%)(Straus *et al.,* 2002). Forty-four patients who quit would need to be treated to prevent one event a year, which is less than the number needed to treat for other recommended secondary prevention measures such as antihypertensive therapy (requiring treatment of 51 patients to avoid an event), statins (57 treated patients) or antiplatelet therapy (64–77 treated patients).

What is the time course of the change in risk?

The studies examining the effect of smoking cessation on the risk of stroke are less numerous than the studies on the risk of coronary heart disease, though the time course of risk reduction after cessation seems to be fairly similar. A marked risk reduction is observed in the 2–5 years after quitting, and in most studies the risk is at the same level with never smokers in 10 years (Wolf *et al.,* 1988; Kawachi *et al.,* 1993; Burns *et al.,* 1997; Iso *et al.,* 2005). However, in some studies the risk reduction has been incomplete after longer durations of cessation, 10–15 years (Abbott *et al.,* 1986, Wannamethee *et al.,* 1995).

Even though the reduction of stroke risk after cessation seems to be fairly fast and complete in general, in some sub-groups of the population the risk may not subside to the level of never smokers. In the British Regional Heart Study, light smokers (<20 cigarettes daily) experienced a risk reduction to the level of those who had never smoked within five years of quitting, but quitters with past heavier smoking history retained a risk more than two-fold that of never smokers. In the Nurses Health Study the age of smoking initiation affected the risk after quitting, and the risk decline was smaller among those who had started smoking before 18 years of age compared with those who had started at an older age (Kawachi *et al.,* 1993). Age at the time of cessation may also influence the timing and magnitude of risk reduction, and the reduction is faster and more complete among younger quitters compared with those who quit at older age (Doll *et al.,* 2004; Iso *et al.,* 2005). However, the age of starting and stopping smoking and the duration of smoking and abstinence are inextricably linked, and their effect cannot be completely separated in the analyses.

Limitations of the data reviewed

Because our knowledge about the association between smoking cessation and the risk of stroke is based on observational studies, some critical considerations are needed. Even though in most of the studies results were adjusted for hypertension and other known cardiovascular risk factors, the adjustment is never complete and some residual confounding may remain. Quitters may differ from those who continue smoking in many ways; they may be lighter smokers, have shorter smoking history and be less nicotine-dependent, be more health conscious and better informed on health matters, e.g. having a healthier diet with a general lifestyle that is healthier, and their educational level and socio-economic background may differ from that of persistent smokers. All these factors most probably overestimate the risk reduction. On the other hand, subjects with sub-clinical cardio- and cerebrovascular symptoms may be more prone to stop smoking, which causes an underestimation in the reduction of stroke risk. Similarly, if only those subjects who have overt cerebrovascular disease are excluded at baseline, but the study population includes coronary heart disease patient, the results may be biased towards underestimation. The true reduction may also be underestimated due to misclassification if some smokers give up smoking (when the former smokers are compared with smokers) or if some subjects recorded as former smokers start to smoke again during the follow-up.

Summary

Smoking is a strong risk factor for stroke incidence and mortality. Based on the data from large prospective studies, current smokers have relative risk for stroke of 1.5 to 4 compared with never smokers. Former smokers have markedly lower risk than do current smokers. Many studies, which did not stratify by duration of abstinence, showed relative risks that differed from never smokers only slightly.

Studies that have assessed the relationship of the duration of smoking abstinence on stroke risk report a marked risk reduction in 2–5 years after cessation, and the risk reduction continues up to 15 years after quitting. In some studies the risk declines to the level of never smokers within 5–10 years, but some studies report increased risk—though markedly lower than among continuous smokers—even after 15 years of abstinence, but. The risk reduction can be observed after controlling for other major risk factors, and both in normotensive and hypertensive persons. No study has assessed the effect of smoking cessation on the long-term prognosis among cerebrovascular disease patients. However, among stroke patients smoking was a strong predictor of survival in 7.5 years of follow-up.

Abdominal Aortic Aneurysm (AAA)

Introduction

Cigarette smoking is the strongest independent risk factor for AAA and accounts for about 75% of AAA (USDHHS, 1989; Lederle et al., 1997). A strong and consistent dose-response relationship between smoking and the risk of AAA has been documented in the literature (USDHHS, 1983), including increased risk with greater daily amount of smoking (Doll et al., 1994) and longer duration (Vardulaki et al., 2000; Singh et al., 2001). Other important risk factors for AAA include male gender, age, atherosclerosis and a family history of AAA. There is an inverse relationship with diabetes (Lederle et al., 1997; Blanchard et al., 2000; Lederle et al., 2000). The relationships between hypertension and hyperlipidemia and AAA are less established (Blanchard et al., 2000).

AAA has traditionally been attributed to atherosclerosis, but atherosclerosis and its various disease manifestations (e.g. coronary artery disease, cerebrovascular disease and peripheral arterial disease) are more prevalent than AAA, contributing to the hypothesis that the pathogenesis of AAA may be different from other forms of vascular disease (Patel et al., 1995; Powell & Greenhalgh, 2003). The magnitude of AAA risk associated with smoking is 2–3 times greater than the association of smoking with other atherosclerotic diseases (except peripheral arterial disease) (Lederle et al., 2003), and in contrast to coronary artery disease and stroke, the risk of AAA declines more slowly after smoking cessation, and does not reach the risk of a never smoker, even after many years. (Rogot & Murray, 1980; USDHHS, 1989; Doll et al., 1994; Alcorn et al., 1996; Wilmink et al., 1999 ; Vardulaki et al., 2000; Singh et al., 2001; Lederle et al., 2003). These observations on the relationship of smoking and AAA also suggest that etiological factors other than atherosclerosis contribute to AAA.

To evaluate the relationship between smoking cessation and AAA, we describe findings from prospective cohort studies that report associations of smoking status and death from AAA in the general population (Table 7) and ultrasonography screening studies for AAA in high-risk (older) populations (Table 8). Two large AAA intervention trials are also described, as they contribute information about screening and associations with smoking cessation in patients with AAA. There is evidence that patients with AAA who smoke have poorer outcomes, such as death from AAA (UKSATP, 2002) or aneurysm expansion (MacSweeney et al., 1994; Brady et al., 2003), than those who do not smoke. In contrast, however, there are relatively little data to evaluate the effect of smoking cessation on the natural history of AAA disease, or surgical outcomes of AAA repair. The effect of smoking cessation on the rate of aneurysm expansion is important, as aneurysm size increases exponentially, and size is the major risk factor for rupture, which frequently causes death.

Publications between 1966 and 2005, in English, that reported 50 or more aneurysms are included. Smaller studies were excluded because of low statistical power to compare subgroups of current, former and never smokers.

Table 7. Cohort studies: risk of death from abdominal aortic aneurysm (AAA) and smoking cessation

Reference Country	Study	Number of Aneurysm deaths	Duration of Follow-up (Years)	Relative risk of death from AAA Versus never smokers (95% confidence interval)		Comments
				Current smoker	Former smoker	
Rogot & Murray (1980) USA	U.S. Veterans Study 293 958 veterans	1318	16	5.2	2.6	Ratio of observed to expected number of deaths
US DHHS (1989) USA	CPS I >1 million men and women	396	6	4.1 (3.1, 5.4)	2.4 (1.7, 3.3)	
Doll et al. (1994) UK	British Doctors Study 34 440 male physicians	331	40	[4.1]	[2.2]	Values shown are ratios of mortality rates. Death rates in current, former and never smokers were 62, 33 and 15 per 100 000 men respectively.
Tang et al. (1995) Lederle et al. (2003) UK	Whitehall Study, British United Provident Association Study and United Kingdom Heart Disease Prevention Study 56 255 men	143	15	Plain cigarettes [8.5] Filtered cigarettes [7.4]	[1.8]	
Nilson et al. (2001) Sweden	Survey on smoking on a random sample of Swedish census population 41 544 men and women	196	33	Men 3.3 (2.1, 5.2) Women 3.4 (2.1, 5.6)	Men 1.6 (0.9, 2.6) Women 0.4 (0.06, 3.0)	
Lederle et al. (2003) USA	CPS II >1.2 million men and women	1296	14	6.0	2.4	

In brackets [ ]: values calculated by the Working Group.

Table 8. Screening studies: Association of abdominal aortic aneurysm (AAA) and smoking cessation

Reference Country	Study Population Description	Number Screen	AAA cases	Current Smokers (95% CI)	Former Smokers (95% CI)	Never Smokers	Comments
Alcorn et al. (1996) USA	Cardiovascular Health Study Medicare population 1956 men 2785 women 65-90 years	4741	451	% with AAA = 14.4% (66 / 457)	% AAA = 11.5% (237 / 2058)	% with AAA = 6.8% (145 / 2136)	Adjustment by age, sex, height and weight.
Wilmink et al. (1999) UK	Nested case-control study from a population-based screening program Men 50 years or older	Cases 210 Controls 237	210	7.6 (3.3, 17.8) Large AAA 5.8 (1.0, 34.0) Small AAA 12.2 (4.4, 34.0)	3.0 (1.4, 6.4) Large AAA RR = 4.2 (0.9, 19.0) Small AAA 3.9 (1.6, 9.8)	OR=1	Smoking status defined by cotinine assay rather than self-report.
Vardulaki et al. (2000) UK	2203 men 2832 women 65-79 years Screened in controlled randomized trial	5050	127	Rate of AAA = 6.8% 2.7 (1.7, 4.4)	Rate of AAA = 4.2% OR = 1.5 (1.0, 2.3)	Rate of AAA = 1.6% OR= 1 (reference)	OR adjusted for age and sex.
Singh et al. (2001) Norway	Tromso Study population-based 2962 men 3424 women ≥25 years	6386	337	Men 7.4 (3.7, 14.7) Women 5.8 (2.9, 11.6)	Men 3.6 (1.9, 7.0) Women 1.64 (0.8, 3.6)	OR=1 OR=1	Age and cardiovascular risk factors adjustment done.

Is the risk of disease lower in former smokers than in current smokers?

Prospective cohort studies, screening studies and the data from the screening phase of one clinical trial contribute information on this question.

Prospective cohort studies

Details from individual prospective cohort studies regarding population size, number of aneurysms detected, length of follow-up, and risk of AAA in current and former smokers compared with never smokers are presented in Table 7. Prospective cohort studies report the risk of death from a number of health conditions, including AAA, by smoking status. Methodological limitations include that smoking status data is generally provided by self-report, and data are often incomplete with regard to the duration of smoking cessation and amount of past smoking. In addition, it is not possible to determine the potential temporal relationship between smoking cessation and course of disease.

Early data comparing the risk of death from AAA in current, former and never smokers were reviewed in the 1990 U.S. Surgeon General's Report on the Benefits of Smoking Cessation (USDHHS, 1990). The excess risk of death from AAA was approximately 50% lower among former smokers than current smokers, but remained 2–3 times higher than that among never smokers.

This report included data from the Cancer Prevention Study (CPS) I and CPS II. In CPS I, current male smokers had a relative risk of death from AAA of 4.11 (95% CI = 3.13–5.40) compared to 2.4 (95% CI = 1.73–3.34) in former smokers (USDHHS, 1989). CPS II reported a higher risk in current smokers (6.0) but a similar relative risk in former smokers (2.4) (Lederle et al., 2003). In 1994 Doll found the death rate from AAA in current male smokers (any tobacco) to

be 62/100 000, compared to 33/100 000 in former smokers and 15/100 000 in never smokers after 40 years of follow-up (Doll et al., 1994). There were 1318 reported deaths from AAA in the U.S. Veterans Health Study, and the observed to expected (O:E) ratio was 5.23 for current smokers and 2.58 for former smokers.

Data not available in the 1990 Surgeon General's Report include a Norwegian study showing a relative risk of death from AAA among men of 3.30 (95% CI = 2.1–5.2) in current smokers and 1.6 (95% CI = 0.9–2.6) in former smokers. The risk among women was 3.4 (95% CI = 2.1–5.6) in current smokers and 0.42 (95% CI = 0.06–3.0) in former smokers; however, there was only one death reported among women (Nilsson et al., 2001). Results from a study of four combined cohorts by Tang et al. show a similar pattern (Table 7) (Lederle et al., 2003; Tang et al., 1995).

In the general or high-risk populations
Screening studies

Screening studies with ultrasonography have been conducted to determine the prevalence of AAA in both general and selected populations, and some protocols included detailed smoking histories. Screening studies report prevalent AAA disease; since AAA may be present for a long, asymptomatic period prior to diagnosis, it is difficult to evaluate the relationship between smoking cessation and risk reduction from the prevalence data. With rare exceptions, studies determine smoking status by self-report, and there is a variable amount of information about the duration of cessation and amount of past smoking. Other methodological limitations include a lack of agreement about the aortic dimensions that define AAA at the small end of the spectrum, and these different definitions of what constitutes an AAA can dramatically affect the reported rates of disease.

Alcorn et al. screened 4741 participants in the Cardiovascular Health Study, a population-based longitudinal study of cardiovascular risk factors in individuals 65 years of age or older (Alcorn et al., 1996). They found a total of 451 aneurysms: 14.4% in current smokers, 11.5% in former smokers and 6.8% in never smokers (unadjusted and adjusted p-values <0.0001). Singh reported similar results from men and women screened in Tromso, Norway (Singh et al., 2001). Among men, former smokers had an OR of 3.6 (95% CI=1.9–7.0, p<0.001) of AAA compared with current smokers (OR=7.4, 95% CI=3.7–14.7, p<0.001). A similar pattern of results was observed in women (former smokers, OR=1.6, 95% CI=0.8–3.6; current smokers, OR=5.8, 95% CI=2.9–11.6). Simoni and co-workers also reported results from a screening trial where nonsmokers had the highest likelihood of normal aortic dimensions (comprising 11.3% of AAA cases), followed by former smokers (49.5%) and current smokers (39.2%, p<0.001) (Simoni et al., 1995).

Lederle et al. have conducted a large randomized controlled trial to test the effect of early surgical intervention compared with surveillance for small AAA. They have published two reports of the screening process that describe the prevalence of and risk factors for AAA, including the effect of smoking and smoking cessation (Lederle et al., 1997; Lederle et al., 2000). The data contribute information regarding the number of years since smoking cessation among former smokers, and the association of smoking status with aneurysm size. In the combined group, 18.4% of participants were current smokers, and 74.8% reported ever smoking regularly (ex-smoking rate 56.4%). The first publication describes 1 031 aneurysms diagnosed in 73 451 veterans screened. The OR of smoking for aortic diameter 3.0–3.9 cm was 2.7 (95% CI=2.4–3.1) and for aortic diameter 4.0 cm or greater was 5.6 (95% CI=4.2–7.3) compared with subjects with normal aortic diameter.

In patients with AAA
Intervention trials
Two large randomized controlled trials designed to test surgical interventions for AAA have been completed (UKSATP, 2002; Lederle *et al.*, 2002). Screening results and baseline data from these studies provide measures of AAA prevalence, and trial protocols provide an opportunity to follow aneurysms over time by smoking status. Both trials collected detailed smoking histories at baseline; one followed smoking status in a subgroup of patients with AAA 12 months after randomization (UKSATP, 2002).

The United Kingdom Small Aneurysm Trial showed that early, prophylactic elective surgery did not improve short-term survival in 1090 patients with small abdominal aneurysms compared with surveillance; however, long-term survival was improved in the early surgery group (at eight years of follow-up the early surgery group showed a survival advantage of 7.2 percentage points over the surveillance group, p=0.03)(UKSATP, 2002). Of note, there was a significant increase in the rate of smoking cessation in the early surgery group (the prevalence of smoking decreased from 58% to 28% compared with 58% to 48% in the surveillance group, p=0.002). The adjusted risk of death in continuing smokers was significantly elevated over that of former smokers (1.25, 95% CI=1.0–1.5). Former smokers had risk similar to that of never smokers (1.25, 95% CI=0.88–1.0). Surgical repair of AAA was the only factor independently positively associated with smoking cessation (OR=12.8, 95% CI=4.2–38.9, p<0.001). The investigators speculate that improved long-term survival in the early surgery group may be due to lifestyle changes such as smoking cessation.

This trial also reported the rate of aneurysm expansion and rupture by smoking status, including 1167 patients with aneurysms who were not enrolled in the trial (total n=2 257). The adjusted hazard ratio for rupture among those with an aneurysm was significantly reduced in former smokers compared with current smokers (HR=0.59, 95% CI=0.39-0.89, p=0.01)(UKSATP, 1999). They further reported a significant association between improved survival and decreased AAA rupture rate and former smoking or nonsmoking status (UKSATP, 2000). At randomization 37% of patients smoked, 57% were former smokers and 6% had never smoked. Survival analysis showed that current smokers had worse survival than former smokers (p=0.02), but this finding was no longer significant after adjustment for baseline characteristics. When smoking status was defined by serum cotinine measures rather than self-report, current smoking was associated with increased mortality (adjusted HR=1.08; 95% CI=1.01–1.15, p=0.02), but this method to define smoking status did not permit analysis of the effect of smoking cessation on risk. This analysis documents a considerable rate of misreporting of smoking status in this population.

Is the risk of disease lower with more prolonged abstinence?

Two studies provide insight regarding the relationship between the duration of abstinence from smoking and risk of AAA. In the U.S. Veterans Study there was a dose-response relationship between the amount of past smoking and risk of death from AAA. The mortality ratio for past smokers of 40 or more cigarettes per day was 3.8; 3.1 for 21–39 cigarettes per day, 2.7 for 10–20 cigarettes per day and 1.6 for <10 cigarettes per day (Rogot & Murray, 1980). In addition, mortality ratios were highest for

current smokers (approximately 5), low for those who stopped for less than 5 years (approximately 1), highest for those who had stopped for 5–9 years and 10–14 years (about 3.5 and 4 respectively), and decreased (approximately 2.5) for 15–19 years of cessation; however, the mortality ratio remained elevated as long as 20 years after stopping smoking (1.8) (estimates from bar graph; this manuscript did not provide exact figures or confidence intervals for ratios). The mortality ratio for former smokers with 8.5 years of cessation was 2.75, and 2.58 for those with 16 years duration of cessation (Rogot & Murray, 1980).

A nested case-control study by Wilmink et al. confirms the benefits of smoking cessation and also showed that the duration of smoking cessation is significantly negatively associated with the risk of AAA (Wilmink *et al.*, 1999). Each year of smoking increased the relative risk of AAA by 4% (95% CI=2-6%, p<0.001), but the longer the period since cessation, the smaller the risk of AAA in a model unadjusted for the duration of smoking (p=0.004). Compared with continuous smoking, the relative risk of AAA in former smokers, adjusted for the duration of smoking, was 0.62 for 1–5 years of cessation (95% CI=0.2–1.7), 0.47 for 6–10 years (95% CI=0.2–1.3), 0.61 for 11–20 years (95% CI=0.3–1.3), 0.28 for 21–30 years (95% CI=0.1–0.7) and 0.20 for >30 years (95% CI=0.1–0.4). This finding was not significant after adjustment for the duration of smoking. The magnitude of the relative risks for small and large aneurysms differed in current but not in former smokers (5.8, 95% CI =1.0–34.0 versus 12.2, 95% CI=4.4–34.0 in current smokers and 3.9, 95% CI=1.6–9.8 versus 4.2, 95% CI 0.9–19.0 in former smokers, respectively).

A study by Vardulaki *et al.* shows a similar pattern; however, this analysis confirms a dose-response relationship between the amount of cigarettes smoked in the past and risk of AAA (Vardulaki *et al.,* 2000). The prevalence of AAA in never smokers was 1.6%, compared to 2.4% in past smokers of 1–19 cigarettes per day, 5.0% in past smokers of 20–24 cigarettes per day and 6.2% in past smokers of ≥ 25 cigarettes per day (p<0.001). This study documents a significant trend for increased risk of AAA with increased duration of smoking (p<0.001), notable because the duration of cessation is inversely related to the duration of smoking. The U.S. Veterans Study (Rogot & Murray, 1980) and the nested case-control study by Wilmink *et al.* (1999) strongly suggest that the risk of AAA in former smokers remains significantly greater than that of never smok-

ers as long as 20 years after cessation.

Screening studies by Lederle *et al.* report that the risk of AAA with smoking decreased slowly, but significantly, with the number of years after quitting smoking: for increments of 10 years of cessation, the odds ratios were 0.81 (95% CI= 0.76-0.86) for AAA of 3.0–3.9 cm, and 0.72 (95% CI=0.65-0.79) for AAA of 4.0 cm or more (Lederle *et al.,* 1997). Similar findings were reported for the subsequent 52 475 veterans screened (613 cases of AAA found) (Lederle *et al.,* 2000). The study reported for the first cohort and per increments of 10 years of cessation an odds ratio of 0.78 (95% CI=0.72–0.84) for AAA of 3.0–3.9 cm and 0.73 (95% CI=0.66–0.82) for AAA of 4.0 cm or

larger. Similar values were reported for the second cohort.

Summary

In synthesis, current smokers are more likely to have AAA than are former smokers.

Prospective cohort studies show a higher risk of death from AAA in current smokers compared with never smokers and in former smokers compared with never smokers. The risk of death from AAA in current smokers is greater than that of former smokers.

Peripheral Arterial Disease (PAD)

Introduction

Cigarette smoking is the strongest risk factor for peripheral arterial disease (PAD) in both men and women (USDHHS, 1983). The range of relative risk reported for current smoking and prevalence of PAD is 1.7–13.9 (Willigendael *et al.,* 2004). The prevalence of PAD is greater in men than women and increases with age, duration and intensity of smoking (USDHHS, 1983; Willigendael *et al.,* 2004). Other important risk factors for PAD include hyperlipidemia, diabetes and hypertension (USDHHS, 1983). The association between smoking and PAD is stronger than the association between smoking and cardiovascular or cerebrovascular disease (Fowkes *et al.,* 1992; Leng *et al.,* 1995).

The vast majority of PAD patients who are not current smokers are former smokers, and most studies report the rate of ever smoking in patients with PAD as greater than 90% (USDHHS, 1983).

Due to the high rate of ever smoking, studies of PAD that compare disease risk in current smokers vs. nonsmokers (rather than never smokers) therefore reflect the potential benefits of stopping smoking. In the following discussion of the benefits of smoking cessation for PAD patients, however, we have restricted the review to studies that distinguish between never and former smokers, and compare risks among former smokers to those of current smokers and never smokers unless otherwise noted.

The methods used to define PAD and measure severity of disease are relevant issues to this review. PAD has an asymptomatic phase (that may be diagnosed using physical examination and noninvasive methods) and a symptomatic phase. Symptoms include intermittent claudication (pain with exercise that is relieved by rest), rest pain or manifestations of tissue necrosis (including

ulceration and gangrene). Tissue necrosis is often a precipitating event for revascularization or amputation procedures. Several methods are available to make a diagnosis of PAD. Although physical diagnosis is frequently used in clinical settings, it is relatively insensitive, and research investigations often employ combinations of questionnaire data and objective measures of vascular compromise. Noninvasive measurement methods include calculation of the ankle-brachial index (ABI), a comparison of blood pressures in the lower and upper extremities, and Doppler ultrasound. Invasive methods include traditional or magnetic resonance angiography. The variation in criteria used to establish a diagnosis of PAD likely contributes to some of the heterogeneity of results observed in the studies presented.

Cross-sectional studies and prospective cohort studies have evaluated the relationship between PAD and smoking cessation in the general population. In patients with clinically evident PAD, retrospective and prospective cohort studies contribute data. Follow-up data from prospective cohort studies (and a few randomized controlled trials) that compare medical and surgical outcomes in continuing smokers, former smokers and never smokers are relevant to consideration of the benefits of smoking cessation for risk of PAD.

Only publications that reported on the risk of PAD and include data on current, former and never smoking status are reviewed. Case–control studies that analyzed a minimum of 100 cases and case series that described at least 100 patients are included, unless otherwise noted in the text.

Is the risk of disease lower in former smokers than in current smokers?

In the general or in high risk populations

Cross-sectional studies

Cross-sectional studies confirm the strong risk of current smoking for the prevalence of PAD (range of odds ratios 3.5–16) (Table 9) (Fowkes et al., 1992; Cole et al., 1993; Ingolfsson et al., 1994; Fowler et al., 2002). The odds ratios reported for PAD among former smokers in cross-sectional studies is consistently lower than that for current smoking (range of odds ratios 2.0–7.0) and significantly greater than that of never smokers in some (Fowkes et al., 1992; Cole et al., 1993; Fowler et al., 2002) but not all studies (Lowe et al., 1993; Ingolfsson et al., 1994). The variable methods of diagnosis contribute to the heterogeneous results. For example, PAD is most commonly defined as intermittent claudication, but analyses from the Edinburgh Artery Study (Fowkes et al., 1992; Lowe et al., 1993; Fowkes et al., 1995; Leng et al., 1995; Lee et al.,

1996) include individuals with asymptomatic disease, with a diagnosis established by ABI. In general the risks for current and former smokers obtained in cross-sectional studies are higher than those reported in prospective cohort studies.

Prospective cohort studies in the general population

Two prospective studies compare the risk of former smokers for incident PAD (new cases) to that of never and current smokers (Table 10). Ingolfsson et al. (1994) also calculated the rate ratio for incident PAD (adjusted for blood pressure and total serum cholesterol) among current smokers to that of never smokers to be 2.6 [CI not provided] for 1–14 cigarettes per day, 7.7 for 15–24 cigarettes per day and 10.2 for ≥ 25 cigarettes per day, with the highest rate of disease in current smokers of 15–24 cigarettes per day (p<0.001). Among new cases of PAD (n=96), 94% were current smokers. The ratio of the rate of PAD in former smokers to that in never smokers was 2.3, not statistically significant. In addition, the authors report that the prevalence of PAD declined by 55% from 1968 to 1986 (for patients aged 70 the decline was from 6.7% to 3.1%, and for those aged 60 the decline was from 3.2% to 1.4%). The incidence rate of intermittent claudication declined 66% (for patients aged 70 the decline was from 600 to 204 cases per 100 000 per year, and for those aged 50 the decline was from 166 to 56 cases per 100 000 per year). The decline was attributed to a lower prevalence of smoking and decreased cholesterol levels among Icelandic men (Ingolfsson et al., 1994).

Hooi and colleagues (2001) followed a population of patients who had a positive screen for asymptomatic PAD for 7 years and documented the incidence of developing symptoms by smoking status. Risk was higher in current smokers (OR=2.2, 95%

CI=1.5–3.1) but not in former smokers (OR=0.9, 95% CI =0.6–1.4), adjusted for age, hypertension, diabetes and hypercholesterolemia (Hooi et al., 2001). The authors described additional risk factors including age, hypertension and diabetes, each increasing the likelihood of disease.

In patients with clinically evident PAD

Cohort Studies

A group of cohort studies with varying lengths of follow up (10 months–7 years) has reported on a range of outcomes in patients with PAD (Table 11). Results from many of these early studies were included in the 1990 U.S. Surgeon General's Report on the Benefits of Smoking Cessation (USDHHS, 1990). Quantitative results from several studies are highlighted here. Faulkner et al. reported statistically significant improvement in survival rates over 5 years of follow-up among former smokers compared to continuing smokers (66% vs. 36%, p<0.01) (Faulkner et al., 1983). The progression of intermittent claudication to rest pain, over 6 years, was described by Jonason et al. in two studies (Jonason & Ringqvist, 1985; Jonason & Bergstrom, 1987). No participants who stopped smoking in the cohort progressed to rest pain, compared with 33 of the 156 (21%) who continued to smoke in one cohort (Jonason & Ringqvist, 1985) and 26/315 (8%) in the other cohort (p=0.049) (Jonason & Bergstrom, 1987). Requirement for surgery was more common in smokers than former smokers (p=0.051) (Jonason & Bergstrom, 1987). Similarly, Juergens et al. showed that 11% of continuing smokers required amputation over 5 years from diagnosis, compared to no amputations among those who stopped smoking (Juergens et al., 1960). A small study by Quick et al. of changes in ABI measurements (not included in Table 11) showed that in smokers who stopped, ABI rose

Table 9. Selected cross-sectional studies of peripheral arterial disease (PAD)

Study Reference Country	Study Population	Disease Definition	Cases	Current Smokers	Former Smokers	Comments
				OR (versus Never Smokers) (95% CI)		
Edinburgh Artery Study Fowkes *et al.* (1992) UK	1582 men and women 55–74 years	Intermittent claudication + major and minor asymptomatic disease	418	*Intermittent claudication* 3.7 (1.7, 8.0) *Major asymptomatic* 5.6 (3.0, 10.6) *Minor asymptomatic* 2.4 (1.6, 3.6)	*Intermittent claudication* 3.0 (1.5, 6.3) *Major asymptomatic* 2.8 (1.5, 5.3) *Minor asymptomatic* 1.8 (1.2, 2.7)	Adjusted for age, sex and body-mass index
Reykjavik Study Ingolfsson *et al.* (1994) Iceland	9141 men 34–80 years		96	*Amount smoked* 1–14 cig/d: 10.7 15–24/d: 13.9 25+/d: 8.1	3.5	Adjusted for age
Edinburgh Artery Study Leng *et al.* (1995) UK	1592 men and women 55–74 years	Intermittent claudication + major asympto-matic disease	131	3.9 (2.2, 6.8) *Amount smoked (packs/yr)* < 25 3.7 ≥ 25 6.0	2.2 (1.2, 3.8) *Amount smoked* < 25 1.3 ≥ 25 4.8	Adjusted for age, sex and risk factors (blood pressure, high density lipoprotein)
Fowler *et al.* (2002) Australia	4470 men 65–83 years	Intermittent claudi-cation and/or ABI<0.9	744	3.9 (2.9, 5.1)	2.0 (1.6, 2.4)	Adjusted for age and other risk factors significant in univariate analysis (demo-graphic, lifestyle and medical)

ABI= Ankle brachial systolic pressure index
OR = odds ratio
CI = confidence interval

Table 10. Association of peripheral arterial disease and smoking status: prospective cohort studies reporting incidence

Study Reference Country	N	PAD Cases	Duration Follow-up (Years)	Current Smokers vs. Never Smokers	Former Smokers vs. Never Smokers
				Ratio[2] of Rates (95% confidence interval)	
Reykjavik Study Ingolfsson et al. (1994) Iceland	8045 men	76	18.0	*Cigarettes/day* 1–14 2.6 15–24 7.7** 25 10.2**	2.3
Limburg PAOD Study Hooi et al. (2001)[1] The Netherlands	2327 men and women	245	7.2	2.2 (1.5, 3.1)	0.9 (0.6, 1.4)

**p<0.001

[1]Screening study for asymptomatic and symptomatic PAD in the Netherlands. Incidence reported for new cases diagnosed at follow-up.
[2]Adjusted for other risk factors.

by 8.7 mmHg (change not significant) but decreased by 10.2 mmHg among continuing smokers (p<0.001) (Quick & Cotton, 1982).

Studies of Outcomes of Surgical Intervention

The increasing use of bypass grafts performed to reduce symptoms of PAD and to salvage limbs has provided an opportunity to follow the outcomes of surgical intervention by smoking status. These studies, conducted in patients with existing disease, are of particular interest because factors that alter surgical outcome may be the same as or different from than those that cause PAD. In addition, surgical intervention is important because it is associated with an increased rate of smoking cessation compared with medical management. In a study by Powell et al., patients who underwent vascular reconstruction were more likely to stop smoking (80/121 versus 41/135, p<0.02) than patients who did not (Powell & Greenhalgh, 1990). One-year graft patency was significantly better in the group with

lower thiocyanate level (non-smokers, 84%), than in the group with thiocyanate levels consonant with smoking (63% patent grafts).

A large number of studies compare surgical results in smokers to nonsmokers (including former smokers and never smokers), and the effect of smoking on patency of lower extremity grafts is the topic of a recent meta-analysis (Willigendael et al., 2005). Continued smoking was associated with a threefold (95% CI=2.34–4.08, p<0.0001) increase in graft failure compared with those who quit at the time of surgery or those who had quit prior to surgery. There was no difference in patency rate between autogenous and synthetic grafts in the group of smokers (OR=0.9, 95% CI=0.6–1.5). There was an increase in risk among heavy smokers compared with moderate smokers, and the authors found that smoking cessation (motivated at the time of bypass surgery) was associated with graft patency rates (80%–92%) similar to those of never smokers (70%–100%) and significantly better than those of smokers (38%–85%, p=0.003).

The majority of studies do not distin-

guish between never smokers and former smokers, but these data are nevertheless relevant to the benefits of smoking cessation, because the majority of nonsmokers are former smokers. Also, some surgical studies group patients with PAD who reduce smoking with those who become abstinent, making it impossible to formally measure the benefit of cessation. For example, Ameli et al. reported that the rate of limb loss in continuing smokers of >15 cigarettes per day compared with that in never smokers and smokers of 15 cigarettes per day or less was five times greater at two years of graft reconstruction, and three times greater at five years (p=0.013) (note that the reference group includes low-level smokers, former smokers and never smokers) (Ameli et al., 1989).

A relatively small number of studies specifically report surgical outcome results by current, former and never smoking status (Table 12). With one exception that showed no independent effect of smoking on graft patency rates (Green et al., 2000), these studies suggest smokers who quit during the follow-

Table 11. Observational studies of patients with peripheral artery disease (PAD) and smoking cessation

Study Type Reference	Study Population	Duration Follow-up	Number Smokers	Number Quitters	Findings	Statistical Testing
Cohort						
Juergens et al. (1960)	520 men and women Arteriosclerosis obliterans	5	159	71	• 11% of continuing smokers required amputation compared to none in quitters	Not reported
Faulkner et al. (1983)	133 men and women Symptomatic PAD	5	114	42	• Survival in former smokers 66% vs 36% in continuing smokers	p<0.01
Jonason & Bergstrom (1987)	354 men and women Intermittent claudication	7	343	39	• All who developed rest pain (n=26) were smokers compared to none in the former smoker group	p=0.049
					• 31% of smokers and 8% of former smokers underwent surgery	p=0.051
					• In multivariate analysis smoking was only variable significantly associated with surgery	p=0.025
Cross-sectional						
Gardner (1996)	PAD patients	Not applicable	38	100*	• Smokers had more severe claudication (occurred more quickly and persisted longer)	p<0.05
					• At peak exercise, smokers had lower oxygen uptake	p<0.01

*average duration of cessation was 7 days

up period have occlusion rates similar to never smokers. Provan et al. describe the results of 5-year follow-up of 326 patients with aorto-femoral and femoro-popliteal grafts. The patency rate in continuing smokers was 46% (n=130), compared with 80% in former smokers (n=67) and 70% (n=12) in never smokers (p<0.001) (Provan et al., 1987). Robicsek et al. calculated graft occlusion rates per observation month to be 0/502 months in never smokers, 1/448 months in former smokers, 1/342 months in light

smokers and 1/137 months in heavy smokers (Robicsek et al., 1975). A report of 217 patients, 91% of who smoked prior to operation, found that smoking reduction to less than 5 cigarettes per day was associated with a higher graft patency rate than continued smoking (of more than 5 cigarettes per day) (Myers et al., 1978). In this study, post-operative smoking, but not the amount of smoking prior to surgery, had a significant effect on the graft patency rate.

Is the risk of disease lower with more prolonged abstinence?

A study by Fowler et al. describes the relationship of the duration of smoking cessation among former smokers and risk of PAD (Fowler et al., 2002). Overall, former smokers (n=478) had an odds ratio of 2.0 (95% CI 1.6–2.4) compared with never smokers (n=129). Those who had stopped smoking within one year had a persistent elevated risk (OR=5.4, 95% CI=2.4 –11.9) that declined steadily as the number of years since stopping

Table 12. Follow-up of lower extremity bypass grafts in PAD by smoking status

Study	Study design and population	Duration Follow-Up in years	Smokers N	Quitters N	Findings	Statistical Testing
Robicsek et al. (1975)	Prospective cohort Aorto-iliac or aorto-femoral grafts	< 1 to 10	177	95	• Graft occlusion rates Never smokers 0/502 months Former smokers 1/448 months Continuing smokers <1 pack/day : 1/342 months Continuing smokers >1 pack/day : 1/137 months • Patency Never smokers (n=10): 100% Former smokers (n=86): 90% Continuing <1 pack/day (n=44): 85% Continuing >1 pack/day (n=180): 69%	Not reported
Myers et al. (1978)	Retrospective cohort study 217 men and women	5	198	37	• Moderate or heavy smokers before the operation who stopped or reduced to < 5 CPD had higher patency rates than those who continued at >5 CPD • Patency rates for those who stopped smoking 90–95% vs. 65-75% in continuing smokers	$p<0.01$
Provan et al. (1987)	Prospective cohort study 326 men and women	5	314	67	• Patency rates Continuing smokers (n=130): 46% Former smokers (n=67): 80% Never smokers (n=12): 70%	$p<0.01$
Green et al. (2000)	Randomized Clinical Trial 240 patients with pros-thetic above-knee bypass grafting	5	80	Not reported	• Smoking status had no independent effect on patency rates	

CPD = cigarettes per day

Table 13. Case series of thromboangiitis obliterans and smoking cessation

Study	N	Mean Duration Follow-up	Smokers* N (%)	Smokers Who Quit (%)	Findings
Olin *et al.* (1990)	112	92 months	74/89 (83)	43/74 (58.1)	• 2/48 who stopped smoking had amputations vs. 22/48 who continued to smoke, p<0.0001 • Continued disease activity (claudication, rest pain, ulceration, thrombophlebitis) observed in 64% of continuing smokers and in 33% of those who stopped (p=0.001)
Borner & Heidrich (1998)	69	10.7 years	48 (20 not classified)	8/48 (20)	• Among patients who continued to smoke 65% required an amputation; twice the rate required in those who stopped
Shigematsu & Shigematsu (1999)	287	19 years	287	171/287 (59.6)	• No significant difference in continuation of clinical symptoms in smokers vs. former smokers • Amputation rate higher in smokers
Sasaki *et al.* (2000)	850	Not reported	792/850 (93.2)	582/729 (79.8)	In those who continued smoking compared to those who stopped: • OR ulcer formation 1.71 (95% CI 1.19, 2.47), p=0.004 • OR amputation 2.73 (95% CI 1.86, 4.0), p<0.0001 • Fontaine's classification significantly improved (p<0.0001)
Wysokinski *et al.* (2000)	377	3–6.8 years	377	110/236 (46.6)	• Patients who quit smoking had a 50% decrease in disease recurrence compared to period when they smoked

* Note that in some cases patients had to be a smoker as a diagnostic criterion for the diagnosis of thromboangiitis obliterans, therefore the number of smokers equals the number in the cohort.
OR, odds ratio

smoking increased (OR=3.8 for 1–4 years (95% CI=2.5–5.7), OR=3.7 for 5–9 years (95% CI = 2.5–5.3), OR=2.7 for 10-19 years (95% CI=2.0–3.6) and OR =1.3 (95% CI=1.0–1.7) for 20 or more years). This suggests that the risk for PAD in former smokers does not return to that of never smokers, even after prolonged abstinence.

In addition, Leng *et al.* showed that the amount (amount and duration of exposure) of smoking prior to cessation had an important effect on risk reduction. Former smokers who had a smoking history of 25 pack-years or more retained a high odds ratio for disease (OR=4.8) compared with never smokers, while former smokers who had a history of 24 pack-years or less had an odds ratio virtually identical to that of never smokers (OR=1.3) (Leng *et al.*, 1995).

The cohort studies following patients with clinically evident PAD suggest the benefits of smoking cessation in patients with disease, especially those who undergo surgery, are evident in 1–5 years of follow-up (Tables 11 and 12), a relatively short time period.

Thromboangiitis Obliterans

Thromboangiitis obliterans (Buerger disease) is an inflammatory obliterative disease of small and medium arteries, and is not related to atherosclerosis. The disorder is uncommon (0.5–5% as common as occlusive arterial disease) but of considerable interest because of its close relationship with smoking. It is typically a disease of young men who use tobacco; in fact, most diagnostic criteria preclude making the diagnosis of thromboangiitis obliterans in non-smokers. It is more common in men than women, and more common in Asia (and

Japan in particular) than in Western Europe and the United States. It is characterized by a relatively early onset (in the thirties or forties) and rapid progression to claudication, rest pain, ulceration, and tissue necrosis which often necessitates minor and major amputations. Pathological examinations show inflammatory cellular infiltrates in segmental arterial lesions that lead to thrombosis and vascular occlusion.

The literature provides data from case series that address the effect of smoking cessation on the course of thromboangiitis obliterans. Some series are from convenience samples (and therefore subject to selection bias), and others follow patients entered in national registries. The studies report variable lengths of follow-up, and some are limited by small sample sizes and poor response rates at the time of follow-up. Detailed smoking histories, including the time course and duration of smoking cessation, are generally not available.

In spite of these methodological limitations, these studies show a consistent benefit of smoking cessation (Table 13). Evidence of benefit includes a lower rate of symptoms of ischemia such as claudication (Olin *et al.,* 1990; Sasaki *et al.,* 2000; Wysokinski *et al.,* 2000), ulceration

(Olin *et al.,* 1990; Sasaki *et al.,* 2000) and amputation (Olin *et al.,* 1990; Borner & Heidrich, 1998; Shigematsu & Shigematsu, 1999; Sasaki *et al.,* 2000; Wysokinski *et al.,* 2000). In aggregate these descriptive studies suggest a benefit of smoking cessation for patients with clinically evident thromboangiitis obliterans, but their small sizes preclude estimation of the amount of risk reduction. In addition it is not possible to assess the time course of attaining benefit, the role of other contributing factors or the importance of the duration or intensity of smoking. Anecdotally, however, many authors comment that disease activity quickly becomes quiescent in patients who stop smoking.

Summary

In synthesis, in populations without clinically evident disease, current smoking has a consistent and strong relationship with PAD. Former smokers have a reduced risk compared with current smokers, and former smokers are at higher risk than never smokers. Estimates of risk among former smokers vary, in part due to heterogeneous study methods.

Data that address the time course of the change in risk with cessation are very limited, and the time course is different for populations with and without clinically evident disease. They suggest the reduction in risk of development of disease occurs over an extended period (at least 20 years). Prospective cohort studies suggest that the risk of PAD in former smokers remains greater than that of never smokers.

Although there are important limitations to prospective cohort studies conducted in patients with clinical evidence of PAD, results suggest an improvement in clinical outcomes among former smokers compared to continuing smokers. In contrast to populations without clinically evident disease, patients with PAD who stop smoking experience complication rates that are similar to nonsmokers in a relatively short period of time. The benefits of smoking cessation for patients with disease have been observed in studies with 1–5 years of follow-up. This suggests there are important benefits of smoking cessation for patients with established PAD.

References

Abbott RD, Yin Y, Reed DM, et al. (1986). Risk of stroke in male cigarette smokers. *N Engl J Med,* 315(12):717-720.

Aberg A, Bergstrand R, Johansson S, et al. (1983). Cessation of smoking after myocardial infarction. Effects on mortality after 10 years . *Br Heart J,* 49(5):416-422.

Alcorn HG, Wolfson SK, Jr., Sutton-Tyrrell K, et al. (1996). Risk factors for abdominal aortic aneurysms in older adults enrolled in The Cardiovascular Health Study. *Arterioscler Thromb Vasc Biol,* 16(8):963-970.

Ameli FM, Stein M, Provan JL, et al. (1989). The effect of postoperative smoking on femoropopliteal bypass grafts. *Ann Vasc Surg,* 3(1):20-25.

Anderson CS, Feigin V, Bennett D, et al. (2004). Active and passive smoking and the risk of subarachnoid hemorrhage: an international population-based case-control study. *Stroke,* 35(3):633-637.

Anthonisen NR, Skeans MA, Wise RA, et al. (2005). The effects of a smoking cessation intervention on 14.5-year mortality: a randomized clinical trial. *Ann Intern Med,* 142(4):233-239.

Asia Pacific Cohort Studies Collaboration (2005). Smoking, quitting, and the risk of cardiovascular disease among women and men in the Asia-Pacific region. *Int J Epidemiol,* 34(5):1036-1045.

Baughman KL, Hutter AM, Jr., DeSanctis RW, et al. (1982). Early discharge following acute myocardial infarction. Long-term follow-up of randomized patients. *Arch Intern Med,* 142(5):875-878.

Bednarzewski J (1984). [Does stopping tobacco smoking affect long-term prognosis after myocardial infarction?]. *Wiad Lek,* 37(8):569-576. [in Polish]

Ben Shlomo Y, Smith GD, Shipley MJ, et al. (1994). What determines mortality risk in male former cigarette smokers? *Am J Public Health,* 84(8):1235-1242.

Blanchard JF, Armenian HK, Friesen PP (2000). Risk factors for abdominal aortic aneurysm: results of a case-control study. *Am J Epidemiol,* 151(6):575-583.

Bonita R, Duncan J, Truelsen T, et al. (1999). Passive smoking as well as active smoking increases the risk of acute stroke. *Tob Control,* 8(2):156-160.

Borner C, Heidrich H (1998). Long-term follow-up of thromboangiitis obliterans. *Vasa,* 27(2):80-86.

Bosetti C, Negri E, Tavani A, et al. (1999). Smoking and acute myocardial infarction among women and men: A case-control study in Italy. *Prev Med,* 29(5):343-348.

Brady AR, Thompson SG, Greenhalg RM, et al. (2003). Cardiovascular risk factors and abdominal aortic aneurysm expansion: only smoking counts. *Br J Surg,* 90(492):493.

Burns DM, Shanks TG, Choi W, et al. (1997). The American Cancer Society Cancer Prevention Study I: 12-Year Follow-up of 1 Million Men and Women. In: Burns DM, Garfinkel L, Samet J, eds., *Changes in cigarette-related disease risk and their implication for prevention and control.* Bethesda, MD, National Cancer Institue: 113-304.

Burr ML, Holliday RM, Fehily AM, et al. (1992). Haematological prognostic indices after myocardial infarction: evidence from the diet and reinfarction trial (DART). *Eur Heart J,* 13(2):166-170.

Cederlof R, Friberg L, Hrubec Z, et al. (1975). *The Relationship of Smoking and Some Social Covariables to Mortality and Cancer Morbidity. A ten year follow-up in a probability sample of 55,000 subjects, age 18–69.* Stockholm, The Karolinska Institute, Department of Environmental Hygiene.

Colditz GA, Bonita R, Stampfer MJ, et al. (1988). Cigarette smoking and risk of stroke in middle-aged women. *N Engl J Med,* 318(15):937-941.

Cole CW, Hill GB, Farzad E, et al. (1993). Cigarette smoking and peripheral arterial occlusive disease. *Surgery,* 114(2):753-756.

Cook DG, Shaper AG, Pocock SJ, et al. (1986). Giving up smoking and the risk of heart attacks. A report from The British Regional Heart Study. *Lancet,* 2(8520):1376-1380.

Corrigan M, Cupples ME, Stevenson M (2002). Quitting and restarting smoking: cohort study of patients with angina in primary care. *BMJ,* 324(7344):1016-1017.

Critchley JA, Capewell S (2003). Mortality risk reduction associated with smoking cessation in patients with coronary heart disease: a systematic review. *JAMA,* 290(1):86-97.

Critchley J, Capewell S (2004). Smoking cessation for the secondary prevention of coronary heart disease. *Cochrane Database Syst Rev,* (1):CD003041.

Dagenais GR, Yi Q, Lonn E, et al. (2005). Impact of cigarette smoking in high-risk patients participating in a clinical trial. A substudy from the Heart Outcomes Prevention Evaluation (HOPE) trial. *Eur J Cardiovasc Prev Rehabil,* 12(1):75-81.

Daly LE, Mulcahy R, Graham IM, et al. (1983). Long term effect on mortality of stopping smoking after unstable angina and myocardial infarction. *Br Med J,* 287(6388):324-326.

Dobson AJ, Alexander HM, Heller RF, et al. (1991). How soon after quitting smoking does risk of heart attack decline? *J Clin Epidemiol,* 44(11):1247-1253.

Doll R, Peto R (1976). Mortality in relation to smoking: 20 years' observations on male British doctors. *BMJ,* 2(6051):1525-1536.

Doll R, Peto R, Wheatley K, et al. (1994). Mortality in relation to smoking: 40 years' observations on male British doctors. BMJ, 309(6959):901-911.

Doll R, Peto R, Boreham J, et al. (2004). Mortality in relation to smoking: 50 years' observations on male British doctors. *BMJ,* 328(7455):1519.

Donnan GA, McNeil JJ, Adena MA, et al. (1989). Smoking as a risk factor for cerebral ischaemia. *Lancet,* 2(8664):643-647.

Faulkner KW, House AK, Castleden WM (1983). The effect of cessation of smoking on the accumulative survival rates of patients with symptomatic peripheral vascular disease. *Med J Aust,* 1(5):217-219.

Fowkes FG, Housley E, Riemersma RA, et al. (1992). Smoking, lipids, glucose intolerance, and blood pressure as risk factors for peripheral atherosclerosis compared with ischemic heart disease in the Edinburgh Artery Study. *Am J Epidemiol*, 135(4):331-340.

Fowkes FG, Dunbar JT, Lee AJ (1995). Risk factor profile of nonsmokers with peripheral arterial disease. *Angiology*, 46(8): 657-662.

Fowler B, Jamrozik K, Norman P, et al. (2002). Prevalence of peripheral arterial disease: persistence of excess risk in former smokers. *Aust N Z J Public Health*, 26(3):219-224.

Friedman GD, Tekawa I, Sadler M, et al. (1997). Smoking and mortality: The Kaiser Permanente experience. In: Burns D, Garfinkel L, Samet J, eds., *Changes in Cigarette-related Disease Risks and their Implications for Prevention and Control*. Bethesda MD, National Cancer Institute: 477-497.

Godtfredsen NS, Osler M, Vestbo J, et al. (2003). Smoking reduction, smoking cessation, and incidence of fatal and non-fatal myocardial infarction in Denmark 1976-1998: a pooled cohort study. *J Epidemiol Community Health*, 57(6):412-416.

Goldenberg I, Jonas M, Tenenbaum A, et al. (2003). Current smoking, smoking cessation, and the risk of sudden cardiac death in patients with coronary artery disease. *Arch Intern Med*, 163(19):2301-2305.

Green RM, Abbott WM, Matsumoto T, et al. (2000). Prosthetic above-knee femoropopliteal bypass grafting: five-year results of a randomized trial. *J Vasc Surg*, 31(3):417-425.

Greenwood DC, Muir KR, Packham CJ, et al. (1995). Stress, social support, and stopping smoking after myocardial infarction in England. *J Epidemiol Community Health*, 49(6):583-587.

Gupta R, Gupta KD, Sharma S, et al. (1993). Influence of cessation of smoking on long term mortality in patients with coronary heart disease. Indian Heart J, 45(2):125-129.

Hallstrom AP, Cobb LA, Ray R (1986). Smoking as a risk factor for recurrence of sudden cardiac arrest. *N Engl J Med*, 314(5):271-275.

Hamsten A (1993). The hemostatic system and coronary heart disease. *Thromb Res*, 70(1):1-38.

Hasdai D, Garratt KN, Grill DE, et al. (1997). Effect of smoking status on the long-term outcome after successful percutaneous coronary revascularization. *N Engl J Med*, 336(11):755-761.

Hedback B, Perk J, Wodlin P (1993). Long-term reduction of cardiac mortality after myocardial infarction: 10-year results of a comprehensive rehabilitation programme. *Eur Heart J*, 14(6):831-835.

Herlitz J, Bengtson A, Hjalmarson A, et al. (1995). Smoking habits in consecutive patients with acute myocardial infarction: prognosis in relation to other risk indicators and to whether or not they quit smoking. *Cardiology*, 86(6):496-502.

Hjermann I, Holme I, Leren P (1986). Oslo Study Diet and Antismoking Trial. Results after 102 months. *Am J Med*, 80(2A):7-11.

Hooi JD, Kester AD, Stoffers HE, et al. (2001). Incidence of and risk factors for asymptomatic peripheral arterial occlusive disease: a longitudinal study. *Am J Epidemiol*, 153(7):666-672.

Hrubec Z, McLaughlin JK (1997). Former cigarette smoking and mortality among U.S. Veterans: A 26-year followup, 1954 to 1980. In: Burns DM, Garfinkel L, Samet J, eds., *Changes in Cigarette-related Disease Risks and Their Implication for Prevention and Control*. Bethesda MD, National Institutes of Health, National Cancer Institute: 501-530.

Hurley SF (2005). Short-term impact of smoking cessation on myocardial infarction and stroke hospitalisations and costs in Australia. *Med J Aust*, 183(1):13-17.

Ingolfsson IO, Sigurdsson G, Sigvaldason H, et al. (1994). A marked decline in the prevalence and incidence of intermittent claudication in Icelandic men 1968-1986: a strong relationship to smoking and serum cholesterol--the Reykjavik Study. *J Clin Epidemiol*, 47(11):1237-1243.

Iso H, Date C, Yamamoto A, et al. (2005). Smoking cessation and mortality from cardiovascular disease among Japanese men and women: the JACC Study. Am J Epidemiol, 161(2):170-179.

Jacobs DR, Jr., Adachi H, Mulder I, et al. (1999). Cigarette smoking and mortality risk: twenty-five-year follow-up of the Seven Countries Study. *Arch Intern Med*, 159(7):733-740.

Jee SH, Suh I, Kim IS, et al. (1999). Smoking and atherosclerotic cardiovascular disease in men with low levels of serum cholesterol: the Korea Medical Insurance Corporation Study. *JAMA*, 282(22):2149-2155.

Johansson S, Bergstrand R, Pennert K, et al. (1985). Cessation of smoking after myocardial infarction in women. Effects on mortality and reinfarctions. *Am J Epidemiol*, 121(6):823-831.

Johnston SC, Gress DR, Browner WS, et al. (2000). Short-term prognosis after emergency department diagnosis of TIA. *JAMA*, 284(22):2901-2906.

Jonason T, Ringqvist I (1985). Factors of prognostic importance for subsequent rest pain in patients with intermittent claudication. *Acta Med Scand*, 218(1):27-33.

Jonason T, Bergstrom R (1987). Cessation of smoking in patients with intermittent claudication. Effects on the risk of peripheral vascular complications, myocardial infarction and mortality. *Acta Med Scand*, 221(3):253-260.

Juergens JL, Barker NW, Hines EA, Jr. (1960). Arteriosclerosis obliterans: review of 520 cases with special reference to pathogenic and prognostic factors. Circulation, 21:188-195.

Kawachi I, Colditz GA, Stampfer MJ, et al. (1993). Smoking cessation and decreased risk of stroke in women. *JAMA*, 269(2):232-236.

Kawachi I, Colditz GA, Stampfer MJ, et al. (1994). Smoking cessation and time course of decreased risks of coronary heart disease in middle-aged women. *Arch Intern Med*, 154(2):169-175.

Kawachi I, Colditz GA (1997). Smoking cessation and decreased risk of total mortality, stroke and coronary heart disease incidence in women a prospective cohort study. In: Burns DM, Garfinkel L, Samet J, eds., *Changes in cigarette related disease risks and their implications for prevention and control. Bethesda MD, National Institutes of Health.* 531-565.

Kiechl S, Werner P, Egger G, et al. (2002). Active and passive smoking, chronic infections, and the risk of carotid atherosclerosis: prospective results from the Bruneck Study. *Stroke,* 33(9):2170-2176.

Kuller LH, Ockene JK, Meilahn E, et al. (1991). Cigarette smoking and mortality. MRFIT *Research Group. Prev Med*, 20(5):638-654.

LaCroix AZ, Lang J, Scherr P, et al. (1991). Smoking and mortality among older men and women in three communities. *N Engl J Med,* 324(23):1619-1625.

Lederle FA, Johnson GR, Wilson SE, et al. (1997). Prevalence and associations of abdominal aortic aneurysm detected through screening. Aneurysm Detection and Management (ADAM) Veterans Affairs Cooperative Study Group. *Ann Intern Med,* 126(6):441-449.

Lederle FA, Johnson GR, Wilson SE, et al. (2000). The aneurysm detection and management study screening program: validation cohort and final results. Aneurysm Detection and Management Veterans Affairs Cooperative Study Investigators. *Arch Intern Med,* 160(10):1425-1430.

Lederle FA, Wilson SE, Johnson GR, et al. (2002). Immediate repair compared with surveillance of small abdominal aortic aneurysms. *N Engl J Med,* 346(19):1437-1444.

Lederle FA, Nelson DB, Joseph AM (2003). Smokers' relative risk for aortic aneurysm compared with other smoking-related diseases: a systematic review. *J Vasc Surg,* 38(2):329-334.

Lee AJ, Fowkes FG, Rattray A, et al. (1996). Haemostatic and rheological factors in intermittent claudication: the influence of smoking and extent of arterial disease. *Br J Haematol ,* 92(1):226-230.

Leng GC, Lee AJ, Fowkes FG, et al. (1995). The relationship between cigarette smoking and cardiovascular risk factors in peripheral arterial disease compared with ischaemic heart disease. The Edinburgh Artery Study. *Eur Heart J,* 16(11):1542-1548.

Lowe GD, Fowkes FG, Dawes J, et al. (1993). Blood viscosity, fibrinogen, and activation of coagulation and leukocytes in peripheral arterial disease and the normal population in the Edinburgh Artery Study. *Circulation,* 87(6):1915-1920.

MacSweeney ST, Ellis M, Worrell PC, et al. (1994). Smoking and growth rate of small abdominal aortic aneurysms. *Lancet,* 344(8923):651-652.

Mannami T, Iso H, Baba S, et al. (2004). Cigarette smoking and risk of stroke and its subtypes among middle-aged Japanese men and women: the JPHC Study Cohort I. *Stroke,* 35(6):1248-1253.

Mast H, Thompson JL, Lin IF, et al. (1998). Cigarette smoking as a determinant of high-grade carotid artery stenosis in Hispanic, black, and white patients with stroke or transient ischemic attack. *Stroke,* 29(5):908-912.

McElduff P, Dobson A, Beaglehole R, et al. (1998). Rapid reduction in coronary risk for those who quit cigarette smoking. *Aust N Z J Public Health,* 22(7):787-791.

Multiple Risk Factor InterventionTrial Research Group (1990). Mortality rates after 10.5 years for participants in the Multiple Risk Factor Intervention Trial. Findings related to a priori hypotheses of the trial. *JAMA,* 263(13):1795-1801.

Myers KA, King RB, Scott DF, et al. (1978). The effect of smoking on the late patency of arterial reconstructions in the legs. *Br J Surg,* 65(4):267-271.

Myint PK, Welch AA, Bingham SA, et al. (2006). Smoking predicts long-term mortality in stroke: The European Prospective Investigation into Cancer (EPIC)-Norfolk prospective population study. *Prev Med,* 42(2):128-131.

Neaton JD, Broste S, Cohen L, et al. (1981). The multiple risk factor intervention trial (MRFIT). VII. A comparison of risk factor changes between the two study groups. *Prev Med,* 10(4):519-543.

Negri E, La Vecchia C, D'Avanzo B, et al. (1994). Acute myocardial infarction: association with time since stopping smoking in Italy. GISSI-EFRIM Investigators. Gruppo Italiano per lo Studio della Sopravvivenza nell'Infarto. Epidemiologia dei Fattori di Rischio dell'Infarto Miocardico. *J Epidemiol Community Health,* 48(2):129-133.

Nilsson S, Carstensen JM, Pershagen G (2001). Mortality among male and female smokers in Sweden: a 33 year follow up. *J Epidemiol Community Health,* 55(11): 825-830.

Ockene JK, Kuller LH, Svendsen KH, et al. (1990). The relationship of smoking cessation to coronary heart disease and lung cancer in the Multiple Risk Factor Intervention Trial (MRFIT). *Am J Public Health,* 80(8):954-958.

Olin JW, Young JR, Graor RA, et al. (1990). The changing clinical spectrum of thromboangiitis obliterans (Buerger's disease). *Circulation,* 82(5 Suppl):IV3-IV8.

Osler M, Prescott E, Godtfredsen N, et al. (1999). Gender and determinants of smoking cessation: a longitudinal study. *Prev Med,* 29(1):57-62.

Patel MI, Hardman DT, Fisher CM, et al. (1995). Current views on the pathogenesis of abdominal aortic aneurysms. *J Am Coll Surg,* 181(4):371-382.

Perkins J, Dick TB (1985). Smoking and myocardial infarction: secondary prevention. *Postgrad Med J,* 61(714):295-300.

Peters RW, Brooks MM, Todd L, et al. (1995). Smoking cessation and arrhythmic death: the CAST experience. The Cardiac Arrhythmia Suppression Trial (CAST) Investigators. *J Am Coll Cardiol,* 26(5):1287-1292.

Powell JT, Greenhalgh RM (1990). Changing the smoking habit and its influence on the management of vascular disease. *Acta Chir Scand Suppl,* 555:99-103.

Powell JT, Greenhalgh RM (2003). Clinical practice. Small abdominal aortic aneurysms. *N Engl J Med,* 348(19):1895-1901.

Prescott E, Hippe M, Schnohr P, et al. (1998a). Smoking and risk of myocardial infarction in women and men: longitudinal population study. *BMJ*, 316(7137):1043-1047.

Prescott E, Osler M, Andersen PK, et al. (1998b). Mortality in women and men in relation to smoking. *Int J Epidemiol*, 27(1):27-32.

Provan JL, Sojka SG, Murnaghan JJ, et al. (1987). The effect of cigarette smoking on the long term success rates of aortofemoral and femoropopliteal reconstructions. *Surg Gynecol Obstet*, 165(1):49-52.

Quick CR, Cotton LT (1982). The measured effect of stopping smoking on intermittent claudication. *Br J Surg*, 69 Suppl:S24-S26.

Quist-Paulsen P, Bakke PS, Gallefoss F (2005). Predictors of smoking cessation in patients admitted for acute coronary heart disease. *Eur J Cardiovasc Prev Rehabil*, 12(5):472-477.

Rea TD, Heckbert SR, Kaplan RC, et al. (2002). Smoking status and risk for recurrent coronary events after myocardial infarction. *Ann Intern Med*, 137(6):494-500.

Robbins AS, Manson JE, Lee IM, et al. (1994). Cigarette smoking and stroke in a cohort of U.S. male physicians. *Ann Intern Med*, 120(6):458-462.

Robicsek F, Daugherty HK, Mullen DC, et al. (1975). The effect of continued cigarette smoking on the patency of synthetic vascular grafts in Leriche syndrome. *J Thorac Cardiovasc Surg*, 70(1):107-113.

Rogot E, Murray JL (1980). Smoking and causes of death among U.S. veterans: 16 years of observation. *Public Health Rep*, 95(3):213-222.

Rose G, Hamilton PJ, Colwell L, et al. (1982). A randomised controlled trial of anti-smoking advice: 10-year results. *J Epidemiol Community Health*, 36(2):102-108.

Rose G, Colwell L (1992). Randomised controlled trial of anti-smoking advice: final (20 year) results. *J Epidemiol Community Health,* 46(1):75-77.

Rosenberg L, Kaufman DW, Helmrich SP, et al. (1985). The risk of myocardial infarction after quitting smoking in men under 55 years of age. *N Engl J Med*, 313(24):1511-1514.

Rosenberg L, Palmer JR, Shapiro S (1990). Decline in the risk of myocardial infarction among women who stop smoking. *N Engl J Med*, 322(4):213-217.

Salonen JT (1980). Stopping smoking and long-term mortality after acute myocardial infarction. *Br Heart J,* 43(4):463-469.

Sasaki S, Sakuma M, Yasuda K (2000). Current status of thromboangiitis obliterans (Buerger's disease) in Japan. *Int J Cardiol,* 75 Suppl. 1:S175-S181.

Sato I, Nishida M, Okita K, et al. (1992). Beneficial effect of stopping smoking on future cardiac events in male smokers with previous myocardial infarction. *Jpn Circ J,* 56(3):217-222.

Shigematsu H, Shigematsu K (1999). Factors affecting the long-term outcome of Buerger's disease (thromboangiitis obliterans). *Int Angiol,* 18(1):58-64.

Shinton R, Beevers G (1989). Meta-analysis of relation between cigarette smoking and stroke. *BMJ,* 298(6676):789-794.

Simoni G, Pastorino C, Perrone R, et al. (1995). Screening for abdominal aortic aneurysms and associated risk factors in a general population. *Eur J Vasc Endovasc Surg,* 10(2):207-210.

Singh K, Bonaa KH, Jacobsen BK, et al. (2001). Prevalence of and risk factors for abdominal aortic aneurysms in a population-based study : The Tromso Study. *Am J Epidemiol,* 154(3):236-244.

Sparrow D, Dawber TR (1978). The influence of cigarette smoking on prognosis after a first myocardial infarction. A report from the Framingham study. *J Chronic Dis,* 31(6-7):425-432.

Stegmayr B, Asplund K, Kuulasmaa K, et al. (1997). Stroke incidence and mortality correlated to stroke risk factors in the WHO MONICA Project. An ecological study of 18 populations. *Stroke,* 28(7):1367-1374.

Straus SE, Majumdar SR, McAlister FA (2002). New evidence for stroke prevention: scientific review. *JAMA,* 288(11): 1388-1395.

Tang JL, Morris JK, Wald NJ, et al. (1995). Mortality in relation to tar yield of cigarettes: a prospective study of four cohorts. *BMJ,* 311(7019):1530-1533.

Tell GS, Howard G, McKinney WM, et al. (1989). Cigarette smoking cessation and extracranial carotid atherosclerosis. *JAMA,* 261(8):1178-1180.

Tofler GH, Muller JE, Stone PH, et al. (1993). Comparison of long-term outcome after acute myocardial infarction in patients never graduated from high school with that in more educated patients. Multicenter Investigation of the Limitation of Infarct Size (MILIS). *Am J Cardiol,* 71(12):1031-1035.

Ueshima H, Choudhury SR, Okayama A, et al. (2004). Cigarette smoking as a risk factor for stroke death in Japan: NIPPON DATA80. *Stroke,* 35(8):1836-1841.

United Kingdom Small Aneurysm Trial Participants (1999). Risk factors for aneurysm rupture in patients kept under ultrasound surveillance. UK Small Aneurysm Trial Participants. *Ann Surg,* 230(3):289-296.

United Kingdom Small Aneurysm Trial Participants (2002). Long-term outcomes of immediate repair compared with surveillance of small abdominal aortic aneurysms. *N Engl J Med,* 346(19):1445-1452.

United States Public Health Service Office of the Surgeon General. (1983). *The Health Consequences of Smoking - Cardiovascular Disease: A report of the Surgeon General.* Rockville, Md. Public Health Service, Office on Smoking and Health. No.84-50204:1–385.

United States Public Health Service Office of the Surgeon General. (1989). *Reducing the Health Consequences of Smoking: 25 Years of Progress. A report of the Surgeon General.* Rockville, Md, Public Health Service, Centers for Disease Control and Prevention, Office of Smoking and Health. No. (CDC)89-8411:1–684.

United States Department of Health and Human Service (USDHHS). (1990). *The Health Benefits of Smoking Cessation. A Report of the Surgeon General.* Rockville, Md. centers for Disease Control, Office of Smoking and Health.

van Domburg RT, Meeter K, van Berkel DF, et al. (2000). Smoking cessation reduces mortality after coronary artery bypass surgery: a 20-year follow-up study. *J Am Coll Cardiol,* 36(3):878-883.

Vardulaki KA, Walker NM, Day NE, et al. (2000). Quantifying the risks of hypertension, age, sex and smoking in patients with abdominal aortic aneurysm. *Br J Surg,* 87(2):195-200.

Vlietstra RE, Kronmal RA, Oberman A, et al. (1986). Effect of cigarette smoking on survival of patients with angiographically documented coronary artery disease. Report from the CASS registry. *JAMA,* 255(8):1023-1027.

Voors AA, van Brussel BL, Plokker HW, et al. (1996). Smoking and cardiac events after venous coronary bypass surgery. A 15-year follow-up study. *Circulation,* 93(1):42-47.

Wannamethee SG, Shaper AG, Whincup PH, et al. (1995). Smoking cessation and the risk of stroke in middle-aged men. *JAMA,* 274(2):155-160.

Wen CP, Cheng TY, Lin CL, et al. (2005). The health benefits of smoking cessation for adult smokers and for pregnant women in Taiwan. *Tob Control,* 14 Suppl. 1:i56-i61.

Whisnant JP, Homer D, Ingall TJ, et al. (1990). Duration of cigarette smoking is the strongest predictor of severe extracranial carotid artery atherosclerosis. *Stroke,* 21(5):707-714.

WHO (1999). Making a difference. The World Health Report 1999. *Health Millions,* 25(4):3-5.

WHO (2002). From the World Health Organization. Reducing risks to health, promoting healthy life. *JAMA,* 288(16):1974.

WHO (2006). Why is tobacco a public health priority? *World Health Organization. (http:WHO.INT/tobacco/health-priority). Accessed 13 December 2006.*

Willett WC, Hennekens CH, Bain C, et al. (1981). Cigarette smoking and non-fatal myocardial infarction in women. *Am J Epidemiol,* 113(5):575-582.

Willett WC, Green A, Stampfer MJ, et al. (1987). Relative and absolute excess risks of coronary heart disease among women who smoke cigarettes. *N Engl J Med,* 317(21):1303-1309.

Willigendael EM, Teijink JA, Bartelink ML, et al. (2004). Influence of smoking on incidence and prevalence of peripheral arterial disease. *J Vasc Surg,* 40(6):1158-1165.

Willigendael EM, Teijink JA, Bartelink ML, et al. (2005). Smoking and the patency of lower extremity bypass grafts: a meta-analysis. *J Vasc Surg,* 42(1):67-74.

Wilmink TB, Quick CR, Day NE (1999). The association between cigarette smoking and abdominal aortic aneurysms. *J Vasc Surg,* 30(6):1099-1105.

Wilson K, Gibson N, Willan A, et al. (2000). Effect of smoking cessation on mortality after myocardial infarction: meta-analysis of cohort studies. *Arch Intern Med,* 160(7):939-944.

Wolf PA, D'Agostino RB, Kannel WB, et al. (1988). Cigarette smoking as a risk factor for stroke. The Framingham Study. *JAMA,* 259(7):1025-1029.

Wysokinski WE, Kwiatkowska W, Sapian-Raczkowska B, et al. (2000). Sustained classic clinical spectrum of thromboangiitis obliterans (Buerger's disease). *Angiology,* 51(2):141-150.

Change in Risk of Chronic Obstructive Pulmonary Disease (COPD) After Smoking Cessation

Introduction

It is generally believed that 15–20% of all long-term regular smokers will develop clinically overt chronic obstructive pulmonary disease (COPD), and most COPD cases worldwide are attributable to cigarette smoking. The prevalence of COPD increases with age and smoking habits, and the available data suggest that prevalence is rising in many parts of the world (Mannino et al., 2002 ; Menezes et al., 2005). Studies of the global prevalence of COPD have generally been lacking, but the existing evidence and mortality statistics from the United States demonstrate that COPD will remain a major morbidity and mortality burden for many decades to come. The prevalence of, and death rates due to, COPD are probably underestimated because COPD, in contrast to diseases such as cancer and coronary heart disease, is widely under-diagnosed. The beneficial effects of smoking cessation on reducing chronic respiratory symptoms and slowing the accelerated loss of lung function seen in smokers have been fully demonstrated. However, the effect of smoking cessation in patients with severe COPD and on COPD-related mortality has not been studied extensively.

Effects of smoking cessation on respiratory symptoms

In a study of the natural history of COPD, Fletcher and Peto showed that the presence of respiratory symptoms such as chronic cough and mucus hyper-secretion in subjects without airway limitation was a benign condition that did not progress to COPD (Fletcher & Peto, 1977), and this finding was recently confirmed by data from Copenhagen (Vestbo & Lange, 2002). Nevertheless, the presence of chronic symptoms in subjects with normal lung function is by definition classified as COPD Global Initiative for Chronic Obstructive Lung Disease (GOLD) stage 0, or "subjects at risk for COPD" (NHLBI/WHO, 2003).*

The impact of smoking cessation on respiratory symptoms has been addressed in many studies. In published cross-sectional studies including subjects unselected for chronic respiratory symptoms, the reported prevalence in former smokers have ranged as follows: intermittent cough 5–21%, phlegm 5–30% and wheeze 1–19%; while in smokers the corresponding figures are 10–40%, 10–40% and 7–32% respectively (Rijcken et al., 1987; Sparrow et al., 1987; Viegi et al., 1988; Brown et al., 1991; Lundback et al., 1991; Sherman et al., 1992; Sherrill et al., 1993; Bjornsson et al., 1994; Enright et al., 1994). In these studies, former smokers reported less frequent symptoms than did current smokers, but the prevalence of these symptoms still remains greater than that reported by never smokers. For instance, the Scottish Heart Health Study analysed cross-sectionally the impact of smoking cessation on chronic cough and phlegm in 10 359 men and women by length of tobacco abstinence (Brown et al., 1991). Within a year of quitting smoking, symptom rates were substantially lower than in current smokers, and the symptom rates in former smokers of more than 2-4 years were comparable to those in never smokers. Longitudinal studies support this observation, showing that cough, phlegm and wheeze decrease rapidly after smoking cessation (Wilhelmsen, 1967; Comstock et al., 1970; Buist et al., 1976; Leeder et al., 1977; Buczko et al., 1984; Tashkin et al., 1984; Lange et al., 1990; Barbee et al., 1991), in some studies within a few months.

Dyspnoea is a cardinal symptom of established COPD, but its assessment in studies of the general population imposes several problems. First, the validity of self-reported dyspnoea can be questioned; second, grading of the symptom varies across the studies; and third, dyspnoea can have causes that are other than pulmonary, e.g. heart disease and lack of physical fitness. Thus, the impact of smoking cessation on dyspnoea is not uniform across the studies that have evaluated this symptom, and some studies have shown no effect of stopping smoking compared with continuing smoking (Tashkin et al., 1984; Israel et al., 1988; Krzyzanowski et al., 1993). Disease severity or an increase in body weight after giving up

---

*The GOLD guidelines were revised in November 2006 and are available online at http://www.GOLDCOPD.org.

cigarettes may be a factor in the lack of improvement in dyspnoea. In a cross-sectional study, dyspnoea was found to be more common in severe COPD, while cough and phlegm were more common in milder COPD (von Hertzen *et al.,* 2000). In the Lung Health Study, in which 5887 heavy smokers with mild-to-moderate COPD were followed over 5 years, sustained quitters had the lowest prevalence of 4 symptoms: cough, phlegm, wheezing and dyspnoea (Kanner *et al.,* 1999) compared with continuing smokers and intermittent quitters, and the changes in symptoms occurred mainly in the first year after smoking cessation (Pride, 2001).

Reduction in risk of COPD compared with continuing smokers

More than 20 years have passed since the Surgeon General's Report summarised evidence, which had been emerging since the 1950s, on the harmful effects of smoking on lung function (USDHHS, 1984). Six years later, another report reviewed the health benefits of smoking cessation and identified that substantial reductions in disease risks and disease progression accrue with tobacco abstinence (USDHHS, 1990). When smoking cessation intervention programmes were first initiated, researchers evaluated the impact of quitting smoking on respiratory symptoms and on objective measures of pulmonary function including spirometry and diffusing capacity. Although the evidence in favour of smoking cessation was already overwhelming in the 1990 report, most of the available studies were cross-sectional, small, included selected populations or had short follow-up (less than 2 years).

According to the GOLD criteria for diagnosis and staging of COPD (described earlier in the chapter on Mechanisms) airflow limitation can sim-

ply be assessed using forced expiratory volume in one second (FEV_1) and forced vital capacity (FVC). Fortunately, even the earliest papers describing lung function in relation to smoking cessation used spirometry, which is still considered the "gold standard" for measuring ventilatory capacity in an individual. However, the interpretation of epidemiological evidence concerning changes in lung function after smoking cessation is complicated by factors such as varying standardisation and adjustment in spirometric measurements, different thresholds for defining airway obstruction and failure to adjust for initial level of lung function and cumulative smoking in continuing smokers and for subjects who quit smoking (discussed in detail below). Even though only a minority of smokers get COPD, many smokers have accelerated loss of FEV_1 compared to never smokers. One of the four main conclusions of the 1990 USA Surgeon General's Report was as follows:

"Cigarette smoking accelerates the age-related decline in lung function that occurs among never smokers. With sustained abstinence from smoking, the rate of decline in pulmonary function among former smokers returns to that of never smokers."

Evidence from cross-sectional studies

Data comparing lung function measurements in never smokers, former smokers and current smokers go back more than 40 years (USDHHS, 1990). Cross-sectional surveys based on the general population as well as selected cohorts have uniformly shown that the level of lung function (expressed as either age- and height-adjusted FEV_1 or percentage of predicted value) in former smokers is in between that of never smokers and current smokers. For instance, this was shown in the US Six Cities Study as calculation of residual FEV_1 in never, former and current smokers which

amounted to, respectively, -34 ml, -257 ml and -506 ml for men; and -24 ml, -54 ml and -234 ml for women (Dockery *et al.,* 1988). In the Whitehall Study comprising more than 18 000 male British civil servants, mean FEV_1 levels adjusted for age and height were 3.3, 3.2 and 3.1 in never, former and current smokers respectively and were negatively affected in ever smokers by amount smoked (Higenbottam *et al.,* 1980). Only one study found lower FEV_1 values in former smokers compared to continuing smokers, concluding that this was probably explained by the "healthy smoker effect" (Xu *et al.,* 1994a). It is, however, not possible to draw any definitive inferences about causality from cross-sectional studies.

Evidence from clinical trials and longitudinal, population-based studies

For decades, the continuously emerging results from smoking intervention trials with various lengths of follow-up and large, long-term cohort studies have contributed to a firm base of evidence for assessing the health benefits of stopping smoking on lung function. The major advantage of these studies is repeated measurements of FEV_1 in the same individuals over time, thus allowing calculations of the annual rate of decline in FEV_1, ΔFEV_1 or FEV_1-slope for various degrees of smoking exposure. Furthermore, many of these studies include detailed information on smoking history and habits as well as a number of baseline characteristics, including initial lung function. Those studies that were well-prepared and well-conducted also controlled for other recognized risk factors for COPD or factors known to affect pulmonary function measurement. This section presents a brief description of the most important studies along with their overall results. More specific and detailed effects of smoking cessation on the airways are discussed in subsequent sections. However, while the impact of smoking cessation on the course of FEV_1 has been studied extensively, this is not the case for the increased bronchial hyperresponsiveness that often accompanies COPD or the inflammatory changes in the airways of smokers. An overview of the longitudinal studies of changes in FEV_1 following smoking cessation is given in Table 1.

Further evidence from epidemiologic observational studies supports the cross-sectional hypotheses and findings from the smaller clinical trials that smoking cessation is associated with a less steep FEV_1-decline compared to persistent smoking regardless of the presence of COPD. The best well-known studies are the West London Study (Fletcher & Peto, 1977), the Normative Aging Study (Bossé et al., 1981), the Whitehall Study (Rose et al., 1982), the UCLA study (Tashkin et al., 1984), the Tucson study (Camilli et al., 1987; Sherrill et al., 1994), the Copenhagen City Heart Study (Lange et al., 1989), the Six Cities Study (Xu et al., 1992), the Vlagtwedde-Vlaardingen study (Xu et al., 1994b), the Honolulu Heart Program (Burchfiel et al., 1995), the Finnish cohorts of The Seven Countries Study (Pelkonen et al., 2001), and the European Community Respiratory Health Survey or ECRHS II (Chinn et al., 2005).

In addition, much of our knowledge of smoking cessation and lung function during the last decade comes from the Lung Health Study (LHS) (Table 1). The relevant papers from this ongoing multi-center clinical trial will be addressed in forthcoming sections. Briefly, in 1986–1988 LHS enrolled 5887 asymptomatic smokers with mild to moderate airway obstruction ($FEV_1/FVC < 0.7$ and FEV_1 55-90% of predicted normal value) and randomised them in two groups: one third to receive usual care (UC) and two thirds to receive special intervention (SI), which consisted of intensive smoking cessation assistance. Further, the SI group was split in two groups on the

basis of double-blind prescription of either inhaled bronchodilator (ipratropium bromide) or placebo. Participants were followed with annual spirometry for five years, and 11 years after the first LHS, a new phase (LHS 3) was conducted with repeat spirometry in over 4000 of the original subjects. Cross-sectional and sustained quit rates at five years were 39% and 22% in the SI group and 22% and 5% in the UC group (Anthonisen et al., 1994).

The main outcome variable of interest— annual change in post-bronchodilator FEV_1— was not affected by the inhaled bronchodilator, whereas smoking cessation increased FEV_1 during the first study year; at subsequent visits, the rate of FEV_1-decline in sustained quitters was half the rate observed in continuing smokers (Scanlon et al., 2000). At the 11-year follow-up, results were essentially the same (Anthonisen et al., 2002a; Figure 1). The advantages of this study besides its methodology included the high participation rate in follow-up visits and the ability to identify and adjust for other risk factors for excess loss of lung function (Table 2). Recently, one of the founders of LHS summarized the most important conclusions from the study, stating that smoking cessation largely prevented development of clinically significant COPD and that the beneficial effects were present for both men and women, at all ages and across all levels of baseline lung function (Anthonisen et al., 2004).

A few studies failed to show an overall effect of quitting smoking and smoking cessation intervention, respectively, on FEV_1-decline. The Kaiser-Permanente medical care program was a large study of 9392 persistent smokers and 3825 persons who quit smoking between two multiphasic health checkups (Friedman & Siegelaub, 1980). Self-reported chronic cough improved in those who quit smoking, but there was no difference in change in FEV_1 between the two

groups. The authors concluded that the short follow-up (mean 1.5 years) was responsible for the lack of effect of quitting. MRFIT was a randomised, controlled risk factor intervention trial originally comprising 12 866 men at high risk for coronary heart disease (Browner et al., 1992). Men with doctor-diagnosed COPD were excluded. Spirometry was not standardized in the first two of the 6–7 years of follow-up, which restricted analyses to the latter half of the study (three annual FEV_1-measurements or two measurements two years apart, N = 6347). Overall, the researchers found no difference in rate of loss of FEV_1 in the special smoking cessation intervention group (SI) and the usual care group (UC). However, they found that smokers of 40+ cigarettes/day or 65+ pack-years at study entry in the SI group had a 16% reduction in the rate of FEV_1-decline and a higher final FEV_1 at the 10% significance level compared with the UC group. The authors inferred that reasons for the apparent underestimation of the impact of quitting in lung function included confounding due to usage of β-blocking medication in the SI-group and to the almost equal quit rates in SI and UC participants (33% and 20%, respectively, p<.0001). However, misclassification of tobacco smoking status may also play a role.

Another publication from MRFIT limited the analyses to men who never used β-blocking drugs (N = 4926) and concentrated on comparison of permanent quitters during the first year of the study with continuing smokers (Townsend et al., 1991). The results showed a slower rate of FEV_1-decline of approximately 8 ml/year in quitters compared to sustained smokers. Cross-sectionally, gradually decreasing level of FEV_1 was observed across never smokers, former smokers, quitters, intermittent quitters and continuing smokers (Figure 2).

Another longitudinal study including data on 759 men and 1065 women in

Table 1. Effects of smoking cessation on lung function

Author, reference	Study location Age	No. of subjects	Follow-up after smoking cessation	Effect on FEV$_1$ (ml/yr)	Other lung function tests and comments
Comstock et al, 1970	Baltimore New York Washington DC	670 males 40–59 years	5 years	Loss of FEV$_1$ is less in subjects who quit smoking	
Martin et al, 1975	Quebec	52 subjects 12 subjects studied after smoking cessation	8 weeks	Not examined	Less frequency dependence of dynamic compliance
Bode et al, 1975	Montreal	50 healthy smokers 10 subjects studied after smoking cessation 29-61 years	6–14 weeks	Not examined	Improvements in MEF and lung volumes on cessation
Buist, 1976	Portland Montreal Winnipeg	75 subjects 21–63 years	52 weeks	No significant change	Closing volume /vital capacity (CV/VC) significant improve; Decrease in respiratory symptoms
McCarthy et al, 1976	Manitoba	131 subjects attending a smoking cessation clinic 17–66 years	48 weeks	Significant improvement in FEV$_1$ after 24 weeks	Improved nitrogen washout curve. Improved closing volume & capacity, FVC
Barter & Campbell, 1976	Victoria, Australia	34 subjects with mild chronic bronchitis 45–66 years	5 years	Loss of FEV$_1$ is less in former smokers	
Fletcher & Peto, 1977	London	792 subjects 30–59 years	8 years at 6mo intervals (initial)	% loss of FEV$_1$ similar in former smokers and never smokers	
Bake et al, 1977	Gothenburg	17 subjects 24–77 years	5 months	Significant improvement in FEV$_1$	Significant improvement in VC
Zamel et al, 1979	Toronto	26 healthy smokers 27–45 years	2 months	Significant increase in FEV$_1$	Significant increase in VC & improvement in frequency dependence of lung dynamic compliance
Buist et al, 1979	Portland	15 subjects 21–63 years	30 months	FEV$_1$ improved	VC, CV and slope of single breath N$_2$ test improved
Michaels et al, 1979	Winnipeg	16 never smokers 19 smokers 32–46 years	18 months	Non-significant increase after smoking cessation	Pulmonary elastic recoil decreases after smoking cessation
Friedman et al, 1980	Oakland (Kaiser Permanente)	9392 smokers 3825 quitters 20–79 years	18 months	No sig. difference in FEV$_1$ and FVC between smokers and quitters	Self-reported respiratory symptoms decreased in quitters
Higenbottam et al, 1980	London	18,000 male civil servants 40–64 years	Cross-sectional	Level of FEV$_1$ similar in ex- and never smokers and higher than in current smokers	After smoking cessation: Reduced phlegm Initial improvement in lung function
Bossé et al, 1981	Boston (Normative Aging Study)	850 healthy men aged 20+ years	5 yrs	Greater FEV$_1$ decline in smokers than quitters	No effect of years since quitting on rate of decrease in FEV$_1$ and FVC
Nemery et al, 1982	Brussels	105 current smokers 51 formers smokers 54 never smokers 45–55 years	Cross-sectional	Observed FEV$_1$ in short- and long term former smokers close to never smokers	

Table 1. Effects of smoking cessation on lung function (contd)

Author, reference	Study location	No. of subjects Age	Follow-up after smoking cessation	Effect on FEV_1 (ml/yr)	Other lung function tests and comments
Hughes et al, 1982		56 males with emphysema 45–63 years	3 years	Greater FEV_1 decline in smokers than ex-smokers	Greater VC decline in smokers than former smokers
Tashkin et al, 1984	Los Angeles	2401 subjects 25–64 years	5 years	Improvement in FEV_1	Significant lessened decline in indexes of small airway lung function; Significant improvement in symptoms of cough, wheeze and phlegm production
Postma et al., 1986	Netherlands	81 subjects with chronic airway obstruction 35–60	2–21 years	Slower rate of FEV_1-decline in former than current smokers	
Camilli et al, 1987	Tucson Arizona	General population sample of 1705 subjects 20–90 years	Mean 9.4 years	Former smokers had similar rates of FEV_1 decline as never smokers, whereas quitters (35+ years) had rates in between current smokers and never smokers	In subjects younger than 35 quitting smoking was associated with an increase in FEV_1
Postma & Sluiter, 1989	Netherlands	Group 1: 129 subjects with severe chronic airflow obstruction Group 2: 138 subjects with less severe airflow obstruction Group 3: 81 subjects out of group 2 with a decline of FEV_1 over time 40–63 years	Group 1: 8-12 years Group 2: 2.8-20 years	Regular therapy and smoking cessation showed slower decline in FEV_1	
Lange et al, 1989	Copenhagen	7764 grouped according to self-reported smoking habits 20–93 years	5 years	Demonstrable beneficial effect in FEV_1 decline	
Townsend et al, 1991	Minneapolis (MRFIT)	Multicenter trial of 4926 men 35–57 years at risk for heart disease	6-7 years	Quitters during the first year had less steep rates of decline in FEV_1 than continuing smokers	Analyses were carried out in the latter half of the trial
Sherrill et al, 1993	Arizona	633 males 891 females > 55 years (mean 67)	14 years	FEV_1-decline rates similar in male former and never smokers but faster in female former smokers	Former smokers had better lung function values than current smokers
Leader et al, 1994	Kentucky	18 with mild-to-moderate COPD enrolled; 7 completed study 40–65	28 weeks	No sig changes in FEV_1	Sig decrease in COPD symptomology
Xu et al, 1994b	Netherlands	4554 men and women 15–54 years	24 years	Less steep rates of decline in FEV_1 in quitters compared to continuing smokers	Compared to non-smokers, female former smokers had significant faster FEV_1 decline, whereas male former smokers had slower decline (non-significant)
Burchfiel et al, 1995	Honolulu Richmond Portland	4451 subjects 45–68 years	6 years	Less steep rates of decline in FEV_1 over a short period of time	

Table 1. Effects of smoking cessation on lung function (contd)

Author, reference	Study location	No. of subjects Age	Follow-up after smoking cessation	Effect on FEV_1 (ml/yr)	Other lung function tests and comments
Pelkonen et al, 2001	Seven Countries Study Finland	1711 men Middle-aged (mean 50 years)	30 years	Quitters had a slower decline in $FEV_{0.75}$ than continuous smokers and never smokers	
Chinn et al, 2005	European Community Respiratory Health Survey in 27 countries across Europe	6654 subjects 20-44 years	7-11 years	Decline in FEV_1 lower in male sustained quitters and those who quit between surveys and greater in smokers.	Maximum benefit needs control of weight gain especially in men
Knudson et al, 1989	Tucson	Asymptomatic subjects 190 current smokers 210 former smokers 463 never smokers 15+ years	Single measurement	FEV_1 not measured	Cigarette smoking results in decrease in D_L Reversible and irreversible elements Improvement in D_L following smoking cessation
Sansores et al, 1992	British Columbia Mexico City	16 smokers before and after smoking cessation 29-52 years	Varies between 24 hours to 3 months		Rapid improvement in DL_{CO} in most subjects following smoking cessation. In some subjects, DL_{CO} remain abnormal.
Watson, 1993	London	Cohort of white middle aged men recruited in 1974. 122 men restudied in 1985. 42 current smokers 21 former smokers 17 quitting smokers 42 never smokers	10 years		Smoking cessation reverses reduction in TL_{CO} and TL_{CO}/VA
Watson et al, 2000	London	Changes over 22 years in 84 men: 42 current smokers 42 never smokers Mean 40.5 years	22 years		
Anthonisen et al, 1994	**Lung Health Study** 11 clinical centres in the USA and Canada:	5887 smokers male and female 35-60 yrs Early COPD (FEV_1 55-90%)	5 years	Significant smaller declines in FEV_1 in intervention groups than in control group	
Murray et al, 1998	Cleveland	As above	5 years	As above	Multiple attempts and relapses provides benefits
Scanlon et al, 2000	Detroit Baltimore Rochester Portland Birmingham Los Angeles	3926 smokers with mild-to-moderate airway obstruction	5 years	Improvement in FEV_1	Respiratory symptoms do not predict lung function.
Kanner et al, 2001	Winnipeg Minneapolis Pittsburgh Salt Lake	5887 subjects	5 years	As above	Lower respiratory illnesses promote FEV_1 decline in current (not former) smokers.
Anthonisen et al, 2002a		4517 subjects	Follow up after 11 years	Less decline in FEV_1 in sustained quitters compared to other groups	At 11 years 38% of continuing smokers had an $FEV_1 < 60\%$, compared with 10% of sustained quitters
Connett et al, 2003		3348 men, 1998 women	5 years	FEV_1 improved more in women (3.7% predicted) than in men (1.6%)	Smoking cessation has greater benefits for women with mild COPD

MEF = mean expiratory flow; FVC = forced vital capacity; CV = closing volume; D_L and DL_{CO} = diffusing capacity of carbon monoxide

A

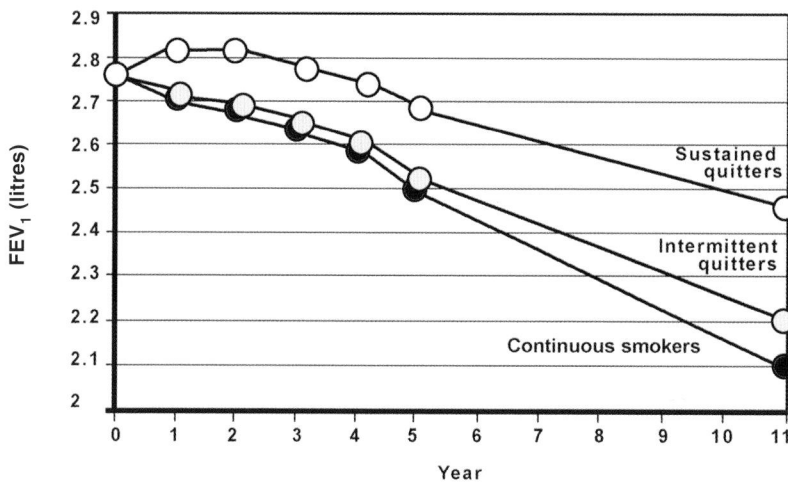

B

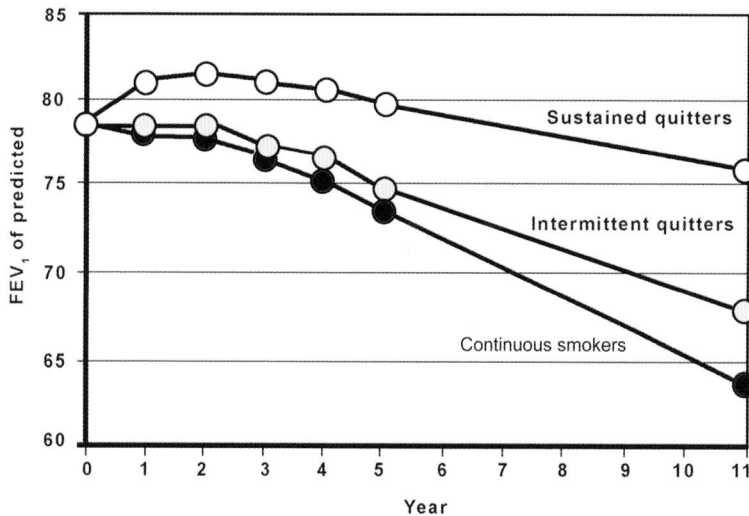

Figure 1. FEV₁ (A) and FEV₁ % (B) predicted value for sustained quitters, intermittent quitters and continuing smokers from the eleven year follow-up of the Lung Health Study

The figures show loss of lung function over the years of the LHS in sustained quitters (open circles), intermittent quitters, (grey circles) and continuing smokers (solid circles). Reported values are average post-bronchiolidator absolute FEV₁ estimates (A) and percentage of predicted normal values (B).

From Anthonisen *et al.* (2002a) Smoking and lung function of Lung Health Study participants after 11 years, *American Journal of Respiratory and Critical Care Medicine*, Vol. 166 (5): 675–679. Official Journal of the American Thoracic Society.

Poland examined twice in 13 years of follow-up found the fastest FEV₁-decline in men who gave up smoking closer to the second examination survey (within 8 years) (Krzyzanowski *et al.*, 1986). Only women who stopped smoking during the first five study years (closer to the baseline examination) experienced a slower rate of loss of FEV₁. These findings were attributed to the fact that many smokers quit due to respiratory or other illnesses.

In conclusion, there is consistent and powerful evidence that smoking cessation slows the smoking-induced accelerated loss of lung function seen in continuing smokers.

The role of intermittent smoking cessation

Some prospective studies have observed that a substantial proportion of the study participants who report quitting smoking subsequently report relapsing or report several more or less successful quit attempts. In a number of papers these subjects are analysed as intermittent quitters, relapsers, recidivists or variable smokers. The effect of this smoking behaviour on lung function decline compared to sustained smokers or quitters is not clear. Comparison of the studies is somewhat hampered by differences in adjustment for cumulative tobacco consumption. In a small sub-sample of the Tucson study, the 71 intermittent quitters actually had a faster FEV₁-decline than consistent smokers after controlling for amount smoked (Sherrill *et al.*, 1996). Also, a study in the Netherlands found that intermittent smokers did not differ from continuing smokers in terms of lung function loss (Xu *et al.*, 1994b). In contrast, the LHS, the Finnish study and the Hawaii study found that intermittent smoking was associated with slower FEV₁-decline compared with that among continuing smokers (Figure 1) (Burchfiel *et al.*, 1995; Murray *et al.*, 1998; Pelkonen *et al.*, 2001). Hence, at present it seems

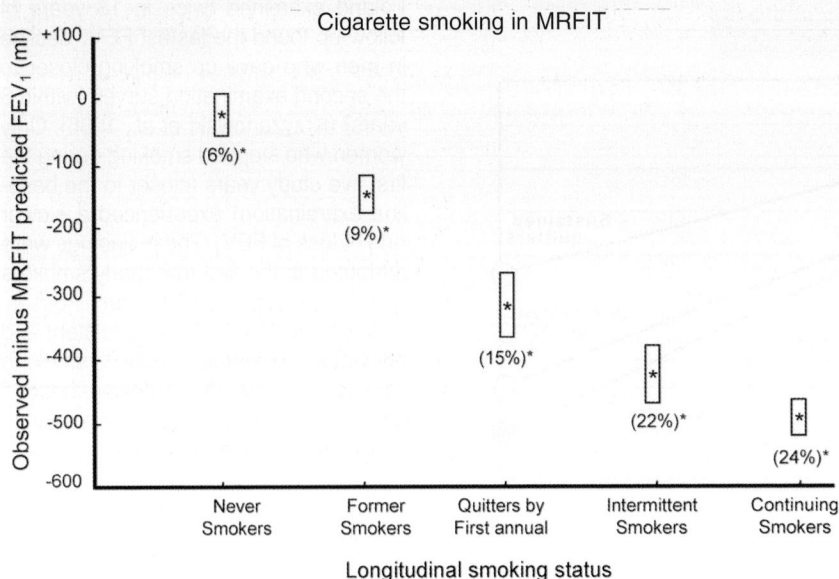

Figure 2. Adjusted FEV$_1$ by smoking status for MRFIT participants

Boxes represent mean FEV$_1$ (star) taken at trial midpoint and 95% confidence intervals (height of box). Adjustment made by substracting prediced FEV$_1$ by age and height in asymptomatic non-smokers, non beta-block treated participants from observed FEV$_1$.

*Percentage of group more than 1.65 standard deviations (797 ml) below predicted FEV$_1$

Reprinted with permission from Townsend *et al.* (1991).

in ml per year, which makes comparisons among different smoking habits readily accessible and understandable from a public health perspective. Table 3 provides an overview of the change in FEV$_1$ or ΔFEV$_1$ (ml/year) after smoking cessation (former smokers and quitters) when compared to continuing smokers for those studies reporting this determination.

Except for results from the general population sampled in the Tucson study (Camilli *et al.,* 1987), which showed that in subjects younger than 35 years smoking cessation increased FEV$_1$ by 21 and 27 ml in men and women respectively when compared to never smokers, cohort studies have not confirmed that smoking cessation in healthy subjects actually increases lung function. However, it can be concluded on the basis of these studies that smoking cessation reduces the rate of FEV$_1$-decline by approximately 10 ml/year, corresponding to a 15–30% slower decline than continued smoking. In contrast, subjects with impaired lung function, as in the LHS, displayed significant improvement in FEV$_1$ in the first year of the study when quitting smoking, and in subsequent years a reduction in the rate of decline of 50% or higher was seen in quitters. A similarly large reduction in ΔFEV$_1$ was observed in the group of middle-aged men with mild COPD in the study by Fletcher and Peto (1977). Furthermore, as will be discussed later, long-term former smokers in most cases have a ΔFEV$_1$ not significantly different from never smokers, and although the lost lung function is generally not regained, the FEV$_1$ slopes in subjects who quit smoking approach the slopes of never smokers (Figure 3). To summarize, the absolute risk of COPD is reduced by smoking cessation.

that it is not possible to establish consistent evidence regarding intermittent smoking and lung function changes.

Change in absolute risk after smoking cessation

One of the four main conclusions of the Surgeon General's 1990 Report was as follows:

"For persons without overt chronic obstructive pulmonary disease (COPD), smoking cessation improves pulmonary function about 5 percent within a few months after cessation."

The report stated that this improvement corresponded to an actual increase in FEV$_1$ of approximately 100 ml, and that the finding was based on clinical studies with a small number of subjects and a short duration of follow-up.

Among non-smoking healthy persons, lung function declines linearly beginning at approximately 25 years of age, at a rate of 20-30 ml/year (Fletcher & Peto, 1977). Older persons, smokers and patients with COPD or emphysema have larger declines, with up to 200 ml/year having been reported (Kerstjens *et al.,* 1996). Fortunately, the longitudinal studies described above have assessed change in lung function as decline in FEV$_1$ expressed as an absolute number

Table 2. Baseline characteristics by final smoking status of the participants in the Lung Health Study

Baseline characteristics	Sustained Quitters Q (n = 559)	Intermittent Quitters I (n = 991)	Continuing Smokers S (n = 2268)	Significance (p < 0.05)
Age, yr	49.1 (6.8)	48.6 (6.9)	48.3 (6.8)	Q,S
Sex. % female	32.9	38.1	36.1	NS
Married, %	74.1	72.6	69.6	NS
Years of education	13.8 (2.9)	13.9 (2.9)	13.5 (2.8)	Q, S; I,S
Nonwhite, %	3.3	4.2	4.6	NS
Cigarettes per day	30.1 (12.6)	29.8 (12.3)	32.0 (12.8)	Q, S; I,S
Salivary cotinine, ng/ml	332.4 (199.8)	334.8 (187.0)	389.0 (207.5)	Q, S; I,S
Age started smoking, yr	17.6 (3.6)	17.8 (3.9)	17.3 (3.8)	I,S
Pack-years	40.1 (18.8)	39.4 (18.2)	40.8 (19.0)	NS
Smoke pipes, cigars, %	5.4	4.3	7.5	I, S
Use alcohol, %	70.8	71.1	70.2	NS
Drinks per week among alcohol users	6.4 (5.7)	6.0 (5.3)	6.2 (5.7)	NS
Body mass index, kg/m^2	26.0 (3.9)	25.9 (3.9)	25.4 (3.9)	Q, S; I,S
FEV$_1$ (post-BD), L	2.82 (0.64)	2.74 (0.64)	2.75 (0.61)	NS
FEV$_1$ %predicted (post-BD)	79.4 (9.1)	78.4 (9.2)	78.1 (8.9)	Q, S
FEV$_1$/FVC (post-BD), %	63.1 (5.6)	62.9 (5.5)	63.0 (5.4)	NS
Bronchodilator response, %	4.5 (4.9)	4.6 (4.8)	4.1 (5.1)	I, S
Log methacholine reactivity				
(LMCR), %mg/ml	0.442 (0.388)	0.478 (0.406)	0.444 (0.373)	Q, I
Men	0.344 (0.349)	0.376 (0.382)	0.353 (0.350)	
Women	0.613 (0,382)	0.615 (0.370)	0.595 (0.379)	
Respiratory symptoms				
Chronic cough, %	39.7	40.6	44.3	NS
Chronic phlegm, %	32.2	35.8	37.7	Q, S
Chronic bronchitis, %	26.1	26.5	30.3	NS
Wheezing grade 1 or higher, %	74.4	76.8	76.9	NS
Dyspnea grade 1 or higher, %	39.0	41.3	44.1	NS

BD = bronchodilator, FEV$_1$ = forced expiratory volume in 1 sec; FVC = forced vital capacity; Q= sustained quitters; I= intermittent quitters; S= continuing smokers; NS=not significant difference

Reproduced with permission from: Scanlon et al. (2000), Smoking cessation and lung function in mild-to-moderate chronic obstructive pulmonary disease. The Lung Health Study. American Journal of Respiratory and Critical Care Medicine, 161:381-390.

Table 3. Rate of decline in FEV_1 (ml/year) for former smokers, quitters and continuing smokers in longitudinal studies

	Rate of Decline in FEV_1 (ml/year)			
Study Reference	**Smokers** men/women	**Quitters** men/women	**Former smokers** men/women	**Comments**
West London Fletcher & Peto (1977)	55/80	30/37	Not reported	Values are for men without/with mild COPD
Respiratory Study Los Angeles (UCLA) Tashkin, *et al.* (1986)	350/270	300/190	260/190	Values are for a period of 5 years
Krakow Study of COPD Krzyzanowski, *et al.* (1986)	60/42	68/37	63/38	
Tucson (General Population) Camilli, *et al.* (1987)	42	35	21	Values are for men aged 50–69
Copenhagen City Heart Study Lange, *et al.* (1989)	56/48	43/too few subjects	36/32	Values are for men and women > 55 years
MRFIT Townsend, *et al.* (1991)	59	50	44	Values are for men aged 38-63
Six US Cities Xu, *et al.* (1992)	53/38	41/29	34/30	
Vlagtwedde-Vlaardingen Study Xu, *et al.* (1994b)	33/30	20/15	20/19	
Honolulu Heart Program Burchfiel, *et al.* (1995)	33.5	22.6 (Exams 1-2) 29.7 (Exams 2-3)	21.7	Values are for men aged 45-68; quitters during the first 2 years (Exam 1-2; next 2-6 years (Exam 2-3); are adjusted for age and height.
Lung Health Study Scanlon, *et al.* (2000)	62 ±55	47± 57/31± 48	Not reported	FEV_1 increased in quitters during the first year in males and females combined
Finnish Seven Countries Study Pelkonen, *et al.* (2001)	66.0	55.5	49.3	Values are for men aged 40–59, and correspond to $FEV_{0.75}$
Lung Health Study Anthonisen, *et al.* (2002a)	66.1/54.2	30.2/21.5	Not reported	Values at the 11-years follow-up
ECRHS II (European Comm. Respiratory Health Survey) Chinn, *et al.* (2005)	35/27	31/22	31/27	Values are for men and women aged 20-44 Unadjusted values reported

*Values in Table are mean ± standard deviations

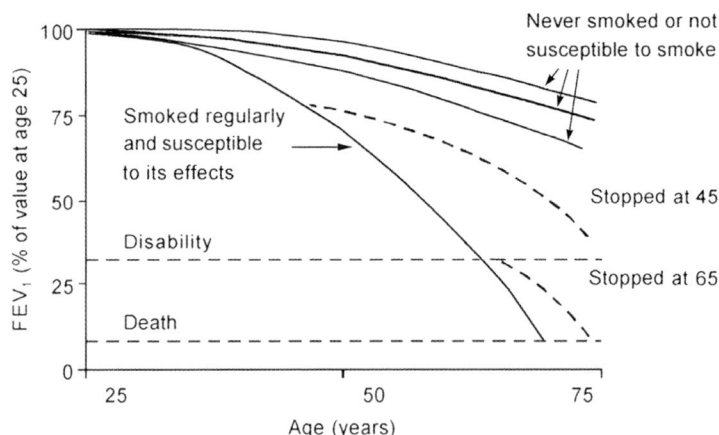

Reprinted by permission of BMJ, 1977, Vol. 1 (6077): 1645–1648, Fletcher & Peto.

Figure 3. Smoking and rate of loss of FEV$_1$ for susceptible smokers

Reduction in risk for those with abnormal lung function

No study has been designed to compare rates of FEV$_1$-decline in COPD patients who quit smoking with the decline in never smokers, but some studies have examined the effect of smoking cessation versus continuing smoking in COPD patients and in those with asymptomatic airflow obstruction. An important problem in detecting asymptomatic airflow obstruction is the fact that COPD is usually not diagnosed before symptoms (dyspnoea, mucus production) are present, and at this stage the airflow limitation is frequently considerable, with an FEV$_1$ < 50-60% of predicted value.

Clinical trials

In the 1990 Surgeon General's Report, only three studies concerning the effect of smoking cessation on FEV$_1$-decline in patients with established COPD were evaluable. Postma and coworkers studied a group of 81 patients with moderate–severe COPD followed for 2–21 years (Postma et al., 1986). The 22 patients who stopped smoking at enrol-

ment or during the study experienced a ΔFEV$_1$ of -49 ml/year, which is still faster than the decline in never smokers in the general population, whereas the sustained smokers declined 85 ml/year. Another previous study followed 56 men with emphysema for 3-13 years to assess ΔFEV$_1$ in smokers and former smokers (Hughes et al., 1982). Of the 19 former smokers, 13 had stopped smoking less than 2 years before study entry. Duration of smoking and cumulative tobacco consumption were equal in the two groups. ΔFEV$_1$ was 15 ml/year in former smokers and –57.7 ml/year in the continuing smokers. Fletcher and Peto also stratified their sample comprising 792 working men according to prevalence of mild airway obstruction and found FEV$_1$-declines of 37 ml/year, 62 ml/year, and 80 ml/year in former smokers, light smokers and heavy smokers, respectively (Fletcher & Peto, 1977). In a small trial (n=57) lasting 30 months, Buist and co-workers found that subjects with impaired lung function at baseline had greater improvement in FEV$_1$% predicted following smoking

cessation than subjects with normal lung function at baseline (Buist et al., 1979).

Population-based studies

In the Honolulu Heart Program, separate analyses were performed in men with impaired lung function (n=216) defined as either being in the lowest baseline tertile of FEV$_1$ or having a Z-score for FEV$_1$ < -1.64 (Burchfiel et al., 1995). The 17 men with impaired pulmonary function who quit within the first two years of the study had a slower FEV$_1$ decline than those who continued to smoke (ΔFEV$_1$ 1.8 ml vs. 31.4 ml), whereas this was not the case in the 47 men who quit later during follow-up (2 to 6 years after baseline examination) (ΔFEV$_1$ 25.1 ml vs. 31.4 ml). The study also indicated that participants in the low or middle tertile of FEV$_1$ benefited more from quitting than those with the best lung function. More recently, the 30-year follow-up from the Finnish cohorts of the Seven Countries Study (Pelkonen et al., 2001) confirmed that quitting smoking during the study was associated with slower FEV$_1$-decline across all tertiles of baseline FEV$_1$ as compared to continuing smokers (Table 4). A study from Copenhagen, Denmark analysed changes in smoking habits and risk of a first hospital admission for COPD, finding a gradient in relative risk (RR) with increasing tobacco exposure (Godtfredsen et al., 2002a). Compared with continuing smokers, the RR estimates were 0.25 (95% confidence interval (95% CI) = 0.20-0.31) for former smokers, 0.36 (95% CI = 0.26-0.49) for smokers of <15 cigarettes/day and 0.58 (95% CI = 0.43-0.80) for quitters who smoked >15 cigarettes/day. Smokers belonging to the lowest baseline tertile of FEV$_1$ who quit during the study showed a lower risk of hospital admissions than continuing smokers. In the LHS, the rates of FEV$_1$-decline of 30 and 21 ml/year for male and female quitters, respectively, at the 11-year follow-up are

Table 4. Mean annual decline in $FEV_{0.75}$ during the first 15 years by smoking status and baseline tertile of $FEV_{0.75\ \tau}$ in the Finnish cohort of the Seven Countries Study

Tertile of baseline $FEV_{0.75}$	N	Quitters** Baseline (ml)γ	Decline (ml/year)*	N	Continuous Baseline (ml)γ	Decline (ml/year)*
Low	111	2565	-48.4	152	2662	-62.9
Middle	129	3259	-51.7	123	3253	-65.0
High	116	3805	-57.6	101	3806	-67.2

τ Tertile limits are < 3019 ml, 3019–3478 ml, and > 3478 ml achieved by dividing height adjusted baseline $FEV_{0.75}$ values of 1007 study subjects into three tertiles.

γ At baseline, adjusted for age and height.

* Adjusted for age; $p<0.001$ for smoking, $p=0.044$ for tertile of baseline $FEV_{0.75}$, $p=0.003$ for age, $p=0.018$ for duration of smoking, $p=0.765$ for smoking tertile of $FEV_{0.75}$ (all ANCOVA).

** Including baseline past smokers and permanent quitters. Reprinted from Thorax, 2001, Vol. 56(9):703-707, Pelkonen, *et al.* with permission from BMJ Publishing Group.

comparable to rates for middle-aged, healthy never smokers in the general population (Anthonisen *et al.,* 2002a).

In contrast, the UCLA study did not find any difference in FEV_1-decline among male quitters and continuing smokers with airflow obstruction, but women with airflow obstruction who quit had slower decline than continuing smokers of the same sex (Tashkin *et al.,* 1984). However, it is not clear whether this subset analysis controlled for cumulative tobacco exposure. The same trend was found in the Tucson study, which reported an analysis of longitudinal data with time-dependent covariates for smoking status and using each study subject as his/her own control when modelling FEV_1 (Sherrill *et al.,* 1994).

In summary, results from smoking cessation trials and prospective population studies support the observation that the rate of FEV_1-decline in people with impaired lung function who cease smoking returns to that of never smokers within a varying time frame (a few months to several years after cessation).

Reduction in risk of COPD for those with normal lung function or who are asymptomatic

To date, no study has followed a sufficiently large number of individuals from birth through old age to assess growth, plateau and decline in lung function. Such a study would be informative since the range of normal lung function, defined as $FEV_1/FVC > 70$ and FEV_1 predicted value (predicted for age, height, gender and race) between 80-120%, is very wide. Different theories exist as to what extent genetic, socio-economic, environmental and behavioural (active and passive smoking, respiratory infections, air pollution, diet, physical activity etc.) factors determine maximal lung growth in children, adolescents and young adults (Lebowitz *et al.,* 1987; Twisk *et al.,* 1998; Jackson *et al.,* 2004). It is however clear that initiating smoking as a teenager negatively affects the maximum attained lung function (Samet & Lange, 1996).

Furthermore, as observed in studies of young asthmatics, most studies

hypothesize that a healthy smoker effect exists also in terms of smoking onset: i.e. smoking prevalence is higher among people with initially better lung function whereas subjects with presence of respiratory symptoms or impairment tend not to take up smoking or quit sooner. Hence, cross-sectional data on lung function, smoking and smoking cessation will tend to produce results that are biased towards not finding a beneficial effect of smoking cessation, since smokers will tend to have better lung function at baseline than quitters.

However, the above-mentioned recent longitudinal studies of samples of the general population clearly show that the reduction in risk of COPD, estimated as the attenuated FEV_1-decline, is remarkably consistent and reproducible. The 1990 Surgeon General's Report reviewed 11 longitudinal studies of healthy people (general or working population) published between 1969 and 1985. The percentage reduction in FEV_1-decline in former smokers/quitters compared with continuous smokers were quite similar to that reported in the newer studies, indicating that secular smoking trends (cigarettes with filters, low nicotine/tar yield) have not influenced lung function changes in smoking cessation. Lastly, not very many studies have explicitly explored the relationship between smoking cessation and the exact timing of signs of reversibility in lung function measures.

Clinical and cross-sectional studies

A study of 10 healthy male smokers (mean age 27 years, mean cigarette consumption of 9 pack-years) showed significant recovery from abnormal pulmonary epithelial permeability after three weeks of smoking abstinence, indicating reversibility in the small airways function. However, there was no effect of short-term smoking cessation on any other tests of ventilatory function (Minty *et al.,* 1981). Small studies conducted in smoking cessation clinics show diverging results for groups with different lengths of follow-up, with improvement in FEV_1 after 5–7 months but no change from baseline value at one or two years (McCarthy et al., 1976; Bake et al., 1977). However, in these studies the participants were compared with themselves and not with continuing smokers, and as such the results are subject to regression to the mean (i.e. with re-testing, values tend to get closer to the average rather than to the original higher or lower individual values). Buist and coworkers (1979) conducted a similar small study with 30 months of follow-up and with a stronger methodology, finding an increase in FEV_1 and FVC during the first 6–8 months after smoking cessation (Figure 4). A cross-sectional study examined the

relationship between timing of smoking cessation and reversibility of carbon monoxide diffusing capacity (DL_{CO}) in 749 healthy individuals (Knudson et al., 1989). Mean duration of smoking cessation was 12.4 years, and there was no significant difference in predicted DL_{CO} or FEV_1 between former smokers and never smokers. This was already apparent for women who had quit within 2 years prior to the study and in men within 2-3 years after quitting. Nemery and colleagues also cross-sectionally assessed observed and "expected" changes in lung function with time since quitting smoking, and showed that early quitting (within 5 years) was associated with slower FEV_1-decline (Nemery et al., 1982). As described earlier, the LHS found a rapid positive effect on ΔFEV_1 within a year of quitting smoking.

Population-based studies

Not all the longitudinal studies agree on the timing of the observed benefits of smoking cessation, but again this is in part due to different methodological approaches. A drawback in general population surveys is that the reasons for giving up smoking are often unknown, increasing the risk of the so-called reversed causality. If a substantial proportion of study participants quit smoking due to sub-clinical disease, this will dilute estimated differences between quitters and continuing smokers, especially in studies with a short duration of follow-up. In the Normative Aging Study, former smokers stopped smoking after study entry, during the 5-year study period and quit rates were evenly distributed throughout the follow-up interval. Regression analysis found no effect of years since quitting on the rate of decline of FEV_1 and FVC; both were significantly lower than in continuing smokers, indicating an onset of benefits soon after cessation (Bossé et al., 1981). However, in other general population samples there were significant differences in ΔFEV_1 or relative risk of COPD between early and late quitters (Tashkin et al., 1984; Camilli et al., 1987; Burchfiel et al., 1995; Godtfredsen et al., 2002a), as illustrated in Tables 5 and 6. However, these studies seem to indicate that at least 4–5 years must elapse before the rate of FEV_1-decline returns to that of never smokers.

Timing of effect of smoking cessation on airway inflammation and hyper-responsiveness

It is well known that smoking causes airway inflammation and that increased bronchial hyperreactivity is negatively associated with the course of FEV_1, especially in patients with COPD (Wise et al., 2003). However, the order of causality in these pathological changes is still poorly understood, which impedes interpretation of changes in these

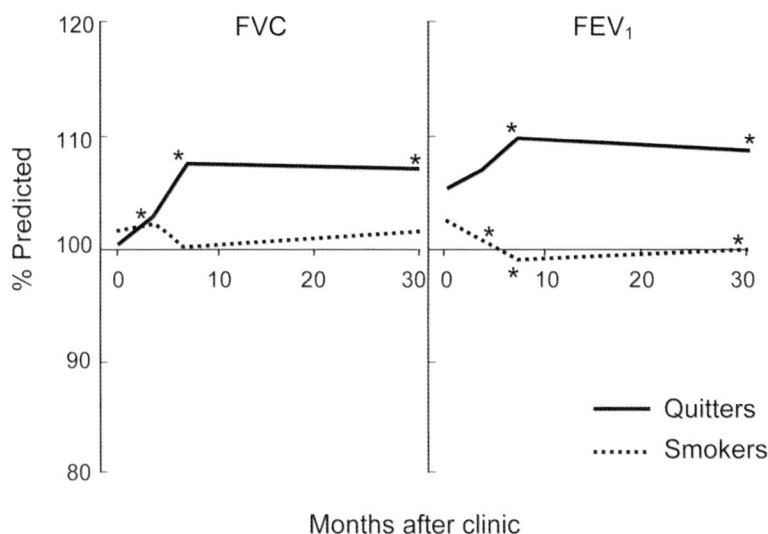

Figure 4. Lung function in quitters and continuing smokers from two smoking cessation clinics

Comparison of mean forced vital capacity (FVC) and forced expiratory volume in one second (FEV) expressed as percentage of predicted values in a group of subjects who attended two smoking cessation clinics and succeeded to quit smoking (n=15; solid line) or failed to quit for more than a month (n=42; dash line) during 30 months follow-up. Asterisk indicate significant differences (p < 0.05) from baseline values

From Buist et al. (1979).

Table 5. Average annual rate of FEV$_1$ decline by smoking status during 6-yr interval

| Smoking status | N | Baseline FEV$_1$ (ml) | Annual FEV$_1$ Decline (ml/yr)* | | | P Value** |
			Exam 1–2	Exam 2–3	Exam 1–3	
Continuous	1400	2702	–34.1	–33.2	–33.5(-34.3)	0.0001
Past at Exam 1	1064	2817	–18.7	–22.8	–21.7(-21.4)	0.90
Quit Exam 1–2	118	2799	–31.7	–19.3	–22.6(-22.4)	0.75
Quit Exam 2–3	268	2653	–33.3	–26.1	–29.7(-31.4)	0.0003
Variable	353	2759	–30.9	–23.5	–25.5(-25.8)	0.054
Never	1248	2888	–21.2	–21.5	–21.6(-20.3)	–

* Adjusted for age at baseline and mean height at three exams using mean values from this population. Values in parentheses are rates of FEV$_1$ decline that have been adjusted for the same variables plus baseline FEV$_1$.

**Two-tailed p values from general linear model for the difference in overall (Exam 1–3) rates of FEV$_1$ decline between each smoking status group and never smokers.

Reprinted with permission from Burchfiel *et al.* (1995). Effects of smoking and smoking cessation on longitudinal decline in pulmonary function. American Journal of Respiratory and Clinical Care Medicine, Vol 151(6):1778–85. Official Journal of the American Thoracic Society

measures after smoking cessation. A recent review concluded that, while cross-sectional studies of subjects with symptoms of chronic bronchitis or overt COPD did not find any change in airway hyperresponsiveness (AHR) between former smokers and continuous smokers, the LHS found a highly significant improvement in AHR with smoking cessation that was largely mediated through the beneficial effect on FEV$_1$-decline (Willemse *et al.*, 2004a). The author of the review subsequently showed in a study of 33 COPD patients that the 15 subjects who were tobacco abstinent for 1 year exhibited significantly less AHR to metacholine challenge and adenosine-5'-monophosphate compared to baseline challenge. This improvement was not associated with changes in FEV$_1$ or sputum inflammation (Willemse *et al.*, 2004b). A study of long-term smoking cessation on airway inflammation (mean abstinence of 13 years prior to study entry) in 16 subjects with chronic bronchitis found no differences between former and continuing smokers in terms of markers of inflammation assessed in bronchial biopsies (Turato *et al.,* 1995). In contrast, a 1-year study of 83 healthy smokers

attending a one-week cessation program showed that smoking abstinence significantly reduced markers of inflammation (macrophages and neutrophils) in sputum compared to continuing smoking (Swan *et al.*, 1992). Recently, two Dutch studies examined the effects of smoking cessation on inflammation in healthy and in symptomatic smokers. Willemse and colleagues (2005) studied a group of 25 smokers with normal lung function and 28 smokers with COPD attending a smoking cessation program, finding that inflammation persisted after smoking cessation in biopsy specimens and inflammatory cells increased in sputum specimens in the COPD patients, whereas inflammation significantly decreased in the asymptomatic smokers who quit. In the second study (Lapperre *et al.*, 2006), only T-lymphocytes and plasma cells from bronchial biopsies were related to duration of smoking cessation; the presence of other inflammatory cells was similar in continuing smokers, short (<3.5 years) and long-term (≥ 3.5 years) former smokers. The clinical implications of these findings are uncertain.

In conclusion, in healthy population samples there is a gradually increasing

benefit of smoking cessation within 4–5 years since quitting in lowering of the excess decline in FEV$_1$. For individuals with symptoms or a diagnosis of COPD, the improvement with smoking cessation occurs sooner, within 1–2 years. Evidence also suggests that smoking cessation rapidly reduces the AHR seen in COPD; but among smokers and COPD-patients with mucus hypersecretion, airway inflammation persists for a substantial period, perhaps lifelong, after smoking cessation.

Intensity of Smoking on Risk Reduction

Development of COPD and severity of the disease is related to duration of smoking and the amount smoked (Antó *et al.*, 2001). However, a lower limit under which smoking is considered "safe" has never been established. All the studies described in the sections above have to some extent considered the participants' cumulative tobacco exposure measured as years of smoking, daily number of cigarettes or pack-years (years as smoker times daily number of cigarettes/20). Table 6 provides an overview of cross-sectional and longitudinal studies that have analysed

Table 6. Cross-sectional and longitudinal studies reporting the effects of smoking cessation and past smoking history on lung function

Study	Smoking duration	Heavy vs. light	Pack-years	Age at quitting	Baseline FEV_1	Other factors
LHS		More improvement in FEV_1 in heavy smokers in Year 1		More improvement in FEV_1 in youngest quintile in Year 1	Not predictive of changes in FEV_1 from Year 1-Year 5	ΔFEV_1 and FEV_1 % predicted smaller in women than men from Year 1 Year 5
MRFIT		Heavy smokers (40+) had slower FEV_1 decline	More pack-years (65+) had slower FEV_1 decline	Younger age (35–39 yrs) had slower FEV_1 decline		
Honolulu Heart Progam	Recent quitters (<4 yrs) had faster FEV_1 decline	Non-significant slower FEV_1 decline in heaviest smokers		Same level of improvement in ΔFEV_1 across all age groups (45–49, 50–59, 60–68)	Low and medium but not high tertile had slower FEV_1 decline	
Tucson General Population Sample from the Epidemiological COPD study (1987)	Early quitting (within 6 yrs after baseline) in men aged 50–69 had ΔFEV_1 similar to never smokers			Improvement in FEV_1 at age < 35 years, men aged 35–49 had ΔFEV_1 similar to never smokers, ages 50–69 had intermediate values		
Copenhagen City Heart Study	No significant differences in ΔFEV_1 with more or less than 5 years since quitting	No significant differences in ΔFEV_1 with more or less than 15 cig/day		No significant differences in ΔFEV_1 below or over age 55 yrs		
Normative Aging Study	No effect on ΔFEV_1 of years since quitting smoking		More pack-years had faster FEV_1 decline	No difference in ΔFEV_1 from never smokers across all age groups (20–34, 35–42, 43+)	High baseline value associated to faster FEV_1 decline	
Tucson General Population Study (1994)			More pack-years had faster FEV_1 decline in women	Smaller improvement in ΔFEV_1 with increasing age		ΔFEV_1 smaller in women than men
Los Angeles Respiratory Study (UCLA)	No significant differences in ΔFEV_1 with >/< 2.5 years since quitting but former smokers > 7 yrs had slower FEV_1 decline	No significant differences in ΔFEV_1 with more or less than 15 cig/day				

Table 6. Cross-sectional and longitudinal studies reporting the effects of smoking cessation and past smoking history on lung function (contd)

Study	Smoking duration	Heavy vs. light	Pack-years	Age at quitting	Baseline FEV$_1$	Other factors
The Whitehall Study*	No effect on FEV$_1$ of $\leq$ 6 yrs, 7–13 years or >13 years of cessation		Lower FEV$_1$ with increasing cumulative exposure			Phlegm production more prevalent in smokers than in former smokers
Cardiovascular Health Study*				FEV$_1$ level when quitting <40 years of age similar to never smokers, but decreased when quitting >40 years		Results were similar in men and women and when analyses were restricted to healthy subjects
Vlagtweede-Vlaardingen Study		Heavy smokers (25+) had slower FEV$_1$ decline (not significant)		Younger age (<45 years) had slower FEV$_1$ decline		ΔFEV$_1$ in female/ male quitters larger/ smaller than never smokers, respectively

*Cross-sectional studies

the effect of smoking cessation in relation to amount smoked. Interestingly, most studies find that although heavier smoking is associated with a steeper FEV$_1$-decline, heavier smokers seem to benefit more from smoking cessation in terms of a slower FEV$_1$-decline compared to lighter smokers. Two studies found a similar effect on ΔFEV$_1$ after quitting according to past smoking intensity (more or less than 15 cigarettes/day) (Tashkin et al., 1984; Lange et al., 1989). However, cross-sectional data from the Whitehall Study revealed that among former smokers, cumulative cigarette consumption but not years since quitting smoking had a negative impact on FEV$_1$ (Higenbottan et al., 1980). In the LHS, baseline smoking rate among sustained quitters was predictive of change in lung function during the first year only, where a larger improvement was observed in the heaviest-smoking quintile (Scanlon et al., 2000). Only three studies specifically assessed pack-years of smoking

and quitting, and the results are conflicting (MRFIT (Browner et al., 1992); the Normative Aging study (Bossé et al., 1981); and the Tucson study (Camilli et al., 1987; Sherrill et al., 1994)).

COPD is rare in persons under 40 years of age. Table 6 shows studies that have addressed the effect of smoking cessation on lung function according to age at quitting and duration of smoking. Age at quitting smoking and duration of smoking/smoking cessation are highly correlated, and comparison of these studies is complicated by the different analytical approaches employed, differences in baseline assessments and varying adjustment for associated covariates. Nevertheless, most studies find that smoking cessation before middle age (40-45 years) is associated with a decline in FEV$_1$ that is not different from that observed in never smokers and shows an improvement in lung function over that of smokers who quit at older age. The prospective Cardiovas-

cular Health Study (Higgins et al., 1993), which included a cross-sectional study of smoking and lung function in 5 201 elderly men and women >65 years of age, found that subjects who reported quitting smoking when younger than 40 years had FEV$_1$ levels comparable to never smokers, whereas those quitting in the age interval 40-60 or 60+ had FEV$_1$ levels that were 7% and 14% lower, respectively. However, a slower rate of FEV$_1$-decline was seen after smoking cessation regardless of age at quitting when compared to continuing smokers. Indeed, some studies have detected no differences in ΔFEV$_1$ according to age at cessation (Bossé et al., 1981; Lange et al., 1989; Burchfiel et al., 1995).

Other factors affecting the effect of smoking cessation on lung function
Sex differences

For equal amounts of tobacco exposure, women are reported to be more susceptible to the deleterious effects of tobacco smoke on the lungs than men (Prescott *et al.,* 1997,1998; Chapman *et al.,* 2004). Hence, it could be anticipated that reversal of the changes in lung function after smoking cessation affects men and women differently. Several studies have explored this issue. In the LHS, the annual FEV_1-decline was only slightly larger among women than men who continued to smoke (Connett *et al.,* 2003). In contrast, female sustained quitters had a more than twice as great improvement in FEV_1% predicted value during the first year of the study, which amounted to a net increase of 1.9% by year 5 versus a 0.4% net increase in men (Connett *et al.,* 2003). Furthermore, female intermittent smokers lost less lung function than their male counterparts.

In a recent report from the European Community Respiratory Health Survey (ECRHS) comprising 6654 participants aged 20-44, sustained male, but not female, quitters had FEV_1-declines that were significantly lower than in never smokers (Chinn *et al.,* 2005). The sex difference was not significant, however. The Tucson study found results comparable to the LHS with a larger age-span (20–80 years), but the results were reversed when subjects with lung function in the lowest quartile were excluded (Sherrill *et al.,* 1994). In the UCLA study, considerable sex differences were also noted (Tashkin *et al.,* 1984). Former smokers of both sexes had FEV_1-slopes comparable to never smokers during the 5-year follow-up, and women who quit between baseline and follow-up also had FEV_1-slopes comparable to never smokers despite a lower baseline FEV_1. In contrast, ΔFEV_1 for male quitters was intermediate between never or former smokers and continuing smokers. Furthermore, this study showed that in subjects with chronic airflow obstruction only women profited from quitting smoking compared to continued smoking in terms of ΔFEV_1 and ΔFVC.

Xu and colleagues examined gender differences in smoking and smoking cessation in the Netherlands' Vlagtwedde-Vlaardingen study (Xu *et al.,* 1994b). The rate of FEV_1 decline in former smokers as compared to never smokers was more pronounced in females than in male participants.

In summary, no consistent pattern on sex differences in effect of smoking cessation emerges, likely due to secular changes in smoking habits between men and women and disparities in the studies' adjustment for gender differences in smoking prevalence, cumulative exposure, inhalation habits and other related factors.

Weight gain
A few studies have analysed whether the favourable effect of smoking cessation on lung function is possibly attenuated by the weight gain accompanying smoking cessation. Weight gain during follow-up was associated with increased FEV_1-decline in quitters, intermittent smokers and continuing smokers in the LHS (Wise *et al.,* 1998). However, weight gain was more pronounced in quitters during the first year (about 5 kg in both men and women) and associated with an estimated loss in FEV_1 of 11.1 ml/kg of weight gain for men and 5.6 ml/kg of weight gain for women. Similarly, two population-based studies reported an analogous effect of weight gain in FEV_1, suggesting that the initial benefit of quitting smoking on FEV_1 may be reduced with excessive weight gain, especially in men (Carey *et al.,* 1999; Chinn *et al.,* 2005).

Respiratory infections/illnesses
Whether lower respiratory tract infections, which are common in exacerbations of COPD, aggravate the course of FEV_1-decline remains controversial. Only the LHS has reported on frequency of self-reported respiratory illnesses in relation to FEV_1-decline (Kanner *et al.,* 2001). Results showed that during the entire study, sustained quitters had fewer respiratory illnesses than continuing smokers without influencing FEV_1-decline, whereas in continuing smokers a decline in FEV_1 was reported with increasing number of yearly infections.

Occupational exposure to dust/fumes
Occupationally exposed individuals from the general population included in ECRHS did not show a steeper FEV_1-decline than those with white-collar occupations during the nine-year follow-up (Sunyer *et al.,* 2005). However, the study population was relatively young, 20–45 years at baseline, and hence had a reduced occupational cumulative exposure. Some studies have examined the concomitant effects of smoking cessation and occupational exposure on lung function decline. In a recently published study of French workers occupationally exposed to respiratory pollutants participating in a smoking cessation programme, smoking abstinence was associated with a small but significant improvement in FEV_1 compared with continuing smokers after 1 year (Bohadana *et al.,* 2005). A recent study of the general population in Norway found that the remission of respiratory symptoms after smoking cessation was considerably less in subjects who reported previous occupational exposure to dust or fumes (Eagan *et al.,* 2004). Another paper from Norway of 231 asbestos-exposed men, of whom only 10 ceased smoking, also found reductions in respiratory symptoms and FEV_1-decline over 2 years after quitting smoking (Waage *et al.,* 1996). A recent, large longitudinal study with almost 30 years of follow-up found increased COPD mortality among dust-exposed construction workers independent of smoking (Bergdahl *et al.,* 2004).

Effect of smoking cessation on mortality and morbidity from COPD

Mortality

Low lung function is an independent predictor of all-cause mortality. In the United States, for example, death rates from COPD have increased in recent decades while trends for other diseases have shown gradual declines (Figure 5). COPD is predicted to become the third leading cause of death worldwide by 2020 (Murray & Lopez, 1997; Chapman *et al.*, 2006). The 1990 Surgeon General's Report evaluated studies of the effect of smoking cessation on COPD mortality in the general population and in COPD patients, including results from landmark studies such as the British Doctors Study, the Whitehall Study, the American Cancer Society's CPS II and several other large prospective studies. In these studies the absolute reductions in mortality risk after quitting smoking were between 32–84% compared with continuing smokers, and were highly dependent on duration of smoking and amount smoked. Even in studies with up to 25 years of follow-up, former smokers have elevated risk of COPD mortality compared with never smokers. In addition, a few studies analysed COPD mortality in former smokers by years since quitting smoking. Also, in apparently healthy quitters the risk of dying from COPD remains higher than in continuing smokers for up to 10 years following tobacco abstinence (Rogot & Murray, 1980).

Since 1990, further evidence from recent studies (Table 7) has strengthened the conclusions described above. Owing to the underdiagnosis and inaccuracy in coding of COPD as underlying or contributing cause of death, many recent studies of smoking and mortality have focused on mortality from all causes, cardiovascular disease and/or cancer. Recently the LHS pub-

lished 14.5-year mortality results (Anthonisen *et al.*, 2005): Mortality from respiratory disease other than cancer constituted 7.8% of all deaths, and mortality rates from these diseases were significantly lower in the intervention group than in the usual care group and did not differ depending on placebo or active treatment (Ipratropium). After 40 years of follow-up on male British doctors, Doll and colleagues found that mortality rates for COPD in former smokers were in between those for never and current smokers (Doll *et al.*, 1994). Similar results were found in the Whitehall Study and MRFIT studies (Kuller *et al.*, 1991; Ben Shlomo *et al.*, 1994), and in a large cohort from Norway (Tverdal *et al.*, 1993). By contrast, a study from Finland, a Spanish study of men aged 65 years or older and the Copenhagen City Heart Study found COPD mortality rates (RR) in quitters similar to rates in continuing smokers (Lange *et al.*, 1992; Sunyer *et al.*, 1998; Pelkonen *et al.*, 2000). However, in the Danish study this was only seen in women. These studies included, however, few deaths from COPD.

Results from a pooled analysis of population studies in Denmark showed a gradual increase in mortality rates from respiratory disease with fewer years since quitting and greater amount smoked (Godtfredsen *et al.*, 2002b), but the adjusted hazard ratio for COPD mortality was not significantly lower in quitters compared with continuing smokers. Lastly, a study of 139 young patients (<53 years of age) with very severe COPD followed for up to 8 years showed that intensity of cigarette smoking and smoking since study entry (as opposed to stopping smoking) were associated with poorer survival (Hersh *et al.*, 2004). Patients who remained quitters during the duration of the study (n=79) had significantly higher survival rates than patients who took up smoking (n=28).

Morbidity

The effect of smoking cessation on hospital admission for COPD has not been extensively studied. In the LHS there were no differences between the groups in hospitalisation due to respiratory disease (Anthonisen *et al.*, 2002b). In the Copenhagen City Heart study and in the Glostrop Population study, the adjusted relative risks of hospitalisation from COPD in former smokers, as compared to never smokers, were 2 (95% CI = 1.5–2.7) and 1.6 (95% CI = 0.8–3.4) respectively (Prescott *et al.*, 1997). Both estimates were substantially lower than those reported in continuing smokers. In the study by Godtfredsen and others (2002a), which pooled data from three prospective population studies in Copenhagen, with up to 23 years of follow-up, the relative risks of admission to the hospital for COPD were 0.14 (95% CI = 0.08–0.25) in never smokers, 0.30 (95% CI = 0.18–0.5) in former smokers, 0.40 (95% CI = 0.29, 0.55) in quitters who smoked <15 grams of tobacco per day (g/day), and 0.66 (95% CI = 0.47–0.93) in quitters who smoked ≥ 15 g/day when compared to heavy smokers.

Does the risk return to that of never smokers with long duration of cessation?

Based on evaluation of the evidence in the preceding sections, this question can be answered for the following outcomes:

 a) Lung function decline
 b) Morbidity
 c) Mortality

a) Lung function

Sufficient documentation exists to conclude that among smokers who quit the habit after ages 40-45, the excess loss of lung function is not regained. However, prospective studies based on

Table 7. Effects of smoking cessation on mortality

Reference	Study location	No. of subjects	Comments
Rogot & Murray,1980	USA	Aproximately 200 000 U.S. veterans (men) followed for 16 years	COPD mortality rates larger in former smokers than current smokers until 10 years after smoking cessation; hereafter lower rates in former smokers than current smokers
Ben-Shlomo et al., 1994	Britain	19 018 men from the Whitehall Study followed for 18 years	COPD mortality rates in never, former and current smokers were 0.68/1000, 0.95/1000 and 2.2/1000 per year
Lange et al.,1992	Denmark	14 214 men and women from the Copenhagen City Heart Study followed for 13 years	Compared to never smokers RR for COPD mortality in women former smokers was 11 (95% CI = 2.5–53), in continuing smokers 15 (95% CI = 3.1–65); for men RR in former smokers 3.0 (95% CI = 0.9–10), in continuing smokers 6.4 (95% CI = 2.0–20).
Tverdal et al., 1993	Norway	68 000 men and women aged 35–49 years and followed for mean 13 years	Mortality rates for former smokers were intermediate between rates for never smokers and current smokers in both men and women .
Sunyer et al.,1998	Spain	477 men from Barcelona aged above 65 years and followed for 8 years	There was similar prevalence of self-reported respiratory illness in former- and current smokers, and similar mortality rates as well (6.0/1000 compared to 1.7/1000 per year in never smokers).
Pelkonen et al., 2000	Finland	1582 middle-aged men followed for up to 30 years	There was lower total mortality in never smokers, past smokers and quitters. The relative risk of COPD mortality was 2.5 (95% CI = 0.7–9.7) compared to continuing smokers.
Godtfredsen et al., 2002b	Denmark	19 732 subjects from 3 population studies in Copenhagen followed for mean 15.5 years	The relative risk of mortality of COPD after smoking cessation is 0.77 (95%CI = 0.4–-1.4) compared to continuing smokers. There was no comparison with never smokers.
Hersh et al., 2004	USA	139 men under 53 years with severe COPD followed from 1994–2002	Recent smoking status predicts mortality independent of the effects of lifetime smoking intensity. Smoking cessation confers a survival benefit even in patients with very severe COPD.
Doll et al., 1994 and 2005	Britain	34 439 male British doctors 50 years of observations	Mortality rates from COPD in former smokers were intermediate between never smokers and continuing smokers.
Anthonisen et al., 2002b	Eleven clinical centres in the USA and Canada	5887 smokers, men and women 35–60 years Early COPD (FEV$_1$ 55–90%)	There were 149 deaths during the study, caused largely by lung cancer and cardiovascular disease. Smoking cessation was associated with significant reductions in fatal cardiovascular and coronary artery disease. Too few COPD deaths to allow a well-powered analysis.
Anthonisen et al., 2005			After 14.5 years of follow-up 731 patients died. All cause mortality was significantly lower in the special intervention group than in the usual care group. This was despite only 21.7% of individuals giving up smoking after 5 years in the special intervention group.

The 2 studies from Denmark included some patients in common.

the general population have shown that the accelerated FEV_1-decline decreases within a few years of smoking cessation, and with more than approximately 5 years abstinence the subsequent rate of decline is comparable to people who have never smoked. The large, randomised, multicenter smoking cessation trial, The Lung Health Study, recruited predominantly asymptomatic, middle-aged smokers with mild to moderate COPD determined by abnormal lung function test results in 1986-1988. In this study, smoking cessation but not administration of a bronchodilating drug was associated with an initial rise in FEV_1 during the first study year and subsequently a decline rate comparable to never smokers throughout the remaining

4 study years. At a follow-up survey 11 years after entry, the results were the same. Furthermore, beneficial effects on lung function after stopping smoking were established in all "sub-group" analyses, i.e. for both sexes, at all ages, across all levels of baseline lung function and amount smoked at baseline.

b) COPD morbidity
Evidence is sparse, and when it comes to hospital admission for COPD there is substantial uncertainty in registration of the discharge diagnosis. In the cohort studies from Copenhagen, risk of hospital admission for COPD in former smokers was still twice that of never smokers even after many years of follow-up. However, with more detailed analyses of

smoking habits, former smokers, quitters who were baseline light smokers and quitters who were baseline heavy smokers had excess risks of 10, 20 and 40%, respectively, compared to never smokers for hospitalisation. Overall, the risk of COPD morbidity appears to be slightly elevated even after many years of sustained smoking cessation.

c) COPD mortality
Sufficiently large studies with mortality from COPD as primary or contributing cause of death in relation to smoking cessation are in part lacking, due to the under-diagnosis of COPD on death certificates. The results from studies discussed previously indicate that mortality rates from COPD decline

Compared to 1965 Rate

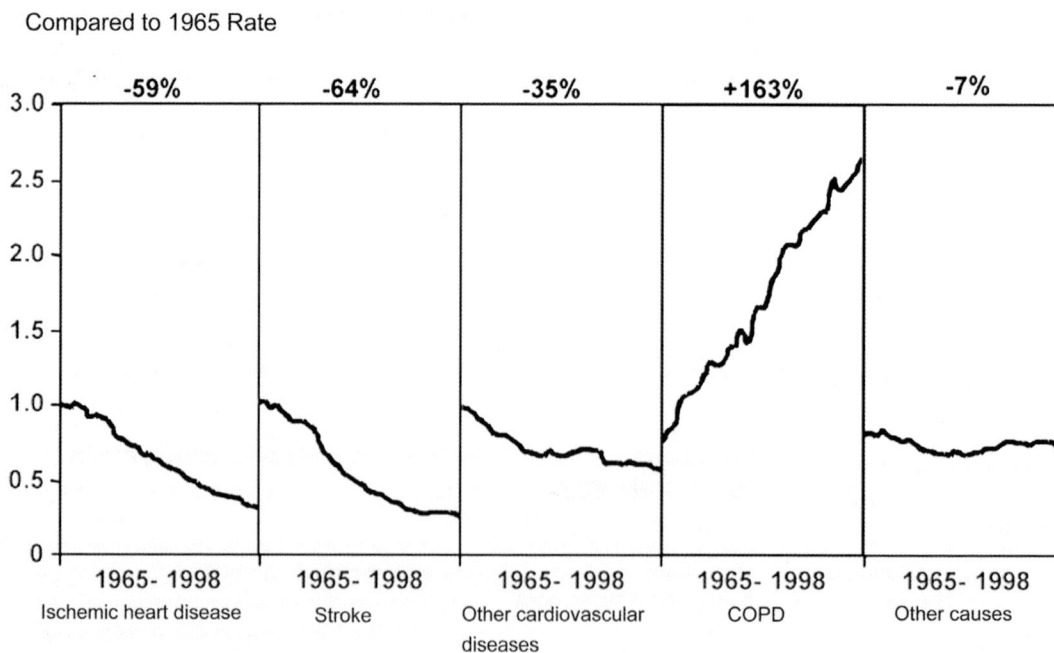

Figure 5. Age-adjusted disease specific mortality rates in the USA between 1965–1988
Change in age-adjusted death rates in the USA, between 1965 and 1998, for a) coronary heart disease (59% decline), b) stroke (65% decline), c) other cardiovascular diseases (35% decline), d) chronic obstructive pulmonary disease (163% increase) and e) all other causes (7% decline).
Adapted from www.GOLDCOPD.org

progressively after smoking cessation compared with sustained smoking, but that risk of mortality from COPD and all causes is still elevated in comparison with never smokers. The most comprehensive study in this respect is the large study of male British doctors, which published results from 50 years of observation in 2004 (Doll *et al.*, 2004). Age-standardised mortality rates per 1000 men/year for COPD, assessed between 1951 and 2001, were 0.11, 0.64, and 1.56 for never smokers, former smokers and current smokers, respectively. Survival analyses were carried out for all-cause mortality for never smokers, continuing smokers and former smokers by age at stopping smoking. Evidence of

reverse causality (the "ill quitter" effect) was present when comparing mortality ratios for equal age groups of quitters and continuing smokers obtained cross-sectionally, as revealed by higher mortality rates among quitters. On the other hand, even one year after quitting, rates were lower than in continuing smokers. For smokers in the oldest age-group, 75–84 years (longest duration follow-up), the following mortality ratios were found (per 1000 men): 51.7, 53.1, 69.1, 78.9 and 112.2 for never smokers, former smokers quitting at age 35-44, 45-54, 55-64 and in continuing smokers, respectively. The authors concluded that for men born around 1920 smoking cessation at age 50 halved the risk of

premature death, and quitting at age 30 conveyed the same risk as that in life-long non- smokers.

In conclusion, while there is a rapid improvement in terms of normalising the rate of loss of lung function after quitting smoking, for endpoints such as morbidity and mortality from COPD, the risk does not seem to decline to the level of never smokers, even after long term cessation. This is not likely due to misclassification of smoking status in the studies but may reflect "reverse causality", meaning that some smokers quit because of symptoms of disease. For COPD, which has a long latency period before clinical manifestations emerge, this is a plausible explanation.

References

Anthonisen NR, Connett JE, Kiley JP, et al. (1994). Effects of smoking intervention and the use of an inhaled anticholinergic bronchodilator on the rate of decline of FEV_1. The Lung Health Study. *JAMA,* 272(19):1497-1505.

Anthonisen NR, Connett JE, Murray RP (2002a). Smoking and lung function of Lung Health Study participants after 11 years. *Am J Respir Crit Care Med,* 166(5):675-679.

Anthonisen NR, Connett JE, Enright PL, et al. (2002b). Hospitalizations and mortality in the Lung Health Study. *Am J Respir Crit Care Med,* 166(3):333-339.

Anthonisen NR (2004). Lessons from the Lung Health Study. *Proc Am Thorac Soc,* 1(2):143-145.

Anthonisen NR, Skeans MA, Wise RA, et al. (2005). The effects of a smoking cessation intervention on 14.5-year mortality: a randomized clinical trial. *Ann Intern Med,* 142(4):233-239.

Antó JM, Vermeire P, Vestbo J, et al. (2001). Epidemiology of chronic obstructive pulmonary disease. *Eur Respir J,* 17(5):982-994.

Bake B, Oxhoj H, Sixt R, et al. (1977). Ventilatory lung function following two years of tobacco abstinence. *Scand J Respir Dis,* 58(6):311-318.

Barbee RA, Halonen M, Kaltenborn WT, et al. (1991). A longitudinal study of respiratory symptoms in a community population sample. Correlations with smoking, allergen skin-test reactivity, and serum IgE. *Chest,* 99(1):20-26.

Barter CE, Campbell AH (1976). Relationship of constitutional factors and cigarette smoking to decrease in 1-second forced expiratory volume. *Am Rev Respir Dis,* 113(3):305-314.

Ben Shlomo Y, Smith GD, Shipley MJ, et al. (1994). What determines mortality risk in male former cigarette smokers? *Am J Public Health,* 84(8):1235-1242.

Bergdahl IA, Toren K, Eriksson K, et al. (2004). Increased mortality in COPD among construction workers exposed to inorganic dust. *Eur Respir J,* 23(3):402-406.

Björnsson E, Plaschke P, Norrman E, et al. (1994). Symptoms related to asthma and chronic bronchitis in three areas of Sweden. *Eur Respir J,* 7(12):2146-2153.

Bode FR, Dosman J, Martin RR, et al. (1975). Reversibility of pulmonary function abnormalities in smokers. A prospective study of early diagnostic tests of small airways disease. *Am J Med,* 59(1):43-52.

Bohadana AB, Nilsson F, Westin A, et al. Smoking cessation-but not smoking reduction-improves the annual decline in FEV(1) in occupationally exposed workers. *Respir Med* 2005, in press.

Bossé R, Sparrow D, Rose CL, et al. (1981). Longitudinal effect of age and smoking cessation on pulmonary function. *Am Rev Respir Dis,* 123(4 Pt 1):378-381.

Brown CA, Crombie IK, Smith WC, et al. (1991). The impact of quitting smoking on symptoms of chronic bronchitis: results of the Scottish Heart Health Study. Thorax, 46(2):112-116.

Browner WS, Du Chene AG, Hulley SB (1992). Effects of the multiple risk factor intervention trial smoking cessation program on pulmonary function. A randomized controlled trial. West *J Med*, 157(5):534-538.

Buczko GB, Day A, Vanderdoelen JL, et al. (1984). Effects of cigarette smoking and short-term smoking cessation on airway responsiveness to inhaled methacholine. *Am Rev Respir Dis*, 129(1):12-14.

Buist AS, Sexton GJ, Nagy JM, et al. (1976). The effect of smoking cessation and modification on lung function. *Am Rev Respir Dis*, 114(1):115-122.

Buist AS, Nagy JM, Sexton GJ (1979). The effect of smoking cessation on pulmonary function: a 30-month follow-up of two smoking cessation clinics. *Am Rev Respir Dis*, 120(4):953-957.

Burchfiel CM, Marcus EB, Curb JD, et al. (1995). Effects of smoking and smoking cessation on longitudinal decline in pulmonary function. *Am J Respir Crit Care Med*, 151(6):1778-1785.

Camilli AE, Burrows B, Knudson RJ, et al. (1987). Longitudinal changes in forced expiratory volume in one second in adults. Effects of smoking and smoking cessation. *Am Rev Respir Dis*, 135(4):794-799.

Carey IM, Cook DG, Strachan DP (1999). The effects of adiposity and weight change on forced expiratory volume decline in a longitudinal study of adults. Int *J Obes Relat Metab Disord*, 23(9):979-985.

Chapman KR (2004). Chronic obstructive pulmonary disease: are women more susceptible than men? *Clin Chest Med*, 25(2):331-341.

Chapman KR, Mannino DM, Soriano JB, et al. (2006). Epidemiology and costs of chronic obstructive pulmonary disease. *Eur Respir J*, 27(1):188-207.

Chinn S, Jarvis D, Melotti R, et al. (2005). Smoking cessation, lung function, and weight gain: a follow-up study. *Lancet*, 365(9471):1629-1635.

Comstock GW, Brownlow WJ, Stone RW, et al. (1970). Cigarette smoking and changes in respiratory findings. *Arch Environ Health*, 21(1):50-57.

Connett JE, Murray RP, Buist AS, et al. (2003). Changes in smoking status affect women more than men: results of the Lung Health Study. *Am J Epidemiol*, 157(11):973-979.

Dockery DW, Speizer FE, Ferris BG, Jr., et al. (1988). Cumulative and reversible effects of lifetime smoking on simple tests of lung function in adults. *Am Rev Respir Dis*, 137(2):286-292.

Doll R, Peto R, Wheatley K, et al. (1994). Mortality in relation to smoking: 40 years' observations on male British doctors. BMJ, 309(6959):901-911.

Doll R, Peto R, Boreham J, et al. (2004). Mortality in relation to smoking: 50 years' observations on male British doctors. *BMJ*, 328(7455):1519.

Doll R, Peto R, Boreham J, et al. (2005). Mortality from cancer in relation to smoking: 50 years observations on British doctors. *Br J Cancer*, 92(3):426-429.

Eagan TM, Gulsvik A, Eide GE, et al. (2004). Remission of respiratory symptoms by smoking and occupational exposure in a cohort study. *Eur Respir J*, 23(4):589-594.

Enright PL, Kronmal RA, Higgins MW, et al. (1994). Prevalence and correlates of respiratory symptoms and disease in the elderly. Cardiovascular Health Study. *Chest*, 106(3):827-834.

Fletcher C, Peto R (1977). The natural history of chronic airflow obstruction. *Br Med J*, 1(6077):1645-1648.

Friedman GD, Siegelaub AB (1980). Changes after quitting cigarette smoking. *Circulation*, 61(4):716-723.

Godtfredsen NS, Vestbo J, Osler M, et al. (2002a). Risk of hospital admission for COPD following smoking cessation and reduction: a Danish population study. *Thorax*, 57(11):967-972.

Godtfredsen NS, Holst C, Prescott E, et al. (2002b). Smoking reduction, smoking cessation, and mortality: a 16-year follow-up of 19,732 men and women from The Copenhagen Centre for Prospective Population Studies. *Am J Epidemiol*, 156(11):994-1001.

Hersh CP, DeMeo DL, Al Ansari E, et al. (2004). Predictors of survival in severe, early onset COPD. *Chest*, 126(5):1443-1451.

Higenbottam T, Clark TJ, Shipley MJ, et al. (1980). Lung function and symptoms of cigarette smokers related to tar yield and number of cigarettes smoked. *Lancet*, 1(8165):409-411.

Higgins MW, Enright PL, Kronmal RA, et al. (1993). Smoking and lung function in elderly men and women. The Cardiovascular Health Study. *JAMA*, 269(21):2741-2748.

Hughes JA, Hutchison DC, Bellamy D, et al. (1982). The influence of cigarette smoking and its withdrawal on the annual change of lung function in pulmonary emphysema. *Q J Med*, 51(202):115-124.

Israel RH, Ossip-Klein DJ, Poe RH, et al. (1988). Bronchial provocation tests before and after cessation of smoking. *Respiration*, 54(4):247-254.

Jackson B, Kubzansky LD, Cohen S, et al. (2004). A matter of life and breath: childhood socioeconomic status is related to young adult pulmonary function in the CARDIA study. *Int J Epidemiol*, 33(2):271-278.

Kanner RE, Connett JE, Williams DE, et al. (1999). Effects of randomized assignment to a smoking cessation intervention and changes in smoking habits on respiratory symptoms in smokers with early chronic obstructive pulmonary disease: the Lung Health Study. *Am J Med*, 106(4):410-416.

Kanner RE, Anthonisen NR, Connett JE (2001). Lower respiratory illnesses promote FEV(1) decline in current smokers but not ex-smokers with mild chronic obstructive pulmonary disease: results from the lung health study. *Am J Respir Crit Care Med*, 164(3):358-364.

Kerstjens HA, Brand PL, Postma DS (1996). Risk factors for accelerated decline among patients with chronic obstructive pulmonary disease. *Am J Respir Crit Care Med*, 154(6 Pt 2):S266-S272.

Knudson RJ, Kaltenborn WT, Burrows B (1989). The effects of cigarette smoking and smoking cessation on the carbon monoxide diffusing capacity of the lung in asymptomatic subjects. *Am Rev Respir Dis,* 140(3):645-651.

Krzyzanowski M, Jedrychowski W, Wysocki M (1986). Factors associated with the change in ventilatory function and the development of chronic obstructive pulmonary disease in a 13-year follow-up of the Cracow Study. Risk of chronic obstructive pulmonary disease. *Am Rev Respir Dis,* 134(5):1011-1019.

Krzyzanowski M, Robbins DR, Lebowitz MD (1993). Smoking cessation and changes in respiratory symptoms in two populations followed for 13 years. *Int J Epidemiol,* 22(4):666-673.

Kuller LH, Ockene JK, Meilahn E, et al. (1991). Cigarette smoking and mortality. MRFIT Research Group. *Prev Med,* 20(5):638-654.

Lange P, Groth S, Nyboe GJ, et al. (1989). Effects of smoking and changes in smoking habits on the decline of FEV$_1$. Eur Respir J, 2(9):811-816.

Lange P, Groth S, Nyboe J, et al. (1990). Phlegm production in plain cigarette smokers who changed to filter cigarettes or quit smoking. *J Intern Med,* 228(2):115-120.

Lange P, Nyboe J, Appleyard M, et al. (1992). Relationship of the type of tobacco and inhalation pattern to pulmonary and total mortality. *Eur Respir J,* 5(9):1111-1117.

Lapperre TS, Postma DS, Gosman MM, et al. (2006). Relation between duration of smoking cessation and bronchial inflammation in COPD. *Thorax,* 61:115-121.

Leader WG, Wolf KM, Cooper TM, et al. (1994). Symptomatology, pulmonary function and response, and T lymphocyte beta 2-receptors during smoking cessation in patients with chronic obstructive pulmonary disease. *Pharmacotherapy,* 14(2):162-172.

Lebowitz MD, Holberg CJ, Knudson RJ, et al. (1987). Longitudinal study of pulmonary function development in childhood, adolescence, and early adulthood. Development of pulmonary function. *Am Rev Respir Dis* , 136(1):69-75.

Leeder SR, Colley JR, Corkhill R, et al. (1977). Change in respiratory symptom prevalence in adults who alter their smoking habits. *Am J Epidemiol,* 105(6):522-529.

Lundback B, Nystrom L, Rosenhall L, et al. (1991). Obstructive lung disease in northern Sweden: respiratory symptoms assessed in a postal survey. Eur Respir J, 4(3):257-266.

Mannino DM, Homa DM, Akinbami LJ, et al. (2002). Chronic obstructive pulmonary disease surveillance - United States, 1971-2000. *MMWR Surveill Summ,* 51(6):1-16.

Martin RR, Lindsay D, Despas P, et al. (1975). The early detection of airway obstruction. *Am Rev Respir Dis,* 111(2):119-125.

McCarthy DS, Craig DB, Cherniack RM (1976). Effect of modification of the smoking habit on lung function. *Am Rev Respir Dis,* 114(1):103-113.

Menezes AM, Perez-Padilla R, Jardim JR, et al. (2005). Chronic obstructive pulmonary disease in five Latin American cities(the PLATINO study): a prevalence study. *Lancet,* 366:1875-1881.

Michaels R, Sigurdson M, Thurlbeck S, et al. (1979). Elastic recoil of the lung in cigarette smokers: the effect of nebulized bronchodilator and cessation of smoking. *Am Rev Respir Dis,* 119(5):707-716.

Minty BD, Jordan C, Jones JG (1981). Rapid improvement in abnormal pulmonary epithelial permeability after stopping cigarettes. *Br Med J,* 282(6271):1183-1186.

Murray CJ, Lopez AD (1997). Alternative projections of mortality and disability by cause 1990-2020: Global Burden of Disease Study. *Lancet,* 349(9064):1498-1504.

Murray RP, Anthonisen NR, Connett JE, et al. (1998). Effects of multiple attempts to quit smoking and relapses to smoking on pulmonary function. Lung Health Study Research Group. *J Clin Epidemiol,* 51(12):1317-1326.

Nemery B, Moavero NE, Brasseur L, et al. (1982). Changes in lung function after smoking cessation: an assessment from a cross-sectional survey. *Am Rev Respir Dis,* 125(1):122-124.

NIH/NHLBI/WHO. (2003). Global Initiative for Chronic Obstructive Lung Disease (GOLD): Global Strategy for the Diagnosis, Management, and Prevention of Chronic Obstructive Pulmonary Disease. p. 1-111.

Pelkonen M, Tukiainen H, Tervahauta M, et al. (2000). Pulmonary function, smoking cessation and 30 year mortality in middle aged Finnish men. *Thorax,* 55(9):746-750.

Pelkonen M, Notkola IL, Tukiainen H, et al. (2001). Smoking cessation, decline in pulmonary function and total mortality: a 30 year follow up study among the Finnish cohorts of the Seven Countries Study. *Thorax,* 56(9):703-707.

Postma DS, de Vries K, Koeter GH, et al. (1986). Independent influence of reversibility of air-flow obstruction and nonspecific hyperreactivity on the long-term course of lung function in chronic air-flow obstruction. *Am Rev Respir Dis,* 134(2):276-280.

Postma DS, Sluiter HJ (1989). Prognosis of chronic obstructive pulmonary disease: the Dutch experience. *Am Rev Respir Dis,* 140(3 Pt 2):S100-S105.

Prescott E, Bjerg AM, Andersen PK, et al. (1997). Gender difference in smoking effects on lung function and risk of hospitalization for COPD: results from a Danish longitudinal population study. *Eur Respir J,* 10(4):822-827.

Prescott E, Osler M, Andersen PK, et al. (1998). Mortality in women and men in relation to smoking. *Int J Epidemiol,* 27(1):27-32.

Pride NB (2001). Smoking cessation: effects on symptoms, spirometry and future trends in COPD. *Thorax,* 56 Suppl. 2:ii7-10.

Rijcken B, Schouten JP, Weiss ST, et al. (1987). The relationship of nonspecific bronchial responsiveness to respiratory symptoms in a random population sample. *Am Rev Respir Dis,* 136(1):62-68.

Rogot E, Murray JL (1980). Smoking and causes of death among U.S. veterans: 16 years of observation. *Public Health Rep,* 95(3):213-222.

Rose G, Hamilton PJ, Colwell L, et al. (1982). A randomised controlled trial of anti-smoking advice: 10-year results. J Epidemiol Community Health**,** 36(2):102-108.

Samet JM, Lange P (1996). Longitudinal studies of active and passive smoking. *Am J Respir Crit Care Med,* 154(6 Pt 2):S257-S265.

Sansores RH, Pare P, Abboud RT (1992). Effect of smoking cessation on pulmonary carbon monoxide diffusing capacity and capillary blood volume. *Am Rev Respir Dis,* 146(4):959-964.

Scanlon PD, Connett JE, Waller LA, et al. (2000). Smoking cessation and lung function in mild-to-moderate chronic obstructive pulmonary disease. The Lung Health Study. *Am J Respir Crit Care Med*, 161(2 Pt 1):381-390.

Sherman CB, Xu X, Speizer FE, et al. (1992). Longitudinal lung function decline in subjects with respiratory symptoms. *Am Rev Respir Dis,* 146(4):855-859.

Sherrill DL, Lebowitz MD, Knudson RJ, et al. (1993). Longitudinal methods for describing the relationship between pulmonary function, respiratory symptoms and smoking in elderly subjects: the Tucson Study. *Eur Respir J,* 6(3):342-348.

Sherrill DL, Holberg CJ, Enright PL, et al. (1994). Longitudinal analysis of the effects of smoking onset and cessation on pulmonary function. *Am J Respir Crit Care Med,* 149(3 Pt 1):591-597.

Sherrill DL, Enright P, Cline M, et al. (1996). Rates of decline in lung function among subjects who restart cigarette smoking. *Chest,* 109(4):1001-1005.

Sparrow D, O'Connor G, Colton T, et al. (1987). The relationship of nonspecific bronchial responsiveness to the occurrence of respiratory symptoms and decreased levels of pulmonary function. The Normative Aging Study. *Am Rev Respir Dis,* 135(6):1255-1260.

Sunyer J, Lamarca R, Alonso J (1998). Smoking after age 65 years and mortality in Barcelona, Spain. *Am J Epidemiol,* 148(6):575-580.

Sunyer J, Zock JP, Kromhout H, et al. (2005). Lung function decline, chronic bronchitis, and occupational exposures in young adults. *Am J Respir Crit Care Med,* 172(9):1139-1145.

Swan GE, Hodgkin JE, Roby T, et al. (1992). Reversibility of airways injury over a 12-month period following smoking cessation. *Chest,* 101(3):607-612.

Tashkin DP, Clark VA, Coulson AH, et al. (1984). The UCLA population studies of chronic obstructive respiratory disease. VIII. Effects of smoking cessation on lung function: a prospective study of a free-living population. *Am Rev Respir Dis*, 130(5):707-715.

Townsend MC, DuChene AG, Morgan J, et al. (1991). Pulmonary function in relation to cigarette smoking and smoking cessation. MRFIT Research Group. *Prev Med,* 20(5):621-637.

Turato G, Di Stefano A, Maestrelli P, et al. (1995). Effect of smoking cessation on airway inflammation in chronic bronchitis. *Am J Respir Crit Care Med,* 152(4 Pt 1):1262-1267.

Tverdal A, Thelle D, Stensvold I, et al. (1993). Mortality in relation to smoking history: 13 years' follow-up of 68,000 Norwegian men and women 35-49 years. *J Clin Epidemiol,* 46(5):475-487.

Twisk JW, Staal BJ, Brinkman MN, et al. (1998). Tracking of lung function parameters and the longitudinal relationship with lifestyle. *Eur Respir J,* 12(3):627-634.

United States Public Health Service Office of the Surgeon General (1984). *The health consequences of smoking: Chronic obstructive lung disease. A report of the Surgeon General.* Rockville, MD, U.S. Dept. of Health and Human Services, Public Health Service, Office on Smoking and Health; Washington, D.C.

United States Department of Health and Human Service (USDHHS) (1990). *The Health Benefits of Smoking Cessation. A Report of the Surgeon General.* Rockville, MD, Centers for Disease Control, Office on Smoking and Health.

Vestbo J, Lange P (2002). Can GOLD Stage 0 provide information of prognostic value in chronic obstructive pulmonary disease? Am J Respir Crit Care Med, 166(3):329-332.

Viegi G, Paoletti P, Prediletto R, et al. (1988). Prevalence of respiratory symptoms in an unpolluted area of northern Italy. *Eur Respir J,* 1(4):311-318.

von Hertzen L, Reunanen A, Impivaara O, et al. (2000). Airway obstruction in relation to symptoms in chronic respiratory disease - a nationally representative population study. *Respir Med,* 94(4):356-363.

Waage HP, Vatten LJ, Opedal E, et al. (1996). Lung function and respiratory symptoms related to changes in smoking habits in asbestos-exposed subjects. *J Occup Environ Med,* 38(2):178-183.

Watson A, Joyce H, Hopper L, et al. (1993). Influence of smoking habits on change in carbon monoxide transfer factor over 10 years in middle aged men. Thorax, 48(2):119-124.

Watson A, Joyce H, Pride NB (2000). Changes in carbon monoxide transfer over 22 years in middle-aged men. Respir Med, 94(11):1103-1108.

Wilhelmsen L (1967). Effects on bronchopulmonary symptoms, ventilation, and lung mechanics of abstinence from tobacco smoking. *Scand J Respir Dis,* 48(3):407-414.

Willemse BW, Postma DS, Timens W, et al. (2004a). The impact of smoking cessation on respiratory symptoms, lung function, airway hyperresponsiveness and inflammation. *Eur Respir J,* 23(3):464-476.

Willemse BW, Ten Hacken NH, Rutgers B, et al. (2004b). Smoking cessation improves both direct and indirect airway hyperresponsiveness in COPD. *Eur Respir J,* 24(3):391-396.

Willemse BW, Ten Hacken NH, Rutgers B, et al. (2005). Effect of 1-year smoking cessation on airway inflammation in COPD and asymptomatic smokers. *Eur Respir J,* 26(5):835-845.

Wise RA, Enright PL, Connett JE, et al. (1998). Effect of weight gain on pulmonary function after smoking cessation in the Lung Health Study. *Am J Respir Crit Care Med,* 157(3 Pt 1):866-872.

Wise RA, Kanner RE, Lindgren P, et al. (2003). The effect of smoking intervention and an inhaled bronchodilator on airways reactivity in COPD: the Lung Health Study. *Chest,* 124(2):449-458.

Xu X, Dockery DW, Ware JH, et al. (1992). Effects of cigarette smoking on rate of loss of pulmonary function in adults: a longitudinal assessment. *Am Rev Respir Dis*, 146(5 Pt 1):1345-1348.

Xu X, Li B, Wang L (1994a). Gender difference in smoking effects on adult pulmonary function. *Eur Respir J,* 7(3):477-483.

Xu X, Weiss ST, Rijcken B, et al. (1994b). Smoking, changes in smoking habits, and rate of decline in FEV1: new insight into gender differences. *Eur Respir J,* 7(6):1056-1061.

Zamel N, Leroux M, Ramcharan V (1979). Decrease in lung recoil pressure after cessation of smoking. *Am Rev Respir Dis,* 119(2):205-211.

Websites

Global Initiative for Chronic Obstructive Lung Disease:
http://www.GOLDCOPD.org

The Effects of Smoking Cessation on Chronic Lung Diseases in China

This section presents the findings of a systematic review of published papers in Chinese to assess whether smoking cessation results in benefits to lung function or affects mortality due to chronic obstructive pulmonary disease (COPD) among Chinese populations.

The Chinese tobacco industry sold 1.95 trillion cigarettes in 2005, generating US$20 billion in taxes. The Chinese Center for Disease Control and Prevention estimates that smoking-related diseases kill about 1 million people in China every year (Jiao, 2006).

In 1990, tobacco caused about 0.6 million Chinese deaths, a figure that is expected to rise to 3 million per year by the middle of this century. Of the Chinese deaths caused by tobacco, the major disease was COPD (45%), followed by lung cancer (15%), oesophageal cancer, stomach cancer, liver cancer, stroke, ischaemic heart disease, and tuberculosis (5-8% each) (Liu et al., 1998). This pattern of tobacco-attributable mortality is very different from those in countries such as the United States and the United Kingdom, where ischaemic heart disease is the major cause of tobacco deaths.

Although the relative risks for the major tobacco-induced diseases, especially COPD, are lower in China than in North America and Europe, the background rates of such diseases (except ischaemic heart disease) in never smokers are much greater in China.

Hence, the absolute risk for COPD is substantial among the smokers, producing a greater absolute number of COPD deaths and a greater proportion of COPD among all deaths attributable to tobacco.

Furthermore, there is evidence that the relative risk of COPD deaths among quitters is higher than that in continuing smokers (Lam et al., 2002). Although this can be explained by reverse causality, such results, together with the layman observation that some smokers died quickly soon after quitting, could reinforce the misbelief of the public (and some healthcare professionals) that quitting may be harmful for people with chronic lung disease.

Literature search

The literature search for papers published in China was done in December 2005 by a team in the Department of Epidemiology, 4th Military Medical University, Xi'an, China. Three scientists independently assessed the papers for inclusion in this review, and disagreements were resolved by discussion with a senior fourth scientist. The databases searched included the MEDLINE, PubMed, CBM disc, CNKI and VIP databases and the China Proceedings of Conference Database. All studies that examined smoking, quitting and lung function in China published before October 2005 were identified by using the following medical subject headings: "Mainland China", "smoking cessation", "smoking", "quitting", "obstructive lung diseases", "chronic obstructive pulmonary diseases", "lung function", "FVC" and "intervention measure" in English or Chinese. The reference list of relevant articles and reviews were examined for additional references. Only papers which reported lung function values to allow assessment of benefits of smoking cessation (quitting) on lung function and related health effects, and on mortality due to COPD or respiratory diseases were included. Of the 169 items found initially, 13 papers were included.

Studies from Taiwan identified in Pub Med using the terms "smoking cessation and Taiwan" were also searched, yielding 17 items, of which one paper was relevant (Hsu & Pwu, 2004). Similarly, the Taiwan National Central Library National Periodical Centre database was examined using the Chinese term for smoking cessation, which yielded 17 items. Only two papers, both in English, were included (Hsu & Pwu, 2004 and Yang & Yang, 2002); one of them had already been found in PubMed. The PubMed search also yielded two papers in English on smoking, quitting and mortality, one from a Xi'an cohort study (with a similar paper in a Chinese journal) and the other from a Hong Kong cohort study. No papers on the effects on symptoms were found, but there was one study on inflammation. The final list of 17 papers was determined by the Hong Kong scientist invited to the Handbook's Working Group.

Critical appraisal of the literature reviewed

- Most of the papers from China were written in Chinese, mostly published in local journals and a few in national journals. Only one Xi'an-Hong Kong and one Hong Kong paper were in English and published in international journals. The 2 papers from Taiwan were in English but were published in local journals.

- All of the papers in Chinese were short (mostly 1-3 pages). This was, and still is, quite common for papers in Chinese journals.

- Because of this limitation in the length of the papers, detailed information on methods was lacking. The results were usually presented briefly in a few tables (mostly 1-3). The discussion was also short. The number of references was small (mostly fewer than 5) and mostly restricted to papers in Chinese.

- The present review included 6 prospective and 7 cross-sectional studies on lung function, one paper on inflammation and 3 prospective studies on mortality.

- We identified four papers from 2 prospective studies that included former smokers and never smokers but did not include current smokers. Such studies could show that ex-smokers had poorer lung function than never smokers but could not provide evidence on the benefits of quitting, as there was no comparison

between former smokers and continuing smokers. Hence they were excluded from the present review.

- The sources of subjects and the methods of sampling or subject selection were reported inadequately if at all in most of the China papers. The representativeness of the subjects was unclear and selection bias could not be assessed. Some papers had some obvious selection bias, which could have resulted in under- or over-estimation of the effects of quitting.

- The sample size was often small, and statistical power was uncertain (but should be low). Sample size calculations were not reported.

- Validation of quitting was not done in any of the papers. Only self-reported data were available.

- Publication bias (papers showing benefits of quitting) for papers which were primarily aimed to assess the benefits of quitting is likely to be present, which can result in over-estimation of the benefits.

Effects of smoking cessation on lung function

Effects on large airway obstruction

Prospective studies/data:
In China, there were 4 prospective studies on healthy subjects, the largest and longest in terms of follow-up was carried out by Wang *et al.* (1999) in Beijing and was based on the North China Lung Function Normal Values project, in which over 500 subjects were examined in 1984. At baseline, 150 retired subjects (130 men and 20 women) with no history of heart and lung diseases and no recent respiratory infec-

tions were selected for further follow-up. This group included 32 current smokers, 58 former smokers and 60 never smokers. Among former smokers, the length of abstinence varied between 6 and 26 years. At 13-year follow-up examination in 1997, all lung function indices in the 3 groups declined from the baseline values.

Smokers had greater declines in ventilatory function (forced vital capacity (FVC) and forced expiratory volume in one second $(FEV_1\%)$), small airway function (V50, V25, V75) and diffusion capacity than did never smokers ($p<0.01$). Former smokers showed declines in $FEV_1\%$ similar to that in never smokers but a smaller decline than observed in smokers (p-value not shown). FEV_1 results were not reported. Note that $FEV_1\%$ can mean FEV_1 observed/FEV_1 predicted or FEV_1/FVC. Although some authors in China recommended the latter, the authors of this paper did not specify the definition used when referring to $FEV_1\%$, probably meaning FEV_1/FVC.

Another prospective study in Nanjing (Jiang *et al.*, 1994) included 38 male smokers and 30 male former smokers, who had no symptoms and normal large airway function on lung function tests (vital capacity (VC) >80% of predicted, $FEV_1\%$ >75% or maximum voluntary ventilation (MVV) >80% of predicted) but abnormal small airway function (defined as closing volume/vital capacity – CV/VC%, closing capacity/total lung capacity -CC/TLC% >125% of normal predicted values or/and V50, V25 <75% of normal predicted values). At 7-year follow-up, the smokers were aged 43–63 years, had smoked for ≥ 15 years or 14 pack-years and were still smoking. Former smokers were those who had stopped within a half-year after baseline lung function test and hence had stopped for at least 6.5 years. They had smoked for a mean duration of 20.9 years and were aged 38–66 years (mean 58) at follow-up. After 6–7 years, there were no significant differences in pre- and post-quitting FEV_1% among former smokers. However, the 29 continuing smokers showed deterioration in small airway function and a varying degree of large airway disorders (with significant reduction of FEV_1% and MVV; p <0.01).

A study with a short follow-up in Lanzhou (Yang, 1999) examined 100 healthy workers aged 22–45 (sex not reported). Of the 50 smokers with normal chest X-ray, 20 quit smoking. At 1 year follow-up, recent quitters (with quitting for ≤ 1 year) had similar FEV_1 (L) to that of non-quitters (3.72±0.57 versus 3.68±0.78; p > 0.05). However, declines in FEV_1 between baseline and 1-year follow-up were not reported.

A study in Baotou (Wang & Wang, 2000) examined 134 male smokers who intended to quit and followed up 67 who had quit for ≥ 3 months. The quitters were aged 14–46, and had smoked for 0.5 to 31 years. Fifty never smokers were used as controls. After quitting, there were improvements in FEV_1, and FEV_1/FVC (p values not reported), and post-quitting values were similar to those in never smokers. There were no significant reductions in prevalence of excessive morning phlegm and other nonspecific symptoms (p >0.05). Smokers were not included; hence, there were no data for comparison purposes in this study. The duration of quitting was short. The duration between the beginning of cessation and the lung function measurements (i.e. duration of follow-up) was over 3 months. A description of this and previous studies is shown in Table 1.

The largest prospective study in China on subjects with chronic cough/phlegm but no COPD (with FEV_1/FVC ≥ 70%) at baseline was based on a large community intervention study involving smoking cessation and other treatments (Xie et al., 2001). In 1992, 67 251 farmers were first exam-

ined in three districts in Beijing, Qianjiang (Hubei Province) and Shenyang (Liaoning Province). Of these, 1999 farmers were found to have chronic obstructive pulmonary symptoms (cough and/or phlegm for ≥ 2 years and cough and/or phlegm for 3 months every year) but no airway obstruction (FEV_1/FVC ≥ 70%). In 2000, 1114 were selected by stratified random sampling; 869 (78%) had complete data. Nonresponders were mainly those who had died or were not at home. There were 218 never smokers, 487 smokers and 164 quitters (Table 1). Quitters were defined as those who smoked at baseline but had stopped for one month or more at follow-up, and smokers were defined as those who smoked at baseline (smoking years times cigarettes per day >1) and had not quit during follow-up. At 8-year follow-up, significant differences in annual FEV_1 and FEV_1/FVC decline were found among never smokers, quitters and smokers, with p <0.05 for a smaller FEV_1 decline in quitters compared with smokers. In multivariate analysis of variance, the declines in both indices were still smaller in quitters than in smokers (p <0.05). COPD was defined by FEV_1/FVC <70%. During the 8-year follow-up, the cumulative incidence of COPD was 18.1%. The crude 8-year incidence rates of COPD in never smokers, quitters and smokers were, respectively, 13.5%, 15.3%, 23.7% in men; 8.3%, 13.2%, 20.5% in women; and 9.2%, 14.6% and 23.2% in total, with p <0.05 between quitters and smokers in the comparison grouping both genders. Although there were clear trends, tests for trends and crude odds ratios were not calculated. The adjusted odds ratio for COPD in the whole group was 2.50 for smokers versus never smokers (p=0.005), and 1.06 for quitters versus never smokers (p=0.87). Compared with smokers, quitters showed reduced risks of developing COPD (adjusted OR=0.45,

p=0.005). Note that because quitting was defined as smoking at baseline and stopping for at least 1 month, the relationship between duration of quitting and its benefits could not be assessed. It is not clear whether there were any quitters at baseline.

A hospital intervention study in Shandong by Wang et al. (2002) included 310 patients with respiratory symptoms and small airway abnormalities but normal large airway function (FEV_1 observed/predicted ≥ 80%; FEV_1/FVC ≥ 70%; V50, V25 observed/predicted <70%). Of the 115 smokers, 72 quit smoking (≤ 6 months) (Table 1). The quitters showed no significant changes in FEV_1/FVC% and FEV_1 observed/predicted %, but their small airway functions improved. It should be noted that FEV_1/FVC and FEV_1 observed/predicted % were slightly greater after quitting (p >0.05).

Cross-sectional studies/data:

In China, cross-sectional data were reported in the prospective study by Wang et al. (1999) (Table 1). At baseline, in 1984, and at 13-year follow-up in 1997, FEV_1% and FVC showed a trend of increasing values across the groups of smokers, former smokers and never smokers (tests for trend not reported).

There were 4 cross-sectional studies which showed lung function data by smoking status of healthy middle-aged subjects. The largest, by Zhang & Li (1993) in Nanjing, was on healthy 55–70 year old men and included 100 subjects for each of the 3 groups, with mean ages of 64, 64 and 57, in current, former and never smokers respectively. The smokers smoked 20–40 cigarettes per day for 15–40 years, and the former smokers had similar smoking history but had quit for 5–30 years. Peak flow, FVC and FEV_1/FVC were different (p<0.01) with increasing magnitude for smokers, former smokers and never smokers

Table 1. Prospective or intervention studies on the effect of smoking cessation on FEV_1 or large airway function in China

Reference, Location	No of subjects, Age (years), Health Status	Duration Follow-up and Cessation	Effects on FEV_1	Other lung function tests Comments
Jiang *et al.* (1994) Nanjing	Current smokers: 38 (43-63 years) Former smokers: 30 (38-66 years) No symptoms, normal large airway function, abnormal small airway function at baseline	7 years Quit for $\geq$ 6.5 years	Former smokers: no significant decline in post-versus pre- quitting FEV_1% (observed/predicted) 29 current smokers with small airway function decline: FEV_1 observed/predicted decline ($p<0.01$)	Former smokers: 63% with small airway function improved. Current smokers: 76% with small airway function deterioration ($p<0.01$). FEV_1 changes not reported for 11 current smokers with no small airway function decline.
Yang, (1999) Lanzhou	Current smokers: 50 Never smokers: 50 (22-45 years) 20 of 50 current smokers quit at 1 year follow-up Healthy subjects	1 year Quit $\leq$ 1 year	At 1 year follow-up, no significant differences in FEV_1 between former and never smokers	Declines in FEV_1 not reported; data were cross-sectional
Wang *et al.* (1999) Beijing	Current smokers: 32 Former smokers: 58 Never smokers: 60 55-65 years Healthy subjects	13 years Quit 6-26 years	Former and never smokers similar decline in FEV_1/FVC but smaller decline than current smokers ($p=$not available)	Former and never smokers: similar decline in small airway function, but smaller decline than current smokers. Decline in DL_{CO}: current smoker>former smoker>never smoker. At follow-up selected sample of 150 healthy subjects of original 500
Wang & Wang (2000) Baotou	Current smokers: 134 64 quit 64 continuing Never smokers: 50 14-64 years	Duration not reported Quit > 3 months	Post-quitting FEV_1 and FEV_1/FVC greater than pre-quitting values ($p=$not available) Post-quitting FEV_1 and FEV_1/FVC not significantly different from values in never smokers	Data of continuing smokers not reported

Table 1. Prospective or intervention studies on FEV_1 (contd)

Author, Reference, Location	No of subjects, Age (years), Health Status	Duration Follow-up and Cessation	Effects on FEV_1	Other lung function tests Comments
Xie *et al*, (2001) Beijing Qianjiang (Hubei Province) Shenyang (Liaoning Province)	Current smokers: 487 Former smokers: 164 Never smokers: 218 15 years or older (mean age: 45 years ± 11) Had chronic bronchitis symptoms (cough/phlegm) but no COPD	8 years Quit 1 month to < 8 years	Unadjusted annual FEV_1 decline: Current smokers = 41.4 Former smokers = 30.4 Never smokers = 32.8 Former versus current smokers: $p<0.05$ Current versus never smokers: $p<0.05$ Former versus never smokers: $p>0.05$ Adjusted: Current smokers = 37.3 Former smokers = 28.1 Never smokers = 39.5	8 year incidence of COPD (FEV_1/FVC <70%): Current smokers = 23.2% Former smokers = 14.6% Never smokers = 9.2% COPD Odds Ratio = 0.45, $p=0.005$ Comparing former to current smokers. Adjusted value.
Wang *et al.* (2002) (Shandong Province)	Current smokers: 115 72 quit 43 continuing 18-64 years Patients with cough, phlegm or dyspnoea; with abnormal small airway function but no COPD, chronic bronchitis or lung disease	6 month Quit for ≤ 6 months	Post-quitting FEV_1 observed/predicted and FEV_1/FVC greater than pre-quitting values, but not statistically different	Post-quitting small airway function greater than pre-quitting, $p<0.05$ 25% quitters with abnormal small airway function returned to normal; none of non-quitters had a similar experience ($p<0.05$)

(p value for trend not reported); former smokers had significantly greater peak flow and FVC than smokers (p <0.01).

Another cross-sectional study on middle-aged subjects by Zhao (1989) in Leshan, Xichuan Province included 38 smokers (37 men; age 35–55) without symptoms and with normal chest X-ray and ECG; 38 never smokers matched by sex, occupation, residential district and age (± 5 years) to the smokers; and 29 men who had quit for at least 1 year. Smokers had significantly smaller FVC and FEV_1/FVC than never smokers (p <0.01 and <0.001). Former smokers had

greater FEV_1/FVC than smokers (p <0.001).

The third cross-sectional study on healthy middle aged and older men by Wang *et al.* (2001) in Shenyang included 24 subjects in each of the 3 smoking status groups with mean ages of 67–68 years. The smokers were healthy and had no history of chronic lung diseases, and had smoked for 12–51 years (mean 29.8±6.2). The former smokers had quit for 10–23 years (mean 17±6.2). Both former smokers and never smokers had significantly better lung function (FVC, FEV_1, FEV_1/FVC) than did smokers

(p <0.05 to <0.01). Never smokers had better indices than former smokers, but the differences were not significant.

The fourth cross-sectional study, by Huang & Tan (1995) in Nanning, Guangxi Province, included male employees of a steel factory with no respiratory symptoms, no history of respiratory and lung diseases, no history of exposure to toxic substances and with normal chest X-ray and ECG. There were 17 former smokers who had smoked 15–20 cigarettes per day for 6–8 years and 14 former smokers who had smoked over 20 cigarettes per day for

11–15 years; both groups had quit for over 2 years. They were matched with the same number of smokers and non-smokers by work and living environment, age (± 5 years), height (± 5 cm) and weight (± 5 Kg). Former smokers and current smokers had similar mean age at first smoking and mean daily cigarette consumption. Former smokers who quit after smoking for 6-8 years had no significant differences from non-smokers or from current smokers in the lung function indices recorded (including FVC, FEV_1, FEV_1/FVC). However, former smokers who quit after smoking for 11-15 years had significantly better FEV_1/FVC than smokers (p <0.05) and no significant differences in FVC, FEV_1, and FEV_1/FVC from those of non-smokers. There was an increasing trend (p for trend not shown) for FEV_1/FVC across the 3 groups (smokers for 11–15 years, quitters after smoking for 11–15 years and non-smokers), and former smokers' FEV_1/FVC was significantly greater than that of smokers (p <0.05). These results suggest that smoking for many years is likely to induce irreversible damages that are not completely reversible following cessation.

There were two cross-sectional studies on healthy elderly subjects. The cross-sectional study on the elderly by Li *et al.* (2004) in Hubei Province included 40 subjects (sex not reported; likely all men) aged ≥ 60 years with no heart or lung diseases, normal ECG, and a chest X-ray showing no tuberculosis or cancer. There were 10 healthy never smokers, 15 former smokers who had quit for 10+ years, and 15 smokers who had smoked more than 20 pack-years. Increasing trends in VC, FVC, FEV_1 and peak expiratory flow (PEF) were found across smokers, former smokers and never smokers (p value for trend not shown). Former smokers had significantly better FVC, FEV_1 and PEF than smokers (p <0.05).

The second cross-sectional study was a lung function study in Nanjing

(Jiangsu Province) by Dai (1997), which included 61 men and 8 women aged 61–72 who had no respiratory symptoms, normal physical examination and chest X-ray, and had smoked 15–20 cigarettes per day for 28–32 years. Eighteen participants (16 men) were current smokers, while former smokers were 28 (25 men) who had quit for 6 years and 23 (21 men) who had quit for 3 years. There were no significant differences in age or years of smoking among the groups. Decreasing trends in FEV_1, FEV_1/FVC, and PEF across the groups (6-year quitters, 3-year quitters and smokers) were observed (p for trend not shown). The 6-year quitters had significantly better PEF than the 3-year quitters. The results suggest that quitting for a longer duration can have greater benefits on large airway function than quitting for a shorter duration. Because non-smokers were not included, it was not clear whether the lung function of the 6-year quitters had returned to that of non-smokers.

A cross-sectional study in Taipei, Taiwan by Yang & Yang (2002) included 109 current smokers (78% smoked <20 cigarettes per day and 29% for <20 years), 82 former smokers (having quit for ≥ 6 months, mean 5.6 ±1.7 years) and 180 never-smokers from 737 subjects randomly selected from the general population. The 371 subjects (mostly men; gender distribution not reported) had no past history of cardiopulmonary diseases, no occupational exposure, no airway infections in the previous 2 weeks, had normal chest X ray and ECG and had, as well, completed lung function tests, measurements of total respiratory resistance (Rrs) and a bronchial challenge test. Those who had cough and phlegm but otherwise had "healthy respiration" were included.

There were no significant differences in mean age (40–43 years) or body size among the 3 smoking status groups and the duration and intensity of smoking did

not differ significantly between current and former smokers. FVC and FEV_1 were similar in the 3 groups. FEV_1/FVC in non-smokers were significantly higher than those in smokers and former smokers, but no significant differences were found between smokers and former smokers.

The 4 prospective studies described earlier showed consistent evidence that among healthy subjects, smoking reduced large airway function, and smoking cessation resulted in improved function or smaller decline with age as compared to continued smoking. Results of the two intervention studies were consistent (Xie *et al.*, 2001; Wang *et al.*, 2002). The cross-sectional studies all showed a trend of increasing large airway function across smokers, former smokers and non-smokers, which also suggested that smoking cessation was beneficial. Specifically for FEV_1, among middle-aged asymptomatic smokers, smoking cessation delayed the decline of FEV_1 when compared to continuing smokers, and the decline became similar to nonsmokers after cessation for 6 years or more. Among young and healthy smokers, the benefits can be observed after cessation for a few months. Among smokers with chronic cough and phlegm but no COPD, cessation for at least one month to 8 years delayed decline of FEV_1 and reduced the risk of developing COPD compared with continuing smokers.

Effects on small airway function

Prospective studies or data
In China, the largest prospective study, by Wang *et al.* (1999) on 150 healthy retired cadres, showed that smokers had a significantly greater decline in small airway functions (V50, V25, V75; p <0.01) compared with never smokers, and former smokers (quitting for 6-26 years) showed smaller declines than smokers (p values not reported (Table 1)). There were 8

former smokers who quit before the age of 40, and there were no significant differences in their small airway function changes compared with those of never smokers (data not shown).

The Nanjing prospective study by Jiang et al. (1994) described earler included 38 smokers and 30 former smokers with asymptomatic small airway obstruction. At 7-year follow-up, 76.3% (29/38) of the smokers had deterioration of small airway function (V50, V25; p <0.01) whereas 63.3% (19/30) of the former smokers had improvements.

The Lanzhou study by Yang (1999) showed no significant differences in small airway function between former smokers (quitting for ≤1 year) and persistent smokers. Former smokers had greater V75, V25 and maximum mid-expiratory flow (MMEF) than persistent smokers but smaller V50; the latter appeared anomalous as it went in the opposite direction (p >0.05). However, smokers had worse small airway function (V25, V50, V75 and MMEF) than never smokers (p <0.01). The Baotou study (Wang & Wang, 2000) also found improvement in MMEF after quitting for ≥ 3 months (p value not shown).

An intervention study in Shandong by Wang et al. (2002) included 310 patients with no history of chronic bronchitis or lung diseases but with cough, phlegm or chest tightness and small airway abnormalities (V50 and V25 < 70% of predicted values) but no large airway obstruction (FEV$_1$≥ 80% predicted; FEV$_1$/FVC ≥ 70%). There were 115 smokers, and after smoking cessation counseling, 72 had quit smoking. At 6-month follow-up, lung function returned to normal in 18 quitters. Of the 43 who did not quit, none had lung function back to normal (25% versus 0%; p <0.05). Although the authors attributed the significant improvement of small airway function (V50, V25 observed/predicted %) to quitting (p <0.05), some could have improved due to relief of respiratory symptoms. The duration of quitting was too short (≤ 6 months), and the smoking history was not reported.

Cross-sectional studies/data:
Cross-sectional data from the prospective study by Wang et al. (1999) at baseline and follow-up showed consistently increasing trends in smokers, former smokers and never smokers for small airway function (V50, V25 and V75) (p for trend not reported).

The largest cross-sectional study (Zhang & Li, 1993) showed significant differences in V75, V50 and V25 among the 3 groups defined by smoking status (p for 3 groups <0.01) and increasing trends. These were significantly greater in former smokers compared to smokers (p <0.01), and in never smokers compared to former smokers (p <0.01).

The second cross-sectional study by Zhao (1989) showed that smokers had significantly smaller small airway function indices (V25, V50, V75, MMEF) than did never smokers, and former smokers had better values than smokers (p <0.01 to <0.001).

The third cross-sectional study by Wang et al. (2001) showed that former smokers and never smokers had significantly better MMV and MMEF than smokers (p <0.05 to <0.01), and never smokers had significantly better values than did former smokers (p <0.05).

Another cross-sectional study by Huang & Tan (1995) showed increasing MMEF across smokers who had smoked for 6–8 years, former smokers after smoking for 6–8 years and quitting for 2 years or longer, and non-smokers; and also across smokers who had smoked for 11–15 years, former smokers after smoking for 11–15 years and non-smokers (p for trend not shown). Smokers who had smoked for 11-15 years had significantly lower MMEF than former smokers and former smokers had significantly lower MMEF than non-smokers (p <0.05).

The study by Li and co-workers (2004) on elderly subjects showed increasing trends in MMEF across smoking status groups (p for trend not shown). Former smokers had significantly better MMEF than smokers (p <0.05) but worse MMEF than never smokers (p < 0.05).

The other study that included elderly subjects (Dai, 1997) showed decreasing trends in MMEF, MEF75, MEF50 and MEF25 across the 3 smoking groups considered, quitters for 6 years, quitters for 3 years and current smokers (p value for trend not shown).

The study by Yang & Yang (2002) found that FEF 25–75 and FEF75 (mean forced expiratory flow at middle half and at 75% FVC respectively) in non-smokers were significantly higher than those in smokers and former smokers, but no significant differences were found between smokers and former smokers (with former smokers having slightly better values than smokers).

The results of the prospective and cross-sectional studies reviewed showed that smoking cessation resulted in improved, or a smaller decline in, small airway function compared with that of continuing smokers.

Effects on hyperinflation
Only 4 cross-sectional studies reported data on hyperinflation (residual volume (RV), functional residual capacity (FRC), RV/TLC). Zhao (1989) reported that smokers had significantly greater RV, FRC and RV/TLC than never smokers, and former smokers had smaller values than smokers (p <0.01 and <0.001), with decreasing trends in smokers, former smokers and never smokers (p for trend not reported). Wang et al. (2001) also showed decreasing trends of RV and RV/TLC across the 3 groups (p for trend not reported). The differences between former smokers and smokers, never smokers and smokers, and never smokers and former smokers were all

significant (p <0.05). Similar trends were reported by Li *et al.* (2004) for RV and RV/TLC, with significant differences between former smokers and smokers (p<0.05).

The study by Dai (1997) did not include non-smokers. Decreasing trends of RV and RV/TLC across the groups of smokers, 3-year quitters, and 6-year quitters (p for trend not reported), and the differences between the 2 groups of quitters were significant (p<0.05). However, both groups of quitters had greater FRC than smokers, and the difference between the quitters was not significant. This latter result was inconsistent with the expected benefits of reduction of FRC in quitters.

Overall, the results of the 4 studies were consistent, especially for RV and RV/TLC, suggesting some reduction in hyperinflation in those who quit smoking as compared with continuing smokers. The values of TLC were not reported in all 4 studies.

Effects on gas transfer

Only one prospective study in China reported data on carbon monoxide (CO) diffusion. The cross-sectional data from the prospective study by Wang *et al.* (1999) in 1984 and 1997 showed increasing trends of DL_{CO} (carbon monoxide diffusing capacity) – across the 3 groups of current smokers, former smokers and never smokers. The prospective data showed that the declines in each of the 3 groups during the 13 years of follow-up were significant (p <0.05), and such declines were attributed to aging. The declines were the greatest in smokers and smallest in never smokers, with former smokers in between. Although tests for trend were not reported, the trends in both cross-sectional and prospective data were consistent. The methods of DL_{CO} measurement were not reported.

The cross-sectional study by Yang & Yang (2002) measured DL_{CO} using an

integrated and automated Chestac-65 lung function analyser (CHEST Corporation, Tokyo, Japan) finding significantly lower DL_{CO} and DL_{CO}/VA (VA: alveolar volume) in smokers than non- and former smokers (p<0.001); former smokers had significantly greater values than smokers (p <0.001).

After correction for age and body size, the % predicted DL_{CO} and % predicted DL_{CO}/VA of current smokers were still lower than those of non-smokers and former smokers (p <0.005). VA was not significantly different in the 3 groups (p=0.63). Furthermore, the % predicted DL_{CO} of 46 men who quit within the past 5 years and of 36 who quit for longer than 5 years were 106% and 105% respectively, suggesting that the improvement in DL_{CO} after quitting was rather rapid.

Hence, both studies above were consistent, with prospective and cross-sectional data showing that smoking cessation in healthy individuals can improve or reduce the decline in gas transfer with age. It should be noted that the values of DL_{CO} (ml/min/mmHg) in the non-smokers in Yang's study (age 39.9±14.1) and in Wang's study in both 1984 (age 55–65) and 1997 (13 years older) were 26.6±5.5, 22.5±3.1, and 20.7±3.1 respectively.

Effects on inflammation

An intervention study conducted in Jinan by Wang *et al.* (2005) randomly selected 50 subjects (42 smokers and 8 non-smokers; 45 men and 5 women; age 25–70) with confirmed small airway disease (SAD) and 40 without SAD (34 men, 5 women; age 23–72; smoking status not specified) from employees of the Jinan Railway Company who had health examinations in 2002. Smoking cessation counseling was provided to the smoking SAD subjects with follow-up in 1 and 3 months. At baseline, the 50 SAD subjects had significantly higher values of TNF-α, TGF-β1 and IL-8 than did the

40 subjects without SAD (p <0.05). Of the 42 smoking SAD subjects, 36 had quit smoking at 1-month follow-up, and post-quitting values of TNF-α and IL-8 were significantly lower than pre-quitting values (p <0.05); there was no significant difference in TGF-β1. At 3-month follow-up, 32 employees had remained abstinent, and post-quitting values of inflammation were significantly lower than values before quitting (p <0.05 for TGF-β1; p <0.01 for TNF-α and IL-8). No comparisons by smoking status are provided in the group without SAD.

This study suggests that SAD is associated with increased levels of cytokines and that smoking cessation for 1–3 months can reduce non-specific inflammation as evidenced by lower cytokine levels. TNF-α and IL-8 levels decreased more rapidly than TGF-β1, suggesting that short-term cessation is first associated with changes in infiltration and exudation and later on with pathological changes in structural remodeling.

Effects on bronchial responsiveness

The study by Yang & Yang (2002) assessed the effects of cigarette smoking and cessation on bronchial reactivity by measuring bronchial responsiveness to methacholine. Three indices of bronchial responsiveness were derived: baseline respiratory resistance (Rrs); the cumulative dose of methacholine (DA) causing an increase in Rrs by twice the baseline values (bronchial sensitivity); and the slope of the linearly decreased respiratory conductance (SGrs), representing bronchial reactivity. Current smokers had significantly higher baseline Rrs (p <0.001) and bronchial responsiveness than did non-smokers and former smokers. Rrs increased twofold or more by the highest dose of methacholine in 24.7% of current smokers (p <0.0001), in 19.5% of former smokers (p=0.28), and in none of never smokers. Smokers had significantly lower DA than former smokers. These results suggest that smoking cessation can partially reverse the adverse effects of smoking, but the study could not examine the effects of duration of cessation.

Effects of smoking cessation on mortality

There were only three studies on cessation, COPD and respiratory mortality in Chinese, and all were cohort studies (Table 2). Lam *et al* (2002) followed up 1268 retired male subjects aged 60 or older from 1987 to 1999 in Xi'an. At baseline, 388 were never smokers, 461 were former smokers and 419 were current smokers; the prevalence of COPD was 12.6%, 30.4% and 25.3%, respectively. During the 12-year follow-up, 299 had died, including 30 due to COPD.

The relative risk (RR) and 95% confidence interval for ever smoking, after adjusting for potential confounders for COPD, was 3.23 (95% confidence interval (95% CI) = 0.95–10.91) (p=0.06). The risk of death for ever smoking increased with the amount smoked per day and duration of smoking (p for trend <0.001). Compared with current smokers, former smokers had lower risks of coronary heart disease mortality but higher risks of COPD mortality. The RR of COPD in former versus never-smokers was 4.10 (95% CI = 1.18–14.28) and 2.13 (95% CI = 0.55–8.30) in current smokers. This was the first report on Chinese showing higher risks of COPD death in former smokers (with or without existing diagnosed COPD at baseline) than those in current smokers. These results could be explained by the "ill quitter effect" or reverse causality, as smokers who were ill due to COPD would be more likely to quit smoking and would die earlier than smokers who were healthier, even with COPD. This is more

remarkable for COPD than coronary heart disease or lung cancer because COPD tends to have an insidious onset with symptoms slowly worsening and undiagnosed over many years before becoming irreversible and resulting in death. Because of the small sample size and small number of deaths, even though the proportion of former smokers was high at baseline (36.4%), analysis of the effects of duration of quitting on mortality was not possible. Furthermore, changes in smoking status during the 12-year follow-up were not reported.

In Taiwan, a prospective study by Hsu & Pwu (2004) followed 4049 subjects (2311 men and 1738 women) aged 60 years or older from 1989 to 1993 and 1996. There were 2033 never smokers, 616 former smokers and 1399 current smokers. In men, 55.3% and 24.4% were current and former smokers, respectively, while in women these percentages were only 7.0% and 3.0% respectively. For former smokers, about 40% had quit within the past 5 years and 25.5% had quit over 20 years previously; the duration of cessation was not specified for the remaining subjects in the group. The outcomes included self-reported chronic diseases and mortality. COPD was not used as an outcome; instead, "lower respiratory tract diseases" including asthma, bronchitis and tuberculosis was reported. From 1989 to 1996, compared with never smokers, current and former smokers were more likely to have lower respiratory disease (RR=1.6, 95% CI =1.3–2.0 and 1.4, 95% CI =1.0–1.9 respectively). Among former smokers, there was no clear trend of increasing RR by years of smoking and no relationship was found for years since quitting (RR for 1–5 years = 1.0; 6–20 years = 0.9 (95% CI = 0.4–2.3); ≥ 21 years = 0.9 (0.4–2.4)). Former (RR=1.3, 95% CI =1–1.7) and current smokers (RR=1.2, 95% CI=1–1.5) had increased risk of death (all cause) over that of never smokers. Potential reasons for not

finding any benefits from quitting included: smoking behaviour could have changed during follow-up; the data collection procedures were not reported, and although the sample was claimed to be nationally representative the sample size and duration of follow-up appeared inadequate, and the authors did not report the number of events (incidence of disease and mortality); and it is not clear how the missing subjects due to loss in follow-up were handled in the analysis.

A population-based prospective study initiated in Hong Kong in 1991 by Ho *et al.* (1999) followed up 2032 subjects (999 men and 1033 women) aged 70 years or older for three years. At baseline, the number of never, former and current smokers in men was 302, 444 and 248, and in women, 763, 185 and 85 respectively. The mean duration of ever smoking was 44.5 years in men and 40.9 years in women, and the mean duration of quitting was 14.2 and 15.6 years respectively. The baseline prevalence of COPD in the 3 groups was 6.6%, 12.4% and 13.3% in men and 3.9%, 8.6% and 12.9% in women respectively. At 36-month follow-up, 1156 were re-contacted: 534 (280 men and 254 women) had died and 342 were lost to follow-up. COPD deaths (ICD9 code: 490-496) were pooled with pneumonia (485, 486) into "respiratory diseases", with 89 deaths in men and 68 deaths in women.

Both male (RR=1.4, 95% CI = 0.9–1.9) and female current smokers (RR=1.6; 95% CI=1.0–2.5) had increased all-cause mortality compared with never smokers; and similar results were observed for former smokers (men, RR=1.2; 95% CI=0.9–1.6; women, RR=1.7; 95% CI=1.2–2.4), with significant trend with amount smoked daily in women (p=0.028) but not in men. For respiratory diseases, the RR was 1.1 (0.6–2.1) and 1.1 (0.6–2.0) in current and former smokers in men, and 0.5

Table 2. Effects of smoking cessation on mortality due to COPD or respiratory diseases in China

Reference Location	No of subjects, smoking status, number of deaths, duration of follow-up	Results
Ho, *et al,* (1999) Hong Kong	2030 (999 men, 1033 women) ≥ 70 years Men Women Current smokers: 248 85 Former smokers: 444 185 Never smokers: 302 763 534 deaths: 157 due to "respiratory diseases" (including COPD) 3 years of follow-up	RR for respiratory disease death Former smokers versus never smokers: Men 1.1 (95% CI: 0.6, 2.1) Women 2.3 (95% CI: 1.3, 4.0) Current smokers versus never smokers: Men 1.1 (95% CI: 0.6, 2.0) Women 0.5 (95% CI: 0.1, 2.1) Short follow-up Small number of current and former smokers among women
Lam *et al.* (2002) Xian	1268 men ≥ 60 years Current smokers: 419 Former smokers: 461 Never smokers: 388 299 deaths: 30 due to COPD 12 years of follow-up	RR for COPD death Ever smokers versus never smokers: 3.2 (95% CI: 0.95, 10.9) Increasing trend with amount and duration of smoking (p<0.001) RR for COPD Former smokers versus never smokers: 4.1 (95% CI: 1.2, 14.3) Current smokers versus never smokers: 2.1 (95% CI: 0.6, 8.3) First report in Chinese showing reverse causality Small number of COPD deaths 12 years of follow-up not long enough
Hsu & Pwu (2004) Tawain	4049 (2311 men, 1738 women) ≥ 60 years Current smokers: 1400 Former smokers: 616 Never smokers: 2033 7 years of follow-up Lower respiratory tract disease incidence and mortality	RR for lower respiratory tract disease incidence and death: Former smokers versus never smokers: = 1.4 (95% CI: 1.0–1.9) Current smokers versus never smokers: = 1.6 (95% CI: 1.3–2.0) Current smokers: no clear trend of increasing risk for years of smoking Former smokers: no clear trend of decreasing risk for years since quitting Short follow-up; number of COPD deaths not reported (probably small)

RR = Relative Risk; 95% CI = 95 % confidence interval on the RR estimate.

(0.1–2.1) and 2.3 (1.3–4.0) in women, respectively. The significantly increased RR in female former smokers suggested reverse causality. It should be noted that this cohort study had only a short follow-up, and the subjects were older than those in the Xi'an and Taiwan cohorts.

All three of the above studies had small numbers of COPD deaths, and the 95% confidence intervals of the relative risks were wide. However, the increased risks of deaths from COPD or respiratory diseases due to smoking were consistent with other large Chinese studies (Liu et al., 1998; Niu et al., 1998; Lam et al., 2001), confirming that smoking causes increased COPD deaths in Chinese people. Because of the short duration of follow-up (except for the Xi'an study, though its duration was probably not long enough), reduced risks of COPD deaths in former smokers versus smokers were not found; instead, there is some evidence of reverse causality, which is consistent with studies in Europe and North America.

Conclusions

Various limitations, including the uncertain quality of most papers, have been acknowledged in this section. Results from the Chinese prospective and cross-sectional studies examined showed beneficial effects of smoking cessation on large and small airway function in healthy middle-aged and older subjects and in subjects with respiratory symptoms and/or some lung function deficits. There is good evidence of benefits on hyperinflation, gas transfer and bronchial responsiveness as shown by a few studies, which can add to the scarce evidence available in the literature. Whereas smoking can clearly increase the risk of COPD deaths, the benefits of cessation on COPD mortality have not been observed in the Chinese population. Instead, excess risks among older quitters were found, probably due to reverse causality.

The extent of the benefits before and after quitting, in terms of absolute values or percentages, is uncertain, especially in relation to the amount and duration of smoking before quitting, duration of quitting, age at quitting and follow-up. Most of the data were in men, as the prevalence of smoking is very low in Chinese women. It should be noted that the epidemic of smoking-related morbidity and mortality in China is still at an early stage relative to North American and European countries, and the prevalence of former smokers is also low in Chinese men. Relapse to smoking among quitters is not uncommon, but there are no data on the extent of relapse and its effect on chronic lung disease (and other diseases) in China.

Public Health Recommendations

The mistaken belief that quitting could be harmful, especially among elderly smokers in China and perhaps in other developing countries, is common and based on an understandable misinterpretation of the observation that some smokers had died from COPD soon after quitting. The lack of awareness of the seriousness of having COPD symptoms and the benefits of cessation and other such mistaken beliefs, if not appropriately handled, could lead to a reluctance of smokers with chronic respiratory symptoms and/or COPD to quit smoking. Health care professionals should be prepared to correct the misunderstanding.

Larger prospective studies on healthy middle-aged subjects with information on cessation during several time points over a follow-up period of over 10 years are needed for both lung function and mortality and morbidity studies. Long-term follow-up studies on smoking cessation among smokers with varying degree of COPD are also needed to clarify how reverse causality can mask the benefits of cessation.

References

References with titles in brackets are in Chinese.

Dai Z (1997). [The effect of smoking cessation and duration of cessation on lung function in healthy elderly]. Acta Academiae Medicine Nanjing, 17(2):185.

Ho SC, Zhan SY, Tang JL, et al. (1999). Smoking and mortality in an older Chinese cohort. J Am Geriatr Soc, 47(12):1445-1450.

Hsu HC, Pwu RF (2004). Too late to quit? Effect of smoking and smoking cessation on morbidity and mortality among the elderly in a longitudinal study. Kaohsiung J Med Sci, 20(10):484-491.

Huang B, Tan H (1995). [Changes of lung function in ex-smokers]. Chin J Prev Med, 29(6):354-355.

Jiang J, Tang Z, Tao S, et al. (1994). [A 7 year follow-up survey of ventilation function in 38 male adult smokers]. Prev Med J Chin PLA, 12(5):372-374.

Jiao Xiaoyang. (2006). Ban proposed on new cigarette factories. China Daily, National . (02/09/2006)

Lam TH, Ho SY, Hedley AJ, et al. (2001). Mortality and smoking in Hong Kong: case-control study of all adult deaths in 1998. BMJ, 323(7309):361.

Lam TH, He Y, Shi QL, et al. (2002). Smoking, quitting, and mortality in a Chinese cohort of retired men. Ann Epidemiol, 12(5):316-320.

Li J, Zhu X, Gao G, et al. (2004). [The signifi-cance of lung function test in the elderly by smoking status]. *JYMC,* 23(6):364-365.

Liu BQ, Peto R, Chen ZM, et al. (1998). Emerging tobacco hazards in China: 1. Retrospective proportional mortality study of one million deaths. *BMJ, 3*17(7170): 1411-1422.

Niu SR, Yang GH, Chen ZM, et al. (1998). Emerging tobacco hazards in China: 2. Early mortality results from a prospective study. *BMJ,* 317(7170):1423-1424.

Wang J, Wang J, Shen C, et al. (2005). [The study of machine-made and interference that give up smoking in small airway dis-ease (SAD)]. *Qilu J Med Lab Sci,* 16(3):21-23.

Wang L, Zhang X, Li Y, et al. (2002). [Effect of etiological therapy to pulmonary func-tion recovery of the patient with small air-way disease]. *J Shandong Univ* (Health Sciences), 40(2):135-137.

Wang M, Wang B (2000). [A survey of health status in ex-smokers before and after quit-ting smoking]. *J Baotou Med Coll,* 16(1):16-17.

Wang P, Lei Q, Li Y, et al. (1999). [The rela-tionship between dynamic changes of pul-monary function in 13 years and smoking in 150 elderly people]. *Health Med J Chin PLA,* 3:22-23.

Wang X, Song L, Wu L, et al. (2001). [The relationship between improvements in lung function after smoking cessation and changes in nitrogen oxide in middle aged and older adults. *Railway Med J,* 29(4):240-241.

Xie G, Cheng X, Xi X, et al. (2001). [Risk fac-tors of chronic obstructive pulmonary dis-ease in patients with chronic bronchitis]. *Natl Med J China,* 81(22):1356-1359.

Yang F (1999). [A survey on the damages of small airway function by smoking]. *Acta Academiae Medicine Suzhou,* 19(6):648.

Yang SC, Yang SP (2002). Bronchial respon-siveness and lung function related to ciga-rette smoking and smoking cessation. *Chang Gung Med J,* 25(10):645-655.

Zhang H, Li Y (1993). [The effect of smoking and smoking cessation on lung function]. *People's Military Surgeon,* 10:43-44.

Zhao C (1989). [A matched study on lung function in asymptomatic smokers]. *J Tuberc Respir Dis,* 12(6):361-363.

Trends in Lung Cancer Mortality in Selected Countries

This section aims to examine the contribution of differences in both current smoking prevalence and smoking cessation to observed divergences in lung cancer mortality rates across countries. To illustrate these relations, smoking and lung cancer mortality data from the US and Japan will be presented. These two countries were selected for comparison because of the availability of data on smoking prevalence and cessation by birth cohort for long enough periods to allow comparisons to mortality data. Observed lung cancer rates are influenced both by the peak smoking prevalence for a cohort and the amount of cessation in that cohort and both of these measures change substantially across cohorts. In addition, these two countries are in different stages of their tobacco epidemic.

Trends of lung cancer mortality by calendar time

Recent trends in lung cancer mortality rates differ by country, even among developed countries (WHO database of mortality and population estimates: http://www-dep.iarc.fr / WHO; Marugame & Yoshimi, 2005). Given that 70–90% of lung cancer is attributable to cigarette smoking in the countries where smoking prevalence is high (USDHHS, 2001; Vineis *et al.*, 2004), trends in birth-cohort specific lung cancer mortality rates generally follow the trends in smoking

behavior by birth cohort with an appropriate time lag of approximately 20 years. However, since the rate of lung cancer for a cohort is heavily influenced by the duration of smoking, it is important to observe country-specific rates of both initiation and cessation when examining lung cancer rates in different countries.

For most developed countries, age-specific male lung cancer mortality rates first began to decrease among younger age groups, and these decreasing trends gradually extended to older age groups (Figure 1). Examples of countries with these trends include the United Kingdom, the United States, Italy, Finland, the Netherlands, Canada, Australia and New Zealand. In a number of developed countries, however, these trends were not observed, including France, Spain and Japan (Figure 1). In these countries, decreasing trends were observed among some older age groups, but younger age groups showed increasing mortality rates with time.

Trends in female lung cancer mortality rates generally followed the patterns observed in males with a delay of several decades (Figure 2). In several developed countries, female lung cancer mortality rates began to decrease in younger age groups, then extended to older age groups. Countries with this pattern include the United Kingdom, the USA, Canada,

Australia and New Zealand (Figure 2). In other developed countries, however, these trends were not observed. In Italy, France, Spain and Japan, lung cancer rates for younger age groups are either flat or increasing (Figure 2), illustrating that many countries are in different stages of the tobacco epidemic (see Figure 2, page 4), and some of them are still in a progressing stage that may result in the influence of smoking being under-estimated.

Lung cancer risk increases with increasing cumulative exposure to smoking, but there is a time lag between exposure and occurrence or death from lung cancer. Because each birth cohort has a specific history of exposure to smoking, and this history varies from cohort to cohort, the relationships between smoking and lung cancer in population trends can be most clearly seen when data are presented by birth cohort.

Trends in lung cancer mortality by birth cohort

For countries such as the United Kingdom, the USA and Italy showing decreasing lung cancer mortality rate trends in men (Figure 3), peak age-specific mortality rates occurred in the same birth cohort, often up to the age groups in their 50s or 60s. For older age groups, the birth cohort in which

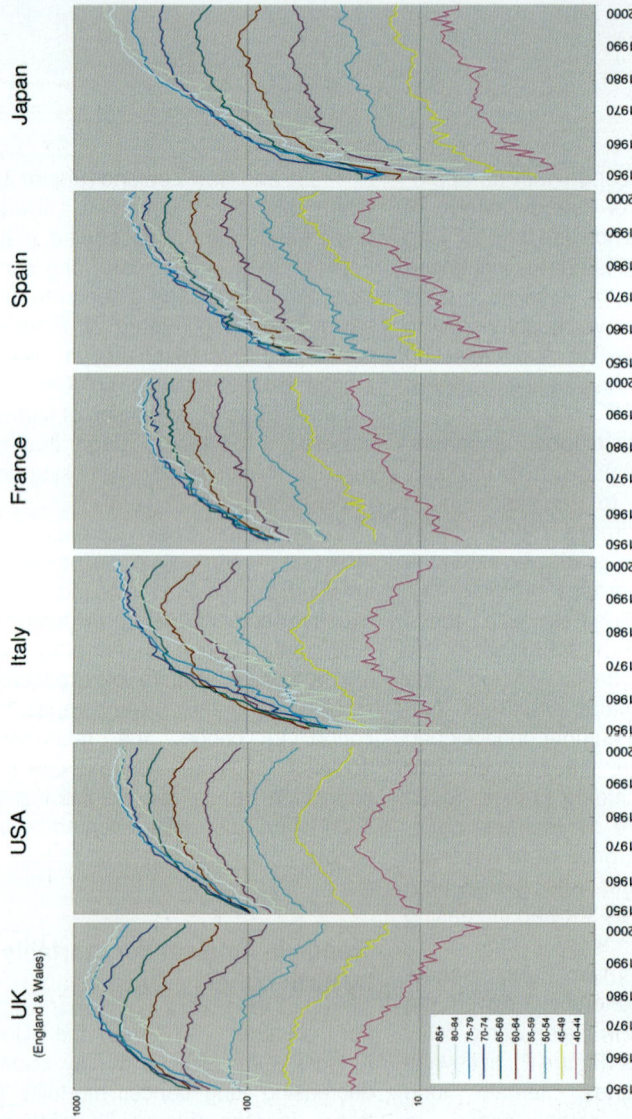

Age specific rates per 100 000 for males 40 to 85+ years of age by year of death in six selected countries.
Data source: WHO Mortality Database

Figure 1. Trends of lung cancer mortality by age group and year of death: males

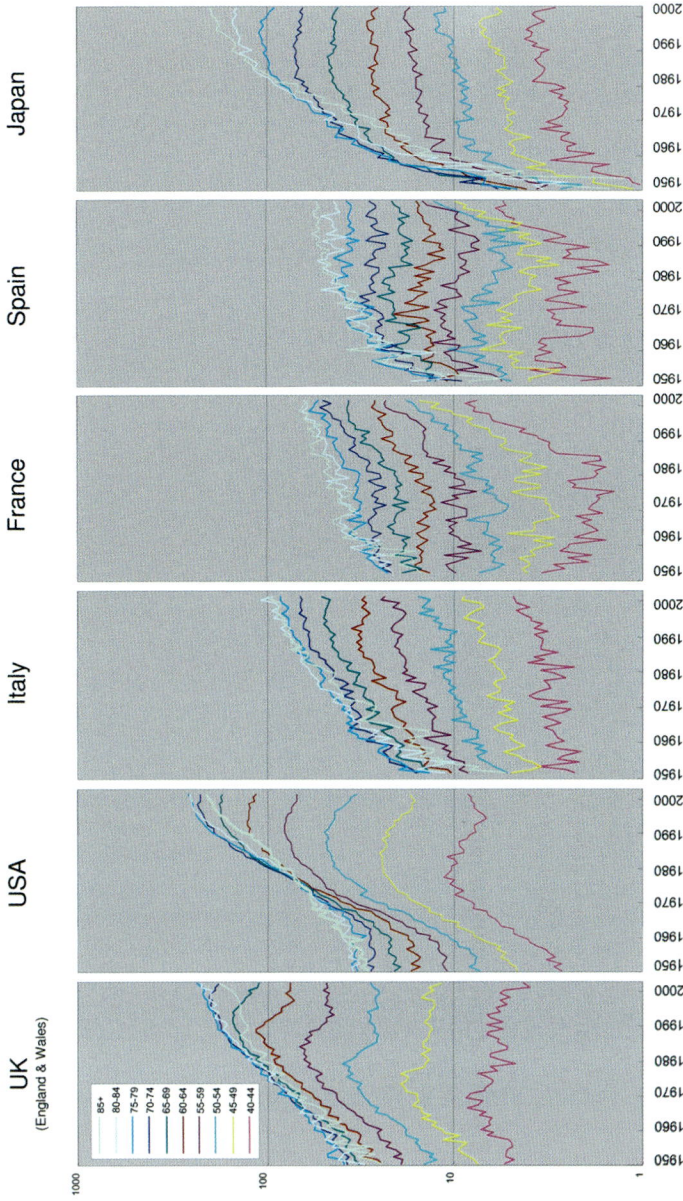

Age specific rates per 100 000 for females 40 to 85+ years of age by year of death in six selected countries.
Data source: WHO Mortality Database

Figure 2. Trends of lung cancer mortality by age group and year of death: females

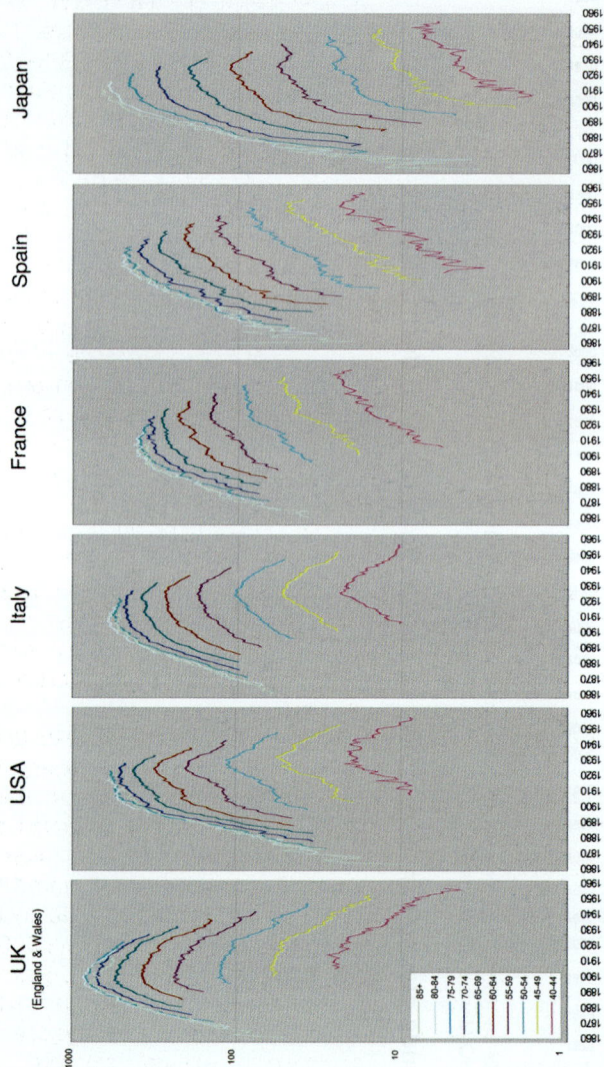

Age specific rates per 100 000 for males 40 to 85+ years of age by year of birth in six selected countries.
Data source: WHO Mortality Database

Figure 3. Trends of lung cancer mortality by age group and year of birth: males

mortality rates peaked tended to shift to earlier birth cohorts. In contrast, Japanese male age-specific mortality rates by birth cohort show a different pattern. The age-specific rates increase in more recent cohorts with a decline noted for the 1930–34 cohort across all age groups. For those born in cohorts after 1935, an increasing trend of age-specific rates is demonstrated. Age-specific rates for age groups over age 70 may be leveling off, but have not shown clear decreasing trends so far.

Age-specific lung cancer mortality rates have different pattern for females in both the USA and Japan (Figure 4). When US female age-specific mortality rates are compared by birth cohort, peak mortality rates are observed in the 1940 birth cohort in the age groups up to 45–49 years. At ages 50–59, the birth cohort at which peak mortality occurred shifts to earlier birth cohorts, at ages 60–69 rates may be leveling off, and above age 70–74 rates continue in an upward trend. Female age-specific mortality rates in Japan at younger ages show a generally increasing trend, in contrast to the decline for more recent cohorts observed among US women. Although the trends are not clear, the rates for Japanese women over age 60 years may be leveling off for cohorts born after 1920.

Peak age-specific mortality rates occurred in the same birth cohort for young age groups, and the peaks shift to earlier birth cohorts for older age groups. One possible explanation for this observation is that lung cancer mortality rates for younger age groups are mainly affected by reductions in rates of smoking initiation, while those for older age groups are also affected by increases in rates of smoking cessation as well as changes in smoking initiation. For countries where the pattern of lung cancer mortality rates did not follow a pattern of decreasing trends for all age groups, including Japan, France and

Spain, rates of smoking initiation have not decreased as markedly and may even have increased among females. In addition, the increases in rates of cessation observed in countries with decreasing mortality trends may have been delayed or blunted.

Trends in smoking prevalence for the USA and Japan in relation to lung cancer mortality trends by birth cohort

Compared to the data availability on the trends of lung cancer mortality, data on smoking prevalence were rather limited for long-term trends by birth cohort for the majority of the countries examined. Since the USA and Japan had relatively sufficient data on long-term trends for smoking prevalence, further analysis is focused in these two countries.

Cigarette consumption per capita in the USA and Japan

Cigarette consumption per capita is a crude index of the population burden of smoking. Figure 5 shows trends in cigarette consumption per capita (in individuals 18 years old or older) in the USA and Japan. In the USA, per capita cigarette consumption started to increase rapidly after the first decade of the 1900s, and continued an upward trend until the early 1960s. It then stayed at a level of approximately 4000 cigarettes/year for a decade, began a downward trend in the mid-1970s and today has reached a level of approximately 2000 cigarettes/year. In Japan, per capita cigarette consumption slowly increased from 1920 to 1940, temporarily dropped after the end of World War II (1945), and increased again from the late 1940s to early the 1970s, reaching a peak of approximately 3500 cigarettes/year. It then began a downward trend in the early 1980s that has reached a level below 3000 cigarettes/-

year by the year 2000. The decreasing trend in Japan started much later than in the USA and has progressed more slowly, at least as of the year 2000.

Data source of smoking prevalence by birth cohort

In this section, we report US age-specific prevalence of current and ever-smokers by birth cohort estimated from a dataset that combines the 1965–2001 National Health Interview Surveys containing smoking information (http://cisnet.cancer.gov; available as an electronic appendix to the Handbook at http://www.IARC.fr). The age-specific estimates of ever-smoking prevalence are based on age of smoking initiation and adjusted for the differential mortality between ever- and never smokers using the cross-sectional prevalence of ever-smokers by cohort from consecutive surveys. Since ever-smokers tend to die at a higher rate than never smokers, the prevalence of ever-smokers by cohort declines in later surveys as they pass age 50. Thus, the estimated age-specific ever-smokers' prevalence decreases after middle age (Figures 6 and 7). The prevalence of former smokers was calculated by subtracting the prevalence of current smokers from the prevalence of ever-smokers.

Estimates of age-specific prevalence of smoking by birth cohort in Japan have been recently reported by Marugame et al. (2006). The authors estimated the age-specific prevalence of current smoking for each cohort born from 1900 to 1952, using the baseline data pooled from four prospective studies (242 330 men and 274 075 women). Using the same data, courtesy of Marugame, the Working Group calculated age-specific prevalence of current smokers and ever-smokers for each birth cohort born from 1900 to 1950 (by 10-year birth cohorts) by counting the number of current smokers and ever-smokers at each age based on individual data on

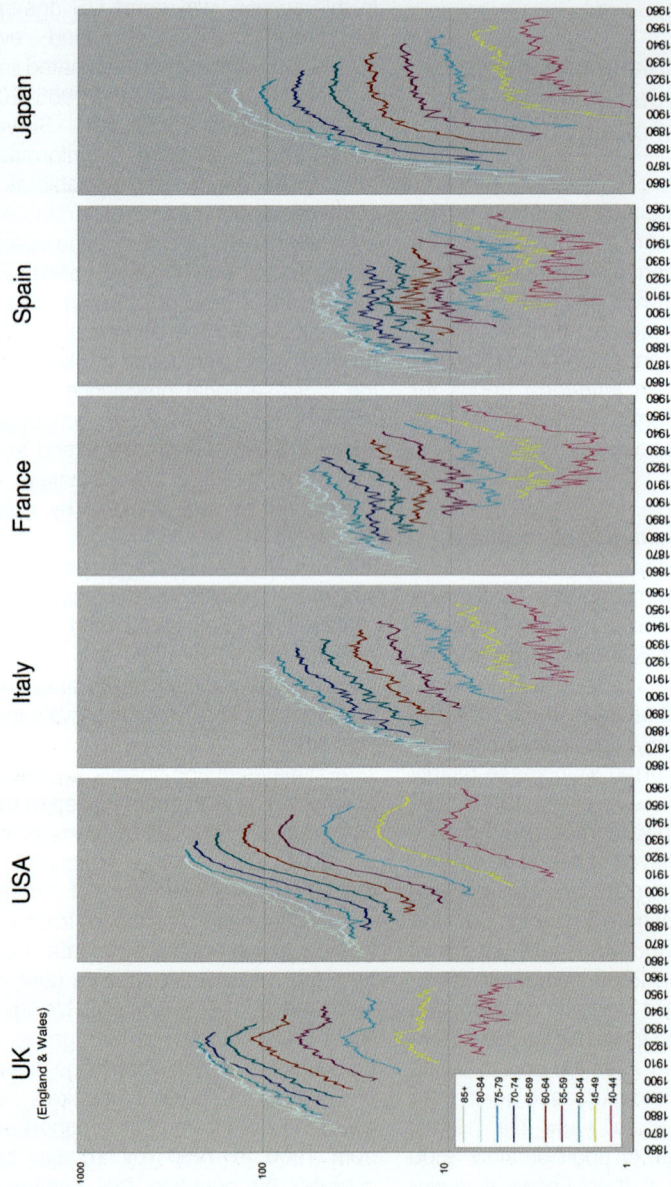

Age specific rates per 100 000 for females 40 to 85+ years of age by year of birth in six selected countries.
Data source: WHO Mortality Database

Figure 4. Trends of lung cancer mortality by age group and year of birth: females

Per capita cigarette consumption (18 years or older)

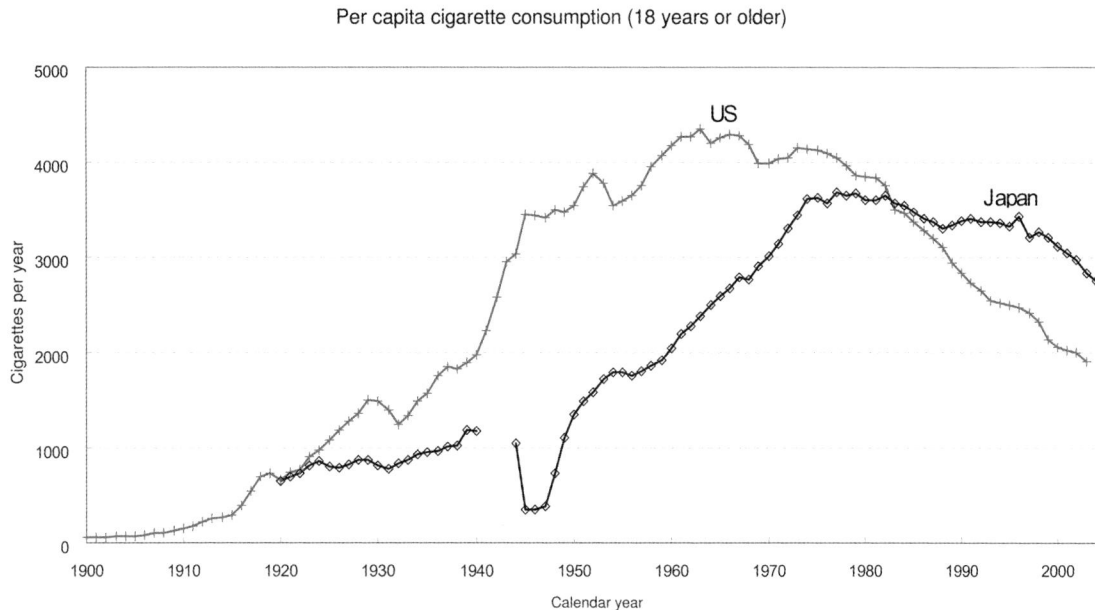

Data are not available for 1941–43 in Japan because of the Second World War.
Data sources: US Department of Agriculture Economic Research Service (http://usda.mannlib.cornell.edu/data-sets/specialty/94012)
Health-Net (http://www.health-net.or.jp/tobacco/menu02.html)
Tobacco Institute of Japan (http://www.tioj.or.jp/index.html)

Figure 5. Trends of cigarette consumption per capita in the USA and Japan

age at smoking initiation and cessation. The prevalence of former smokers was calculated by subtracting the prevalence of current smokers from the peak prevalence of ever-smokers. In contrast to US age-specific prevalence of ever-smokers (Figures 6 and 7), Japanese age-specific prevalence of ever-smokers does not move downward, even after middle age (Figures 8 and 9). This is because the estimation of the Japanese prevalence of ever-smokers is based on age at smoking initiation, with data obtained from a single survey for each cohort study and not adjusted for differential mortality. This may lead to a slight underestimation of smoking prevalence for calendar years remote from the time of the survey.

Prevalence of current and former smokers according to attained age by birth cohort US men

For all cohorts examined of US men, the prevalence of current smoking increased rapidly after age 12, peaked at about age 30 and then decreased as the cohort ages (Figure 6). In more recent years of birth, the peak prevalence of current smoking occurs at a younger age. For the 1950 birth cohort, peak current smoking prevalence occurs at around 20 years of age, whereas among those born in 1910 the peak prevalence occurs at around 30 years of age (Figure 6). The absolute level of peak prevalence of current smoking for specific birth cohorts was almost constant for cohorts born from 1900 to 1930, then declined

after the 1930 birth cohort. The prevalence of former smoking increases rapidly after age 30, and recent cohorts tend to show increases in the rates of smoking cessation that begin at earlier ages and are greater in magnitude than those of earlier cohorts.

Japanese men

Among Japanese men the prevalence of current smoking began to rise steeply at age 20 in all cohorts examined, considerably later than the same cohorts of U.S. males (Figure 8). In the 1900 birth cohort, current smoking prevalence peaked at around age 40 and then declined with increasing age. As year of birth advanced, the peak prevalence of

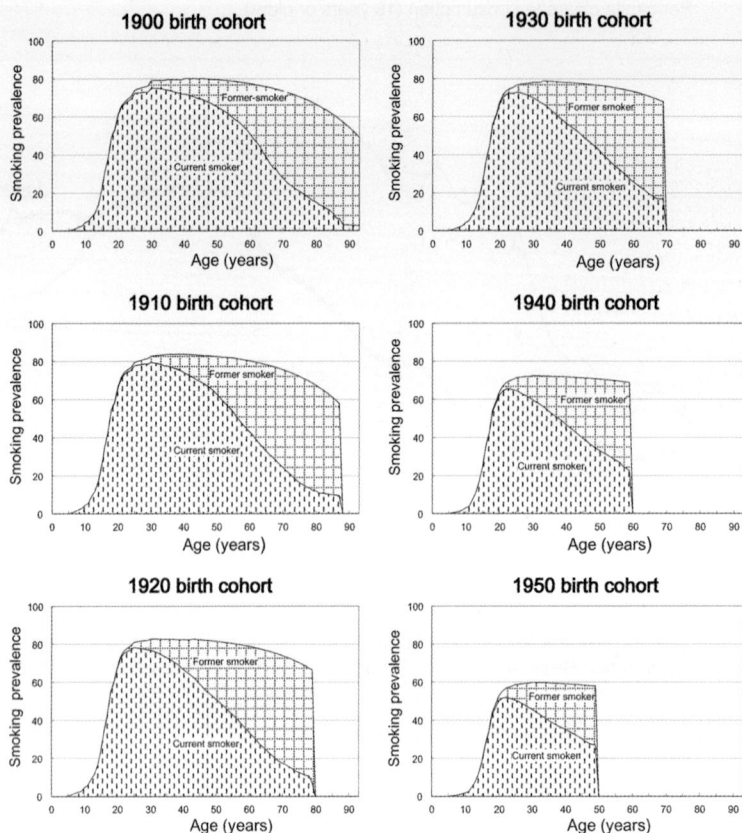

Data source: NCI – CISNET

Figure 6. Age-specific prevalence of current and former smokers by birth cohort in US white males

current smokers was registered at younger ages, and the onset of the steep rise in smoking prevalence also appeared at an earlier age (Figure 8). For the 1950 birth cohort, the peak prevalence of current smoking was seen around 25 years of age. The absolute level of peak prevalence of current smoking increased for cohorts born between 1900 and 1920 and then declined slightly in subsequent cohorts. Prevalence of former smoking started to increase around age of 40 and then increased as the cohort aged, but the prevalence of former smoking at any

given age was low compared with the same cohorts of US men.

US women

The pattern of smoking prevalence across cohorts of US women (Figure 7) is quite different from that of US men (Figure 6). For the 1900 birth cohort, the prevalence of current smokers started to increase at around age 15, peaked around age 50 and then decreased as the cohort aged. As year of birth advanced, age at peak prevalence of current smokers decreased. For the 1950 birth cohort, the peak occurred at

around 25 years of age, at almost the same age as for men. In contrast to the US men, there was a substantial shift in the age of peak prevalence of smoking towards younger ages across the cohorts examined. The absolute level of peak prevalence of current smoking among US women increased with advancing birth cohort from 1900 to 1920, remained constant from 1920–1940, and began to decrease with the 1950 birth cohort. For the 1900 birth cohort, the prevalence of former smokers started to increase around age 50 and then continued to rise as the cohort

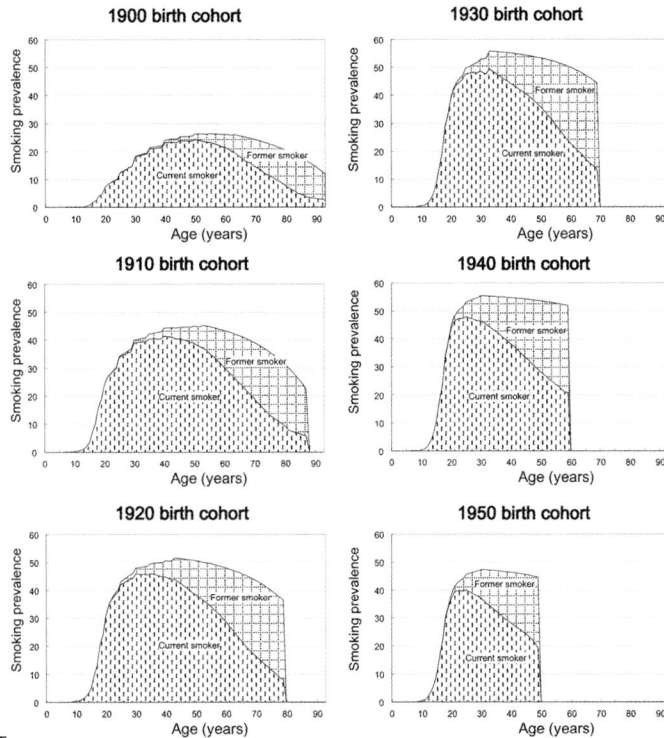

1900 birth cohort · 1930 birth cohort · 1910 birth cohort · 1940 birth cohort · 1920 birth cohort · 1950 birth cohort

Data source: NCI – CISNET

Figure 7. Age-specific prevalence of current and former smokers by birth cohort in US white females

aged. In successive cohorts, the prevalence of former smoking increased rapidly after age 30; more recent cohorts tended to show increases in the rates of smoking cessation at earlier ages and are greater in magnitude than those of earlier cohorts. The variation across cohorts in terms of age at peak prevalence and cessation patterns is more dramatic for US women than for US men.

Japanese women

Among Japanese women born in 1900, there is a slow rise in the prevalence of current smoking beginning around the age of 20 (Figure 9). Smoking prevalence peaked at about ages 50–65 and

then decreased as the cohort aged. Compared with US females (Figure 7), the absolute level of peak prevalence of current smoking was much lower, around 15%. According to Marugame and colleagues (2006), cohorts born after 1950 show an increasing trend of ever-smoking prevalence reaching approximately 20%. In the cohorts examined, the prevalence of former smokers was very small and is likely to have limited impact on female lung cancer trends in the general population. In Japan, no substantial decrease in smoking initiation or increase in smoking cessation occurred, based on the baseline survey of the above cohorts conducted in 1990. More recent trends in

current smoking prevalence up to the year 2002 show a further decrease of current smoking among Japanese men in older age groups, but increasing trends are observed in younger women (Ministry of Health, Labour and Welfare, 2004).

Cumulative exposure to smoking for specific birth cohorts and its relation to lung cancer mortality trends by birth cohort

The cumulative exposure to smoking at any given age for a specified birth cohort is a function of rates of initiation and cessation that occur prior to that

1900 birth cohort

1930 birth cohort

1910 birth cohort

1940 birth cohort

1920 birth cohort

1950 birth cohort

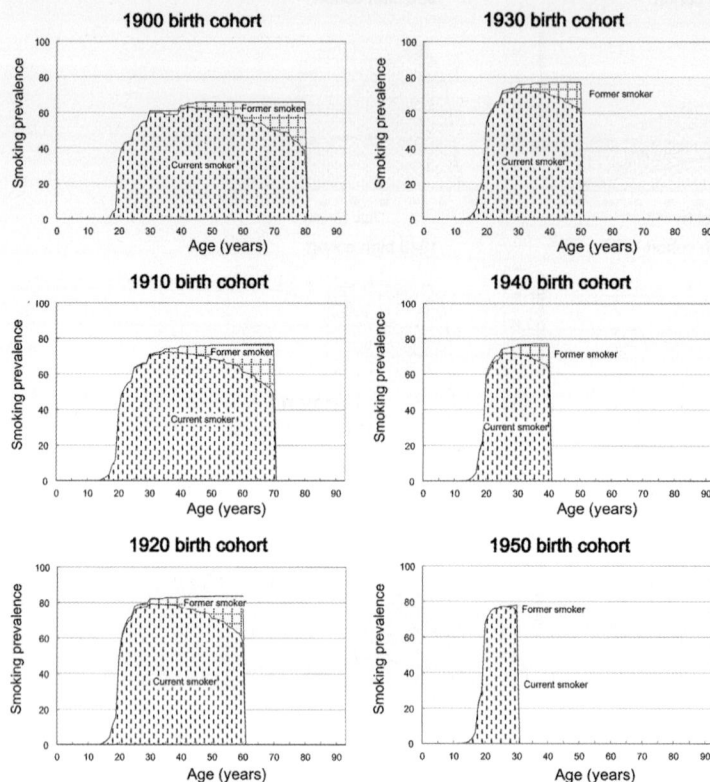

Data source: Marugame *et al.* (2006)

Figure 8. Age-specific prevalence of current and former smokers by birth cohort in males, Japan

age. Cumulative exposure increases with age within the same birth cohort. Linking cumulative exposure to lung cancer risk requires consideration of the appropriate lag time between exposure and manifestation of disease risk.

Figure 10 shows the scheme for determining cumulative prevalence-years for current smokers from age 0 to 29 (or 49) years and cumulative prevalence-years for former smokers from age 0 to 69 years. The former is an indicator of smoking initiation, reflecting both prevalence and age at initiation, and the latter

is an indicator of smoking cessation. For men, age 29 was chosen because most male smokers have initiated smoking by this age. The Working Group believes that this indicator will be associated with the risk of lung cancer in age groups up to 70 years. The combination of indicators for initiation and cessation will be associated with the risk of lung cancer in older age groups, such as those 70 to 80 years of age. In this chapter, data for these two parameters are presented separately in order to examine the differing effects of smoking on lung cancer risk on a population basis when exposure is

increasing in one part of the population and decreasing in another.

For US women, cumulative prevalence-years for current smokers from age 0 to 49 years was chosen since the prevalence of current smokers continued to increase after 30 years of age, especially for earlier cohorts. The level of peak prevalence of current smoking was very low in Japanese women, precluding examination of smoking and lung cancer mortality trends.

Among US male cohorts (Figure 11A), cumulative prevalence-years of

1900 birth cohort

1930 birth cohort

1910 birth cohort

1940 birth cohort

1920 birth cohort

1950 birth cohort

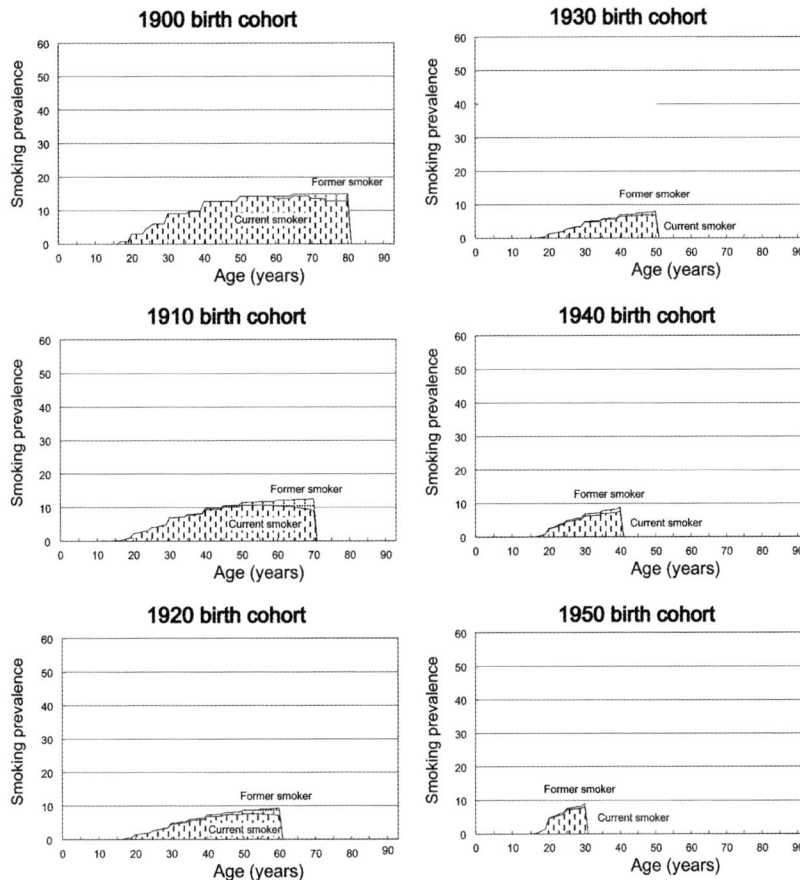

Data source: Marugame *et al.* (2006)

Figure 9. Age-specific prevalence of current and former smokers by birth cohort in females, Japan

current smoking from ages 0 to 29 increased slightly from 1900 to 1905, became almost constant from 1905 to 1925 and then decreased steadily across subsequent cohorts. The increase from 1900 to 1905 was due to a shift of age at smoking initiation to younger ages. The decline after 1925 was mainly due to the decrease in smoking initiation rate. The cumulative prevalence-years for former smokers increased across all of the birth cohorts. When comparing smoking prevalence by birth cohort with trends in lung cancer mortality rates, the deceasing trends of current smokers prevalence-years after the 1925 birth cohort would correspond to decreased lung cancer mortality trends seen after the 1925 birth cohort for the age group below 55–59 years (Figure 11B). However, an increasing trend in the lung cancer mortality rates in the 1905 to 1925 birth cohorts could not be explained by a constant level of cumulative prevalence-years of current smoking in the same birth cohorts.

Lung cancer mortality rates for age groups above 60 years peaked in cohorts born prior to 1925, and the mortality peak rate moved to earlier cohorts with increasing age (Figure 11B). This relationship could correspond to the increasing cumulative prevalence-years for former smokers for the 1905-25 birth cohorts (Figure 11A). For age groups above 70 years, there were slight decreasing trends that could correspond to the effect of increasing prevalence-years for former smokers from 1900 to 1925.

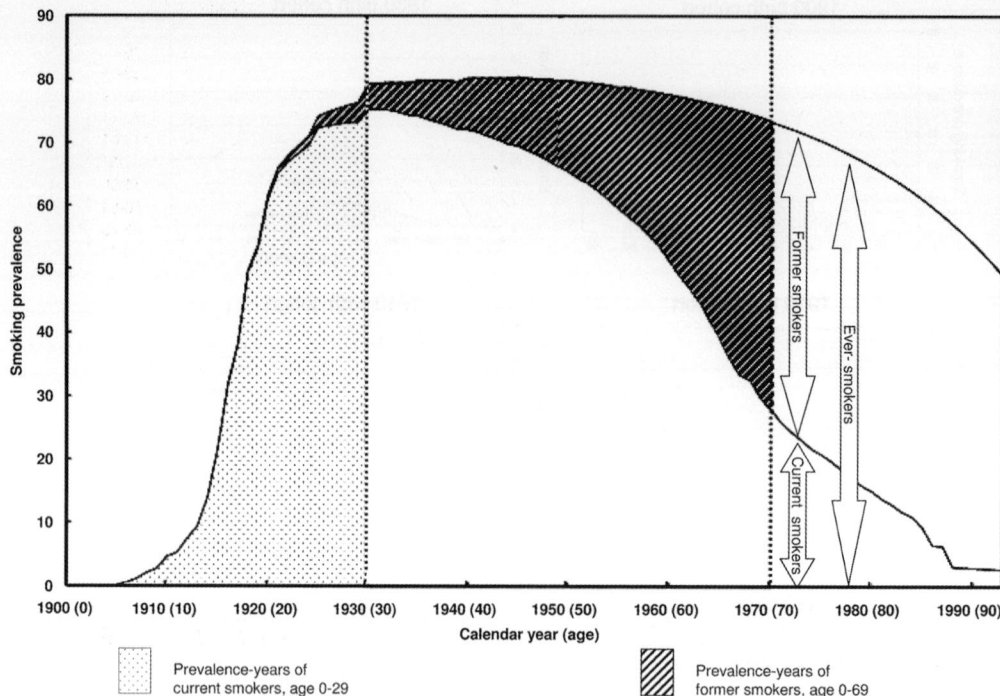

Figure 10. Scheme for calcuating birth-cohort-specific accumulation of current smokers or former smokers (prevalence-years)

Cumulative prevalence-years for Japanese male current smokers for ages 0 to 29 years (Figure 12A) were lower than the levels for US men. Japanese male cumulative prevalence years increased from the 1900–04 to the 1925–29 birth cohort, decreased from the 1925–29 to the 1935–39 birth cohort, then increased in later cohorts. The decrease from 1925–29 to 1935–39 was due to a decreased initiation rate, probably due to a limited supply of cigarettes during and just after World War II. Cumulative prevalence-years for Japa-nese male former smokers gradu-ally increased after the 1900 birth cohort. Compared with US male cohorts, the level of cumulative prevalence-years was substantially lower.

When comparing smoking preva-lence by birth cohort (Figure 12A) with trends in lung caner mortality rates for Japanese men (Figure 12B), the increasing trends of prevalence-years for current smokers for 0 to 29 years of age from the 1900–04 to the 1925–29 birth cohort could correspond to the increas-ing trends of lung cancer mortality for these birth cohorts. Decreasing cumula-tive prevalence-years for current smokers from the 1925–29 to the 1935–39 birth cohorts, and increasing trends afterwards (Figure 12A), offer an explanation for the decreasing and increasing trends for lung cancer mortality in the same cohorts (Figure 12B). The prevalence of former smokers was low, and the effect of the increasing prevalence

was not apparent even in older age groups.

Cumulative prevalence-years for US female current smokers from age 0 to 49 years (Figure 13A) increased from the 1900 cohort to the 1930 cohort, remained almost constant up to the 1935 cohort, and then decreased in subsequent cohorts. Cumulative preva-lence-years for US female former smokers from ages 0 to 69 years increased steadily across all cohorts after the 1900 birth cohort. Compared with US and Japanese men, the level of cumulative prevalence-years for female former smokers was higher than in Japanese men and lower than in US men.

When comparing smoking preva-lence and trends in age-specific lung

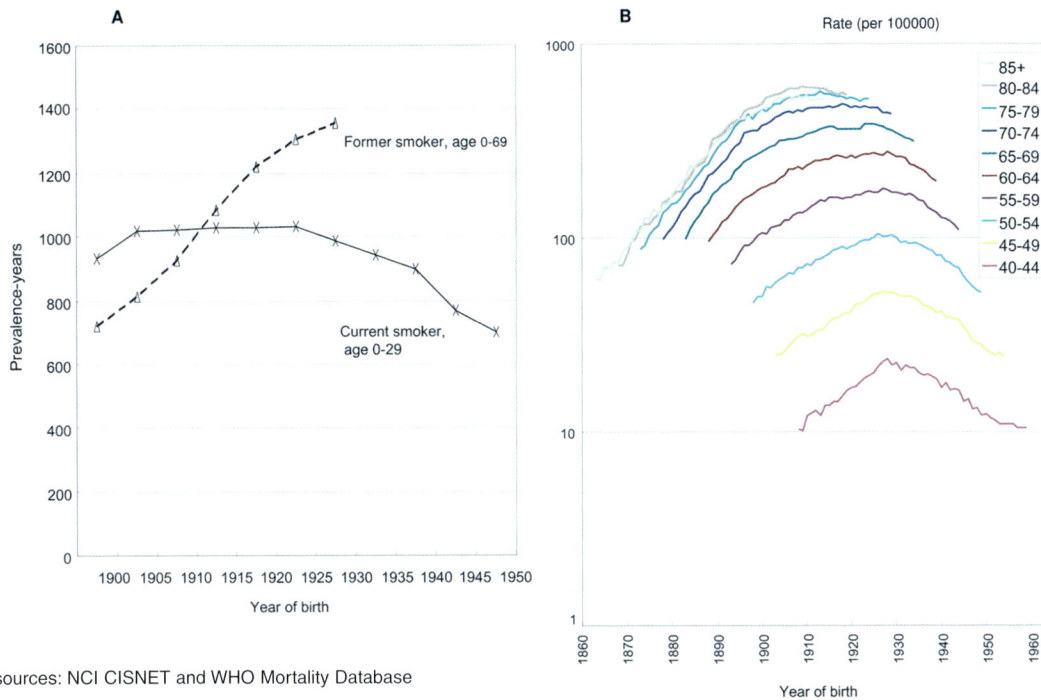

Data sources: NCI CISNET and WHO Mortality Database

Figure 11. Trends of prevalence-years of current and former smokers (A) and age-specific lung cancer mortality rates (B) by year of birth in US white males

cancer mortality rates by birth cohort for age groups below age 55–59 years (Figure 13B), both prevalence-years for current smokers from ages 0 to 49 years and lung cancer mortality trends are similar. Both trends increased for the cohorts born from 1900 to 1930, remained constant for the cohorts born 1930 to 1935, and decreased from the 1940 birth cohort onward.

Lung cancer mortality for the age groups 60 years or older was still increasing for US women. This increase may be due to increasing trends in smoking initiation and cumulative prevalence-years for current smokers from 0 to 49 years. These possible effects may have overwhelmed the effect of increasing smoking cessation in these birth cohorts.

Discussion

For US men, significant change in terms of smoking initiation and cessation occurred during the 20th century. Trends in lung cancer mortality by birth cohort can be explained by parameters related to smoking initiation and cessation, such as cumulative prevalence-years of current smokers from 0 to 29 years of age and cumulative prevalence-years of former smokers from 0 to 69 years of age. Trends in lung cancer mortality below age 70 were affected by smoking initiation and those above age 70 by both initiation and cessation.

Among Japanese men, parameters measuring smoking cessation, such as cumulative prevalence-years of former smokers, are not yet large enough to

affect lung cancer mortality rates. Japanese male lung cancer mortality is mainly explained by the smoking initiation parameter, cumulative prevalence-years of current smokers from ages 0 to 29 years. Restrictions in the cigarette supply during and after World War II explain the temporary decrease of smoking initiation for the 1930-44 birth cohorts, which also translated into a decrease in lung cancer mortality for these cohorts.

Among US women, trends in lung cancer mortality below 60 years of age by birth cohort can be explained by smoking initiation with cumulative prevalence-years of current smokers expanded to ages 0 to 49 years. For those above 60 years of age, the increasing trend of smoking initiation

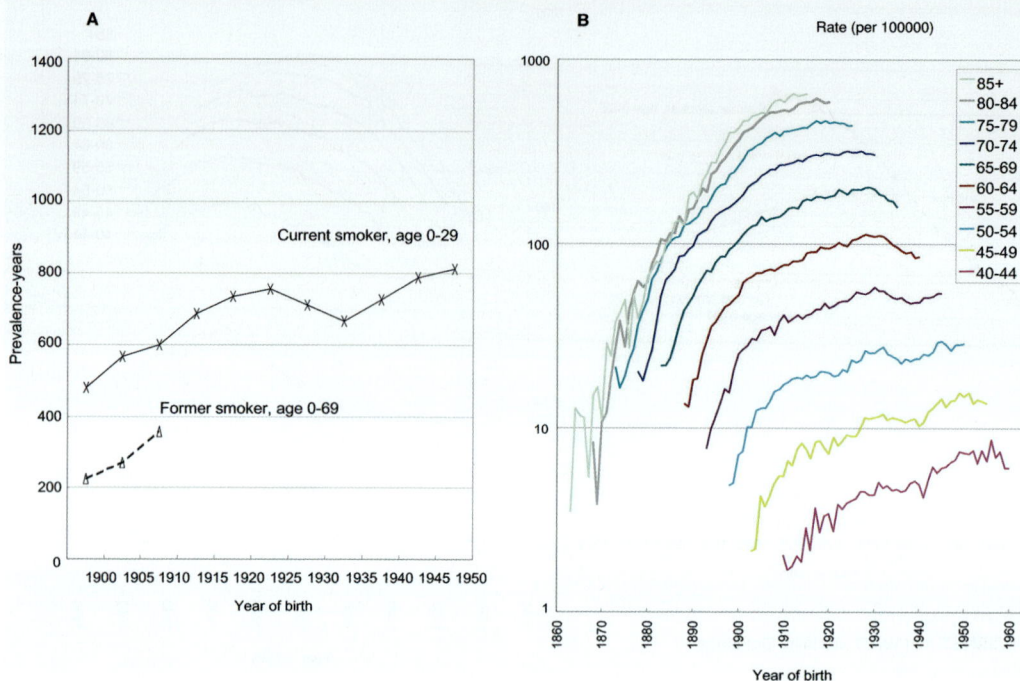

Data sources: Marugame *et al.* (2006) and WHO Mortality Database

Figure 12. Trends of prevalence-years of current and former smokers (A) and age-specific lung cancer mortality rates (B) by year of birth in Japanese males

overwhelmed the effect of increasing smoking cessation.

Among US men, increasing cessation was observed across all birth cohorts and a decrease in initiation occurred with the 1930 and subsequent birth cohorts. Among Japanese men, there was no substantial decrease in initiation or increase in cessation across the birth cohorts. US women experienced simultaneous increases in initiation and in cessation across cohorts born from 1900 to 1930 (though the former effect overshadowed the latter). A decrease in initiation occurred in the 1940 and following birth cohorts. For Japanese females, smoking cessation rates were not large enough to affect lung cancer mortality.

Comparison of US and Japan trends to the experience of other countries is pertinent. In the United Kingdom, Finland, Canada and Italy, where male lung cancer mortality rates began to decrease first in younger age groups and only subsequently extended to older age groups, similar to the trends in the USA, the decrease in smoking initiation occurred within a short interval after rates of smoking cessation began to increase (La Vecchia *et al.*, 1986; Wald *et al.*, 1988; Pelletier *et al.*, 1996; Laaksonen *et al.*, 1999).

In Spain, where lung cancer mortality in younger age groups is still increasing, similar to Japan, the decrease in smoking initiation has not started yet

and an increase in smoking cessation is not yet evident. In France, the prevalence of current smoking is decreasing among males and stable among females in the past 20 to 30 years (Marques-Vidal *et al.*, 2003; Hill & Laplanche, 2004). Lung cancer mortality in younger age groups is increasing for both sexes, and the decreasing trend in male smoking prevalence has not yet been reflected in lung cancer mortality. Different trends in lung cancer mortality from other developed countries can also be explained by differences in the timing of reductions in smoking initiation and increases in smoking cessation (Fernandez *et al.*, 2003). This illustrates that even within developed countries

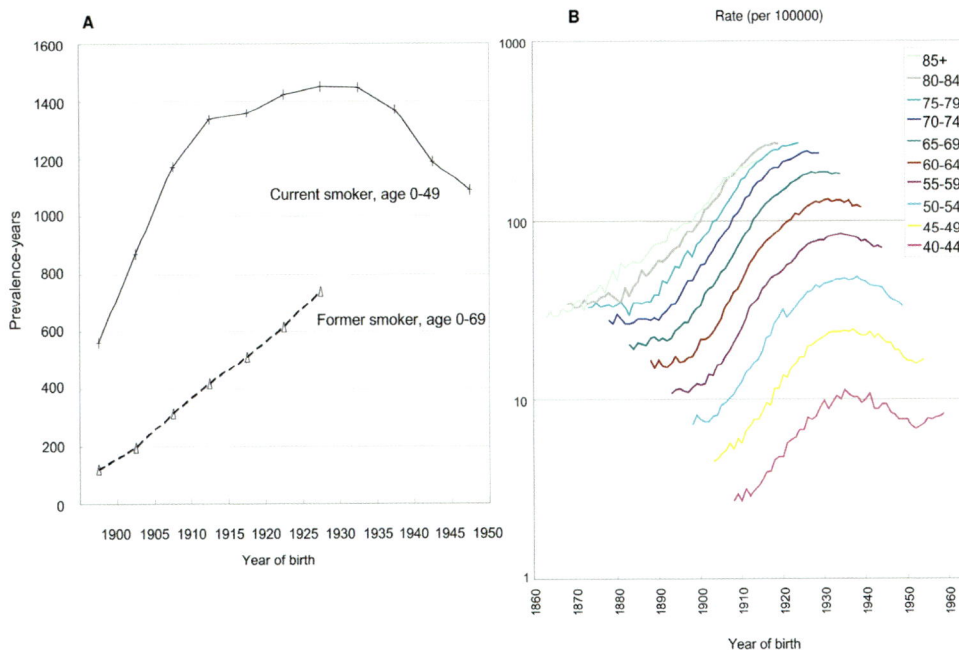

Data sources: NCI – CISNET and WHO Mortality Database

Figure 13. Trends of prevalence-years of current and former smokers (A) and age-specific lung cancer mortality rates (B) by year of birth in US white females

there are substantial differences in both age of onset of smoking and age of onset of cessation among established smokers.

For US women, the trends are similar to those of men in recent cohorts. In earlier cohorts of U.S. females, however, the peak prevalence of current smoking shifted substantially to younger ages in later birth cohorts. This makes it difficult to set the parameters for smoking initiation—specifically, to fix the age range for calculating cumulative prevalence-years for current smokers. In addition, in the case where increases in initiation and cessation occurred simultaneously, as observed for US women, not only timing but also magni-

tude of the effect due to those changes should be considered. More sophisticated statistical modelling will be needed to examine these smoking changes.

In the USA, switch from non-filter to filter cigarettes occurred rapidly from 1950 to 1960 and somewhat more gradually from 1960 to 1985. In Japan, the shift to filters began slightly later but was essentially complete by 1975. The type of filter predominantly used in Japan was a charcoal filter, while plain acetate filters are more widely used in the USA. These factors do not seem to explain the differences in lung cancer rates between the two countries.

Conclusion

Differences in patterns of smoking initiation and cessation have been identified for Japan and the USA. These differences in behaviors by birth cohort underlie some of the variations in lung cancer mortality rates between these countries. When interpreting observed trends of lung cancer mortality and predicting future trends, it is necessary to consider both initiation and cessation. Data documenting smoking behavior are not readily available for many countries at present.

References

Fernandez E, Schiaffino A, Borras JM, et al. (2003). Prevalence of cigarette smoking by birth cohort among males and females in Spain, 1910-1990. *Eur J Cancer Prev,* 12(1):57-62.

Hill C, Laplanche A (2004). *Le tabac en France, les vrais chiffres.* Paris, La Documentation Française.[In French]

La Vecchia C, Decarli A, Pagano R (1986). Prevalence of cigarette smoking among subsequent cohorts of Italian males and females. *Prev Med,* 15(6):606-613.

Laaksonen M, Uutela A, Vartiainen E, et al. (1999). Development of smoking by birth cohort in the adult population in eastern Finland 1972-97. *Tob Control,* 8(2):161-168.

Marques-Vidal P, Ruidavets JB, Cambou JP, et al. (2003). Changes and determinants in cigarette smoking prevalence in south-western France, 1985-1997. *Eur J Public Health,* 13(2):168-170.

Marugame T, Yoshimi I (2005). Comparison of cancer mortality (lung cancer) in five countries: France, Italy, Japan, UK and USA from the WHO Mortality Database (1960-2000). *Jpn J Clin Oncol,* 35(3):168-170.

Marugame T, Kamo K, Sobue T, et al. (2006). Trends in smoking by birth cohorts born between 1900 and 1977 in Japan. *Prev Med,* 42(2):120-127.

Ministry of Health Labour and Welfare (2004). The National Nutrition Survey in Japan 2002. Tokyo, Dai-Ichi Shuppan Publishing Co. Ltd. [In Japanese]

Pelletier F, Marcil-Gratton N, Legare J (1996). A cohort approach to tobacco use and mortality: the case of Quebec. *Prev Med,* 25(6):730-740.

United States Department of Health and Human Service (USDHHS) (2001). Women and Smoking. *A Report of the Surgeon General.* Atlanta,GA, U.S Department of Health and Human Services, Centers for Disease Control and Prevention, Office of Smoking and Health.

Vineis P, Alavanja M, Buffler P, et al. (2004). Tobacco and cancer: recent epidemiological evidence. *J Natl Cancer Inst,* 96(2):99-106.

Wald N, Kiryluk S, Darby S, et al. (1988). *UK smoking statistics.* Oxford, New York, Oxford University Press.

Websites

U.S. Department of Agriculture Economic Research Service: http://usda.mannlib.cornell.edu/data-sets/specialty/94012/

Cigarette consumption data in Japan: Health-Net http://www.health-net.or.jp/tobacco/menu02.html

Tobacco Institute of Japan http://www.tioj.or.jp/index.html

Population data of Japan: Population estimates. Statistics Bureau, Ministry of Internal Affairs and Communications, Japan: http://www.stat.go.jp/english/data/jinsui/index.htm

WHO database of mortality and population estimates http://www-dep.iarc.fr

US National Health Interview Surveys http://cisnet.cancer.gov

Smoking behaviour estimates for the United States (courtesy of David Burns) http://www.IARC.fr

Prediction of Lung Cancer Mortality Rates in Selected Countries

Introduction

This chapter describes a statistical analysis aimed at predicting future rates of lung cancer mortality in selected countries and investigating possible changes in these rates associated with reductions in the percentages of individuals who smoke. These projections are performed in order to give a possible picture to the future morbidity and mortality from persistent smoking. By demon-strating the potential magnitude of the number dying from on-going smoking, it is hoped that this will illustrate the needs to assist in smoking cessation

The predictions are based upon two methods. The first uses Age–Period–Cohort (APC) models (Osmond, 1985; Robertson & Boyle, 1998) to predict future rates and is a simple descriptive prediction of what is expected to happen assuming that past trends and associations in the data continue into the future. This method is exactly the same as that used by Møller *et al.* (2002) and Quinn *et al.* (2003). Within this model the age effects represent the increasing risk of dying from lung cancer in older age groups. Period and cohort both represent time trends in the mortality rates. Period effects represent changes to the trends which affect all age groups at the same calendar time and are often associated with treatment effects, diagnostic

effects or the appearance of a new risk factor which affects everyone at the same time. The cohort effects represent long term behavioural patterns which change over time such that cohorts born in different periods have different patterns. Lifetime cigarette consumption is generally thought of as a cohort effect.

In the second prediction method we investigate the association between the levels of smoking at particular ages and lung cancer mortality. The percentages of individuals in a cohort smoking at the age of 20, 30 or 40 are used as cohort-specific predictor variables to replace the cohort effects in the same general APC model. The percentages of individuals smoking 10, 20 or 30 years in the past are also considered. These can be thought of as period-specific predictor variables and replace the general period effects in the APC model.

There have been a number of previous attempts to predict lung cancer incidence of mortality based upon smoking history. In the most recent, Shibuya *et al.* (2005), lung cancer mortality data from 1950 to 2000 were used to predict mortality up to 2035 in the United States, Canada, the United Kingdom and Australia. The period effects in an APC model were replaced by a continuous explanatory variable, which was the product of the average tar content of cigarettes and tobacco

consumption lagged by 25 years. The available data gave age- and period-specific values for the explanatory variable from 1950 to 1998. Consumption prior to 1950 was estimated using an Age Cohort model, and independent time series models were used to forecast future values of the tobacco variables and the effects for future cohorts. The predictions showed a decrease in lung cancer mortality for men in all countries, but with higher rates in United States and Canada than in Australia and the United Kingdom. For women a rise is forecast in United States, Canada and Australia before a decline. The rates in the United Kingdom have peaked and are forecast to decline.

Brown and Kessler (1988) analysed lung cancer mortality in the United States from 1958 to 1982 replacing the period effects in the APC model by a lagged measure of the population's exposure to tar. They then forecast mortality to 2025. Stevens and Moolgavkar (1979) replaced the cohort parameters in the APC model by a non-linear combination of the proportion of smokers and the cumulative number of cigarettes smoked by specific cohorts and age groups.

The common feature of these studies is that they replace either the period or the cohort effect (but not both) in the APC model with population estimates of some tobacco related consumption. This strategy breaks the inherent linear dependency leading to non-identifiability in APC models (Robertson & Boyle, 1998) provided there is not an exact linear relationship between the tobacco-related variable and period or cohort (Holford, 1992).

The choice of tobacco-related variable does not appear to be exceptionally crucial to the projections, as similar results have been obtained using different variables. For this study data on current smoking prevalence by age group and period or cohort were used for those countries with long series of data. Although tobacco consumption data may be more readily available, attention was focused on prevalence of smoking, as this is related to cessation and initiation of tobacco use. Some data were also available on the percentage of a cohort who were ever smokers as well as the percentage quitting smoking at different ages, but these data were not consistently available for all countries.

Methods

We obtained lung cancer mortality data and population estimates in five-year age groups from the 1950s up to the latest available data for each country from the WHO database (http://www-dep.iarc.fr.WHO). The countries which were selected represent the main groups of North, Central and South America (United States, Costa Rica and Chile), Europe (United Kingdom, France, Spain, Poland and Hungary), and Australasia (Australia, Japan, China, Hong Kong and Singapore) where there are known to be different patterns of smoking behaviour and lung cancer mortality. Furthermore, the selected countries all had long-term series of mortality data with no gaps, and the latest data ranged from 2000 to 2002.

Long-term smoking data were obtained for the United Kingdom, the United States and Japan. For the United States and Japan, cohort-specific estimates of the percentage of males and females smoking at specified ages were available from cohorts born from 1900 to 1980. The Japanese data (Marugame et al., 2006) came from two sources, the first covering the period 1900–1980 and the second 1989–2003. We amalgamated these data and used a generalized additive model using a bivariate smoothing of age and period to interpolate the missing data (Hastie & Tibshirani, 1990; Keiding & Carstensen, 2006). The USA data were derived from National Health Interview Surveys 1965–2001(http://www.cdc.gov/nchs/nhis .htm and http://cisnet.cancer.gov). Detailed documentation of the development of the smoking behaviour estimates for the United States by sex, race/ethnicity, and five-year birth cohorts by Burns and colleagues is available as an electronic appendix to the *Handbook* at http://IARC.fr. The data for the United Kingdom came from the General Household cross sectional survey (GHS) (http://www.statistics.gov.uk/ssd/surveys/general_household_survey.asp) and were available from 1973. The GHS began reporting on smoking every other year in 1973 and yearly since 2000. It is the official source for smoking prevalence figures for Great Britain. The survey covers Great Britain only (i.e. England, Scotland and Wales) and not Northern Ireland.

There is a lack of data on smoking prevalence among the older cohorts at younger ages, and we employed some imputation techniques to try to estimate these missing data, which is needed to relate the lung cancer rates to smoking rates by age group and cohort. There is a strong association between the age-specific smoking patterns in the United States and the United Kingdom over the period when concurrent data were available, which enabled the development of a linear regression prediction model. For men, an adjustment for period was also needed, but not for women, as there was evidence of a lag in age-specific smoking prevalence for men but not for women. The validity of this imputation was checked against historical published data from the United Kingdom (Forey & Lee 2002) which is derived from tobacco company surveys. The estimates in Forey and Lee (2002) had the same pattern as the imputed data but were consistently about 10% to 20% higher.

The mortality rates were modelled as a function of age, calendar period and birth cohort. Birth cohort was calculated as age subtracted from calendar period. Since the data were aggregated into five-year age groups and five-year calendar periods, the birth cohorts are synthetic, and partly overlapping.

Lung cancer mortality in Japan has been forecast using a Bayesian version of the APC model (Kaneko et al, 2003). The model can be written as:

$$R_{ap} = \exp (A_a + D \cdot p + P_p + C_c),$$

where R_{ap} is the mortality rate in age group a in calendar period p, A_a is the age component for age group a, D is the common drift parameter (Clayton & Schifflers, 1987), P_p represents the non-linear period curvatures and C_c is the non-linear cohort curvatures. This Poisson regression model often gives a good fit when modelling cancer mortality rates, though not for lung cancer, where there are large numbers of cases in all age groups; hence extra Poisson models were used (Breslow, 1984).

The exponential multiplicative relationship between the rate and the covariates can produce predictions in which the rates grow exponentially with time. This is especially a problem for long-term predictions. Following Møller et al. (2002), we used a power link instead of the log link to level off the exponential growth in the multiplicative model. Also, current trends can be expected to extrapolate more reliably for the near future than for more distant periods. Consequently, the linear trend (drift) was dampened towards zero in all the prediction periods except the first one. In the second period only 75% of the drift was projected, and 50% in the third. For the fourth and fifth five-year prediction periods only 25% was projected, and for subsequent periods only 20%. This is based on the belief that trends would eventually tend to flatten.

A third problem is that if there is a recent sharp change in the trends, the model would project the average increase based upon all the time periods, which would not reflect the recent change in the trends. If the rates displayed significant curvature in the observed time period, the trend in the last 10 years was used as the drift component to be projected. This allows recent changes in the rates to be used for the predictions and is important where there has been a historic long-term increase in rates but a recent slowing down or decrease.

An empirical evaluation (Møller *et al*, 2003) showed that all these modifications resulted in better predictions for cancer incidence in the Nordic countries in the period 1993–1997. The power model used in the Nordic incidence predictions has therefore also been used for the present mortality predictions:

$$R_{ap} = (A_a + D \cdot p + P_p + C_c)^5, \text{ where}$$

R_{ap}, A_a, P_p and C_c are defined as in the multiplicative model.

Mortality rates were directly age-standardised using the world standard population (IARC, 1976). Truncated rates based upon those aged 40–84 are also presented, as the predictions based upon smoking data can only be made for those aged over 40 in view of the lagged nature of these variables. Predictions of

age-specific cancer mortality were made up to 2050, but the reliability of these long-term projections is very poor. This manuscript concentrates on the results up to 2020. When making the projections, we used the age effects estimated from the data from 1950–2000. Age groups 20–24 to 80–84 were used in the estimation. Furthermore, the period effects for future periods were taken to be the same as the period effect for the last observed period. Similarly for new cohorts, who are too young to be included in the estimation of the effects using data from 1950 to 2000, the estimated effect was taken to be the same as that of the youngest observed cohort. This implies that for future periods and cohorts there is no curvature, and the drift is the most important parameter for the trend in the long-term predictions.

The reason that predictions more than 20 years into the future are considered is that some of the important smoking parameters in the smoking predictions are lagged 20 or 30 years. Consequently, the effects of changes in lung cancer mortality associated with future changes to smoking percentages can only be observed more than 20 years into the future.

The most universally available smoking prevalence data is the percentage of the population currently smoking at specified ages and time periods. When including these data in the prediction models the period effects, P_p or the cohort effects, C_{p-a}, in the APC model, $R_{ap} = \exp(A_a + P_p + C_{p-a})$ are replaced with variables derived from the smoking data. Specifically, the cohort effects are replaced with the percentage of the cohort who were smokers at the ages of 20, 30, 40 or 50. The period effects are replaced by the percentage in the age group who were smokers 10, 20 or 30 years in the past. The latter is similar to the methodology of Shibuya *et al.* (2005). When making predictions based upon these models, various assump-

tions are made about the smoking levels in the future.

The model selection of the appropriate lagged percentage or cohort smoking at a particular age was based upon minimisation of the residual deviance. The models used to predict lung cancer mortality had linear terms for the smoking percentages. The appropriateness of the linear association was investigated using generalised additive models and smoothing splines (Hastie & Tibshirani, 1990). There were no gross deviations from linearity.

Results

Figure 1 shows the truncated 40–84 age-adjusted rates for lung cancer mortality among men from 1970 onwards. This graph shows rates in the United Kingdom declining from their initial high levels. In all other countries there is an initial rise to a peak in the range 1980–2010. Earlier peaks are observed in the United States, Australia, Hong Kong and Singapore. Poland, Hungary, Spain and Japan are the countries where the epidemic has only just peaked or is not predicted to peak until 2010. For women the rates are lower than for men but the peak in the epidemic comes later (Figure 2). The temporal trends in these predictions are primarily influenced by the damped drift and the cohort effects. Beyond 2030 the majority of the cohort effects are assumed to be the same as the youngest cohort during the estimation period, and most of the projections would be mere speculation.

The smoking data (not shown) revealed decreasing rates in all ages in recent periods in the United States and United Kingdom for both men and women. The temporal decline in the age group 20–24 has levelled off, and shows some signs of increasing among men and women in the United Kingdom and

Men - Age Period Cohort
Predicted Rates after 2000

Legend: UK, France, Spain, Poland, Hungary, USA, Australia

Men - Age Period Cohort
Predicted Rates after 2000

Legend: Japan, Hong Kong, Chile, Costa Rica, Singapore

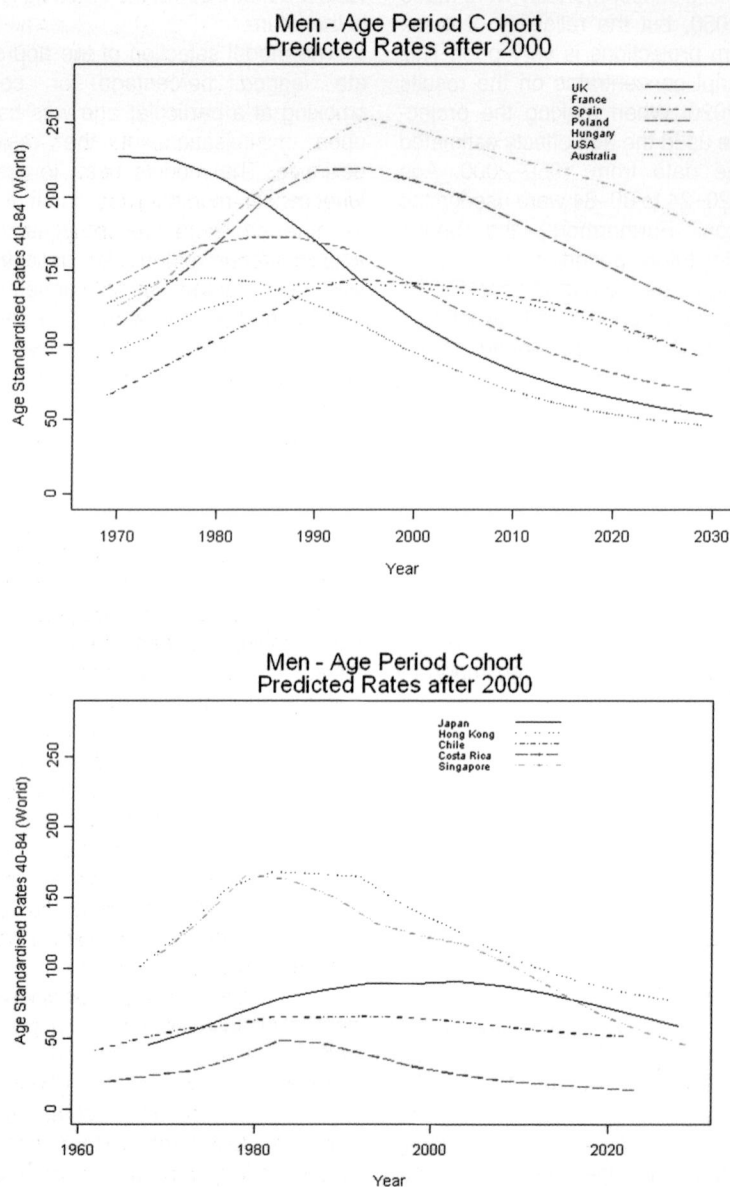

Figure 1. Observed and predicted truncated age 40–84 world standard age adjusted lung cancer mortality rates for men in selected countries

among men in the United States. In Japan there is a clear increase among men aged 20–25. Among women in Japan, the rates of smoking are particularly low, though again there is evidence of an increase among those aged less than 50, especially in the younger age groups.

Predictions based upon smoking data for the United States are presented in Figures 3 and 4, for the United Kingdom in Figure 5, and for Japan in Figure 6. Comparing Figures 4, 5 and 6 with Figures 1 and 2 shows that the predictions based upon the Cohort Smoking model are close to those of the APC predictions. In Figure 4 there is a sharp change in the predicted rates associated with various percentage reductions in smoking at lag 10 years. This arises because there has been a general decline in smoking among the older age groups and assuming no further changes in smoking percentages this decline is halted. A 10% decline in smoking every 10 years continues the trend of the recent past in these age groups. Similar comments apply to men and women in Japan.

As shown in Figure 3, the models fit reasonably well to the data, as measured by the closeness of the observed lines to the fitted points, given that they are quite simple prediction models. This was true for the other countries as well (graphs not shown). The greatest lack of fit arises with the younger age groups. This does not have a great deal of influence on the predicted truncated age-standardised rates in Figure 4, as these groups do not have a high rate. The projected effects of the smoking cessation scenarios are all superimposed in the near future, as these are based upon lagged data and the smoking prevalence is known. For men, strong declines in lung cancer mortality are predicted, but these level off at around 2030 in line with the APC Predictions (Figure 1) as the 1960 cohort reaches 70 and the majority of the cohorts in the projections have not yet begun smoking. Differences among the smoking cessation scenarios appear 10 to 20 years into the future and to maintain the projected decreases in lung cancer mortality among women from 2000 to 2010 further reductions in

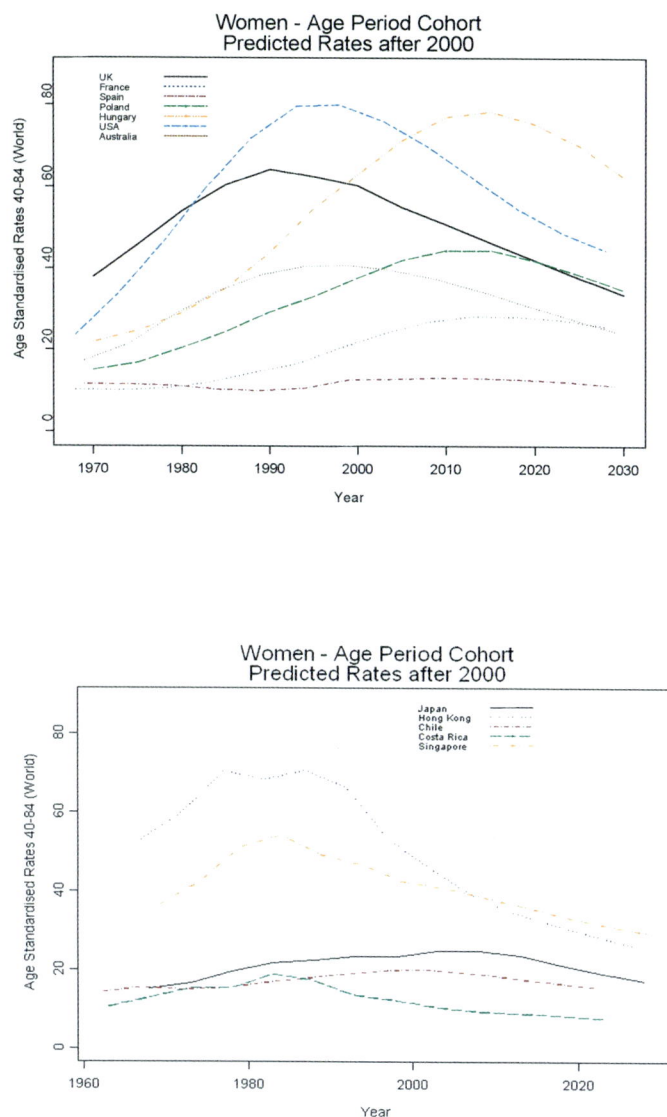

Figure 2. Observed and predicted truncated age 40–84 world standard age adjusted lung cancer mortality rates for women in selected countries

Kingdom than in the USA, as there have been trends toward reduced smoking in the United Kingdom since the 1970's for most age groups. The projections are not heavily influenced by the levels of smoking cessation, as the current levels of smoking prevalence are low relative to what they were in the past.

In Japan, there are abrupt changes when the discounted smoking rates in the future start to have an influence on the projections (Figure 6) especially when the period effect is replaced by smoking at a lag of 20 years. In men this occurs because there have been decreases in smoking among older men; if these decreases are halted then the rates are projected to rise from 2020, although they are projected to level off from 2000 to 2020 at around 85 per 100 000. Among women, smoking is increasing among the young and decreasing among the elderly; this combination leads to a projected increase in 40–84 age-standardised lung cancer mortality rates from 23 per 100 000 in 2000 to 28 per 100 000 in 2020. The projected abrupt change in 2020 occurs because the smoking prediction is based upon keeping the rates as they currently are at the last available date or discounting them by a fixed percentage every five years. Set against the background of steadily increasing smoking percentages among younger women less than 60, these smoking forecasts represent an abrupt change to the previous trends.

In the last two sets of predictions (Figure 7 and Figure 8), both of the temporal variables are replaced with the corresponding smoking variable. Cohort is replaced by the percentage of the cohort smoking at age 20 and period by the percentage of the age group smoking 20 years in the past. While the fit of the model is not as good as either of those based upon one temporal variable (compare the left-hand graphs in Figure 7 to those in Figure 3), this model has no unspecified temporal variables, and the

smoking prevalence on the order of 10% every five years are needed.

For the United Kingdom (Figure 5), the truncated 40–84 age standardised rates are projected to fall from the year

2000 rate of 116 per 100 000 to 40–44 per 100 000 by 2030 for men and from 60 per 100 000 to around 33–37 for women. For women there is less variation in the projections for the United

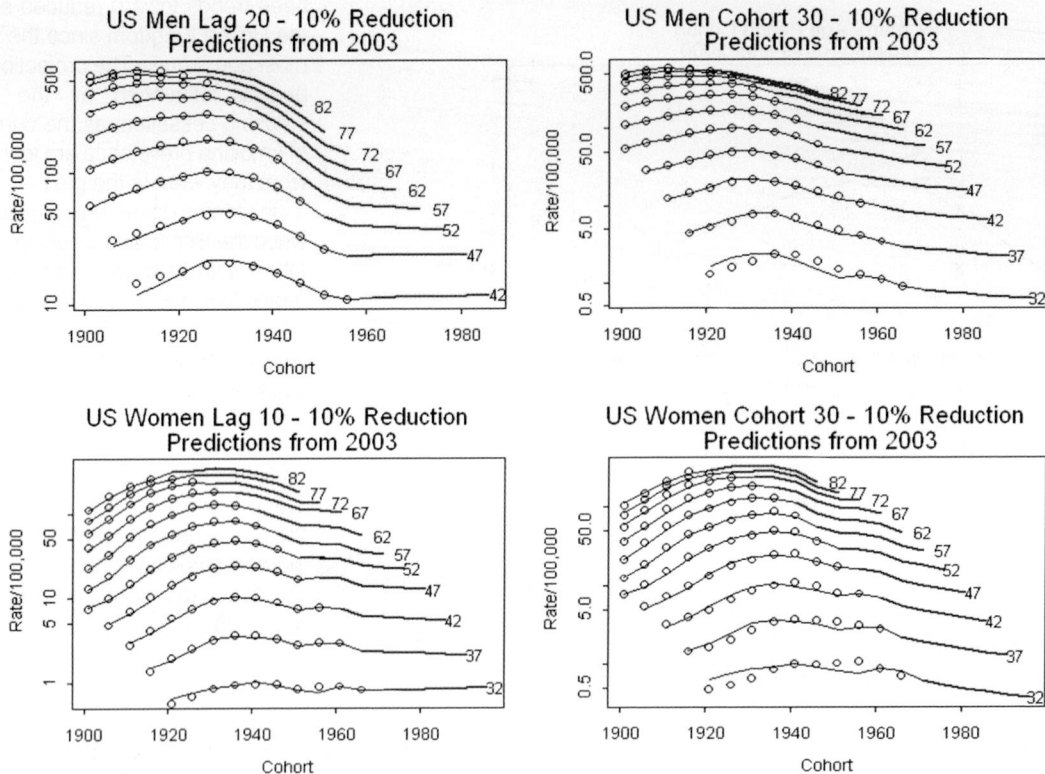

Figure 3. Predicted rates (per 100 000) of lung cancer in the United States by age group and year of birth for men (top graphs) and women (bottom graphs)

The left hand graphs are based upon a model with terms for Age + Cohort + Percentage of the Age Group Smoking 20 Years in the past (10 women). Predictions from 2003 to 2018 (2008 women) are based upon existing smoking data. The smoking percentages used for the predictions from 2023 (2013 women) onwards are based upon the last available data for each age group discounted by 10% every 5 years.

The right hand graphs are based upon a model with terms for Age + Period + Percentage of the Cohort Smoking at age 30. Predictions from 2003 to 2018 are based upon existing smoking data. The smoking percentages used for the predictions from 2023 onwards are based upon the last available data for each cohort discounted by 10% every 5 years.

In each graph the black lines with circles superimposed represent the observed rates. The circles represent the fitted values from the prediction model and the blue lines represent the predictions from the model into the future.

predictions are based solely upon the age effect and smoking data. A similar-model was suitable for men in Japan but not for women, where a big increase was predicted as a consequence of the relatively high rates of smoking among older Japanese women prior to 1970 (now declining slowly) and an increase in smoking among young Japanese women.

Discussion

The predictions of lung cancer mortality in Figures 3–6 are based upon Age–Period–Cohort models in which one, or both, of the temporal variables (period or cohort) are replaced by a smoking-related variable, such as the percentage of a cohort smoking at 20 or 30 years of age or the percentage in the age group smoking 20 years in the past. In the left-hand graphs the predicted changes in the rates over the period

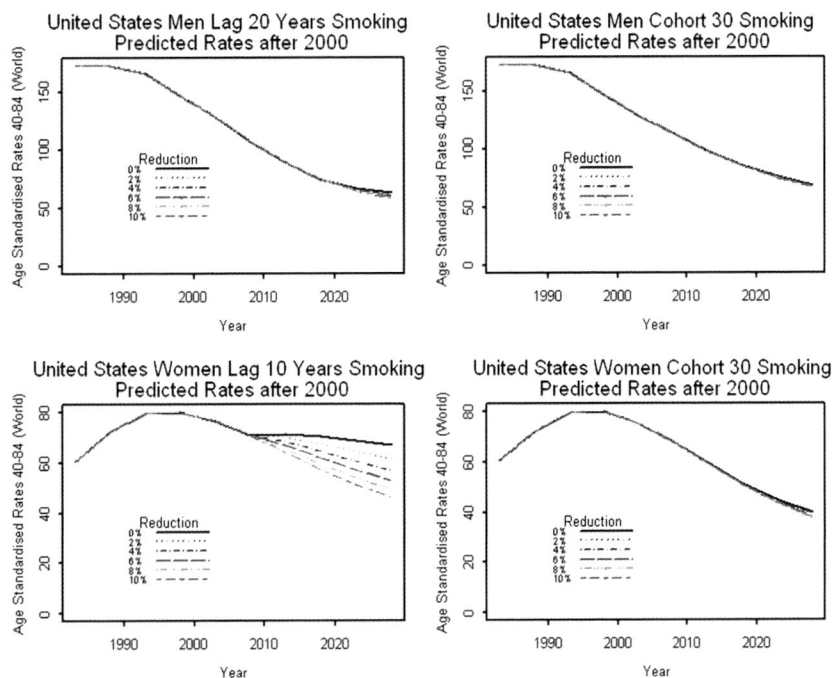

Figure 4. Predicted truncated (40–84) age standardised rates (per 100 000) of lung cancer in the United States by age group and year of birth for men (top graphs) and women (bottom graphs)

The left hand graphs are based upon a model with terms for Age + Cohort + Percentage of the Age Group Smoking 20 Years in the past (10 Years for women). Predictions from 2003 to 2018 (2008 women) are based upon existing smoking data. The smoking percentages used for the predictions from 2023 (2013 women) onwards are based upon the last available data for each age group discounted by 0% to 10% every 5 years.

The right hand graphs are based upon a model with terms for Age + Period + Percentage of the Cohort Smoking at age 30. Predictions from 2003 to 2018 are based upon existing smoking data. The smoking percentages used for the predictions from 2023 onwards are based upon the last available data for each cohort discounted by 0% to 10% every 5 years.

2000–2020 are associated with changes in the smoking pattern which have already taken place over the last 20 years and temporal effects due to cohort. The predicted changes in the rates after 2020 are associated with postulated reductions in smoking over the next 20 years and temporal effects due to cohort. In most cases recent cohorts have a reduced mortality, adjusting for smoking, and the continuation of this effect alone into the future is associated with a reduction in the rates.

In the right-hand graphs the predicted changes in the rates over the period 2000–2020 are associated with changes in the smoking rate at ages 20 or 30 among cohorts born before the 1970s and temporal effects due to period. The predicted changes in the rates after 2020 are associated with predicted reductions in smoking at ages 20 or 30 among cohorts born before the 1970s and temporal effects due to period. In most cases recent periods have a reduced mortality, after adjustment for smoking by cohorts, and the continuation of this effect alone into the future is associated with a reduction in the rates.

The predictions based upon a cohort's smoking rates at a particular age are not greatly affected by changes

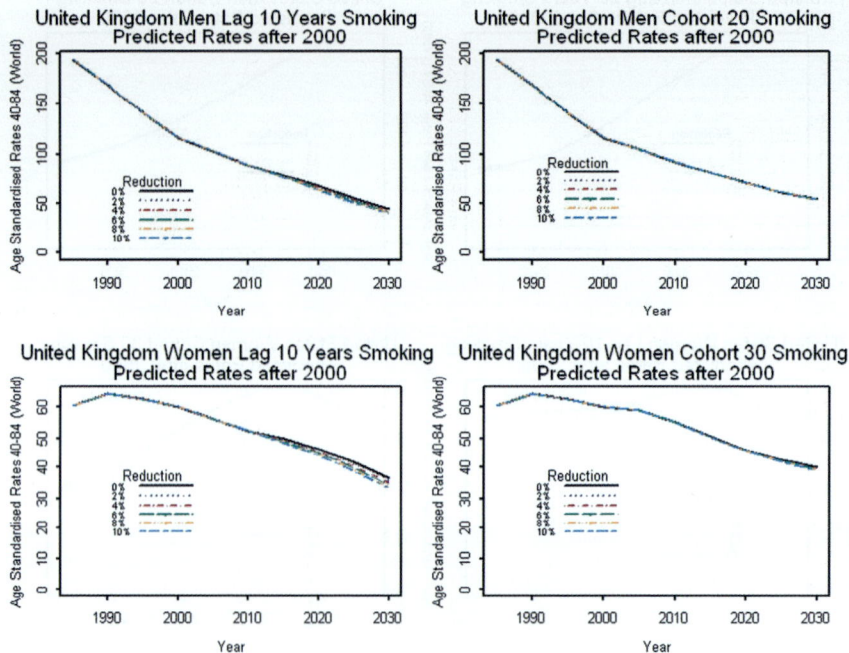

Figure 5. Predicted truncated (40–84) age standardised rates (per 100 000) of lung cancer in the United Kingdom by age group and year of birth for men (top graphs) and women (bottom graphs)

The left hand graphs are based upon a model with terms for Age + Cohort + Percentage of the Age Group Smoking 10 Years in the past. Predictions from 2003 to 2008 are based upon existing smoking data. The smoking percentages used for the predictions from 2013 onwards are based upon the last available data for each age group discounted by 0% to 10% every 5 years.

The right hand graphs are based upon a model with terms for Age + Period + Percentage of the Cohort Smoking at age 30 (20 for men). Predictions from 2003 to 2018 (2028 men) are based upon existing smoking data. The smoking percentages used for the predictions from 2023 (2033 men) onwards are based upon the last available data for each cohort discounted by 0% to 10% every 5 years.

in this variable over time. This is associated with the long time lag; for example, for the cohort born in 1970 smoking at age 30 is known in 2000 and is used to predict mortality at all ages up to 80, which is in 2050. The predictions based upon the lagged percentage of the age group smoking in the past are more affected by changes in this percentage. Within this model the changes in smoking rates now will have predicted effects on all ages 20 years into the future.

In general terms, the predictions here are quite similar to those of Shibuya *et al.* (2005). Indeed, the Age + Cohort + Lagged percentage of the age group smoking model is very similar to the one used by them. The reliability of any forecast of future trends based on historical mortality data also depends heavily on the appropriateness of the statistical model used and the assumptions that are either made explicitly or are built into the statistical processes.

The validity of some of these (power link and damped drift) have been checked for short-term predictions of cancer incidence (Møller *et al.*, 2002, 2003), but there still remains the issue that all predictions depend upon the assumptions that the previously observed trends and associations will continue.

Limitations

This analysis has concentrated on the

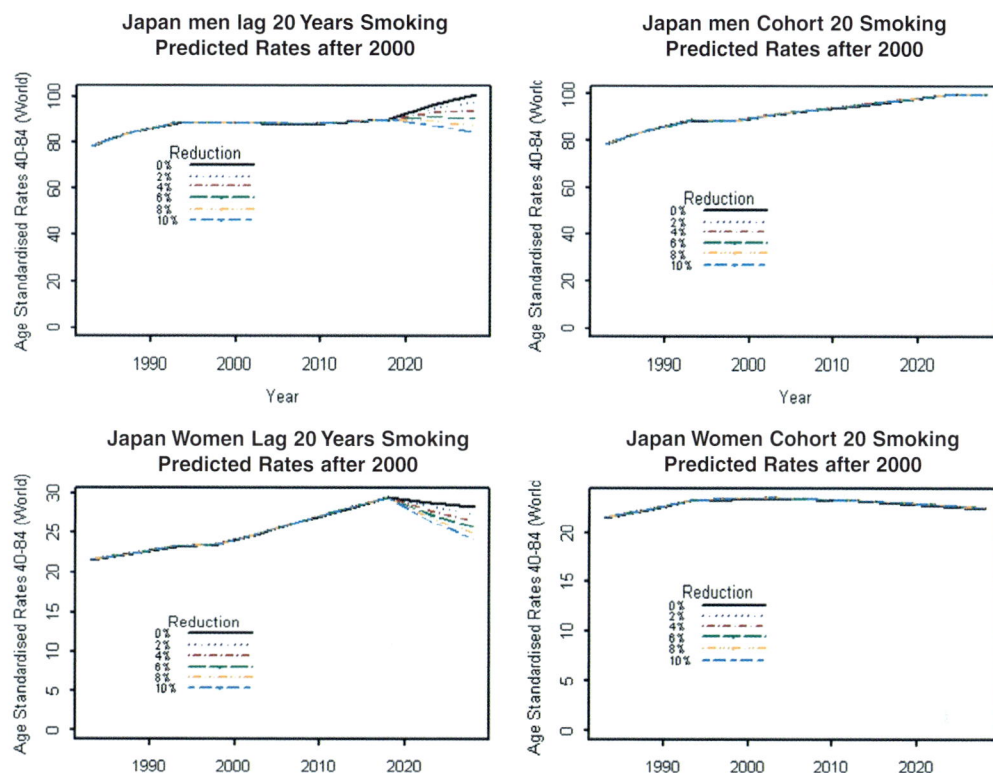

Figure 6. Predicted truncated (40-84) age standardised rates (per 100 000) of lung cancer in Japan by age group and year of birth for men (top graphs) and women (bottom graphs)

The left hand graphs are based upon a model with terms for Age + Cohort + Percentage of the Age Group Smoking 20 Years in the past. Predictions from 2003 to 2018 are based upon existing smoking data. The smoking percentages used for the predictions from 2023 onwards are based upon the last available data for each age group discounted by 0% to 10% every 5 years.

The right hand graphs are based upon a model with terms for Age + Period + Percentage of the Cohort Smoking at age 20. Predictions from 2003 to 2008 are based upon existing smoking data. The smoking percentages used for the predictions from 2013 onwards are based upon the last available data for each cohort discounted by 0% to 10% every 5 years.

effects of lagged smoking prevalence on current lung cancer mortality rates, which are a combination of previous smoking initiation and cessation. The number of countries which have sufficient long-term series of smoking prevalence data is limited; hence this modelling cannot easily be extended to a wide range of countries. In order to carry out this type of predictive modelling it is necessary to have data on smoking prevalence by age group going back at least 20 years before the beginning of the cancer mortality data. For many countries there is cancer mortality data from the 1950's; therefore smoking prevalence data from the 1930's to the present would be required to fully utilise the mortality data.

Implications

Assuming that lung cancer mortality is causally related to smoking prevalence in the past, the implications of these projections for smoking cessation are that continued efforts need to be made in smoking cessation to maintain the projected decline in lung cancer mortality that is likely to occur in the near future in the United Kingdom and United States. Smoking prevalence among men aged 30–34 in the United Kingdom has fallen from 80% in 1945 to 35% in 2000;

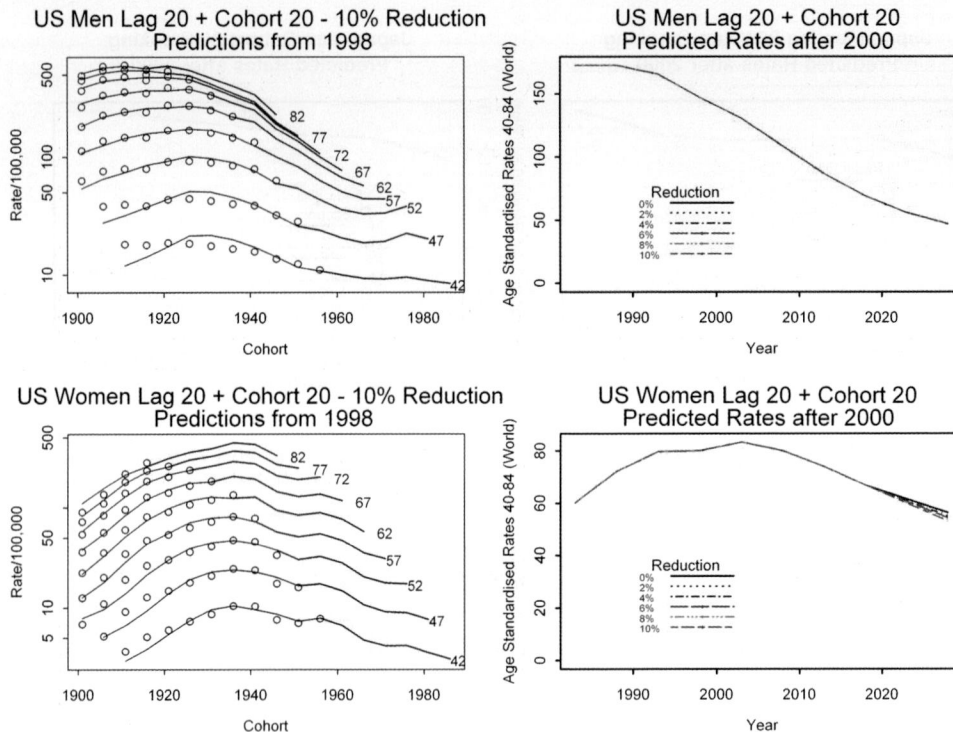

Figure 7. Predicted rates (per 100 000) and truncated (40-84) age standardised rates (per 100 000) of lung cancer in the United States by age group and year of birth for men (top graphs) and women (bottom graphs)

The graphs are based upon a model with terms for Age + Percentage of the Age Group Smoking 20 Years in the past + Percentage of the Cohort Smoking at age 20. Predictions from 2003 to 2013 are based upon existing smoking data. The smoking percentages used for the predictions from 2018 onwards are based upon the last available data for each age group discounted by a fixed percentage every 5 years (10% in left hand graphs).

In each of the left hand graphs the black lines with circles superimposed represent the observed rates. The circles represent the fitted values from the prediction model and the blue lines represent the predictions from the model into the future.

it is dramatic trends such as these which are associated with the large predicted fall in the 40–84 truncated age-standardised rates of lung cancer mortality from 194 per 100 000 in 1985 to about 60 per 100 000 in 2020. Similar comments can be made about women in the United Kingdom and men in the USA, where there are already positive trends in smoking cessation, especially among older age groups. Continuation of these trends will have a positive impact on the projected lung cancer mortality rates.

Of the groups we studied, smoking cessation activities are likely to have the greatest impact among women in the United States and in Japan. The history of smoking cessation is not as long in these communities, and indeed in some age groups there is a strong rise in smoking. Unless there are continued successful efforts at smoking cessation, then the projected recent decline in lung cancer mortality among females in the United States from the peak in 2000 to 2020 may continue but with a much shallower downward gradient. Among Japanese men, cancer rates, rather than levelling off at their peak in 2000–2020,

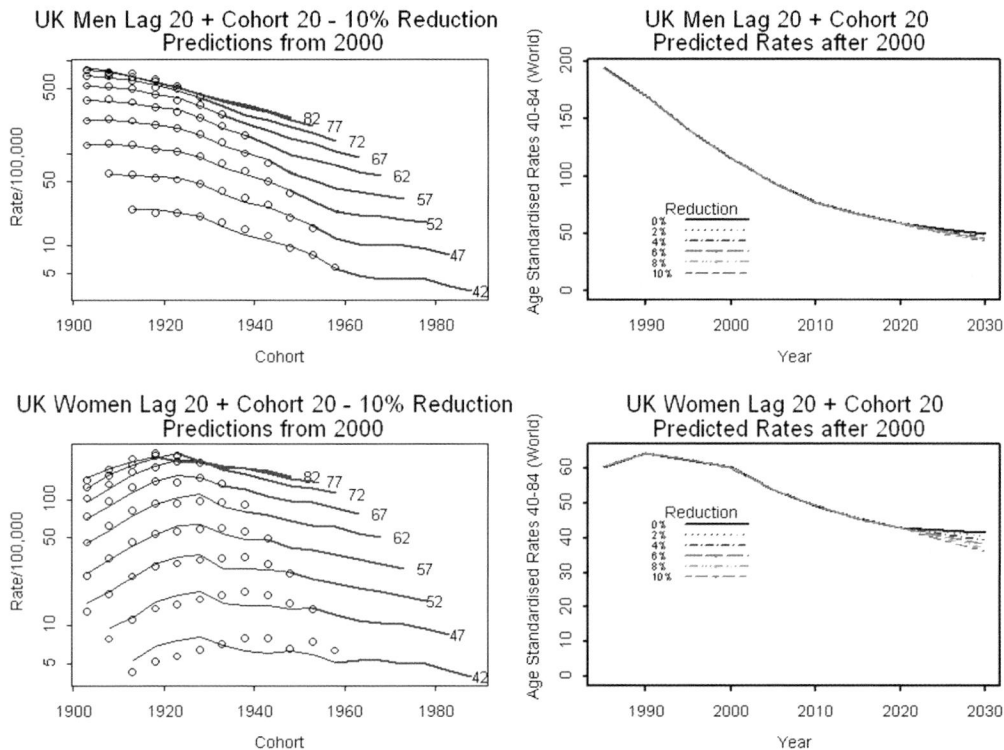

Figure 8. Predicted rates (per 100 000) and truncated (40–84) age standardised rates (per 100 000) of lung cancer in the United Kingdom by age group and year of birth for men (top graphs) and women (bottom graphs)

The graphs are based upon a model with terms for Age + Percentage of the Age Group Smoking 20 Years in the past + Percentage of the Cohort Smoking at age 20. Predictions from 2003 to 2018 are based upon existing smoking data. The smoking percentages used for the predictions from 2023 onwards are based upon the last available data for each age group discounted by a fixed percentage every 5 years (10% in left hand graphs).

In each of the left hand graphs the black lines with circles superimposed represent the observed rates. The circles represent the fitted values from the prediction model and the blue lines represent the predictions from the model into the future.

may continue to rise. Even maintaining the current smoking percentages among Japanese women is projected to have a benefit in reducing projected lung cancer mortality, as rates are projected to increase dramatically from 2000–2020 in association with increased smoking among women currently aged under 60. Smoking cessation policies are a priority and need to be maintained. Similar predictions should hold for other countries where there are also increases in the prevalence of women smoking. Thus, the need to improve smoking cessation and prevention of smoking initiation to reduce the projected increase in lung cancer mortality.

References

Breslow NE (1984). Extra-Poisson variation in log-linear models. *Appl Statist,* 33(1):38-44.

Brown CC, Kessler LG (1988). Projections of lung cancer mortality in the United States: 1985-2025. *J Natl Cancer Inst,* 80(1):43-51.

Clayton D, Schifflers E (1987). Models for temporal variation in cancer rates. II: Age-period-cohort models. *Stat Med,* 6(4):469-481.

Forey B, Hamling J, Lee P, et al. (2002). Estimation of sex specific smoking statistics by standardized age groups and time periods. In: *International Smoking Statistics. A collection of historical data from 30 economically developed countries* London and Oxford, Wolfson Institute of Preventive Medicine and Oxford University Press: 1-204.

Hastie T, Tibshirani R (1990). *Generalized Additive Models.* London, Chapman and Hall.

Holford TR (1992). Analysing the temporal effects of age, period and cohort. *Stat Methods Med Res,* 1(3):317-337.

IARC (1976). *Cancer incidence in five continents,* Vol. III. Lyon, IARC.

Kaneko S, Ishikawa KB, Yoshimi I, et al. (2003). Projection of lung cancer mortality in Japan. *Cancer Sci,* 94(10):919-923.

Keiding N, Carstensen B. (2006). Age-Period-Cohort Models: Statistical inference in the lexis diagram. A report from the Institute of Public Health, Copenhagen. p. 1-76.

Marugame T, Kamo K, Sobue T, et al. (2006). Trends in smoking by birth cohorts born between 1900 and 1977 in *Japan. Prev Med,* 42(2):120-127.

Moller B, Fekjaer H, Hakulinen T, et al. (2002). Prediction of cancer incidence in the Nordic countries up to the year 2020. *Eur J Cancer Prev,* 11 Suppl. 1:S1-96

Moller B, Fekjaer H, Hakulinen, T, et al. (2003) Prediction of cancer incidence in the Nordic countires: Empirical comparison of different approaches.Stat Med, 22:2751–2766

Osmond C (1985). Using age, period and cohort models to estimate future mortality rates. *Int J Epidemiol,* 14(1):124-129.

Quinn MJ, d'Onofrio A, Moller B, et al. (2003). Cancer mortality trends in the EU and acceding countries up to 2015. *Ann Oncol,* 14(7):1148-1152.

Robertson C, Boyle P (1998). Age-period-cohort analysis of chronic disease rates. I: Modelling approach. *Stat Med,* 17(12): 1305-1323.

Shibuya K, Inoue M, Lopez AD (2005). Statistical modeling and projections of lung cancer mortality in 4 industrialized countries. *Int J Cancer,* 117(3):476-485.

Stevens RG, Moolgavkar SH (1979). Estimation of relative risk from vital data: smoking and cancers of the lung and bladder. *J Natl Cancer Inst,* 63(6):1351-1357.

Websites

National Health Interview Surveys 1965-2001
http://www.cdc.gov/nchs/nhis.htm
http://cisnet.cancer.gov

Smoking behaviour estimates for the United States (courtesy of David Burns)
http:/www.iarc.fr
United Kingdom General Household Survey
http://www.statistics.gov.uk/ssd/surveys/general_household_survey.asp

Age-Period-Cohort Models: Statistical inference in the lexis diagram
http://staff.pubhealth.ku.dk/~bxc/APC/notes.pdf

Estimation of sex specific smoking statistics by standardized age groups and time periods
http://www.pnlee.co.uk/ISS2.htm

WHO database of mortality and population estimates
http://www-dep.iarc.fr/WHO Databases

Functions for the prediction of cancer mortality by Björn Möller and Herald Fejkaer
http://www.kreftregisteret.no/software/nord-pred/

Summary

When assessing risk reduction within the first two years after smoking cessation, certain methodological issues of particular concern, including reverse causation and constancy of smoking habits, complicate interpretation of the data. Assessment of risk reduction following long term abstinence is less subject to these methodological concerns and can rely more on the very large observational cohort studies available to shed light on the issue. These methodological challenges in studying the effects of cessation are pertinent to all of the diseases covered in the Handbook and were acknowledged when examining the available evidence.

Lung Cancer

A large number of epidemiologic studies have compared lung cancer risk in persons who stop smoking with the risk of those who continue. The major published studies show lower lung cancer risk in former than in current smokers. The absolute annual risk of developing or dying from lung cancer does not decrease after stopping smoking. Rather, the principal benefit from cessation derives from avoiding the much steeper increase in risk that would result from continuing to smoke. Within five to nine years after quitting, the lower lung cancer risk in former compared with otherwise similar current smokers becomes apparent and diverges progressively with longer time since cessation. There is a persistent increased risk of lung cancer in former smokers compared to never smokers of the same age, even after a long duration of abstinence. Stopping smoking before middle age avoids much of the lifetime risk incurred by continuing to smoke. Stopping smoking in middle or old age confers substantially lower lung cancer risk compared with continuing smokers.

The full benefits of smoking cessation and hazards of continued smoking are underestimated, at least in absolute terms, in studies of populations where the maximum hazards of persistent lifetime smoking have not yet emerged. Individuals and policymakers who live in countries where lung cancer risk is still increasing should recognize that the maximum hazard from continuing to smoke—and the maximum benefits from cessation—have not yet been reached. Studies of cessation in these circumstances will seriously underestimate the long-term benefits of cessation.

Laryngeal Cancer

Four cohort studies and at least 15 case-control studies have reported information on smoking cessation and laryngeal cancer. These studies indicate that the risk of laryngeal cancer is considerably reduced in former smokers compared with current smokers. The relative risk steeply decreases with time since stopping smoking, with reductions of about 60% after 10 to 15 years since cessation, and even larger after 20 years. The favourable effect of stopping smoking is already evident within a few years after cessation. However, after stopping smoking, former smokers still have elevated risks of laryngeal cancer as compared to never smokers for at least twenty years.

Oral Cancer

The results of four cohort studies and at least 25 case-control studies on oral and pharyngeal cancers have shown the risk for former smokers to be intermediate between those of non-smokers and current smokers. In studies where risks were analysed by duration of abstinence, there was generally a decreasing relative risk with increasing duration of abstinence compared with continuing smokers. In several studies, the risk remained elevated compared with never smokers during a second decade of abstinence, but reached the level of never smokers thereafter.

Oesophageal Cancer

The results from at least 10 cohort and 10 case-control studies indicate that former smokers have a lower risk than current smokers of squamous-cell oesophageal cancer. Most investigations have shown that the risk of oesophageal cancer remains elevated many years (at least 20) after cessation of smoking. After 10 years since cessation of smoking, former smokers still have twice the oesophageal cancer risk of never smokers.

A few studies have investigated the effect of smoking cessation on adeno-carcinoma, indicating no clear reduction of risk. The data on oesophageal adenocarcinoma are too limited, however, to provide adequate inference on the relation with time since smoking cessation.

Stomach Cancer

Epidemiological studies show that former smokers have a lower risk for stomach cancer than do current smokers. Increasing number of years since cessation and younger age at cessation were associated with decreasing risk in comparison with continuing smokers in most studies.

Liver Cancer

The risk of cancer of the liver appears to be lower in former than in current smokers, but the data are inconsistent across geographic areas. There is inadequate information to assess the effect of time since cessation.

Pancreatic Cancer

The risk of pancreatic cancer is lower in former than in current smokers. The risk declines with time since cessation compared to continuing smokers, but remains higher than that in never smokers for at least 15 years after cessation.

Bladder Cancer

The risk of cancer of the bladder is lower in former than in current smokers. The relative risk declines with time since cessation in comparison with continuing smokers, but remains higher than that for never smokers for at least 25 years after cessation.

Renal Cell Cancer

The risk of renal cell cancer is lower in former than in current smokers. Based on limited evidence, the relative risk declines with time since cessation in comparison with continuing smokers, but remains higher than that for never smokers for at least 20 years after cessation.

Cervical Cancer

The risk of squamous cell carcinoma of the cervix is lower in former smokers than in current smokers. Following cessation, the risk in former smokers rapidly decreases to the level of never smokers.

Myeloid Leukemia

The risk of myeloid leukemia may be lower in former smokers than in current smokers, but available data are inconsistent. There is inadequate information to assess the effect of duration of abstinence.

Nasopharyngeal and Sinonasal Cancer

The risk in former smokers seems to be lower than in current smokers for nasopharyngeal carcinoma. There is inadequate information to assess the effects of duration of abstinence.

For sinonasal carcinoma as well there is inadequate information to assess the effect of abstinence.

Coronary Heart Disease (CHD)

Cigarette smoking is a major cause of coronary heart disease. The risk is manifest both as an increased risk for thrombosis and as an increased degree of atherosclerosis in coronary vessels. The cardiovascular risk caused by cigarette smoking increases with the amount smoked and with the duration of smoking. Former smokers have considerably reduced risk of CHD compared to smokers.

Evidence from studies of patients with manifest CHD point toward a relative risk reduction in the order of 35% compared with continued cigarette smokers of similar accumulated exposure within the first two to four years of smoking cessation. Findings from case-control studies and cohort studies of subjects without diagnosed CHD are compatible with this conclusion and point toward a similar relative risk reduction following smoking cessation.

Some studies of prolonged abstinence find the risk to be similar to never smokers after 10 to 15 years of abstinence, whereas others find a persistent increased risk of 10-20% even after 10 to 20 years. The main methodological issue in this type of study is misclassification of both current and former smoking status with prolonged follow-up without re-assessment of smoking status. An additional issue is self-selection of former smokers. Taking these methodological issues into account, the body of evidence suggests that the risk of CHD with long-term abstinence approaches the risk of never-smokers asymptotically. The risk reduction is observed after controlling for other major risk factors.

Cerebrovascular Disease

Smoking is a cause of stroke. Data from large prospective studies revealed that current smokers have a relative risk of 1.5 to 4 for stroke compared with never-smokers. Former smokers have markedly lower risk compared to current smokers.

Studies that have assessed the effect of duration of abstinence on stroke risk report a marked risk reduction by two to five years after cessation, and the relative risk decreases for up to 15 years after cessation. In some studies, the risk returns to that of never smokers by five to ten years, but other studies report small increased risks even after 15 years of abstinence; all of these studies show a lower risk for former smokers than for continuing smokers. The risk reduction is observed after controlling for other major risk factors.

There is inadequate evidence to assess the effect of smoking cessation on the long-term prognosis among cerebrovascular disease patients.

Abdominal Aortic Aneurysm (AAA)

Prospective cohort and screening studies show that the risk of death from, and prevalence of, AAA is large (RR: 4.0-8.0) in current smokers compared with never smokers. The magnitude of this relative risk is greater than that observed in other forms of CVD for current smokers. Former smokers have a lower risk of AAA than do continuing smokers. The limited data that address the relationship between the duration of cessation and risk of AAA suggest that cessation is associated with a slow decline in risk that continues for at least 20 years after stopping smoking. The risk remains greater than that of a never smoker, even after a prolonged duration of abstinence. This pattern is different from that observed in patients with coronary heart disease and cerebrovascular disease in that the risk remains significantly higher than that of never smokers. In patients with an established diagnosis of AAA, the single published intervention study concludes that former smoking status is associated with reduced all-cause mortality and AAA rupture compared with continued smoking.

Peripheral Artery Disease (PAD)

Data that address the time course of the change in risk with cessation are very limited, and the time course is different for populations with and without clinically evident disease.

In populations without clinically evident disease

Current smoking is a major cause of PAD. Former smokers have a reduced risk compared with current smokers. In former smokers without clinical evidence of disease, the reduction in risk of development of disease occurs over an extended period (at least 20 years), but the time course of reduction in risk is poorly characterized. Prospective cohort studies suggest that the relative risk of PAD in former smokers remains greater than that of never smokers even after long duration of abstinence (at least 20 years).

In populations with clinically evident disease

In patients with clinical evidence of PAD, the evidence suggests an improvement in clinical outcomes among former smokers compared to continuing smokers. PAD patients who stop smoking experience complication rates that are similar to those who are classified as nonsmokers in the studies in a relatively short period of time following cessation (within one to five years), and the rates are substantially below those of continuing smokers. However, studies in patients with clinically evident PAD often classify smoking status as current smoker, ex-smoker and 'nonsmoker', with nonsmokers including never smokers and smokers who stopped before the beginning of follow-up. The evidence as a whole suggests there are important benefits of smoking cessation for patients with established PAD.

Chronic Obstructive Pulmonary Disease (COPD)

Former smokers have lower risk of accelerated loss of lung function and COPD-related morbidity and mortality than do continuing smokers.

Evidence from cross-sectional and longitudinal studies shows that symptoms of chronic bronchitis (chronic cough, mucus production and wheeze) decrease rapidly within a few months after smoking cessation. Prevalence of these symptoms is the same as that reported by never smokers within five years of sustained smoking abstinence. With respect to lung function loss, cohort studies of the general population show that the accelerated decline in FEV_1 observed in current smokers reverts to the age-related rate of decline seen in never smokers within 5 years of smoking cessation. In people diagnosed with mild to moderate COPD, an increase in FEV_1 during the first year after smoking cessation has been observed; in following years, the rate of decline in FEV1 in sustained quitters has been half the rate of that observed in continuing smokers.

Data on lung capacity and hospital admission for patients with severe COPD are limited, but available evidence suggests that smoking cessation results in a reduction in excess lung function loss and a decrease in risk of hospitalization for COPD in comparison with continuing smokers. Evidence from several long-term studies indicates a substantial reduction in mortality risk in former smokers compared with continuing smokers. Assessment of risk reduction for COPD mortality following smoking cessation is complex because of reverse causality. For example, there is a persistent increased risk of COPD mortality with long duration of abstinence.

COPD in China

China is the world's largest producer of tobacco and cigarettes, with the world's largest number of smokers and largest number of tobacco deaths (about 1 million per year). Of all the diseases contributing to tobacco-related mortality, the most numerically significant is COPD, constituting 45% of tobacco-related deaths. Hence, China has the world's largest number of COPD deaths

due to smoking, about 450,000 per year.

Evidence from 17 studies in the Chinese medical literature on the effects of cessation in COPD, though limited in quality and quantity, supports the finding that among middle-aged asymptomatic subjects, smoking cessation delayed the decline of FEV_1 when compared with continuing smokers. The decline became similar to that in never smokers after cessation for six years or more. In young and healthy smokers, the benefits of smoking cessation (improvements in FEV1, or decline relative to continuing smokers) can be observed after cessation for a few months. Among subjects with chronic cough and phlegm but no COPD, cessation for at least one month to eight years delayed decline of FEV_1 and reduced the risk of developing COPD compared with that of continuing smokers. Whereas smoking can clearly increase the risk of COPD deaths, the benefits of cessation on COPD mortality have not been observed in the Chinese

population. Instead, studies found excess risk among older quitters, probably due to reverse causality. It is not clear why Chinese never smokers have a much higher prevalence of COPD than those in North America; possible explanations are poor indoor air quality from burning of biomass and/or genetic differences. In addition, there is a common belief among the Chinese public that smoking cessation may be harmful in smokers with COPD. Smokers who already have serious COPD, diagnosed or undiagnosed by a doctor, may appear to die from COPD soon after quitting smoking (reverse causality). Because of the higher proportion of COPD among the total tobacco death toll in China, smoking cessation on a large scale is likely to result in greater long-term effects on COPD morbidity and mortality than for other diseases, such as lung cancer and ischaemic heart disease.

Questions and Answers

Cancer

Question 1: Is the risk of cancer lower in former smokers than in otherwise similar current smokers?

- The risk of lung cancer is lower in former smokers than in current smokers.

- The risk of laryngeal cancer is lower in former smokers than in current smokers.

- The risk of oral and pharyngeal cancer is lower in former smokers than in current smokers.

- The risk of squamous cell carcinoma of the oesophagus is lower in former smokers than in current smokers. There is inadequate evidence to evaluate the risk of adenocarcinoma of the oesophagus after stopping smoking.

- The risk of stomach cancer is lower in former smokers than in current smokers.

- The risk of liver cancer appears to be lower in former smokers than in current smokers, but available data are limited and inconsistent across geographic areas.

- The risk of pancreatic cancer is lower in former smokers than in current smokers.

- The risk of bladder cancer is lower in former smokers than in current smokers.

- The risk of renal cell carcinoma is lower in former smokers than in current smokers.

- The risk of squamous cell carcinoma of the cervix is lower in former smokers than in current smokers.

- The risk of myeloid leukemia may be lower in former smokers than in current smokers, but available data are inconsistent.

- The risk in former smokers seems to be lower than in current smokers for nasopharyngeal carcinoma based on the limited available evidence.

- There is inadequate information to determine the change in risk for sinonasal carcinoma in former smokers.

Cancer

Question 2: Among otherwise similar former smokers, is the risk of disease lower with more prolonged abstinence?

- In former smokers, the lower lung cancer risk compared with that in otherwise similar current smokers becomes apparent within five to nine years after quitting and diverges progressively with longer time since cessation.

- For laryngeal cancer, the benefits of cessation relative to continued smoking increase with increasing duration of abstinence.

- The reduction in the risk of oral and pharyngeal cancer for former smokers compared with current smokers, increases with increasing duration of abstinence.

- For former smokers, the reduction in the risk of squamous cell carcinoma of the oesophagus versus that of current smokers increases with increasing duration of abstinence.

- The reduction in the risk of stomach cancer for former smokers versus current smokers increases with increasing duration of abstinence.

- For liver cancer, there is inadequate information to assess whether a reduction in risk for former smokers compared with current smokers increases with increasing duration of abstinence.

- The reduction in the risk of pancreatic cancer for former smokers compared with current smokers increases with increasing duration of abstinence.

- The reduction in the risk of bladder cancer for former smokers compared with current smokers increases with increasing duration of abstinence.

- The reduction in the risk of renal cell carcinoma for former smokers compared with current smokers appears to increase with increasing duration of abstinence based on the limited available evidence.

- For cervical cancer, the benefits of cessation in former smokers compared with current smokers seem to be fully achieved in the first five years of abstinence.

- For myeloid leukemia, there is inadequate information to assess whether the possible reduction in risk for former smokers as compared to current smokers increases with increasing duration of abstinence.

- For nasopharyngeal carcinoma, there is inadequate information to assess whether a reduction in risk for former smokers compared with current smokers increases with increasing duration of abstinence.

Cancer

Question 3: Does the risk return to that of never smokers after a long period of abstinence?

- There is a persistent increased risk of lung cancer in former smokers compared to never smokers of the same age, even after a long duration of abstinence.

- The risk for laryngeal cancer does not return to that of never smokers after a long duration of abstinence: it remains higher than that in never smokers for at least two decades after cessation.

- The relative risk for oral cancer for former smokers who have stopped for at least twenty years is not increased over that of never smokers.

- The relative risk for carcinoma of the oesophagus does not return to that of never smokers after a long duration of abstinence: it remains higher than that in never smokers for at least two decades after cessation.

- There is inadequate information to evaluate whether the risk of stomach cancer for former smokers ever returns to that of never smokers.

- There is inadequate information to evaluate whether the risk of liver cancer for former smokers ever returns to that of never smokers.

- The risk for pancreatic cancer for former smokers who have stopped for at least twenty years appears to return to that of never smokers.

- The risk for bladder cancer does not return to that of never smokers after a long duration of abstinence: it remains higher than that in never smokers for at least twenty-five years after cessation.

- There is inadequate information to evaluate whether the risk for former smokers ever returns to that of never smokers for renal cell carcinoma.

- The relative risk for cervical cancer returns to that of never smokers within five years after smoking cessation.

- There is inadequate information to evaluate whether the risk of myeloid leukemia for former smokers ever returns to that of never smokers.

- There is inadequate information to evaluate whether the risk for former smokers ever returns to that of never smokers for cancers of the nasopharynx.

Cardiovascular Diseases

Question 1: Is the risk of cardiovascular disease (CVD) lower in former smokers than in otherwise similar current smokers?

- There is unequivocal evidence of reduced risk for coronary heart disease (CHD) morbidity and mortality in former smokers compared with continuing smokers. This is true for healthy subjects and patients with already-diagnosed CHD.

- Former smokers have a markedly lower risk of cerebrovascular disease compared to current smokers. No study has assessed the effect of smoking cessation on the long-term prognosis among cerebrovascular or stroke patients. However, among stroke patients smoking was a strong predictor of survival within a decade of onset.

- In the absence of clinically evident disease, former smokers have a lower risk of abdominal aortic aneurysm (AAA) compared with continuing smokers. For patients with AAA, the risk of AAA expansion, rupture or death is reduced in former smokers compared with that in continuing smokers.

- The risk of peripheral arterial disease (PAD) is reduced in former smokers without clinically evident disease compared with that in continuing smokers, but is greater than the risk found in never smokers. In patients with clinical evidence of PAD, the evidence suggests an improvement in clinical outcomes among former smokers compared to continuing smokers.

Question 2: Among otherwise similar former smokers, is the risk of disease lower with more prolonged abstinence?

- In former smokers without CHD there is a substantial reduction in risk of CHD compared with that of continuing smokers within the first two to four years of smoking abstinence, followed by a slower decline of risk, with risk approaching that of never smokers in fifteen to twenty years. For methodological reasons, the assessment of risk reduction is problematic within the first two years of cessation.

- Evidence from studies of patients with manifest CHD point toward a relative risk reduction of recurrent reinfarction or death on the order of 35 percent compared with continuing smokers of similar accumulated exposure within the first two to four years of smoking cessation. The data are inadequate to assess the magnitude of risk reduction with longer duration of abstinence for patients with clinically evident CHD.

- There is a marked reduction in stroke risk with two to five years of abstinence from smoking.

Cardiovascular Diseases

- In the absence of clinically evident disease, the reduction in risk for AAA among former smokers compared with that in continuing smokers shows a decline over at least ten years and probably as long as twenty years after smoking cessation. Former smokers have a slower rate of aneurysm expansion than continuing smokers and a lower rate of rupture, but the time course is not known.

- The decline in risk of PAD in former smokers without clinically evident disease compared with that in continuing smokers occurs over a prolonged period, at least twenty years. The reduction in risk for former smokers with clinically evident disease, compared to continuing smokers, occurs within one to five years.

Question 3: Does the risk return to that of never smokers after a long period of abstinence?

- After a long duration of abstinence, the risk of CHD for former smokers approaches that of never smokers. However, the increased risk for former smokers with a long duration of abstinence, if any, is expected to be too small to be reliably determined.

- For patients with established disease, the question is not applicable.

- In some studies the risk of stroke decreases to the level seen in never smokers within five to ten years, but other studies report small increases in risk even after fifteen years of abstinence. All of these studies show a lower risk for former smokers than for continuing smokers.

- The risk of AAA in former smokers without clinical evidence of disease does not return to the level of risk of never smokers, even after long periods of abstinence.

- For patients with clinical evidence of disease, the question is not applicable.

- The risk of PAD in former smokers without clinically evident disease does not return to the level of risk of never smokers.

- For patients with clinically evident disease, the question is not applicable.

Chronic Obstructive Pulmonary Disease (COPD)

Question 1: Is the risk of COPD lower in former smokers than in otherwise similar current smokers?

• Both chronic cough and phlegm production improve after smoking cessation.

• In unselected populations, smoking cessation slows the smoking-related accelerated decline in lung function, measured as forced expiratory volume in one second (FEV_1).

• The Lung Health Study (LHS) of smokers with mild to moderate airway obstruction showed over eleven years that smoking cessation slowed the rate of FEV_1 decline. Smoking cessation prevented or delayed development of severe COPD irrespective of baseline lung function, smoking intensity, age or gender.

• In severe COPD, limited data indicate that smoking cessation is associated with a lower rate of FEV_1 decline and less risk of hospital admission for a COPD exacerbation compared with continuing smoking.

• Smoking cessation leads to decreased mortality from COPD compared with continued smoking.

Question 2: Among otherwise similar former smokers, is the risk of disease lower with more prolonged abstinence?

• In cross-sectional and longitudinal studies, self-reported symptoms of chronic bronchitis decreased by one to two months after smoking cessation.

• Population based cohort studies show that the rate of FEV_1 decline in former smokers returns to the rate of never smokers within five years after smoking cessation. Smokers with normal lung function who quit before age 40 have a normal age-related FEV_1 decline, and do not generally develop COPD from their past smoking.

• In the LHS of smoking cessation in subjects with mild to moderate COPD there was an increase in FEV_1 during the first year after smoking cessation. In the subsequent eleven years, the rate of FEV_1 decline in sustained quitters was approximately half the rate of decline of the continuing smokers. The decreased rate of FEV_1 decline in former smokers with airway obstruction is confirmed by cohort studies with varying follow-up periods.

• Long-term studies of smoking cessation in more severe COPD show that the rate of FEV_1 decline and relative risk of hospitalization with COPD exacerbation in former smokers decreases over a twenty-year period compared with that of continuing smokers.

Chronic Obstructive Pulmonary Disease (COPD)

- Smoking cessation reduces the risk of COPD mortality, but the data demonstrating the timing of this effect are difficult to interpret. In earlier studies, mortality rates from COPD were paradoxically increased for up to ten years after smoking cessation compared to continued smoking but thereafter rates decreased. Recent studies do not have sufficient size or strength to clarify this issue, and the increased mortality in the early period following cessation may be the result of the population of former smokers containing substantial numbers of smokers who quit because they had developed COPD.

Question 3: Does the risk return to that of never smokers after a long period of abstinence?

- Longitudinal data show that the prevalence of chronic cough and phlegm production returns to the level of never smokers after a long duration of abstinence.

- Population-based cohort studies show that the rate of FEV_1 decline in former smokers becomes the same as in never smokers within five years of quitting smoking.

- While smoking cessation in subjects with mild to moderate COPD decreases the rate of FEV_1 decline, the lung function lost before cessation is not fully recovered. However, there is a greater capacity for recovery of lung function in subjects who stop smoking before age 40.

- In subjects with more severe COPD, the FEV_1 decline and risk of hospital admission for COPD remain higher for former than for never smokers.

- Available data show a permanently elevated COPD mortality risk in former smokers compared with never smokers; however, this effect may be the result of the population of former smokers containing substantial numbers of smokers who quit because they had developed COPD.

Is There Sufficient Evidence to Address Questions on the Effects of Smoking Cessation on Risk of Disease?

1. **Risk for Former Smokers:** Is there sufficient evidence to determine whether the risk of disease is lower in former smokers than in otherwise similar current smokers?

2. **Risk with Prolonged Abstinence:** Is there sufficient evidence to determine whether, among otherwise similar former smokers, the risk of disease is lower with more prolonged abstinence?

3. **Residual Increased Risk:** Is there sufficient evidence to determine whether the risk returns to that of never smokers after long periods of abstinence?

Disease	Risk for Former Smokers (1)	Risk with Prolonged Abstinence (2)	Residual Increased Risk (3)
Cancers			
Lung cancer	■	■	■
Laryngeal cancer	■	■	■
Oral cancer	■	■	■
Squamous cell esophageal cancer	■	■	■
Esophageal adenocarcinoma	☐	☐	☐
Stomach cancer	■	☒	☐
Liver cancer	☒	☐	☐
Pancreatic cancer	■	■	☒
Bladder cancer	■	■	■
Renal cancer	■	☒	☐
Cervical cancer	■	■	■
Myeloid leukemia	+/-	☐	☐
Nasopharyngeal cancer	☒	☐	☐
Sinonasal cancer	☐	☐	☐
Vascular Disease			
CHD incidence and death in subjects without established disease	■	■	■
CHD incidence and death in those with clinical evident disease	■	■	Not applicable
Cerebrovascular disease incidence and death for those without established disease	■	■	☒
Cerebrovascular disease incidence and death for those with clinical disease	☐	☐	Not applicable
Aortic aneurysm incidence and death for those without established disease	■	☒	☒
Aortic aneurysm incidence and death for those with clinical disease	■	☐	Not applicable
PAD incidence and death for those without established disease	■	☒	☒
PAD incidence and death for those with clinical disease	☒	☒	Not applicable
Lung Disease			
Cough and phlegm production	■	■	■
Decline in FEV_1 in healthy subjects	■	■	■
Decline in FEV_1 for those with mild/moderate disease	■	■	Not applicable
Decline in FEV_1 for those with severe disease/Morbidity	■	■	Not applicable
Mortality from COPD	■	■	☒

Level of evidence to address questions:

■ Adequate: The evidence is adequate to draw a clear conclusion on the question; ☒ Limited: The evidence to answer the question is suggestive; the interpretation is considered by the Working Group to be credible, but chance, bias, confounding or other factors cannot be adequately evaluated; +/- Conflicting: The data provide conflicting answers to the question; ☐ Absence of Observations: There is an absence of data or data are inadequate to address the question.

FEV_1: Forced expiratory volume in one second; CHD: Coronary Heart Disease; PAD: Peripheral Artery Disease

Recommendations

Based on the evidence available, the Working Group developed several recommendations. These recommendations are divided into Public Health and more specific disease Research recommendations.

Public Health Recommendations

Cessation of cigarette smoking produces short-term benefits for reducing the disease burden for current smokers, both as individuals and as subgroups of the population. For most countries, existing risk data are likely to underestimate both the magnitude of the disease burden that will occur due to current smoking behaviors and the benefits that might be achieved with increased rates of cessation. This underestimation is likely to be substantively larger for countries in the early stages of the tobacco epidemic.

Public Health Recommendation: Methods for more accurately defining current disease burdens due to tobacco use and predicting the future benefits of cessation are necessary for countries in all stages of the tobacco epidemic (see Figure 2, page 4; Lopez et al., 1994) Accurate estimates of the burden of disease that could be avoided with smoking cessation are invaluable in forming appropriate public policy.

The full benefit of cessation is now evident in the population-based death rates for countries where the tobacco epidemic has progressed to the stage of falling smoking prevalence. However, increased rates of cessation will be required in these countries to sustain the observed disease rates of decline. The effects of quitting could be more rapidly apparent on a population scale than the effects of not starting to smoke.

Public Health Recommendation: Measures of cessation rates and cumulative cessation that can be obtained in countries with limited resources are necessary, as are methods for acquiring and disseminating these measures. Simply tracking smoking prevalence in the population may lead to inaccurate assessment of the current and future disease burden due to tobacco use and the potential to avoid it through increased cessation.

Cessation provides a benefit even for older groups of the population, but much of the disease risk of smoking can be avoided by cessation by middle age. In a similar fashion, countries that are in the middle stages of the tobacco epidemic can avoid much disease risk if they could increase rates of cessation in their populations. Effective control of lung cancer in particular requires effective anti-smoking policies to discourage cigarette consumption and encourage early quitting.

Younger individuals and countries in the early stages of the tobacco epidemic can avoid almost all of the tobacco-related morbidity and mortality that would otherwise occur if the smokers in those countries can be persuaded to quit. Results from the British Doctors Study show that quitting smoking before middle age avoids the majority of the excess risk sustained by continued smoking. Helping large numbers of adult smokers to quit (preferably before middle age, but also in middle age) might avoid one hundred million or more tobacco-related deaths in the first half of this century. Large numbers of deaths during the second half of the century could also be avoided if many of those who, despite warnings, still start to smoke in future years could be helped to stop before they are killed by the habit.

Public Health Recommendation: Besides measuring the prevalence of smoking, with initiation and cessation rates, policymakers in countries at all stages of the tobacco epidemic should take appropriate steps to reduce tobacco use among all age groups.

Appropriate policy measures are outlined in the Framework Convention for Tobacco Control, and numerous organizations, starting with the World

Health Organization, have initiated detailed steps for how to achieve these measures. Experience in initiating these policy measures abounds in various countries – both in the developed and developing countries.

Public Health Recommendation:
Methods to estimate the future tobacco-related disease burden and the benefits of cessation for countries which are both early in the tobacco epidemic and which have limited resources would be helpful, as would the formulation of estimates that are useful in guiding public policy in these countries. For example, the ability to assess the impact of morbidity and mortality from COPD in China could significantly help China recognize the extensive burden of this particular disease on their society.

Various countries have done much work in developing smoking cessation guidelines that follow evidence-based methodologies. However, depending on the regulatory environment and culture, not all methods are applicable or available in all regions of the world.

Public Health Recommendation:
Country-specific and culture-appropriate methods to achieve effective smoking cessation are badly needed in many countries of the world.

The mistaken belief that quitting smoking could be harmful, especially common among elderly smokers in China and perhaps in other developing countries, is based on an understandable misinterpretation of the observation that some smokers had died from chronic obstructive pulmonary disease (COPD) soon after quitting. Such misconceptions, coupled with a lack of awareness of the seriousness of having COPD symptoms and the benefits of cessation, if not appropriately handled, could lead to a reluctance of smokers

with chronic respiratory symptoms and/or COPD to quit smoking.

Public Health Recommendation:
Healthcare professionals should be prepared to correct this type of misunderstanding. Countries should consider ways to educate the public that quitting smoking is beneficial regardless of an individual's state of health.

Recommendations for Future Research

Studies with long-term follow-up requiring repeated assessment of smoking status, specifically of sustained cessation—as opposed to cross-sectional determinations—would augment our understanding of the extent and timing of changes in symptoms, morbidity, hospital admissions and mortality following smoking cessation. These studies could also allow exploration of the degree of reverse causality.

Understanding of the mechanisms by which smoking causes disease is rapidly expanding, and biomarkers useful for examining these mechanisms are available and are increasingly predictive. Evidence examining changes in these biomarkers among former smokers as they quit and as they continue their abstinence is very limited. Research on changes in disease mechanisms among former smokers is likely to offer important insights into disease causation and reveal methods by which the disease burden might be reduced among smokers of long duration.

As prevalence data are being developed globally, it would be helpful to develop cessation data simultaneously (stratified by both gender and age) in the same countries. This information could then be used to develop models for predicting lung cancer mortality (such as those demonstrated in the modeling section in this Handbook). In addition,

the collection of such information would aid in assessing the efficacy of each country's smoking cessation/tobacco control policies as they are implemented.

The number of countries which have sufficiently high-quality long-term series of smoking prevalence data is limited. In order to carry out this type of predictive modeling it is necessary to have data on smoking prevalence by age group going back at least 20 years before the beginning of the cancer mortality data. For many countries there is cancer mortality data from the 1950s, and smoking prevalence data from the 1930s to the present would be required to fully utilize the mortality data. Therefore, if we are to assess the future impact of smoking and its relationship to disease mortality, both pieces of information must be collected.

General Research Recommendations:
Future research should involve studies with long-term follow-up and repeated smoking status assessment. These studies should use newly available biomarkers to assess changes in disease mechanisms among former smokers. Studies of prevalence should collect cessation data simultaneously, as these data can be used to develop models for predicting mortality. Prevalence data should include information by age group that predates mortality data by at least 20 years.

Proposals for studies of specific diseases

The summation of the available data in this Handbook on the changes in risk associated with smoking cessation has highlighted specific gaps in our understanding of the relationship between smoking and certain specific disease states, including chronic obstructive pulmonary disease, cardiovascular disease, and cancer. Further data on the potential role of smoking cessation in the management of other diseases, including tuberculosis and AIDS/HIV, would also have great value.

Chronic Obstructive Pulmonary Disease (COPD)

There is a pressing need for long-term prospective studies of smoking cessation—as opposed to cross-sectional determinations—to be carried out in highly characterized patients with COPD of differing severity and with appropriate control groups, requiring repeated assessment of smoking status, specifically of sustained cessation. These studies could help understanding the extent and timing of changes in symptoms, morbidity, hospital admissions and mortality following smoking cessation.

In those studies, lung function tests should encompass assessment of large and small airways, together with measures of inflation and interstitial gas transfer. It will be important to have CT scans to identify emphysema, while novel techniques such as MRI scanning have the potential to visualise small airways (Hill & van Beek, 2004). The studies should involve biomarkers of translational medicine, including genomic and proteomic analysis that could be performed on blood, breath, and sputum. Especially in more severe COPD, it will be important to assess dyspnoea, exercise response, quality of life, frequency of exacerbations and effects on mortality (Anthonisen et al., 2002; Celli et al., 2004). These large-scale studies of cancer risk could simultaneously evaluate risk of cardio-vascular and respiratory disease.

In countries such as China, and perhaps other developing countries, research questions should include why the incidence of COPD in non-smokers is increased over more developed countries such as the USA or the United Kingdom. This would include studying other potential risk factors that are causative for COPD besides cigarette smoking and how they affect the rates of COPD, and if they modify disease resolution with smoking cessation.

Larger prospective studies on healthy middle-aged subjects with information on cessation during several time points over a follow up period of over 10 years are needed for both lung function and mortality and morbidity in China. Long-term follow-up studies on smoking cessation among smokers with varying degree of COPD are also needed to clarify how reverse causality can mask the benefits of cessation.

Research Recommendations:

Long-term prospective studies involving CT and MRI scans and comprehensive tests of lung function, inflation and interstitial gas transfer, are necessary to increase our understanding of the relation between COPD and smoking cessation. Further research is especially warranted in countries such as China where high rates of COPD present a significant health risk.

Cardiovascular disease (CVD)

In patients with clinically evident coronary heart disease, there is a lack of data to assess the magnitude of risk reduction with longer durations of abstinence (>2–4 years). Few studies have explored the effect of smoking cessation in CVD patients and whether their relative risk ever returns to that of the never smoker.

No study has explored the effect of smoking cessation on the long-term prognosis of the patient with cerebrovascular disease, particularly after 5 years of cessation.

Research Recommendations:

Further studies in CVD should assess risk reduction after long-term smoking abstinence, in particular among patients with cerebrovascular disease.

Mechanisms of Cancer

As the number of former smokers in a population increases, it will become increasingly important to be able to identify the pre-malignant and inflammatory changes that could predict the onset of either malignancy (for example with lung cancer) or reversible/treatable COPD. This work will necessarily require accurate identification of smoking status during long-term follow-up. Biomarkers might then be identified that could distinguish lesions that are not life-threatening from those that are, and gene expression profiles might be found that predict which lung lesions are most likely to change from indolent to malignant.

Research is needed on biomarkers to distinguish latent from aggressive sub-clinical molecular lesions in the lung, and to characterize individual profiles of persistent airway epithelial cell deregulated gene expression. Research also is needed to identify gene expression profiles that result in conversion of lung lesions from indolent to malignant. Discovery of gene pathway-specific interventions would offer the potential to mitigate the specific steps in this conversion.

Whether the changes described in the lung cancer mechanisms section are simply the result of cumulative exposure (similar to the effect of cigarettes per day and duration of smoking on lung cancer risk following cessation) or if they are also affected by repair of the genetic damage or a reversal of the cellular environment that allows normal cells to out-compete damaged cells is not known.

Research Recommendations: Further work in cancer mechanisms should focus on identifying characteristics—such as gene expression profiles or other biomarkers—that predict malignancy. Identification of these characteristics could provide an avenue for preventing the development of cancer. Research is also needed to answer the following questions:

- Do all of the genetic changes that lead to cancer persist to the same extent as cessation duration extends?

- Is there a difference in extent of changes between smokers and former smokers not explained by intensity and duration of exposure?

- Do changes progress in the absence of smoking, and do some progress faster than others?

We know already enough about the impact of smoking to act aggressively to prevent initiation and promote cessation of tobacco use. However, there is still much to be examined to better understand the changes that occur with cessation, their time course and methods to intervene to prevent disease onset. With the information presented in this Handbook, and pursuing the recommendations above, we should be able to mitigate the unacceptable morbidity and mortality that is presently predicted from current models.

References

Anthonisen NR, Connett JE, Enright PL, et al. (2002). Hospitalizations and mortality in the Lung Health Study. *Am J Respir Crit Care Med,* 166(3):333-339.

Celli BR, Cote CG, Marin JM, et al. (2004). The body-mass index, airflow obstruction, dyspnea, and exercise capacity index in chronic obstructive pulmonary disease. *N Engl J Med,* 350(10):1005-1012.

Hill C, Van Beek E.J.R. (2004). MRI of the chest: present and future. Imaging, 16:61-70.

Lopez AD, Collishaw NE, Piha T (1994). A descriptive model of the cigarette epidemic in developed countries. *Tob Control,* 3:242-247.

Working Procedures for the IARC Handbooks of Tobacco Control

Starting in 2006, the series of International Agency for Research on Cancer (IARC) *Handbooks* of Cancer Prevention will add tobacco control as a new area of prevention for their reviews. When appropriate, in addition to cancer, other health outcomes preventable by avoiding tobacco use may be included for evaluation in a *Handbook*.

The text that follows is organized in two principal parts. The first addresses the general scope, objectives and structure of the *Handbooks* of Tobacco Control. The second describes the scientific procedures for evaluating cancer-preventing agents or interventions.

The Working Procedures described herein are largely taken from the *Handbooks* of Cancer Prevention devoted to Chemoprevention and Screening, and from the recently updated IARC Monograph Preamble (January 2006).

The term "exposure" appears repeatedly in these procedures, borrowed from the IARC *Monographs* devoted to the evaluation of carcinogenicity. Epidemiological studies conducted to assess the association between exposure to a given hazard and disease outcome are based on the meaning of the term "exposure" implying increased risk to an undesired health effect. Hence when describing the criteria used to judge the quality of epidemiological studies, the traditional meaning of the term "exposure" is preserved (as opposed to a "protective exposure", assessed in the Chemoprevention *Handbooks*). However, in this series of Handbooks dedicated to the evaluation of the preventive effects of compounds, biological or pharmaceutical products, behaviours, programs and interventions, the traditional meaning of the term "exposure" is unfitting. Therefore in several instances the term "intervention", which lacks a hazardous connotation, is preferred. Examples of interventions with expected benefits in the area of tobacco control are smoking cessation, banning of smoking in public places and taxation on cigarettes. The evaluation of their health effects may be the focus of future *Handbooks*.

Part one:

General principles

General Scope

The prevention and control of cancer are the strategic objectives of the International Agency for Research on Cancer. Cancer prevention may be achieved at the individual level by avoiding cancer-causing agents and at the population level by adopting programs, legislation and regulations to reduce exposure to cancer-causing agents.

The *Handbooks* of Tobacco Control will evaluate the available evidence on the role of chemical compounds, biological and pharmaceutical products, behaviours, programs and interventions in reducing tobacco use and decreasing tobacco-associated morbidity and mortality. The aim of the *Handbook* series is to provide the scientific community, policymakers and governing bodies of IARC member states as well as of other countries with evidence-based assessments of these interventions at the individual and population levels, with the ultimate goal of assisting in the global implementation of tobacco control provisions within national and international programs aimed at reducing tobacco-related morbidity and mortality.

Objectives

The objective of the programme is to prepare, and to publish in the form of *Handbooks*, critical reviews and consensus evaluations of evidence on the preventive effect or risk reduction resulting from interventions focusing on tobacco control, with the help of an internationally formed Working Group. The *Handbooks* may also indicate where additional research efforts are needed, specifically when data immediately relevant to an evaluation are not available. The evaluations in the *Handbooks* are scientific and qualitative judgements of the peer-reviewed published data, conducted during a week-long meeting of peer review and discussions by the Working Group.

Topic for the Handbook

The topic to be evaluated in a *Handbook* is selected approximately twelve months prior to the meeting by the head of the Tobacco Unit after consultation with IARC scientists involved in tobacco research. A Handbook may cover a single topic or a group of related topics.

Meeting Participants

Soon after the topic of a *Handbook* is chosen, international scientists with relevant expertise are identified by IARC staff, in consultation with other experts. Each participant serves as an independent scientist and not as a representative of any organization, government or industry.

Five categories of participants can be present at *Handbook* meetings: Working Group Members, Invited Specialists, Representatives of national and international health agencies, Observers and the IARC Secretariat. Participants in the first two groups generally have published significant research related to the topic being reviewed or in tobacco control in particular. IARC uses literature searches to identify most experts. Consideration is also given to demographic diversity and balance of area of expertise. All participants are listed, with their addresses and principal affiliations, at the beginning of each *Handbook* volume.

1. The *Working Group* is responsible for the critical reviews and evaluations that are developed during the meeting. The tasks of the Working Group are: (i) to ascertain that all appropriate data have been collected; (ii) to select the data relevant for the evaluation on the basis of scientific merit; (iii) to prepare accurate summaries of the data to enable the reader to follow the reasoning of the Working Group; (iv) to critically evaluate the results of epidemiological, clinical, and other type of studies; (v) to prepare recommendations for research and for public health action; and (vi) if the topic being reviewed so permits, to make an overall evaluation of the evidence of a protective effect or reduced risk associated with the exposure or intervention focus of the evaluation. Working Group members are selected based on knowledge and experience pertinent to the topic evaluated and absence of real or apparent conflicts of interest.

2. *Invited Specialists* are experts who also have critical knowledge and experience but have a real or apparent conflict of interest. These experts are invited when necessary to assist in the Working Group by contributing their unique knowledge and experience during subgroup and plenary discussions. They may also contribute text on the intervention being evaluated. Invited Specialists do not serve as meeting chair or subgroup chair, or participate in the evaluations.

3. *Representatives* of national and international health agencies may attend meetings because their agencies sponsor the programme or are interested in the topic of a Handbook. Representatives do not serve as meeting chair or subgroup chair, draft any part of a Handbook, or participate in the evaluations.

4. *Observers* with relevant scientific credentials may be admitted to a meeting by IARC in limited numbers. Priority will be given to achieving a balance of Observers from constituencies with differing perspectives. They are invited to observe the meeting and should not attempt to influence it. Observers serve as sources of first-hand information from the meeting to their sponsoring organizations. Observers also can play a valuable role in ensuring that all published information and scientific perspectives are considered. Observers will not serve as chair or subgroup chair, draft any part of a *Handbook*, or participate in the evaluations. At the meeting, the chair and subgroup chairs may grant Observers the opportunity to speak, generally after they have observed a discussion.

5. The *IARC Secretariat* consists of scientists who are designated by IARC and who have relevant expertise. They serve as rapporteurs and participate in all discussions. When requested by the meeting chair or subgroup chair, they may also draft text or prepare tables and analyses.

The WHO Declaration of Interest form is sent to each prospective participant at the first contact, with the preliminary letter presenting the *Handbook* meeting. IARC assesses the declared interests to determine whether there is a conflict that warrants some limitation on participation. Before an official invitation is extended, each potential participant, including the IARC Secretariat, completes the WHO Declaration of Interests to report financial interests, employment and consulting, and individual and institutional research support related to the topic of the meeting. Working Group Members are selected based on the absence of real or apparent conflicts of interest. If a real or apparent conflict of interest is identified, then the expert is asked to attend as an Invited Specialist. The declarations are updated and reviewed again at the opening of the meeting. Interests related to the subject of the meeting are disclosed to the meeting participants and in the published volume (Cogliano *et al.*, 2004).

Data for the Handbooks

The *Handbooks* review all pertinent studies on the intervention to be evaluated. Only those data considered relevant to evaluate the evidence are included and summarized. Those judged inadequate or irrelevant to the evaluation may be cited but not summarized. If a group of similar studies is not reviewed, the reasons are indicated.

With regard to reports of basic scientific research, epidemiological studies and clinical trials, only studies that have been published or accepted for publication in the openly available scientific literature are reviewed. In certain instances, government agency reports that have undergone peer review and are widely available can be considered. Exceptions may be made ad hoc to include unpublished reports that are in their final form and publicly available, if their inclusion is considered pertinent to making an evaluation. Abstracts from scientific meetings and other reports that do not provide sufficient detail upon which to base an assessment of their quality are generally not considered.

Inclusion of a study does not imply acceptance of the adequacy of the study design or of the analysis and interpretation of the results, and limitations identified by the Working Group are clearly outlined in square brackets (ie, [ ]). The reasons for not giving further consideration to an individual study are also indicated in square brackets. Important aspects of a study, directly impinging on its interpretation, are brought to the attention of the reader. In general, numerical findings are indicated as they appear in the original report; units are converted when necessary for easier comparison. The Working Group may conduct additional analyses of the published data and use them in their assessment of the evidence. These analyses are outlined in square brackets in the *Handbook*.

Working Procedures

(a) Literature to be reviewed

After the topic of the *Handbook* is chosen, pertinent studies are identified by IARC from recognized sources of information such as PubMed and made available to Working Group members and Invited Specialists to prepare the working papers for the meeting. Meeting participants are invited to supplement the IARC literature searches with their own searches. Studies cited in the working papers are available at the time of the meeting.

(b) Chair of the Meeting

A provisional chair of the *Handbook* meeting will be identified soon after the topic of a *Handbook* is chosen. The provisional chair may help develop an outline for the *Handbook* early on, participate on conference calls with Working Group members and Invited Specialists in preparing for the meeting, provide early feedback on working papers and chair the meeting. The provisional chair will be formally elected chair of the meeting on the first day of the event.

(c) Working papers

The first version of the working papers is compiled and formatted by IARC staff about two months prior to the meeting, or as soon as they are received, and made available ahead of time through IARC's Internet to Working Group members, Invited Specialists and the IARC Secretariat. Reception of working papers ahead of the established deadline is encouraged, as it allows review of their content, facilitating identification of information gaps early enough. When possible or when deemed necessary, some working papers may be discussed early on among experts to expedite the review

process to be accomplished during the meeting. A conference call will be scheduled after reception of all working papers and prior to the meeting, with the aim of identifying areas deserving additional work by experts before the meeting.

Acknowledgement of significant contributions to the chapters by colleagues of the invited experts, either at their home institution or elsewhere, can be included in the Handbook under an acknowledgement paragraph to be shown following the listing of the meeting participants.

(d) Meeting

The Working Group members meet at IARC for seven to eight days to discuss and finalize the texts of the *Handbook* and to formulate the evaluations. The Working Group members and Invited Specialists are grouped into sub-groups according to their area of expertise. Sub-groups meet during the first three to four days to review in detail the first versions of their working papers, develop a joint subgroup draft, and write summaries. Scheduling of plenary and sub-group time may change from one *Handbook* meeting to another. Care is taken to ensure that each study summary is written or reviewed by someone not associated with the study being considered. During the last few days the participants meet in plenary session to review the subgroup working papers. Working Group members develop the consensus evaluations.

(e) Post-Meeting

After the meeting, the draft of the *Handbook* composed during the meeting is verified (by consulting the original literature), edited and prepared for publication by IARC staff. The aim is to publish *Handbooks* within six months of the meeting. If applicable, summaries reporting the results of the evaluation may be available on the IARC website (http://www.iarc.fr) soon after the meeting, and a short report may be published in the international literature.

Part two:

Scientific review of the evidence and evaluation

1. Scientific Review

The results of the studies reviewed will constitute the evidence forming the foundation of the evaluation. The validity of these studies should be examined critically to determine the weight of the studies contributing to the assessment. This will entail judging the appropriateness of study design, data collection (including adequate description of the intervention and follow-up), data analysis, and ultimately deciding if chance, bias, confounding or lack of statistical power may account for the observed results. The experts will ascertain how the limitations of the studies affect the results and conclusions reported. The criteria that follow apply to epidemiological and clinical studies and therefore may not be as relevant to studies where other quality criteria would be indicated—for example, those assessing the impact of economic policies.

(a) Quality of studies considered

It is necessary to take into account the possible roles of bias, confounding and chance in the interpretation of epidemiological studies. Bias is the operation of factors in the study design or execution that lead erroneously to a stronger or weaker association than in fact exists between the exposure/intervention being evaluated and the outcome. Confounding is a form of bias that occurs when the association with the disease is made to appear stronger or weaker than it truly is as a result of an association between the apparent causal factor and another factor that is associated with either an increase or decrease in the incidence of the disease. The role of chance is related to biological variability and the influence of sample size on the precision of estimates of effect.

In evaluating the extent to which these factors have been taken into account in an individual study, the *Handbook* considers a number of aspects of design and analysis as described in the report of the study.

First, the study population, disease (or diseases) and exposure/intervention should have been well defined by the authors. Cases of disease in the study population should have been identified independently of the intervention of interest, and the intervention should have been assessed in a way that was not related to disease status.

Second, the authors should have taken into account—in the study design and analysis—other variables that can influence the risk of disease and that may have been related to the intervention of interest. Potential confounding by such variables should have been dealt with either in the design of the study, such as by matching, or in the analysis, by statistical adjustment. In cohort studies, comparisons with local rates of the disease may or may not be more appropriate than those with national rates. Internal comparisons of disease frequency among individuals at different levels of the intervention are also desirable in cohort studies, since they minimize the potential for confounding related to difference in risk factors between an external reference group and the study population.

Third, the authors should have reported the basic data on which the conclusions are founded, even if sophisticated statistical analyses were employed. They should have given the numbers of exposed and unexposed cases and controls in a case-control study and the numbers of cases observed and expected in a cohort study. Further tabulations by time since exposure began and other temporal factors are also important. In a cohort study, data on all cancer sites and all causes of death should have been given to reveal the possibility of reporting bias. In a case-control study, the effects of investigated factors other than the exposure of interest should have been reported.

Finally, the statistical methods used to obtain estimates of relative risk, absolute rates of cancer, confidence intervals and significance tests, and to adjust for confounding should have been clearly stated by the authors. These methods have been reviewed for case-control studies (Breslow & Day, 1980) and for cohort studies (Breslow & Day, 1987).

Aspects that are particularly important in evaluating experimental studies are: the selection of participants, the nature and adequacy of the randomization procedure, evidence that randomization achieved an adequate balance between groups, the exclusion criteria used before and after randomization, compliance with the intervention in the intervention group, and 'contamination' with the intervention in the control group. Other considerations are the means by which the end-point was determined and validated, the length and completeness of follow-up of the groups, and the adequacy of the analysis. Detailed analyses of both relative and absolute risks in relation to temporal variables, such as age at first exposure, time since first exposure, duration of exposure, cumulative exposure, peak exposure (when appropriate) and time since exposure ceased, will be reviewed and summarized when available.

Independent population-based studies of the same exposure or intervention may lead to ambiguous results.

Combined analyses of data from multiple studies may be a means of resolving this ambiguity. There are two types of combined analysis: The first involves combining summary statistics such as relative risks from individual studies (meta-analysis), and the second involves a pooled analysis of the raw data from the individual studies (pooled analysis).

The advantages of combined analyses include increased precision due to increased sample size as well as the opportunity to explore potential confounders, interactions and modifying effects that may explain heterogeneity among studies in more detail. A disadvantage of combined analyses is the possible lack of compatibility of data from various studies due to differences in subject recruitment, data collection procedures, measurement methods and effects of unmeasured covariates that may differ between studies.

Meta-analyses may be conducted by the Working Group during the course of preparing a *Handbook* and are identified as original calculations by placement of the results in square brackets. These may be de-novo analyses or updates of previously conducted analyses that incorporate the results from new studies. Whenever possible, however, such analyses are preferably conducted prior to the *Handbook* meeting. Publication of the results of such meta-analyses prior to or concurrently with the *Handbook* meeting is encouraged for purposes of peer review. The same criteria for data quality that would be applied to individual studies must be applied to combined analyses, and such analyses must take into account heterogeneity between studies.

(b) Criteria for causality

After the quality of each study has been summarized and assessed, a judgement is made concerning the strength of evidence that the exposure or intervention in question reduces the risk of disease or is protective for humans. Hill (1965) lists areas for evaluating the strength of epidemiological associations used in the review of human data when assessing carcinogenesis. These criteria, in many instances, will apply to the assessment included in a *Handbook*:

- Consistency of observed associations across studies and populations;
- Magnitude of the reported association;
- Temporal relationship between exposure/intervention and change in disease;
- Exposure-response biologic gradient;
- Biological plausibility;

- Coherence of results across other lines of evidence; and
- Analogy present in related exposures and their effects on health.

If the results are inconsistent among investigations, possible reasons (such as differences in level of exposure/intervention) are sought, and results of studies judged to be of high quality are given more weight than those of studies judged to be methodologically less sound.

When several studies show little or no indication of an association between a intervention and cancer prevention, the judgement may be made that, in the aggregate, they show evidence of lack of effect. The possibility that bias, confounding or misclassification of exposure or outcome that could explain the observed results should be considered and excluded with reasonable certainty.

2. Summary of the data reviewed (evidence)

This section summarizes the results presented in the preceding sections in a concise manner.

3. Evaluation of the evidence

An evaluation of the strength of the evidence for disease prevention or reduction in morbidity and mortality is made using standard terms. It is conceivable that not every exposure/intervention reviewed in a *Handbook* of tobacco control will permit a formal evaluation of the evidence, as traditionally done in other *Handbooks* of Cancer Prevention and in the *Monographs*. In evaluating the strength of the evidence, a topic may allow a more formal evaluation (i.e. assigning causality or a protective effect in the prevention of cancer).

If assignment of causality is pertinent and possible, the possible outcomes of an evaluation can include:

Sufficient evidence of a reduction in risk:
The Working Group considers that a causal relationship has been established between the intervention under consideration and a reduction in morbidity and mortality. That is, a relationship has been observed between the expo-sure/intervention and disease morbidity and mortality in studies in which chance, bias and confounding could be ruled out with reasonable confidence. A statement that there is sufficient evidence should be followed by a separate sentence that identifies the types of cancer and other diseases where a decreased morbidity and mortality was observed in humans.

Limited evidence of a reduction in risk
An association has been observed between the expo-sure/intervention under consideration and a reduction in disease morbidity and mortality for which a causal interpretation is considered by the Working Group to be credible, but chance, bias or confounding could not be ruled out with reasonable confidence.

Inadequate evidence of a reduction in risk
The available studies are of insufficient quality, consistency or statistical power to permit a conclusion regarding the presence or absence of a causal association between the exposure/intervention and a reduced morbidity and mortality. Alternatively, this category is used when no data are available.

Evidence suggesting lack of effect
There are several adequate studies that are mutually consistent in not showing an association between the exposure/intervention and disease morbidity and mortality. A conclusion of evidence suggesting lack of risk reduction is inevitablylimited to the disease sites, conditions and levels of control, and length of observation covered by the available studies.

4. Overall evaluation
The overall evaluation, usually in the form of a narrative, will include a summary of the body of evidence considered as a whole and summary statements made about the health protective or preventive effect, or adverse effects, as appropriate.

5. Recommendations
After reviewing the data and deliberating on them, the Working Group may formulate recommendations, where applicable, for further research and public health action.

References
Breslow NE, Day NE (1980). *Statistical Methods in Cancer Research,* Vol. 1, The Analysis of Case-Control Studies (IARC Scientific Publications No. 32), Lyon, IARC.

Breslow NE, Day NE (1987). *Statistical Methods in Cancer Research,* Vol. 2, The Design and Analysis of Cohort Studies (IARC Scientific Publications No. 82), Lyon, IARC.

Cogliano VJ, Baan R, Straif K, *et al* (2004). The science and practice of carcinogen identification and evaluation. *Environmental Health Perspectives,* 112: 1269–1274.

Hill AB (1965). The environment and disease: association or causation? *Proceedings of the Royal Society of Medicine,* 58:295–300.